ADDITIONAL PRAISE FOR
CUTTING-EDGE THERAPIES FOR AUTISM

"Lost in the Spectrum? *Cutting-Edge Therapies for Autism* provides a compass and comprehensive map for finding your path to actionable options for your child. The many autistic children who have 'lost their diagnosis' have done so with therapies thoughtfully explained in the pages of this book, which contains plentiful insights from the research, experience, and love of our most thoughtful and articulate scientists, practitioners and parents."
   —Sidney M. Baker, MD, founder, Autism360

"It's like having a parent mentor with you at all times. *Cutting-Edge Therapies for Autism* delivers on so many levels—from practical advice and alternative insights, to the most relevant and high-value information on autism therapies today. A must-have for caregivers, even veteran parents!"
   —Lori McIlwain, executive director, National Autism Association

"This updated edition is so jam-packed with new and useful information that it is a must-have even if you bought last year's edition."
   —Kim Stagliano, author of *All I Can Handle: I'm No Mother Teresa*

"The Autism Society of Illinois supports individuals with autism and their families through the critical stages of early detection and intervention following. *Cutting-Edge Therapies for Autism* offers information on many interventions that have been used by parents who have watched their children improve."
   —Mary Kay Betz, executive director, Autism Society of Illinois

"For parents, *Cutting-Edge Therapies for Autism* is an invaluable resource. Whether you are new to an autism diagnosis or a parent who has been in the trenches for years, Ken Siri and Tony Lyons compile the most current information all in one place to allow parents to research the best options for their child's unique needs. This is a must-have book that you will find yourself consulting over and over."

—Kim Mack Rosenberg, president, National Autism Association New York Metro Chapter, and board member of the Elizabeth Birt Center for Autism Law & Advocacy

"Bioautismo is a non-profit corporation that promotes biomedical interventions to children diagnosed with ASD in Chile. We firmly believe that by detecting environmental insults, removing them from the children's environment and making available the appropriate therapies, we can improve the quality of life of individuals on the spectrum. We encourage parents to make informed decisions in terms of causes, treatments and therapies and to be in control of their child's recovery. The book *Cutting-Edge Therapies for Autism* helps parents do just that."

—Carmen Chaigneau, Bioautismo-Chile

Cutting-Edge Therapies for *Autism*

Fourth Edition

Ken Siri and Tony Lyons

Foreword by Dr. James Jeffrey Bradstreet
Afterword by Teri Arranga

Skyhorse Publishing

Skyhorse Publishing books may be purchased in bulk at special discounts for sales promotion, corporate gifts, fund-raising, or educational purposes. Special editions can also be created to specifications. For details, contact the Special Sales Department, Skyhorse Publishing, 307 West 36th Street, 11th Floor, New York, NY 10018 or info@skyhorsepublishing.com.

Skyhorse® and Skyhorse Publishing® are registered trademarks of Skyhorse Publishing, Inc.®, a Delaware corporation.

Visit our website at www.skyhorsepublishing.com.

10 9 8 7 6 5 4 3 2 1

A record for this title is on file with the Library of Congress.
ISBN: 978-1-62914-174-9

Printed in the United States of America

This book is for Lina, Alex, and all the kids suffering from autism, and for their parents struggling to give them the best possible life.

ACKNOWLEDGMENTS

Ken and Tony are deeply indebted to in-house Skyhorse Publishing editor Joseph Sverchek, without whom we could not possibly have completed this project. We are also indebted to Teri Arranga of AutismOne who spent countless hours going over the manuscript, the jacket, and the press release and gave us excellent editorial advice.

Tony would like to thank his ex-wife Helena who has worked with Lina to the brink of insanity, utilizing many of the therapies described in this book, staying up with her when she can't sleep, calming her down when she is dysregulated, holding, comforting, and carrying her, joining and engaging with her and giving her as much love as any human being has ever received from another human being. She is pulling Lina with both hands out of the abyss of autism.

Ken would like to thank his parents, Ken and Carole, and his sister, Noelle, for standing by him and Alex and for all their support and guidance.

CONTENTS

Foreword *by Dr. James Jeffrey Bradstreet*   xi

Preface *by Ken Siri and Tony Lyons*   xiii

**Navigating the Autism Superhighway: How to Determine if
a Therapy Is Right for Your Child and Family** *by Dr. Mark Freilich*   xxiii

BIOMEDICAL

1. **Allergy Desensitization: An Effective Alternative Treatment for Autism**
   by Dr. Darin Ingels   2

2. **Antiepileptic Treatment for Seizures and Epilepsy in Autism Spectrum
   Disorder** *by Dr. Richard E. Frye*   6

3. **Biofilm: A Cause of Chronic Gastrointestinal Issues in ASD** *by Dr. John H. Hicks* 14

4. **Chelation: Removing Toxic Metals** *by Dr. Michael Elice*   25

5. **Enzymes for Digestive Support in Autism** *by Dr. Devin Houston*   28

6. **How Enzymes Complement Therapeutic Diets** *by Kristin Selby Gonzalez*   32

7. **Flavonoid Formulation for Allergy-Like Symptoms and Brain
   Inflammation in Autism** *by Dr. Theoharis Theoharides and Shahrzad Asadi*   35

8. **Gastrointestinal Disease: Emerging Consensus** *by Dr. Arthur Krigsman*   42

9. **Biome Depletion, Helminths, and Autism** *by Judith Chinitz*   50

10. **Intestine, Leaky Gut, and Autism: Is It Real and How to Fix It
    (Including with Probiotics)** *by Dr. Alessio Fasano*   57

11. **IVIG: Intravenous Immunoglobulin** *by Dr. Michael Elice*   64

12. **Medical Cannabis as a Treatment for Symptoms Associated with
    Autism Spectrum Disorders** *by Nathan Coombs*   71

13. **Methyl-B$_{12}$: Myth or Masterpiece** *by Dr. James Neubrander*   78

14. **Treatments for Mitochondrial Disease and Dysfunction**
    by Dr. Richard E. Frye   84

15. **Neurofeedback for the Autism Spectrum** *by Dr. Siegfried and Susan F. Othmer* 89

16. Using Nutrigenomics to Optimize Supplement Choices *by Dr. Amy Yasko*   95

17. Nutritional Supplementation for Autism *by Larry Newman*   103

18. NeuroField pEMF for the Treatment of Autism *by Dr. Nicholas Dogris*   115

19. Transcranial Magnetic Stimulation for the Treatment of Autism *by Dr. Joshua M. Baruth, Dr. Estate Sokhadze, Dr. Ayman El-Baz, Dr. Lonnie Sears, and Dr. Manuel F. Casanova*   120

20. The Role of the Microbiome/Biome and Cysteine Deficiency in Autism Spectrum Disorder *by Dr. James Jeffrey Bradstreet*   131

21. Effects of Ambient Prism Lenses and Visual-Motor Training on Heart Rate Variability and Behavioral Outcomes in Autism *by Dr. Brynn Dombroski, Dr. Melvin Kaplan, Dr. Barbara Kotsamanidis-Burg, Dr. Stephen M. Edelson, Marie K. Hensley, Dr. Estate M. Sokhadze, and Dr. Manuel F. Casanova*   138

22. Stem Cells and Autism *by Dr. James Jeffrey Bradstreet*   151

23. The Thyroid-Autism Connection: The Role of Endocrine Disruptors *by Dr. Raphael Kellman*   165

24. Hyperbaric Oxygen Therapy—Let's Put the Pressure on Autism for Recovery *by Dr. James Neubrander*   180

25. Cerebral Folate Deficiency in Autism Spectrum Disorders *by Dr. Richard E. Frye and Dr. Daniel A. Rossignol*   186

26. From Preconception to Infancy: Environmental and Nutritional Strategies for Lowering the Risk of Autism *by Dr. David Berger*   195

27. Tetrahydrobiopterin Metabolism in Autism Spectrum Disorder *by Dr. Richard E. Frye*   210

28. Observing the Autism Brain with Real-Time Imaging: The Role of Transcranial Ultrasound (TUS) in Autism, with Implications for the Brain-Immune System Link in Autism and an Exploration of Interventions *by Dr. James Jeffrey Bradstreet*   214

29. Chlorine Dioxide's Role in Healing Autism *by Kerri Rivera*   222

30. Repetitive Transcranial Magnetic Stimulation and Magnetic Resonant Therapy™ for Autism *by Dr. James Jeffrey Bradstreet*   228

COMMUNICATION

31. AutisMate: Personalized for Life *by Jonathan Izak*   236

32. Rapid Prompting Method *by Soma Mukhopadhyay*   240

33. Augmentative and Alternative Communication *by Patti Murphy*   245

34. Feeding and Language Strategies for Mealtime *by Debbie Shiwbalak and Alpin Rezvani*   256

35. Avant Garde Approaches to Language Restoration *by Dr. Harry Schneider*   264

36. Community-Based Speech Language Pathology *by Alpin Rezvani*   272

37. Joint Action Routines (JARS) *by Lerone Kamara, Jessica Goldberg, and Alpin Rezvani*   278

DIETARY

38. Specific Carbohydrate Diet (SCD) *by Judith Chinitz*   290

39. Combined Approaches to Feeding Therapy *by Erica Goss*   299

40. The Healing Power of Fermented Foods *by Dr. John Hicks and Betsy Hicks*   304

EDUCATIONAL

41. How to Recognize a Top-Quality ABA Program *by Dr. Jonathan Tarbox, Dr. Doreen Granpeesheh, and Angela Persicke*   316

42. Emotional Vocal Exploration: A Revolutionary Mode of Communication *by Amanda Friedman and Alison Berkley*   324

43. CARD eLearning™ and Skills®: Web-Based Training, Assessment, Curriculum, and Progress Tracking for Children with Autism *by Dr. Doreen Granpeesheh and Dr. Adel C. Najdowski*   333

44. Drama Therapy *by Sally Bailey*   339

45. The Floortime Center *by Jake Greenspan and Time Bleecker*   343

46. Integrated Play Groups® (IPG) Model *by Dr. Pamela Wolfberg*   349

47. Integrative Educational Care *by Dr. Mary Joann Lang*   353

48. Integrating ABA with Developmental Models: MERIT *by Jennifer Clark*   361

49. Relationship Development Intervention *by Laura Hynes*   369

50. Asynchronous Telehealth Technology for Autism Spectrum Disorder *by Dr. Mary Joann Lang and Ronald Oberleitner*   376

51. The Ramapo Approach—Fostering Relationships That Motivate Behavioral Change *by Lisa Tazartes, Mike Kunin, and Jennifer Buri da Cunha*   384

HOLISTIC

52. The Holistic Approach to NeuroDevelopment and Learning Efficiency (HANDLE®) *by Carolyn Nuyens and Marlene Suliteanu*   392

53. Houston Homeopathy Method for Autism and ASDs: Sequential Homeopathy and Beyond *by Julianne Adams, Lynn Rose Demartini, Cindy L. Griffin, and Lindyl Lanham*   **400**

54. Homotoxicology and Beyond *by Mary Coyle*   **408**

55. Living Energy: Using Therapeutic Grade Essential Oils in the Treatment of Autism *by Dr. Shawn K. Centers*   **414**

56. Stress Reduction for Parents of Children with Autism *by Karen Nourizadeh*   **429**

57. Osteopathy: A Philosophy and Methodology for the Effective Treatment of Children with Autism *by Dr. Shawn K. Centers*   **435**

58. NAET Explained *by Geri Brewster*   **449**

PHYSICAL

59. CranioSacral Therapy and Autism *by Tami A. Goldstein*   **458**

60. Dance/Movement Therapy *by Mariah Meyer LeFeber*   **463**

61. Exercise: The Gateway to Building Relationships, Self-Esteem, and Fitness *by David Geslak*   **468**

62. Early Intervention Physical Therapy *by Dr. Allan Cuevas*   **479**

63. Yoga and Martial Art Therapies for the ASD Child *by Isauro Fernandez*   **491**

SENSORY

64. The Listening Program®: An Effective Treatment for Autism *by Alex Doman*   **498**

65. NACD's Targeted Neurodevelopmental Intervention: Perspectives and Interventions for Those on the Autism Spectrum *by Bob Doman*   **505**

66. Animals in the Lives of Persons with Autistic Spectrum Disorder (ASD): Companions to Co-Therapists *by Dr. Aubrey H. Fine*   **512**

67. Architecture and Autism: Creating a Toxic-Reduced Environment for Your Autistic Child *by Catherine Purple Cherry*   **523**

68. Art Therapy Approaches to Treating Autism *by Nicole Martin and Dr. Donna Betts*   **532**

69. Berard Auditory Integration Training *by Sally Brockett*   **537**

70. Occupational Therapy and Sensory Integration *by Markus Jarrow*   **543**

71. The Davis Model of Sound Intervention℠ *by Dorinne S. Davis*   **554**

72. Vision Therapy *by Dr. Jeffrey Becker*   **565**

Afterword *by Teri Arranga*   572

Autism Organizations   575

Schools for Persons with Autism Spectrum Disorders   589

Recommended Reading   607

References   610

Index   655

FOREWORD

Autism is a disorder in desperate need of better biomedical therapies. The father of one of my patients works in a field of information management called "big data." At the time when he gave me a fabulous book on big data, I didn't really know much about it or how big data was changing the world we live in. To give you a feel for its potential, big data is now capable of analyzing datasets larger than 1 billion gigabytes. As the Internet grows, our cumulative knowledge expands at an amazing rate. The future of solving truly complex issues like autism likely will finds its path through big data analytics.

Like many disorders where the current state-of-the-art medical care falls short of the clinical needs, families work to push the treatments and research to new levels. Generally, this is a good thing. Those with the passion to help their own families are tireless researchers, who often stay up late at night investigating possible interventions through the Web. But filtering out the creative, potential and promising therapies from the ramblings can be very challenging. There are no medications to treat autism; only a handful of powerful and potentially dangerous antipsychotics are approved to treat irritability in autism. Biomedical solutions—immunological, detoxification, nutritional, and hyperbaric oxygen—have been published with varying degrees of success. But for most of the rest, well-controlled studies to support their use is missing. This isn't the fault of parents. Medical research is mainly funded by those interested in patentable and profitable therapies. In the absence of support from their own doctors, parents are abandoned to do nothing or to venture out to try something new.

While some, even most, of these biomedical approaches are logical, and most are likely safer than available psychopharmaceuticals, many in the so-called mainstream of medicine call for caution and express concern. Internet chat rooms, blog sites, Facebook®, and Twitter® often find parents networking with stories of success, setbacks, and novel strategies. Although, ideally, any biomedical intervention or change in biomedical regimen should be done with the oversight of a knowledgeable healthcare practitioner, all of these posts and chats along with the accumulating published scientific data can be assessed efficiently through big data analytical systems. And it is probable that within all of these datasets, some new understanding of the truth will be revealed, and, with that, better therapies will emerge at a much faster pace than in the past.

Despite these concerns, parental-directed therapies are a new reality we in medicine need to accept and help guide as we also learn from everyone's collective and best efforts. 2014 promises to be a year of significant gains for autism therapies. Gastrointestinal issues related to abnormal ecosystems inside the intestines of children with autism spectrum disorders are receiving greater academic attention. Immune abnormalities are becoming better understood and various interventions are being tested to improve the outcomes from immunological interventions. Brain physics (the harmonics of how the brain sends signals) is a subject of intense research with magnetic stimulation and EEG (electroencephalogram) analyses. Publication of imaging of the autism brain with transcranial ultrasound, available by the time this 2014 edition of *Cutting-Edge Therapies for Autism* is in press, will facilitate rapid assessment of the cortex and fluid spaces around the brain and may improve interventional assessments.

More children than ever before are experiencing significant recoveries. Unfortunately, an unprecedented number of new cases challenge us to improve the delivery of quality biomedical therapies.

—**James Jeffrey Bradstreet,** MD, MD(H), FAAFP, FMAPS
Director of the Brain Treatment Center of Atlanta
Adjunct Professor, Western University of Health Sciences, CA

PREFACE

Dear Reader

Welcome to the fourth edition of *Cutting-Edge Therapies for Autism*. Whether this is your first read of *Cutting-Edge* or the fourth, we thank you for your support and attention. We have to say, this edition is very exciting and much new research has come to light over the last two years since we published the Updated Edition. We highly recommend Dr. Bradstreet's chapter on "Observing the Autism Brain with Real-Time Imaging," chapter 29, which represents a true milestone. This work has the potential to move diagnosis and follow-up from subjective clinical observation to medical based data. As the year 2013 came to a close, we also received fascinating research on the gut-brain connection and Ken comments on that in our expanded Preface. Finally, we acknowledge the loss of young Avonte Oquendo, who went missing from his school here in New York during October. We share our sympathies with his family and hope that his memory will lead to improved understanding of the challenges of raising children with special needs. During the summer, Ken's son Alex also ran, but was promptly found after a hectic two hours on his own in Manhattan. Ken comments on that as well.

Autism: A Punch to the Gut?

Autism, Dementia, and Gastrointestinal Issues

At the end of 2013 there were a couple of studies that came out which garnered some modest press. The first was "Dementia Epidemic Looms with 135 million Sufferers Expected by 2050." This particular headline was on Fox, but was similarly reported by multiple outlets (*see* FoxNews.com for December 5, 2013).

The story highlighted the exponential growth expected in dementia, highlighted by Alzheimer's, going from 44 million to 135 million by 2050. Alzheimer's Disease International (ADI) said the study showed a 17 percent increase over two years, which when extrapolated forward gives the 135 million in 2050 figure. This growth rate is significantly higher than the world population growth of about 1.2 percent (US Census Bureau). More telling, the world population growth rate will be cut in half between now and 2050 to .6 percent (US Census again). The ADI called it a "global epidemic" which is only going to get worse. The current global cost of care for dementia is more than $600 billion, equal to about 1.0 percent. By 2050 we are talking about 3 percent of the global population having dementia given the estimates above, which will become a serious drag on global growth.

Now where have we come across numbers similar to this before? A subset of the population that is growing significantly faster than the population as a whole. A subset that should remain constant in percentage terms if it is genetic. And, a subset that seems to be growing along with another subset, or subsets actually. Yes, the autism and dementia growth rates are very similar. Possibly a coincidence. Possibly not. When you figure in the increasing rates of autoimmune conditions (which are also similar) and see that all seem to increase exponentially from the same base, the possibility of coincidence diminishes.

I find it interesting that we are not hearing about better diagnosis in terms of dementia, or autoimmune conditions, only in autism. *So,* what could be causing this?

Well, a few days later, a second study, reported in multiple outlets, indicated that "autism may be linked to gastrointestinal issues" according to a study from Caltech (December 7, 2013).

The study evidenced that behaviors associated with autism are "influenced from gastrointestinal (GI) issues, and could be treated with probiotic therapy." Researchers utilized a particular "good" human bacteria in a mouse model to treat induced GI and autism issues; what resulted was a decrease in GI troubles and in autism-like symptoms. This led the scientists to theorize that behavioral issues on the autism spectrum may be caused by GI issues and can be treated by healing the gut.

The study also pointed out how "leaky gut," the induced GI condition, has also become a target of researchers in Parkinson's, multiple sclerosis, and Alzheimer's as other studies have tied these conditions to GI disease. What Caltech scientists conclude is "this suggests that GI problems could contribute to particular symptoms in neurodevelopmental disorders."

The specific connections investigated between autism and GI were: chronic constipation, diarrhea, reflux, IBD in GI, and defects in social interaction, communication, and repetitive behaviors in autism.

It seems from all this that the increases in the neuro and autoimmune conditions may be linked by GI. Long thought to reside in the brain, perhaps all the trouble or the cause of these conditions lies in the stomach/GI tract. If so, this would also lead one to believe the hypothesis that something, other than better diagnosis, is causing the exponential increase in these conditions. This brings us back to the heavy use of antibiotics, pesticides, drugs, and other chemicals in our food supply, bodies, and environment.

The hope is that this information will result in more research and focus on the gut's impact on autism, dementia, and all the above. The exciting implications of this, according to the researchers, is that the gut is far easier to study and address than the brain and potentially more impactful, as the mice in the study became more communicative and less anxious with treatment (particularly probiotics). Stay tuned.

So My Son Ran Today. September 2013.

More of a stroll really, but I guess the official term is "run." I've written before about how he has "escaped" from my apartment here in NYC, and typically been found by neighbors in the building and or the doormen. Today was different.

I had a sitter here working with Alex; I was out riding my bike in Central Park. When I returned home, my doorman told me Alex was missing and the staff was looking for him. This has happened before, however when he told me how Alex had been gone for over thirty minutes I felt sick. That was new. His adventures before lasted about five minutes or so, before cameras or residents found him. I should say he is quite noisy and tough to miss. Most in our neighborhood know him on sight, luckily (a good reason to stay put, I guess).

Upon learning Alex was gone for such a long time, I quickly joined the hunt. Our high-rise is connected to a smaller building via a stairwell. This smaller "back" building houses mostly retired folks, who in the past have contacted the front desk upon finding Alex wandering their halls (overall this has happened maybe four times). This time he was spotted getting on an elevator (separate elevators for the two buildings). As I searched I learned he had been spotted there and focused on the "back" building. Staff was in both buildings (along with some fellow residents and Alex's worried sitter) climbing stairwells, riding elevators, and checking roofs, back gardens, the street. I ran around the outside of the building, asking dog walkers, doormen, garage attendants, and random passersby if Alex had been spotted. Again, Alex as a fifteen-year-old, curly blonde-haired, noisy yet non-verbal boy is tough to miss. After about an hour—or I should say an HOUR—the front desk of the building got me on my cell and said the police had brought Alex in.

What had happened was that Alex had gotten out though the "back" building to the street and decided to walk towards Second Avenue (we live on Third) and a kindly neighbor in another apartment building realized something was up and actually knew of Alex (just from being in the neighborhood) and took him in (she has a townhome). After giving him a sandwich and banana, she called the police, and they jointly returned him to our building. Police suggest a bracelet with the usual "lost" information, however Alex can easily rip that off (and has). My best bet is to add an inside lock and key. Needless to say it was quite the way to end Labor Day Weekend.

My purpose in sharing this is twofold. One, to just help me unwind! The other, to communicate to those who have experienced similar "runs" that they are not alone, and that people, our neighbors and the police, can be caring and concerned. Some of the neighbors and police officers involved hugged me and slapped my back in a show of support. I thank them all!

What's New in the Fourth Edition?

In this fourth edition we present more than one hundred therapies over the course of seventy-two chapters, including twenty brand-new chapters and another fifteen that have been substantially revised. We maintain our seven therapeutic categories (Biomedical, Communication, Dietary, Educational, Holistic, Physical, and Sensory) to help the reader focus his or her effort.

Teri Arranga of AutismOne returns to provide us with our afterword, and longtime contributor Dr. Jeff Bradstreet, joins the team, providing our foreword in addition to some exciting new research.

We have also added to our resource lists at the back of the book and are happy to take suggestions for other therapies or resources for future editions. Email us at autism@skyhorsepublishing.com with suggestions.

The central purpose of this book is to provide people interested in autism therapies—including parents, grandparents, teachers, therapists, doctors and researchers—with articles about the cutting-edge work being done in the field. This field changes rapidly and we plan to update the book frequently. *Cutting-Edge Therapies for Autism* is for people who want to learn as much as they possibly can about the therapies available, and about how to do everything in their power to help the growing number of children who are suffering.

Autism is the country's fastest-growing medical emergency, affecting more children than cancer, diabetes, Down syndrome and AIDS combined. More than one million people in the United States currently suffer from some form of autism.

Autism is difficult to define. No two kids have the same exact set of symptoms or respond to the same combination of therapies. Each child's treatment plan needs to be unique, taking into consideration the specific symptoms the child exhibits, the results of tests administered, and the observations of the child's doctors, therapists, teachers and, just as importantly, parents.

Case study #1: Lina

My daughter Lina was a bright, happy, talkative, social little girl. She had some ongoing problems with eczema but, other than that, was very healthy. Just before she turned three, she was given a regimen of antibiotics for bronchitis. Shortly thereafter, she received her measles mumps and rubella (MMR) booster shot. About two weeks later, she started to drool uncontrollably. It looked like her lips and jaw muscles had gone totally numb. The pediatrician took some tests and found that she had been exposed to the Epstein-Barr Virus, but couldn't tell us anything more. The drooling episode lasted a couple of weeks, during which time her speech became garbled and she began to stutter. It took an incredible effort for her to push words out of her mouth. She was like a toy running low on batteries, losing steam, losing control. As things inside of her began to disconnect, she was becoming disconnected from the world around her. A friend came over with her daughter for a play date and, after a few minutes with Lina, she asked, with real fear in her eyes: "What's going on with Lina? She seems like a different person." Lina seemed to improve after that, but then gradually deteriorated. She was first diagnosed with Sensory Processing Disorder, then Pervasive Development Disorder (PDD), and then, finally, autism. For some kids autism means screaming, biting, throwing things out the window, breaking everything in sight, even head banging. Life with them and for them can be harsh. When I look at Lina I see a peaceful, loving, gentle girl struggling to get out of a body that isn't functioning correctly. She's the victim—not me, not her mother, not her teachers, not society. The other day after slamming doors, screaming uncontrollably, and throwing things, she was able to calm down and walked over to me. I was sitting in my home office and, exhausted, she put her cheek on my arm, pulled my fingers to her back and said: "Can I please have a tickle, scratch, scratch." Lina clearly has attention deficit hyperactivity disorder (ADHD), she's obsessive compulsive (OCD), she has sensory processing disorder (SPD), is often manic, has gut and sleep issues, and her language is a constant struggle. But her mother, Helena, and I are fighting these symptoms and Lina is fighting them and we'll keep fighting them together and, God willing, we'll continue to see progress.

Case study #2: Alex

My son Alex was born in June of 1998 and developed normally, meeting or exceeding all his milestones until just after the age of 3. He attended daycare early (from age 4 months old) and was a popular and happy kid. While at daycare, Alex was able to pick up some Spanish in addition to his native English and could count to 10 in English, Spanish and Japanese by his second birthday. Medically, Alex was healthy as an infant and toddler, although he did have frequent sinus and ear infections that were treated with inhaled albuterol. He had all his vaccinations on time, the last of which followed his third birthday. By late summer folks at daycare began to comment that Alex was uncharacteristically spending more time on his own, sometimes staring out the window. A visit to his pediatrician produced an all too common "Don't worry, it's just a stage." Then Alex began to lose some speech, though he was still able to say, "Turn that off, that's scary," in response to TV coverage of 9/11. By Christmas 2001, Alex had lost a significant amount of speech, frequently stimmed by clapping his hands loudly (you never heard such a clap) and clearly had ADHD. At a holiday party that season, a person who owned a daycare center told me she thought Alex was autistic. This began our year-long journey into the autism abyss. By the end of 2002 Alex was non-verbal and a fully diagnosed member of the autism epidemic.

There is still no general consensus on what causes autism—either classic Kanner's autism or the regressive kind. Some people think it's entirely genetic, while others think it's caused by Pitocin, fluoride in tap water or tooth paste, GAMT (guanidinoacetate methyltransferase) deficiency, chemicals in foods or household products, parental age, parental weight, stress, treatments for asthma given to pregnant women, vaccines and/or the preservative thimerosal in some vaccines, viruses in the stomach or perhaps a specific retrovirus known as XMRV (which is under investigation by the CDC), gastrointestinal (GI) tract problems, immune problems, impaired intestinal functioning, environmental toxins, vitamin D deficiency, seizures, mobile phone radiation, encephalitis, hypoglycemia, antibiotics, and the list goes on and on. In compiling this book we have noticed a consensus beginning to emerge that the symptoms of autism result from a perfect storm of factors that come together to create a kind of system overload, a tipping point, in a genetically predisposed child's developing immune system. Recent studies point toward this overload causing problems at the cellular level, impairing the ability of nerve cells to transmit information properly through the synapses of the brain. Furthermore, the dramatic and continuing increase in the incidence of autism spectrum disorders points toward environmental factors playing a significant role. Further supporting this is the fact that scientists have found that by introducing environmental toxins or antibiotics they can create autistic symptoms in rats.

So what happened to Lina and Alex? We believe that they were genetically predisposed to contract autism, but required a big push and that the push came from a virus and a high fever, followed by antibiotics and a barrage of vaccines, all of which occurred at a fragile developmental stage. The antibiotics dysregulated the immune system and the vaccines, thrown in as an additional stressor at the worst possible time, were the final straw. We also believe that the dysregulated, hyper-active immune system created an autoimmune response whereby the immune system couldn't tell the difference between healthy tissue and the antigens that it normally fights and then probably attacked the healthy tissue of both the stomach lining and the brain. We believe that this combination of factors created a gut malfunction, a kind of climate change in the stomach that made it difficult for our kids to digest certain proteins that are necessary for healthy blood-cell development and healthy nerve cell activation. The proteins in the blood cells are necessary for the healthy development of the cognitive centers of the brain and in the nerve cells they help the neurotransmitters fire up correctly, send proper messages (like pain, hot and cold, sound etc.) and connect the right and left lobes of the brain. We think that the human body can normally withstand severe complications and stressors but, for the young, predisposed child, this chain of events is just too much. While we're not scientists, like everyone reading this book, we're doing our very best to try to solve the puzzle.

As far as treatments for autism, most doctors still tell parents with absolute certainty that it is an incurable lifelong condition and that treatments simply don't work. Kim Stagliano, author of the book *All I Can Handle: I'm No Mother Teresa* about life with three autistic daughters writes:

> An autism diagnosis can erase a person's ability to get solid medical care. If you brought your 6-year-old to a hospital in the throes of a seizure, the neurologists would run tests and look for the cause. When I brought my 6-year-old in, I was told, "She has autism. She has different circuitry." And then when I requested tests, I was told, "We're just not that aggressive with autism." My child has a brain and a gut and immune system just like any other child. Why does her autism negate that?

In looking at a more than 50% increase in the incidence of autism between 2002 to 2006, Dr. Thomas Insel director of the National Institute of Mental Health (NIMH) and chair of the Interagency Autism Coordinating Committee (IACC) the nation's top autism research coordinator, had this to say in an interview with David Kirby for the *Huffington Post*:

> This tells you that you really have to take this very seriously. From everything they are looking at, this is not something that can be explained away by methodology, by diagnosis.

He goes on to say that we should not be looking at autism as a single thing, with one cause, one treatment, one explanation. There may, in fact, be 10 or 20 or more distinct variations.

> I think this is a collection of many, many different disorders...It's quite believable to me that there are many children who develop autism in the

context of having severe gut pathology, or having autoimmune problems, or having lots of other problems. And some of these kids really do recover. And this is quite different from the autism that was originally described in the 1940s and 1950s—where it looks like you have it and you are going to have it for the rest of your life.

If autism is caused by the comorbidity of the underlying medical conditions, and if there are really endless variations of autism, then why on earth wouldn't we treat these conditions, mandate that insurance companies pay for these treatments, and get on to the business of trying to heal the underlying conditions. Dr. Insel agrees and says: "We've got to be able to break apart this spectrum disorder into its component parts and identify who's going to respond to which interventions." He advocates for genetic mapping as a way to pinpoint the underlying medical conditions so that we can figure out whether an individual had been "exposed to organophosphates, or perhaps to some infection, or some autoimmune process" that interferes with the way the brain develops. Others are beginning to express similar sentiment. Dr. Christopher Walsh, Ballard Professor of Neurology and Chief of the Division of Genetics at Children's Hospital in Boston says: "I would like every kid on the spectrum to have not 'autism' but a more specific disorder. By isolating the genes involved and understanding their functions, researchers can begin to develop particular treatments aimed at particular disorders." Dr. James Gusella, Ballard Professor of Neurogenetics and director of the Center for Human Genetic Research at Massachusetts General Hospital (MGH) says: "Autism is a problem that no one person or discipline can figure out alone."

Throughout the book, we use the word "treatment" in the broadest possible sense. Nevertheless, the therapies included by no means constitute an exhaustive list. Most of the practitioners included can tell you about cases where their therapy helped decrease the symptoms of a specific child, helped the child relate better, speak better, helped minimize gut problems, or helped control behavioral problems. And they have parents to support their claims. On the other hand, most of these therapies have not undergone rigorous trials, the kind of trials that cost substantial amounts of money and often take years to complete and evaluate. As a result, there are some people who contest the claims of the practitioners or parents. In any case, by including a specific treatment, we are not endorsing that treatment or telling you that it will work for your child or patient. Nor are the more than a hundred doctors, teachers, therapists, parents, and other experts who have contributed to this book endorsing any treatment other than the one that they are writing about. Furthermore, practically none of these therapies are endorsed by any state or the federal government or covered by health insurance.

We certainly believe that the government should mandate insurance coverage for extensive genetic, blood and spinal fluid testing before any definitive diagnosis can be given. We have heard of cases where children showed the symptoms of autism or other disorders such as cerebral palsy, multiple sclerosis, or schizophrenia, but in fact had easily treatable disorders and were fully rehabilitated. We believe these kids, like any other kids, deserve the best medical care available, including full coverage for any treatment that is recommended by a specialist in any specific underlying medical condition. Some states have already started heading in this direction. For now, the only FDA approved drugs are Abilify and Risperdal and the only therapy approved by most states is applied behavior analysis (ABA), based on the teachings of B. F. Skinner. Recently, however, practitioners and researchers have begun advocating for approaches that combine the various therapies and scientists are trying to develop ways to measure how particular therapies improve brain connections in a specific individual.

Autism costs families an incredible amount of money. Estimates range from $60,000 to $100,000 per year and that assumes that you can either find an adequate public school in your district or, more likely, a private school that your city will agree to pay for. If you can't get the school paid for, then the cost could be as high as $200,000 per year. Whoever pays, autism is a growing problem and states and the federal government need to address it. Right now, autism costs the United States an estimated 35 billion dollars per year, but that could well be the trickle that turns into a flood. We believe that by funding more research and by agreeing either to pay for a broader range of therapies or to require insurance companies to do that, states and the federal government will save money in the long run.

Dr. Insel admits that when he was in training as a psychiatrist he "never saw a child with autism." He says that he wanted to see kids with autism, but he simply couldn't find any. Now, Insel says, "I wouldn't have to go any further than the block where I live to see kids with autism." This is an epidemic. We've come from a time when 1 in 10,000 babies born in the United States exhibited symptoms of autism to a time when the statistics are 1 in 88. Think about that for a moment: more than 1% of kids born in this country become autistic. And those statistics, which come from the Centers for Disease Control (CDC), are based on data collected four years ago, so given the growth rate in diagnosis, the current incidence is likely greater.

If you were to take the 70% increase in the incidence of autism between 2000 and 2008, as calculated by the CDC (which the CDC itself says cannot be explained away by a shift in diagnostic criteria) and extrapolate forward, then at least half of all children born in the United States will be autistic by 2046. And these statistics fail to differentiate between classic autism, which is characterized by a child sitting in a corner rocking back and forth with little interest in social interaction, and regressive autism, where a normally developing child suddenly loses speech, interest in social interaction with peers and develops various biomedical symptoms. Ten years ago no one talked or wrote about regressive autism and now this is the fastest growing segment of the autistic population.

What if this is just a different disorder? What if it's a disorder that has gone from 1 in 200 million to 1 in 200 in a 10 year period? Then, certainly, we're looking at a medical disaster of unprecedented proportions that is here, now and warrants a response at least as dramatic as the CDCs response to swine flu or the AIDS epidemic. We could well be at the tipping point of a crisis that will soon consume our future.

We are not doctors or scientists or government officials, but dads who love our kids and want to do the very best we can for them. We don't know for sure what caused our kids' autism and maybe we never will. If it was an immune system overload, we think that in most cases the cure is going to come not from a one-off drug, but from a counterassault, an all-out systemic approach, from DIR, from ABA, from dietary interventions, from GI tract treatments, from nutritional supplements, from anti-virals, from physical therapy, from sensory integration therapy, from brain therapy, from whatever fits the individual child. The current unwillingness of insurance companies, states and the federal government to pay for therapies is typical short-term thinking. Costs will only escalate, as untreated children become adults who need to be cared for by the state. A long-term approach will ultimately save money and will undoubtedly lead to at least some children being cured. This is war and if we want these children back, if we want to stop the progress of this disorder, we are going to have to fight. There will be people, lots of people, who will keep pointing out that there is no known cure, that they believe the struggle is hopeless. They will tell you that the best thing to do is to try to protect your own sanity and save your money. Our mission is to give our children, everyone's autistic children, their lives back to the fullest extent possible. We want to be involved in finding a remedy or a series of therapies that act together to bring these kids back to themselves and to their families and to the world.

Lina and Alex may never be typical kids. But perhaps they can be in a position to make informed decisions about their own lives, to communicate with people, to experience friendship and love and passion and hope. And who knows, perhaps if we help cure them, they will be the ones who develop a cure for cancer! Whatever the outcome, until there is a cure, we will do our very best to look for promising therapies for the symptoms of autism and continue to publish *Cutting-Edge Therapies for Autism*.

—**Ken Siri and Tony Lyons**

Find us on Facebook at "Cutting-Edge Therapies."

NAVIGATING THE AUTISM SUPERHIGHWAY: HOW TO DETERMINE IF A THERAPY IS RIGHT FOR YOUR CHILD AND FAMILY

When Cutting-Edge Therapies for Autism was first published in April 2010 the overall prevalence of Autistic Spectrum Disorders was 1:110 children. At that time it was stated that "at no other time in recent history has the need for Autism Awareness been so important". Fast forward to 2014 with the publication of the 4th edition of Cutting-Edge Therapies for Autism and the prevalence has risen to 1:88 (or 1:50 depending on the focus population). Autism Spectrum Disorders have become the fastest growing serious developmental disability in the United States.

What is the cause or causes of autism? Why has the prevalence continued to dramatically increase? Is it a disorder of genetic, environmental and neurologic etiology or do multiple factors come into play? Unfortunately the answers to these questions and many others remain elusive. It is speculated that at the present time everyone in the United States is somehow directly or indirectly connected to someone who is affected by autism. Given these statistics, the assumption can be made that if you are intently reading or just skimming through the chapters of this book, your child or a child you know was recently or at some time in the past diagnosed with an Autism Spectrum Disorder.

At this point you have hopefully, to one degree or another, started to come to terms with the diagnosis and what it means for your child, for you, and for your family. You are now ready to enter the Autism Superhighway, in either the slow or the fast lane.

In either case, it is now time to gather your team of co-navigators who will assist you in putting together a GPS system with the appropriate approaches, methods, and interventions. These should all be based on your child's unique and individual profile. This profile is essential in guiding the course of treatment.

For any child with autism, determining a course of treatment using only information you have read in a book or researched on the internet is ill-advised. One needs a qualified team of specialists to properly evaluate, diagnose, prescribe, and monitor your child's strengths and areas of need.

This book continues to be a valuable resource for families, helping to place a child on the road to recovery from autism. It needs to be said that there continues to be no cure for autism. There are many children, however, who have received timely, individualized and comprehensive interventions who no longer meet the diagnostic criteria for an Autism Spectrum diagnosis. No matter the severity of manifestations, significant benefit can be gained by the child, the family, or both, with early and intensive interventions. However, if any clinician, specialist, or intervention approach promises a cure, be very leery and scrutinize carefully the validity of their claims.

Your primary pediatric care provider should be knowledgeable about the various medical, developmental, and behavioral issues that children with Autism Spectrum Disorders may encounter. They should be aware of the available treatment options and the specialists in your area to whom you need to be referred. They need to be open-minded to ALL treatments, whether they are based on a Western medicine approach or an alternative/complementary medical philosophy. Most importantly, there needs to be close collaboration and communication between your family, your specialists/therapists, and your child's primary care pediatric physician.

Since a common etiology for autism has not been discovered, each child may broadly share common general manifestations but the triggers and causes for these manifestations may vary greatly from one child to another. It appears that the way parents and professionals view autism today is in transition. Although many continue to view it as strictly a psychiatric or a neurologic disorder, newer viewpoints are being embraced. Autism is increasingly being viewed as a disorder with multiple etiologies defined by its behavioral manifestations. These include impairments in communication and social interactions, repetitive behaviors, and sensory processing and regulatory issues. Therefore, autism continues to be considered a "spectrum" disorder that not only is impacted by issues in the brain and nervous system but one that is impacted by dysfunction in the immune, gastrointestinal, and metabolic systems. Since the etiologies as well as the manifestations of autism are influenced by a variety of multiple factors, a cookie-cutter or a one-size-fits-all approach to treatment and intervention programming is steering you onto the wrong road. Creating an individual profile is therefore essential to navigating the Autism Superhighway. This profile must include an assessment of the child's present developmental level. It needs to analyze the child's individual medical, genetic, behavioral, sensory processing, and regulatory profile. Consideration of parenting skills, cultural beliefs, and familial as well as societal expectations need to be factored in.

The child's profile should and will change over time. The key to successful outcomes is establishing a cohesive team approach, with ongoing monitoring of progress to ensure treatments remain relevant and goals are always current and realistic.

One cannot promise that the Autism Superhighway your child and your family will be travelling on will offer a smooth or detour-free trip. There will be bumps, curves, and forks in the road. Remember, this is most likely going to be a long journey, not a short road trip. There will be many moments when you say "are we there yet?" but there will also be many scenic road stops and enjoyable attractions. Be sure to take the time to celebrate even the smallest of accomplishments along the way.

—MARK FREILICH, MD

BIOMEDICAL

ALLERGY DESENSITIZATION: AN EFFECTIVE ALTERNATIVE TREATMENT FOR AUTISM

By Dr. Darin Ingels

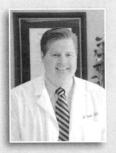

Darin Ingels, ND

2425 Post Road, Ste. 100
Southport, CT 06890
IngelsFamilyHealth.com
WellnessIntegrative.com
dingels@gmail.com

Dr. Darin Ingels is a respected leader in natural medicine with numerous publications, international lectures, and more than 20 years experience in the healthcare field. He received his bachelor of science degree in medical technology from Purdue University and his doctorate of naturopathic medicine from Bastyr University in Seattle, Washington. Dr. Ingels completed a residency program at the Bastyr Center for Natural Health. He is a licensed naturopathic physician in the State of Connecticut and State of California, where he maintains practices in both states. Dr. Ingels is a member of the American Association of Naturopathic Physicians, the Connecticut Naturopathic Physicians Association, the New York Association of Naturopathic Physicians, the American Academy of Environmental Medicine, the American College for Advancement in Medicine, and the Holistic Pediatric Association. He has served on the board of directors for the Naturopathic Physicians Licensing Exam (NPLEX) as the chair of microbiology and immunology. Dr. Ingels' practice focuses on autism spectrum disorders with special emphasis on chronic immune dysfunction, including allergies, asthma, recurrent or persistent infections, and other genetic or acquired immune problems. He uses diet, nutrients, herbs, homeopathy, and immunotherapy to help his children achieve better health.

Allergies and asthma affect more than 50 million people living in the United States and comprise the sixth leading cause of physician office visits. Children with autism often have impaired immune function and may be predisposed to allergy symptoms.[1,2] Studies also show that children with autism have multiple defects in immune function and that the severity of immune dysfunction is proportional to the severity of autism.[3] Unfortunately, allergies are often underdiagnosed and undertreated due to lack of verbal skills of the child or the lack of understanding by parents of what symptoms may be caused by allergy. The immune system produces five different antibodies (also known as immunoglobulins) in response to substances that are recognized as being foreign (e.g., bacteria, viruses, allergens, etc.). Immunologists refer to them as IgG, IgM, IgA, IgD and IgE. Each immunoglobulin serves a primary role in our normal immune function, and IgE is the one most associated with allergies. Common symptoms of allergy, including runny nose, itchy eyes, sneezing, and asthma, are often precipitated by IgE, which triggers the cascade of events leading to allergic symptoms. However, there is good evidence that many allergic reactions do not involve IgE at all and can be mediated by different immune mechanisms. Non-IgE reactions have been identified as causing neuropsychiatric symptoms such as irritability, hyperactivity, mood disorders, or cognitive deficits; gastrointestinal or motility problems; skin rashes; and sleep disturbances.[4] Conventional allergy testing specifically looks mostly at IgE reactions (whether by blood test, intradermal, or scratch testing), so it is not uncommon for a child with autism to get allergy testing and be told they do not have any allergies. However, IgE testing excludes most non-IgE reactions and, therefore, has limited value in diagnosing these types of allergies.

Treatment of allergies usually consists of over-the-counter or prescription oral antihistamines (e.g., Benadryl®, Zyrtec®, or Claritin®), leukotriene inhibitors (Singulair®), or steroids. Nasal and inhaled steroids may also be prescribed to prevent inhaled allergy reactions. While medications may be used to suppress symptoms, they do not treat the underlying cause of allergies. Subcutaneous immunotherapy (SCIT), commonly referred to as "allergy shots" may be used to help desensitize the immune system to specific allergens, such as pollen, mold, or house dust mites. It is rarely used in the United States to treat food allergy due to its risk of triggering life-threatening (anaphylactic) reactions. However, children with autism who suffer from allergies and asthma now have a viable alternative to conventional injection immunotherapy in treating their symptoms. Although injection immunotherapy has been the gold standard for allergy desensitization for almost 100 years, over 300 published studies show that sublingual immunotherapy (SLIT) is equally or more effective than allergy shots in reducing allergy and asthma symptoms.[5,6,7,8] The allergy extracts used in SLIT are identical to those used in injection immunotherapy, but rather than receiving a shot on a weekly or monthly basis, oral drops are administered under the tongue, often on a daily basis.

Recent research shows that during SLIT, the allergen is absorbed into the oral mucosa. The underlying dendritic cells, which are part of the immune system, produce a series of chemicals that ultimately result in a decrease in IgE and other molecules that produce allergy symptoms as well as decreasing inflammation in target tissues.[9,10] This mechanism of action is similar to that observed in conventional immunotherapy.

Although SLIT seems relatively new in the United States, it has been used clinically for more than three decades. Its use has increased steadily in the past 15 years but mostly in other countries, especially those in Europe. There are many advantages to SLIT over injection immunotherapy. SLIT may be used in children who are not eligible to receive conventional allergy injections or who may have sensory issues that would prohibit using injections. There are no reports of SLIT causing anaphylaxis, making it a safer alternative to injections. SLIT is more convenient than injection immunotherapy, since the drops are administered at home by the parent, meaning fewer office visits and no needles. There are no significant medical disadvantages of SLIT treatment; however, many insurance companies in the United States do not reimburse for SLIT, which may be financially limiting for some individuals.

The practical application and successful use of SLIT is dependent on accurate assessment of a child's allergies and sensitivities. Since conventional allergy tests only pick up on the serious types of allergic reactions, other assessment tools may be helpful in identifying more subtle allergic triggers. Environmental medicine physicians have specialized training in some of these alternative methods. Provocation/neutralization is a technique where a small amount of a food substance is injected just under the skin. If a child is allergic or sensitive to the food, then an area of redness will appear on the skin and the child may start to exhibit physical signs of reaction, including red ears, irritability, screaming, head banging, etc. When the neutralizing dose is subsequently injected, the area of redness goes away and the physical symptoms stop. It can be a very powerful tool for the parent to observe how specific foods affect their child. A similar technique is used to test for inhalant allergies, such as mold, pollen, or dust mites.

However, testing most children with autism with a needle technique is difficult and time consuming. Other noninvasive methods may be more suitable for these children. Electrodermal screening (EDS) is an effective method of determining a child's sensitivities. Although there has been little research comparing EDS to conventional allergy testing, many practitioners have found it to be an invaluable tool in identifying hidden sensitivities. EDS is a noninvasive technology that allows the practitioner to measure energy patterns in the body. Dr. Alfred Gilman and Dr. Martin Rodbell won the Nobel Prize in Physiology and Medicine in 1994 by discovering that cells communicate electrically before they communicate chemically. This means we have a way of measuring how the energy of different allergens affects the energy of our own bodies.

EDS has the capacity to assess for sensitivities to foods, molds, pollen, animal dander, and even more subtle triggers, such as chemicals, hormones, and neurotransmitters. While conventional allergy testing looks specifically at IgE or IgG antibodies,

EDS looks at the broader scope of immune reactions, particularly delayed reactions. It is not uncommon for a child with autism to go through allergy testing and be told that they do not have any allergies. Since the term "allergy" has a strict definition of IgE reaction, this may very well be true. However, this does not necessarily mean that the child does not react to various allergens. EDS is an effective means to measure delayed or subtle sensitivities that are often missed through conventional allergy testing.

The author of this article and other physicians have successfully treated thousands of children with autism with SLIT and have not observed any significant side effects or severe reactions to the treatment. Some children do get hyperactive or agitated during their initial course of treatment, but this usually resolves after a couple of weeks. Sometimes the dose has to be adjusted down for very sensitive children. Although injection immunotherapy can take a year or longer to begin controlling allergies or asthma, SLIT will often diminish symptoms within weeks. The combination of EDS and SLIT has enabled our practice to successfully treat children with autism for their various allergies and sensitivities. SLIT is a safe, effective treatment that should be considered as a first line therapy for the treatment of allergies and asthma in children with autism.

ANTIEPILEPTIC TREATMENT FOR SEIZURES AND EPILEPSY IN AUTISM SPECTRUM DISORDER

By Dr. Richard E. Frye

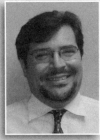

Richard E. Frye, MD, PhD

Arkansas Children's Hospital Research Institute
University of Arkansas for Medical Sciences
Slot 512-41B
Room R4041
13 Children's Way
Little Rock, AR 72202
REFrye@uams.edu

Dr. Richard E. Frye received his MD and PhD in physiology and biophysics from Georgetown University. He completed his residency in pediatrics at University of Miami and residency in child neurology at Children's Hospital Boston. Following residency Dr. Frye completed a clinical fellowship in behavioral neurology and learning disabilities at Children's Hospital Boston and a research fellowship in psychology at Boston University. Dr. Frye also completed a MS in biomedical science and biostatistics at Drexel University. Dr. Frye is board certified in General Pediatrics and in Neurology with Special Competency in Child Neurology. Dr. Frye has been funded to study brain structure function in individuals with neurodevelopmental disorders, mitochondrial dysfunction in autism, and clinical trials for novel autism treatments. Dr. Frye is the Director of Autism Research at the Arkansas Children's Hospital Research Institute and the Director of the Autism Multispecialty Clinic at Arkansas Children's Hospital.

There is a high prevalence of seizures, epilepsy, and subclinical electrical discharges in Autism Spectrum Disorder (ASD). Recent large scale studies have verified the high prevalence of epilepsy in children with ASD and have suggested that the prevalence increases with age, with a higher incidence in adolescence and adulthood. In addition, follow-up studies have suggested that epilepsy is associated with behavioral and intellectual disability into adulthood as well as increased mortality. Thus, epilepsy is an important medical co-morbidity to consider in individuals with ASD. In addition, individuals with ASD have a high rate of seizure-like electrical discharges on electroencephalogram (EEG), which are referred to as subclinical electrical discharges (SEDs). Meta-analyses have suggested that SEDs affect approximately 60 percent of children with ASD. The clinical significance of these SEDs is not clear as they rarely result in classical symptoms of seizure but have been associated with cognitive dysfunction in children with epilepsy and more severe ASD symptoms in children with ASD.

Seizures are commonly treated with antiepileptic drugs (AEDs) but non-AED treatments are used when seizures are cannot be controlled with AEDs. While a wide range of antiepileptic treatments are available to treat epilepsy, few treatments have been specifically studied on children with ASD.

Specific genetic and metabolic syndromes could underlie seizures in children with ASD. Some of these specific diagnoses may respond to specific treatments. Lastly, there are specific epileptic encephalopathies syndromes, such as Landau-Kleffner Syndrome and Continuous Spike-wave Activity during Slow-wave Sleep, which have characteristics of ASD, but the classic form of these syndromes are rare in ASD.

Success Rates

Success with treatment depends on the epilepsy syndrome and/or the underlying cause of the seizures. In some cases, significant improvement in ASD and behavioral symptoms can occur with antiepileptic treatment. For example, dramatic resolution of ASD symptoms has been reported in isolated cases of epilepsy treated with AEDs. However this is very rare. Other children may not tolerate certain AED medications and will require trials of several medications before one is found that does not have significant adverse effects. If the child has a history of allergic reaction to several medications, it may be additives and fillers that the child is reacting to rather than the AED medication itself. In such a case, a compounding pharmacy may help with obtaining AEDs without such additives.

Treatments

Treatments that produce minimal adverse effects are usually the most successful. Many children will respond to AED treatments while others will have refractory epilepsy and seizure-like events that do not respond to AEDs and should be reviewed carefully. A video electroencephalograph is particularly useful for confirming that paroxysmal events are indeed seizures. If seizures are confirmed and do not respond to standard AED therapy for reasons other than adverse effects and compliance with treatment, more extensive metabolic and genetic (see Table below) as well as neuroimaging investigations may be indicated. In addition, alternative non-AED therapies should be attempted as treatments.

Genetic and Metabolic Disorders Associated with ASD and Seizures

Genetic Syndromes	Metabolic Syndromes
• Angelman's	• Mitochondrial Disease
• Down's	• Cerebral Folate Deficiency
• Fragile X	• Succinic Semialdehyde Dehydrogenase Deficiency
• Prader-Willi	• Adenylosuccinate Lyase Deficiency
• Rett's	• Phenylketonuria
• Smith-Lemli-Opitz	• Creatine Metabolism Disorder
• Tuberous Sclerosis	• Pyridoxine dependent & responsive seizures
• Velocardiofacial	• Urea cycle defects

Antiepileptic Drugs: Although AEDs are the first line for treating seizures, no AED has undergone evaluation for efficacy for the treatment of seizures in the ASD population in high-quality clinically controlled study. A few AEDs have been evaluated for control of behavioral ASD symptoms in well-controlled studies. Valproate has been demonstrated in several controlled studies to improve behavioral symptoms in ASD while lamotrigine and levetiracetam have been shown in several controlled studies to neither improve nor worsen behavioral symptoms in ASD. Recently, to determine whether specific treatments were more beneficial than others for individuals with ASD and seizures or SEDs, 733 parents of children with ASD were asked to rate the effect of AEDs on seizures and other clinical factors including sleep, communication, behavior, attention, and mood. Four AEDs, valproate, lamotrigine, levetiracetam and ethosuximide, were rated as providing the best seizure control and worsening other clinical factors the least out of all AEDs examined. As expected, valproate and lamotrigine had the least detrimental effect on mood, although they did not have a positive effect on mood as would be expected from their traditional mood stabilizing effects and from previous clinical studies on the ASD population. Lamotrigine appeared to have the least adverse effects overall. These ratings appear to confirm the clinical experience of many clinicians.

No controlled studies have examined the effectiveness of AEDs on SEDs but several case-series have suggested that valproate and lamotrigine can improve language and cognition in children with ASD that have SEDs. Controlled studies on children with epilepsy but not necessarily ASD have suggested that lamotrigine can improve behavioral and cognitive symptoms. Much research needs to be done to define the subgroup of children with ASD and SEDs as well as their treatments.

Other medications and treatments that have not been specifically development as antiepileptic drugs can be useful in epilepsy that is not well controlled with AEDs.

Steroids: One-time treatment or regular scheduled treatments of steroids (sometimes combined with valproate) may help in refractory epilepsy, particularly epileptic encephalopathy syndromes. Daily steroids may also be effective but are difficult to maintain because of the high risk of adverse effects. Steroids are best used sparingly because of their potential adverse effects.

Intravenous Immunoglobulin: Regularly scheduled infusion of intravenous immunoglobulin may help in refractory epilepsy, particularly epileptic encephalopathy syndromes. The evidence of this treatment is based on several case-series reports.

Magnesium: Magnesium has been shown to be helpful in the control of epilepsy. Magnesium has also been demonstrated in several clinical studies to help with cognition and behavior when combined with pyridoxine. In several forms magnesium is useful for treating constipation—a common gastrointestinal problem associated with autism. Although it has not been evaluated for seizures in children with autism, it has the potential to be very useful.

Omega-3 Fatty Acids: Several clinical studies have suggested that omega-3 fatty acids may be useful in individuals with epilepsy and in individuals with autism. Overall the evidence suggests a weak positive effect of this supplement. Given the positive health benefits of this supplement, it may have a positive effect on individuals with autism and epilepsy.

Dietary treatment can be useful in epilepsy that is not well controlled with medications.

Low Carbohydrate Diets: Low carbohydrate diets, such as the ketogenic diet, have been very effective at controlling seizures in some children with refractory epilepsy. The ketogenic diet is a very restrictive diet, so some have tried the modified Atkins diet and found it to be effective. An interesting case report has demonstrated the effectiveness of a gluten-free casein-free diet combined with the ketogenic in drug resistant epilepsy. Any dietary treatment should be conducted under the guidance of a trained professional.

Milk-Free Diet: A milk-free diet has been shown to lower the level of the folate receptor autoantibody—an autoantibody that is associated with cerebral folate deficiency which is a syndrome that includes autism and seizures as characteristics. Milk-free diets can limit calcium intake so calcium supplements may be needed when instituting a milk-free diet.

Elimination Diets: Isolated cases of improvement in seizures with elimination of certain foods or preservatives have been reported but no large studies have confirmed this practice as effective. Any dietary treatment should be conducted under the guidance of a trained professional.

Surgery can be useful in special types of epilepsy that is not controlled with other treatments or diets. An extensive medical workup to eliminate undiagnosed genetic and metabolic conditions should be performed prior to considering surgery.

Vagus Nerve Stimulator: The vagus nerve stimulator is a small device that is implanted under the skin that has a wire that wraps around the vagus nerve. The device stimulates the vagus nerve which has neural inputs into the brain. It is believed that stimulation of the brain results in changes in several levels of neurotransmitters, particularly gamma-aminobutyric acid, which can help control seizures. The studies on the use of this device in autism demonstrate very variable outcomes.

Corticetomy: If seizures are found to arise from one small area of the brain, it is possible for a neurosurgeon to remove the dysfunctional part of the brain. In order to determine if one portion of the brain is generating seizures a patient must typically go through several extended hospitalizations. Although these procedures can be very successful for controlling the epilepsy, cognitive outcomes have been documented to be very variable and sometime worsen after surgery.

Multiple Subpial Transection: If a dysfunctional portion of the brain is found but cannot be removed, it is possible for a neurosurgeon to make small cuts in the brain areas surrounding the dysfunctional areas. The outcome of autistic patients that have undergone multiple subpial transection is variable but one study that applied multiple subpial transection to carefully mapped multiple active foci along with steroid treatment has demonstrated impressive results.

Individuals with epilepsy, especially those with frequent or prolonged seizures, should have an emergency medication readily available to stop any generalized seizure that is sustained for over 5 minutes.

Adverse Effects

Most antiepileptic treatments can have adverse effects. Adverse effect of AEDs are highly dependent on the medication. In general, newer antiepileptic drugs such as lamotrigine, oxcarbazepine, and levetiracetam have few serious adverse effects as compared to older AEDs, such as phenobarbitol, phenytoin, primidone, carbamazepine. The exception to this is valproate, which is an older antiepileptic medication that appears to have good efficacy for many individuals with ASD. However, the toxicity of valproate acid on the liver, pancreas, and blood cells must be carefully monitored and valproate acid must be avoided in individuals with certain mitochondrial disorders. The adverse effect profiles have not been studied in ASD specifically, so it is not known whether individuals with ASD have a higher incidence of adverse effects than other populations of individuals with epilepsy. However, it is best to avoid older AEDs (phenobarbitol, phenytoin, primidone) that have a high incidence of cognitive and neurological adverse effects as existing behavioral and cognitive abnormalities could be exacerbated. In general, almost all AEDs can cause neurological side-effects (ataxia, tremor, nystagmus), behavioral side-effects (hyperactivity, agitation, aggressiveness), gastrointestinal side-effects (abdominal pain, nausea) and an allergic reaction which can be severe in some cases. Serious side effects can often be avoided with careful monitoring. It is best to have a practitioner with experience in these medications prescribe an AED and monitor the patient. Care should be taken when using multiple AEDs as adverse effects can be additive. Since almost all AEDs elevate the rate to birth defects, it is important to carefully consider the choice of AEDs in females of reproductive age and potentially consider progesterone based oral contraception to prevent the possibility of pregnancy.

There are specific adverse effects that every practitioner should be aware of and should communicate to the patient when prescribing specific antiepileptic drugs:

Valproate: Valproate can result in serious adverse effects. The most serious adverse effects are hepatotoxicity (liver toxicity), hyperammonemia (high ammonia), and pancreatitis (inflammation of the pancreas). Precautions can be taken to prevent these adverse effects from occurring. In general, complete blood count, liver function tests and amylase and lipase should be monitored during the initial period of starting the medication and if the patient experiences gastrointestinal symptoms. Once a stable dose has been selected, the patient can be monitored approximately every 3 months. Hepatotoxicity is believed to be more prevalent in children under 2 years of age, so it is best to avoid prescribing valproate to very young children. In children with Alperts' syndrome, a syndrome caused by depletion of mitochondrial DNA, valproate can be fatal. In general, L-carnitine may mitigate liver damage resulting from valproate and, thus, cotreatment with L-carnitine is recommended. Common adverse effects of valproate include, weight gain and thinning of the hair. The latter is believed to respond to selenium (10-20 mcg per day) and zinc (25-50 mg per day). Long-term use of valproate has been linked to bone loss, irregular menstruation, and polycystic ovary syndrome.

Lamotrigine: Lamotrigine has a low incidence of serious adverse effects and is generally well-tolerated. The most serious adverse effect of lamotrigine is a life threatening whole body rash known as a Steven-Johnson's reaction. Increasing the lamotrigine dose slowly towards the target dose can reduce the risk of this reaction occurring.

Oxcarbazepine: Hyponatremia (low blood sodium) can develop in some individuals.

Topiramate: Common adverse effects include weight loss and cognitive and psychomotor slowing. Topiramate is minimally metabolized by the liver and is excreted mostly unchanged by the kidney. Topiramate can cause a metabolic acidosis (high blood acid), nephrolithiasis (kidney stones), and oligohidrosis (decreased sweating). This medicine should be avoided in individuals with kidney disorders and extra care during hot weather is necessary. Glaucoma (increased eye pressure) has occurred in rare cases, so any vision symptoms should be evaluated.

Levetiracetam: Levetiracetam has a low incidence of serious adverse effects and is probably one of the safest antiepileptic drugs. The most talked about adverse effects which affect very few patients who take the medication (<10%) are behavioral, including agitation, aggressive behavior, and mood instability. Cotreatment with pyridoxine (vitamin B6) helps reduce adverse behavioral effects in some cases.

Vigabatrin: Vigabatrin is associated with a progressive and permanent visual loss. Thus, its use is usually restricted to control of a special type of seizure known as infantile spasms in a specific condition known as Tuberous Sclerosis.

The table below can help guide the selection of a particular antiepileptic drug.

ASD Symptoms	Avoid	Possible Alternative
Gastrointestinal Disorders	Valproate	Levetiracetam, Lamotrigine
Mitochondrial Disorders	Valproate	Levetiracetam, Lamotrigine
Poor growth	Topiramate	Lamotrigine
Overweight	Valproate	Lamotrigine, Levetiracetam
Behavioral problems		Valproate

Steroids: Common adverse effects include weight gain, edema, mood instability, and insomnia. Serious adverse effects include hypertension, immunosuppression, gastrointestinal ulceration, glucose instability, and osteoporosis. Anyone on steroids for an extended period should be closely monitored for serious adverse effects.

Intravenous Immunoglobulin: Common adverse effects include rash, headache, and fever and require prophylactic pretreatment. This treatment is contraindicated in individuals with kidney or heart problems and should be administered by a practitioner familiar with the treatment. Many individuals develop increasingly severe allergic reactions to intravenous immunoglobulin treatment. In such cases, changing the brand may reduce adverse effects.

Low Carbohydrate Diets: The ketogenic diet can cause acidosis (high blood acid), so anyone on this diet needs to be carefully monitored.

Vagus Nerve Stimulator: This device can cause alternations in vocalization, coughing, throat pain and hoarseness. More serious side effects include spasms of the vocal cords, obstruction of the airway and sleep apnea. The studies on the use of this device in autism demonstrate very variable outcomes.

Corticetomy: Brain surgery can have serious adverse effects, so this option is typically reserved for the most refractory patients. Although these procedures can be very successful for controlling the epilepsy, cognitive outcomes have been documented to be very variable and sometime worsen after surgery.

Multiple Subpial Transection: Like corticetomy, this requires brain surgery which can have serious adverse effects and requires an extended in-hospital workup.

Diazepam: The most common adverse reaction is drowsiness. Respiratory depression can occur if high doses or multiple doses are given. If it is necessary to use this medication, medical personnel should be called to evaluate the patient.

For More Information

Autism Research Institute
www.autism.com.

Autism Speaks
www.autismspeaks.org

The Epilepsy Foundation of America
www.epilepsyfoundation.org

American Epilepsy Outreach Foundation
www.epilepsyoutreach.org

BIOFILM: A CAUSE OF CHRONIC GASTROINTESTINAL ISSUES IN ASD

By Dr. John H. Hicks

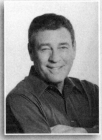

John H. Hicks, MD

Elementals Living
Medical Director
5411 State Road 50
Delavan, WI 53115
262-740-3000

www.elementalsliving.com

A renowned medical doctor and pediatrician for over thirty years, Dr. Hicks offers a unique integrative approach to health, incorporating medical, nutritional, emotional, and vibrational energy philosophies to create a customized treatment plan for each patient. This holistic approach draws clients of every age, in a variety of circumstances and from many different walks of life. As a result Dr. Hicks has gained broad and comprehensive experience in all kinds of health situations. In addition to diagnostic testing and analysis, expertise in natural supplements, and a strong focus on good nutrition, Dr. Hicks combines intuition with compassion for a highly successful program. Adding to his clinical practice as the Medical Director of Elementals Living, Dr. Hicks lectures nationally at workshops, classes, conferences and seminars throughout the country. His belief in the power of healing and good health inspires him to continue to seek out new and progressive methods of achieving good health.

Introduction

Community existence is an instinctive and natural way for species to flourish and survive, even under the most difficult climates and conditions. It is an amazing evolutionary response that sustains life and propagates the group. By forming what are called biofilms, groups of cooperative microscopic entities survive and thrive in environments that would typically destroy a single species. Specifically, biofilm is the term given to a community of microorganisms living together under or within a self-produced polymer matrix. These communities may consist of one species of microbe or a variety of different organisms including bacteria, viruses, yeast, fungi, protozoa, and single-cell microorganisms that live in extreme environments (often referred to as extremophiles).[1] The polymer matrix, which provides rigidity and structure for the microorganisms, is primarily made up of polysaccharides. It adheres firmly to a given surface, providing strong protection to the resident organisms while allowing them to thrive and prosper.

Ubiquitous in nature, biofilms occur in rivers, streams, ponds, and hot acid pools. They are even to be found in the harsh glacial habitats of Antarctica.[2] Biofilms in the natural environment offer constructive potential benefits such as self-purification of streams and rivers, a benefit that could be extended to the treatment of waste water and pollution. Microbes that naturally break down carbon can provide invaluable assistance in breaking down oil particles resulting from accidental oil spills. Using specific bacteria in a controlled manner could conceivably return to a natural state an environment that has been unnaturally polluted and compromised. Additionally, biofilms can be helpful to the mining industry in preventing acid runoff. Biofilms also benefit growing vegetation in the natural environment. Microbes that form a biofilm in the area between the soil and roots of plants can provide increased access to nutrients for themselves and the plant that would otherwise not be available.

Biofilms are not contained exclusively within the external environment of nature, however, nor are their consequences always benign or beneficial. It is now known that biofilm communities are responsible for sundry contamination occurrences. An example is found in clogged and corroded pipes, which often lead to sanitation issues. According to the Center for Biofilm Engineering at Montana State University, biofilm organisms can attach to each other or to any moist, aqueous environment, which provides a highly diverse spectrum of unlimited potential attachments, including soil particles and animal and human tissues.[1-3] Biofilms can also attach securely to the metals and plastics used in implanted medical devices such as joint replacements, heart valves, and indwelling catheters, resulting in many new, invasive, and destructive infections; due to biofilms, joint replacements have had to be removed and replaced. Biofilms can be created from bacteria and other organisms within the human body and survive from food that is consumed. Finally, biofilms are capable of adapting to human environments as varied as plaque on teeth, sinuses, tonsils, Eustachian tubes in the middle ear, and the intestines, where they are creating some of the biggest issues for patients with autism spectrum disorders (ASDs).

How biofilms work

Initially, the organisms structure weak, reversible bonds which, over time, mature and become uncompromisingly firm and secure. Strong protein adhesion molecules hold these more permanent attachments together. At this point, biofilms are far more difficult to control and eliminate. The biofilms secrete extracellular signal molecules within the matrix that act as auto-inducers (chemical signaling molecules) to start up detailed genetic programs. At a particular level of auto-inducer concentration, planktonic microorganisms attract and attach themselves to the cell adhesion areas. The extracellular polymeric matrix provides a proficient pathway for cellular communication between the assorted organisms. When the chemical messages gain sufficient strength, the group begins to function as a unit.

As a symbiotic group, biofilm organisms take on various unique characteristics. One example is the ability to synchronize genetic information through a process called quorum sensing.[4-6] Quorum sensing may take place between a single species or a diverse group of microbes. In addition, quorum sensing helps the organisms communicate more efficiently with each other and further assist in the formation and survival of the biofilm community. As different species of microbes share information back and forth, the individual strains and the group as a whole coordinate gene information, replication, and accept extracellular DNA, which they then incorporate into their own genome. This process allows the organisms living within the biofilm to become more virulent and resistant to antimicrobial agents.[1,4,6,7]

An example of this process is when specific fungi pass resistance against antibiotics onto bacteria sharing the same biofilm. The receiving bacteria cooperate and accept the new cellular information and likewise donate their DNA intelligence. This, in turn, allows the fungi to become more resistant to antifungals. Hence, biofilm organisms create an exchange and division of labor that enables them to develop powerful resistance to antibiotics and antifungal agents by preventing penetration of the antimicrobials and their metabolism or breakdown. This ability to exchange genetic information also allows organisms to more effectively evade the natural immune system defenses of the host.[1] Current research suggests that *E. Coli* bacteria have the ability to form a biofilm in 24 hours and can become virtually immune to antibiotics due to a low level of metabolic activity.[8] Other studies estimate that biofilm organisms are 1000 times more resistant to antibiotics than planktonic or free-living bacteria.[6,9-11]

In short, large varieties of microbes living within a biofilm community hold the potential for diverse genetic information exchange, along with new forms of activity from previously known microbe species.[12] This is one of the most critical issues with biofilms and ASD individuals. In individuals with ASD, cell-mediated immunity is often compromised and their system is producing excess antibodies (see *The body's response to biofilms*). However, this is precisely the system (cytotoxic T cells and natural killer cells) that is needed to protect an individual from the formation of biofilms. The biofilms therefore form quickly and strip nutrients from the host, producing toxins and releasing stronger organisms that, in turn, create more gut overgrowth and further issues with detoxification and neurologic function.

Biofilm adaptation

When free-floating bacteria sense stress in a human host, they will often begin to form a biofilm. The bacteria starting the biofilm will look for a location that has sufficient iron, which is necessary for their survival. At the same time, however, the organisms in a biofilm modulate their virulence because they depend on their host. Generally, biofilms are slow to create overt and debilitating symptoms, though this is dependent on the type and species of organisms and the toxins they produce.[1] The formation of a biofilm enables microorganisms to change their growth rate and metabolic rate and, over time, become more resistant to substances designed to exterminate them. Because of their ability to hide from the host's natural immune defenses, biofilm organisms, therefore, cannot be eradicated without external help and assistance.

Because biofilm organisms are not actively invading the human body but are instead attached to tissues or medical implants (and are protected by their immune-fighting, extracellular matrix), they can easily seed and repopulate new areas. When biofilms naturally mature, they release free-living organisms into central fluid portions of the matrix. The released organisms then seed or swim away in clumps to establish new biofilms elsewhere in the host. As the biofilms persist, they become the source of recurrent fevers and persistent inflammation in the body. In time, through continual overgrowth, some organisms produce toxins that negatively affect the systems of the host.[2,8] In this way, biofilm microorganisms can be responsible for illnesses ranging from mild respiratory infections to pneumonia, and from septic shock to necrotizing fasciitis (flesh-eating disease).[7,13]

Another common example is found when persistent otitis media bacteria create biofilms in the ear that escape through the Eustachian tube to settle in the warm, moist tissues of the gastrointestinal tract. Many ASD children have a significant history of recurrent ear infections that can be a mechanism for the establishment of biofilms in the gastrointestinal tract. As planktonic bacteria, fungi, and parasites are attracted and attach to new adhesion sites, the biofilm grows and changes from its original form. The newly fashioned mix of respiratory and intestinal organisms shares DNA information and different resistance and survival strategies and may become invasive. This, in turn, can lead to recurrent seeding and chronic relapsing infections.[3]

Along with the sharing of DNA, biofilms involve intracellular communication from chemical messengers that signal biofilm formation or resolution (dismantling of the biofilm) and indicate when to produce toxins. For some species, auto-inducers dictate when to produce a biofilm and when to release planktonic bacteria to search out another host.[4] Different varieties of biofilm use many different ways to communicate with the varied organisms in their cluster. In cholera, for example, the main messenger is a compound called CAI-1. Low levels of this compound in the *Vibrio cholerae* produce biofilms, but as the level of CAI-1 increases, pathogenic toxins are released to indicate that it is time to leave the body.[4] Other species collaborate and use other types of molecules for auto-induction communication. Gram-positive bacteria use small peptides, N-acyl homoserine lactones, and furanosyl borate diester.[6] *P. aeruginosa*, often found in the lungs of people with cystic fibrosis, produces two signaling molecules: one that is long and one is that short.[5] The practical implications of these communication differences are that biofilms are not all the same as regards the organisms that are involved and the matrix that is formed. Therefore, their resistance mechanisms will vary, meaning that there is no single protocol or way to treat all biofilms.

The body's response to biofilms

As previously mentioned, the body uses cell-mediated immunity, a specific response dictated by the immune system, to attempt to attack, control, and eliminate biofilms. Cell-mediated immunity activates macrophage cells, natural killer cells, cytotoxic T cells, and antigen-specific T-lymphocytes, which destroy pathogens and stimulate the production of cytokines. Although cytokines recruit more immune assistance, they also increase inflammation. When the immune system is compromised and shifted out of balance (in what is termed a Th2 immune shift), the antibody response side of the immune system is highly overactive, and the opposing/balancing cell-mediated Th1 side is recurrently and persistently suppressed. In this situation, the immune system is unable to activate the necessary response. Contributors to immune system imbalances of this type are numerous and include genetic predisposition, toxic substances, vaccination residuals, and heavy metals.

Biofilms (along with other types of organisms such as cell wall deficient species, L forms, stealth organisms, viruses, and certain spirochetes) have the ability to exploit Th2 immune shifts and debilitate immune system function. Another factor contributing to immune dysfunction is bacterial-induced vitamin D receptor dysfunction. Biofilms and certain other intracellular organisms produce compounds that bind and inhibit vitamin D receptor function. As a result, microbial pathogens increase and cause persistent infection and inflammation, with suppression of the needed cell-mediated immune response. This can cause a wide variety of chronic diseases, increased susceptibility to other infections, and a decline in innate immunity.[14]

Biofilms and autism spectrum disorders

With the increasing incidence of autoimmune diseases, recurrent infections, and chronic illnesses, it has become clear that existing treatment information and protocols are incomplete and that some components of disease are being insufficiently or inadequately addressed. With ASDs, in particular, certain pieces of this mismatched puzzle have been evident for a number of years. Immune dysfunction, heavy metal toxicity, an inability to detoxify waste and toxins, along with the resultant dysbiosis of the gastrointestinal system are well known to be persistent and recalcitrant to modification by current and accepted means of treatment.

Clearly, the role that biofilms play as one of the sources of chronic or recurrent infections that are highly resistant to biocides and antibiotics is an important part of the ASD story.[3,15] The Centers for Disease Control and Prevention and the National Institutes of Health currently report that 65% of all infections are quite possibly caused by biofilms.[1,8,9] Some of the more common organisms related to chronic infections are *Helicobacter pylori, Clostridium* species, *Streptococcus* species, *Bacillus* species, *Pseudomonas* species, *Klebsiella* species, *Proteus* species, *Candida* species, *Enterococcus* species, and *Serratia* species, to name a few. Biofilms are implicated in many diverse, unrelenting, and debilitating infections, some of which overlap with ASD, such as Lyme disease, arthritis, sarcoidosis, Crohn's disease, irritable bowel syndrome, recurrent strep infections, cystic fibrosis, chronic ear infections, chronic sinusitis, periodontal disease, and many others.[1-3,5,8,16] Further examples of biofilm infections include but are not limited to urinary tract infections, osteomyelitis, chronic prostatitis, gingivitis from plaque, relapsing fevers, chronic sinusitis, toxic shock syndrome, kidney stones, and endocarditis.[2,9,11,16]

Because biofilms produce toxins, an extensive and wide variety of cell and tissue abnormalities can result. With toxins traveling freely in the bloodstream, the extent of their penetration is limited only by the protective nature of the blood-brain barrier. However, heavy metal toxicity such as is found in many individuals with ASD (specifically aluminum) renders the blood-brain barrier more permeable and vulnerable to penetration and biofilm influence. In ASD, the consequences of biofilm toxicity can include cognitive impairment, processing abnormalities, and memory problems. In addition, the pathogenic toxins generated by biofilms are highly permeable and can ultimately access all parts of the body to affect any gland, organ, or system.[17,18] It is therefore reasonable to conclude that biofilm toxins affect and influence multiple body systems. In several studies on ASD individuals with gastrointestinal issues, it was found that disordered gut flora contributed to a vast increase of the *Clostridium* and *Ruminococcus* species of bacteria. This particular bacterial overgrowth leads to changes in pH balance, which affects digestion and greatly impairs the proper absorption of minerals and cofactors necessary for cell energy and neurotransmitter production.[19]

Streptococcus also has the ability to form biofilms, and it is evident that biofilms can be a source of persistent and recurrent streptococcal infections in ASD. There are many different species of *Streptococcus,* and they live in a wide variety of environments. By living in biofilms, streptococci can make adaptive changes and survive in a greater variance of pH, thereby tolerating greater levels of cellular acidity than is typical. Studies also show that streptococci living in a biofilm have the ability to incorporate foreign DNA, moderate their metabolism and replication rate, and be highly resistant to antibiotics. *Streptococcus* bacteria have the potential to form biofilms that seed and produce toxins in all areas of the body. As testing techniques continue to improve, it appears likely that a relationship between bacterial biofilms and pediatric autoimmune neuropsychiatric disorders associated with streptococcal infections (PANDAS) will be established. Like heavy metal toxicity, the *Streptococcus* bacterium also appears able to change the permeability of the blood-brain barrier, thereby changing the permeability of the central nervous system. This could lead to the neuropsychological symptoms seen with PANDAS. A 2005 study has shown that *Clostridium histolyticum* can also cause neuropsychiatric symptoms, which can be temporarily eased by the use of the prescription antibiotic vancomycin.[19]

Disrupting and eradicating biofilms

The knowledge base regarding biofilms and awareness of their medical implications have increased rather slowly, in part because microbiology was and is based on the study of pure cultures of planktonic bacteria rather than complex mixed microbial communities. Fortunately, methods of identifying, culturing, and testing microbes are now improving.[13] This will open the door to much-needed information and insights about how to control and eliminate biofilm-related chronic diseases.

In the early formation phase of a biofilm, disruption is relatively straightforward, as the biofilm is more easily detached. However, as the rigid protein matrix structure matures, biofilms become increasingly more difficult to destroy. One solution is to render the matrix softer and more penetrable. Laboratory studies and experiments are being carried out to manipulate the quorum sensing communication process as a way to modify the matrix and eradicate biofilms. Most of this work has not yet reached human trials, however, and many of the compounds under consideration are toxic to humans.[7] Moreover, it is wise to be cautious and prudent, as we do not know the full implications of manipulating quorum sensing. For example, when the entire genome of *P. aeruginosa* was screened, it was discovered that quorum sensing controlled at least thirty-nine genes,[5] showing that intricate and complex interactions occur within different species and may create unanticipated reactions. In some species, manipulation of the quorum sensing molecules will automatically increase their virulence and some species will activate invasion of the tissues.

In looking for a way to treat biofilms, it is obvious that traditional antibiotic therapy is not sufficient, even at atypical high doses. Current antibiotics are proving to be ineffective against these potent communities of microbes. Moreover, antibiotics may negatively contribute to the internal environment by increasing microbial resistance and virulence in certain species.[6,9] Many infections reoccur more powerfully after multiple rounds of different antibiotics, each time with increasingly destructive signs and symptoms.

Beneficial microorganisms living in the gut provide a natural protection against disease-causing microbes, help to develop the immune system, and aid in the digestion and assimilation of food and nutrients. Some types of gastrointestinal biofilms are normal, and use of antibiotics can result in the destruction of our natural beneficial probiotic biofilm. Without this protection, pathogenic bacteria can flourish, destroying gut tissue integrity and increasing gut permeability. Leaky gut tissue then allows movement into the bloodstream of compounds and substances that will create inflammation, generate food and environmental sensitivities, and negatively impact and alter immune function. Additionally, a leaky gut will create a persistent Th2 shift and increase susceptibility to other dangerous pathogens. Weakening of gut motility and function leads to decreased toxin clearance and increased proinflammatory cytokines. This, in turn, can result in diminished absorption of essential nutrients, even in the presence of daily supplementation. With these issues in mind, it is clearly imperative to rid the intestines of pathogenic biofilms to allow for complete healing of the digestive, immune, and all other affected body systems.

The first line of defensive therapy is an effective and potent probiotic, which allows healthy, beneficial, and protective bacteria to repopulate the internal gut environment and prevent the attachment and replication of pathogens that are released as the biofilm regresses. Whenever possible, it is beneficial to identify the specific organisms involved in the biofilm. This can be done through specialized stool testing and culturing as well as antigen and DNA processing. The type of organism determines whether the cell's surface charge is Gram-positive or Gram-negative. Gram-positive bacteria are more sensitive to the destructive effects of antibiotics and the natural defenses of the immune system, whereas Gram-negative bacteria are more resistant. Furthermore, the positivity or negativity determines what ions or elements are attracted or bound to the cell. These ions may be minerals (such as calcium, magnesium, chloride, or potassium) or heavy metals (such as mercury, aluminum, cadmium, and lead). The nature of the bond between cells and ions (or elements), which provide cross bridging, can greatly enhance the complexity of a biofilm matrix.

Secondly, it is necessary to penetrate the matrix of the biofilm to weaken its protective shield and thereby permanently eradicate the resident microorganisms. One of the most effective and beneficial ways to do this is with enzymatic therapy, using enzymes that specifically break apart protein and carbohydrate molecular bonds. There are several brands of enzymes that contain multiple strains and proprietary blends to facilitate biofilm deactivation and penetration. Enzymes have also been shown capable of preventing biofilm formation. Unfortunately, in some biofilms, the process of matrix disruption has the effect of making certain species even more virulent and invasive.[20] In such cases, the organisms move to different locations, increasing the level of infection throughout the body. As the biofilm spreads and matures, different species attach and detach, contributing to and increasing genetic modification through an exchange of extracellular DNA.[21] The choice to use or not use enzymes will depend on the types of organisms that each person has within their biofilm. It cannot be assumed that enzymes alone will completely destroy a biofilm once the matrix has matured and is more resistant to degradation.[7]

In cases where enzymatic therapy is inadequate, chelating agents may be needed to remove iron, which is necessary for microbes' survival and the creation of biofilms. For this process, the use of lactoferrin and ethylenediaminetetraacetic acid (EDTA) compounds that remove iron, minerals, and heavy metals are recommended. These compounds may be the most effective additional therapy to prevent biofilms from forming and to remove them once firmly established.[22] (However, attempting to remove heavy metals at the same time as treating the biofilm may increase activity of some yeast components. This is another reason to proceed cautiously with an experienced practitioner who will monitor the situation—organisms, order of operations, and individualization/timing of each treatment—on a regular basis.) Biofilm studies also show that sub-inhibitory levels of antibiotics, when combined with enzymatic therapy, can assist in reducing the biofilm burden.[23] These are given in low intermittent doses to avoid the increasing resistance typically induced by high doses of antibiotics.[9,10,24,25] Antibiotics that target the cell cycle will not be as effective, given that biofilms often modify cell metabolism and replication.

Thirdly, the innate immune system needs to be balanced and reactivated. In this way, the immune system can most efficiently regulate a defense against pathogenic biofilms and destroy existing biofilms. Because many of the organisms that make up a biofilm become planktonic and move to different locations, it is critical that the overall immune system be addressed to function optimally. Any Th2 shift must be corrected to stimulate and balance the Th1 side of the immune system to clear pathogens. This can be accomplished with specific immune-boosting supplements called transfer factors. Transfer factors, both general and specific, significantly aid in shifting the immune system back to neutral, increasing the activity of the immune system's natural killer cells. Transfer factors also tag or mark cells that harbor pathogenic organisms, thereby boosting the T-lymphocyte cells' ability to remove the pathogens.[26]

It is imperative to make sure that vitamin D levels are normal and that the receptors are functioning properly. Genetic predisposition to polymorphism or gene variance can influence the activity of the vitamin D receptors that are essential to the uptake of vitamin D. Vitamin D plays an essential role in calcium and bone metabolism, induction of cell differentiation, inhibition of cell growth, and modulation of the immune and hormone systems.[14,27] If the vitamin D receptors are shown to be impaired, an agonist that stimulates the receptors to function properly may be used. Some medications given for high blood pressure have the side effect of being a vitamin D agonist.

In devising a therapeutic protocol, it is needful to prepare for the expulsion of free radicals. Some form of cell protection is critical. The level of protection will be dictated by the length of time the biofilm has been present in the body and the organisms involved. Essential fatty acids (such as black currant oil) provide optimal cell membrane protection along with cell-protective antioxidants like glutathione and antioxidants from berries (including blueberries, blackberries, raspberries, and strawberries).

Other biofilm treatment options to be considered include homeopathic and vibrational remedies. These substances offer assistance in both removing and preventing biofilms. Furthermore, the impact that diet has on the various organisms must be recognized and addressed. Sugar, vinegar, simple carbohydrates, and corn act as food for microbes; therefore, intake of these should be limited and their complete digestion should be sought.

It is important to address all of the pathogens residing within a biofilm. Fungi such as *Candida* will not respond to standard antifungal substances when protected in a biofilm. A different approach is needed. The use of natural products such as cellulase enzymes that dissolve yeast and other remedies such as olive leaf extract, uva ursi, cranberry with berberine, or Indian Fire Tree Bark tea can be effective. These substances also provide strong antibacterial protection for the immune system.

As a cautionary note, quickly killing a multitude of organisms all at once may release large quantities of toxins, overwhelming an already compromised detoxification system. This can elicit a Herxheimer reaction, which is typically referred to as "die off." A reaction of this type stems from the release of toxins into the bloodstream, which stimulates the production of inflammatory cytokines and generates temporary hormonal imbalances. It can also prompt diarrhea or nausea as the body strives to clean up and clean out. Activated charcoal can reduce the toxin load on the body and help to eliminate the additional toxic burden, thereby reducing the incidence of Herxheimer reactions.

Conclusion

Attention to biofilms is expanding and gaining momentum. Biofilms have constructive, beneficial potential and yet are also associated with chronic diseases and illnesses that are recurrent and persistent. Nature has gifted biofilms with impressive survival abilities, including group communication and genetic adaptability. These varied communities of organisms are highly resistant to current treatments and protocols, including antibiotics and antifungal substances. Therefore, understanding the role that biofilms play in the human body is critical. Combined therapies are warranted, including probiotics, enzymes, natural immune stimulants, and detoxifying supplements. All of these can lend assistance to the immune system to clear and eradicate these potent and powerful microbes.

CHELATION: REMOVING TOXIC METALS

By Dr. Michael Elice

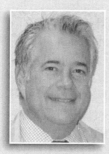

Michael Elice, MD

AIM Integrative Medicine
80 Crossways Park Drive
Woodbury, New York 11797
(516) 802-5028

Dr. Elice is a board-certified pediatrician and has been in practice for thirty years. Dr. Elice is a graduate of Syracuse University and the Chicago Medical School. He completed his pediatric residency at the North Shore University Hospital in Manhasset, New York. He has academic wteaching positions and is on the staff of North Shore University Hospital and Schneider Children's Hospital. He is an associate professor of pediatrics at the New York University Medical School and the Albert Einstein School of Medicine. He is on the medical advisory board of the New York Families for Autistic Children (NYFAC) and is a member of the National Autism Association New York Metro Chapter. He has lectured at Defeat Autism Now! conferences around the country.

Lead, mercury, aluminum, nickel, cadmium, and other metals are common environmental pollutants in industrialized countries. Although measures to control these metals have been put into place during past decades, high levels of pollutants persist in soil, water, and the air we breathe. They seep into our food supply, leading to consequences of environmental exposure of populations living in those areas. Whether it is oil refineries, smelting facilities, or industry in the US or China, these metals are here to stay. Most of the toxicity associated with heavy metals is due to their effects on the mitochondria, whose functions are short-circuited by inhibiting vitamins, enzymes, and depleting glutathione. These metals have cumulative toxicities as they combine together to have a more significant toxic effect, even if their individual levels are below the danger threshold. Metals can affect our central nervous systems, kidneys, and bone. Clinical conditions associated with metal toxicity are cardiovascular disease, cancer, Alzheimer's disease, diabetic neuropathy, renal disease, fibromyalgia, chronic fatigue, and autoimmune diseases.

Children with autism have disorders of immune function which lead to lower levels of glutathione, a major source of removal of toxic metals. These children are more susceptible to symptoms of autism, many of which are consistent with presence of heavy metals. There are several tests that can be considered for testing for exposure to heavy metals. Blood tests may test for recent exposure but not past or prolonged exposure, since most metals have only a short half-life in the blood. Hair and urine are measures of the body's excretion of toxic metals, which is affected by both the body burden and the body's glutathione level, which controls excretion. Since glutathione levels are often low in autism, a decreased level of glutathione can mask a high body burden. The most conclusive method to test for metal toxicity is the use of detoxification agents followed by a collection of urine or stool. This testing reveals if the metal is present in the body and demonstrates that the detoxification (chelation) agent can remove it.

There are different agents that can work to chelate or remove these metals from within the cells. BAL (British Anti-Lewisite) was the first of the chelating compounds and was developed by the British during WWII as an antidote to arsenical war gases. In 1945, it was first used as treatment for lead toxicity. Calcium EDTA, first used in 1933, forms complexes with metal ions such as chromium, iron, mercury, copper, and lead, and are excreted by the kidneys. In 1964 patients with atherosclerotic cardiovascular disease were treated successfully with EDTA. In 1961 it was found that EDTA helps patients with scleroderma, rheumatoid arthritis, and circulatory disease. In the late 1970s publications supported the use of chelation for osteoporosis and improvement in mitochondrial function in the ischemic heart muscle. In 1980 Blumer and Reich found that EDTA reduced cancer incidence by 90 percent in patients over ten years. They also found improvements in fatigue, arterial stenosis, bone density, heart rate, blood pressure, pulmonary function, total cholesterol, and kidney functions.

DMSA (Chemet) reacts with the same group of metals as BAL. It has no clinical effects on essential minerals and can be administered orally where approximately 23 percent is absorbed, intravenously or intramuscularly. DMPS, not approved by the FDA, is an analog of BAL and has similar affinities as DMSA but even more for mercury. Sixty percent is absorbed orally or can be given IV as well.

In 2000 "Position Paper on Diagnosis and Treatment of Heavy Metal Toxicity in Autism Spectrum Disorders" was published along with "Autism: A Unique Type of Mercury Poisoning." The premise is that the characteristics of autism and mercury poisoning, derived from the medical literature, have been found to be strikingly similar and that autism may actually be a form of mercury poisoning. Nelson's Textbook of Pediatrics describes lead poisoning symptoms that also mimic the symptoms of behavioral abnormalities, perseveration, attention and focus problems, language problems, and neurological damage, found in patients with autism.

In 2009 "Safety and Efficacy of Oral DMSA Therapy for Children with Autism Spectrum Disorders" was published. A two-phase study involving a total of 114 children received either DMSA or a placebo. The groups receiving DMSA had significant improvements on all assessment measures. It was safe in children with ASD who had high levels of urinary excretion of toxic metals and was helpful in reducing some of the symptoms of autism in those children. While the DMSA treatment appeared to be beneficial in most cases, there was a small subset that had slight worsening of hyperactivity, which was usually temporary. Age had little effect on the degree of improvement.

The procedure known as chelation usually involves the collection of a urine sample to establish a baseline for the amount of metals that the patient can excrete on their own. A challenge dose of the chelating medication is given either orally or intravenously and is followed by a urine collection to measure the amount of increase in metal excretion. DMSA is given for three days and the cycle can be repeated every seven or fourteen days. DMPS can also be given orally or IV. The dose is calculated based on the weight of the patient. Many practitioners will administer Calcium-EDTA and glutathione in conjunction with IV DMPS or DMSA rather than these agents alone. Libutti and Baker tested over 200 urine samples and found a greater than 3:1 difference in the levels of lead excretion compared to DMSA alone. Alpha Lipoic Acid, an over the counter nutritional supplement, can be administered orally as well. D-Penicillamine, used for copper toxicity, is also used to improve chelation since it can cross the blood-brain barrier and remove toxins from the brain. Many protocols have taken on the names of different doctors and researches, i.e., Cutler, Buttar, et al. In my practice, I have tried to assimilate concepts described in these protocols and those found in the scientific literature to create a customized chelation plan for my patients. The IV infusion is no worse than having blood drawn and takes a short period of time. While there is a small chance of the patient feeling feverish, fatigued, or nauseated, the majority of patients can leave the office after the procedure and return to their normal daily activities. Many parents report that their child will have the best night's sleep on the day of chelation. Often, positive behavioral changes will follow. Since the initial infusion of medication is at a lower dose, the results as measured by urine tests and parental observation are not always apparent. Over time with repetitive infusions done biweekly, clinical improvement in neurological behaviors, sleep, bowel, and bladder function ensue. The duration of these improvements varies from patient to patient. The process of detoxification may take months or even years to rid the body of toxic metals, again dependent upon body burden and glutathione production. Results vary from patient to patient regardless of their age. Chelation is often suspended when clinical improvements plateau. If any form of sensitivity reaction occurs, the procedure should be stopped as well. The decision to end treatment needs to be based on both laboratory and clinical evidence.

ENZYMES FOR DIGESTIVE SUPPORT IN AUTISM

By Dr. Devin Houston

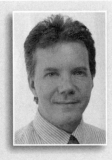

Devin B. Houston, PhD

www.houston-enzymes.com
866-757-8627

Dr. Devin Houston founded Houston Enzymes in 2001 after many years of enzyme research in academia and industry. He invented the first enzyme product targeted to the autism community in 1999, and has since improved on that first effort. Dr. Houston continues to educate the public on enzymes and speaks on a regular basis at many autism conferences and parent groups.

The term "enzyme" refers to a broad class of specialized proteins that catalyze chemical reactions. Without enzymes these reactions would not occur, or they would proceed at a rate not conducive to sustaining life. As catalysts, enzymes are not destroyed during the reaction. This allows a very small amount of enzyme to perform a large amount of work.

Digestive enzymes are a subset of enzymes specialized to break down foods after ingesting. These enzymes are necessary to derive nutrition from food. Specialized enzymes exist for different food proteins, carbohydrates, and triglycerides. The end result of their action is the provision of amino acids, glucose, and short-chain fatty acids to the body for production of compounds required for human metabolism.

The human body provides a fair amount of different enzymes for digestion, mostly from the pancreas and cells lining the gut wall. The bulk of the enzyme work occurs within the first part of the small intestine, or duodenum. It is here that protease enzymes begin the process of breaking proteins into smaller fragments called peptides, and carbohydrase enzymes start cleaving large carbohydrates into simple sugars. The duodenum and rest of the small intestine are also the site of absorption of nutrients into the systemic circulation.

Enzymes are present in raw foods but only in amounts sufficient to degrade the food over a period of several days. Many feel that enzymes in raw foods can supplement the digestion of food. Since digestion occurs within hours, not days, the actual contribution of food enzymes towards digestion is minimal. Enzymes can be supplemented in much more concentrated form. Fermentation of certain non-pathogenic fungi produces prodigious amounts of enzymes. Specific enzymes can be selected for production by altering the conditions under which the fungi are grown. The enzyme is then purified from the fungi through many biochemical procedures resulting in a homogenous enzyme protein containing no fungal residue. The concentration of these enzyme blends is increased some billion-fold over what is found in raw foods.

Many doctors have noted that children with autism often have gut problems. Inflammation can be a major problem. Tissues that are inflamed are damaged. Damaged cells don't produce enzymes; therefore, many children with autism may present deficiencies in some enzymes until the gut is healed and operating normally. Malabsorption may present as well. Food intolerance and outright food allergies may also manifest in these children. However, the vast majority of people with food intolerances have no obvious enzyme deficiency. The pancreas, in most cases, puts out more than enough enzymes to break down foods. The problem is not so much the amount of enzymes available as is the location of protein digestion. The majority of enzymes available for digestive work are located in the intestinal tract. This is also the location of nutrient absorption. The problem for those with food intolerances is that food breakdown occurs in the same area as absorption. This can be altered using acid-stable plant enzymes that can work in the stomach.

The most common food intolerance plaguing those with autism appears to be related to food proteins producing opioid-like peptides during digestion. Wheat and dairy products containing gluten and casein, respectively, are especially noted for producing exorphin peptides after contact with pepsin and elastase enzymes during the digestive process. This is a normal occurrence during digestion; however, some with autism exhibit stereotypical behaviors after ingesting wheat or dairy foods. One school of thought is that an inappropriate interaction between opiate ligands and their receptors exists; however, this has not been substantiated. Many parents found that diets that restrict wheat and dairy seemed to diminish the behavioral problems. The gluten-free/casein-free diet (GFCF diet) is strongly recommended by many health care givers to their patients struggling with autism. The diet is not easy and requires a major lifestyle change for the patient and often the entire family.

Unsuccessful attempts were made in the 1990s to find a single enzyme that would address the "peptide problem." Only when several different protease enzymes were combined with a specific peptidase enzyme called dipeptidyl peptidase IV, or DPP IV, was a degree of success obtained. DPP IV was a known enzyme but not documented in commercially available enzyme blends until 1999. DPP IV specifically degrades exorphin peptides and is produced by human gut cells. The fungal form is acid-resistant, as are most fungal enzymes. The actions of DPP IV provide a possible mechanism of action and rationale for using protease enzyme supplements as a possible alternative to the GFCF diet.

With the exception of alcohol, water, B vitamins, and some drugs, very little is absorbed from the stomach. Proteins and peptides are not absorbed until the food mass enters the small intestine. The stomach does not empty its contents into the duodenum until approximately 2–3 hours after ingestion. This provides a window of opportunity for addressing the problem proteins before their breakdown and absorption can occur in the small intestine. Plant-based enzymes are quite acid-resistant, unlike their pancreatic counterparts, and so may start working on foods within the stomach once in solution. A potent formulation of appropriate protease and peptidase enzymes can alter the pattern of protein break down such that exorphin peptides are not produced. If such peptides are produced, DPP IV peptidase can specifically degrade the exorphin peptides prior to food moving into the gut. However, the proper approach is to combine the DPP IV with other potent proteases to present a two-pronged attack: 1) change the manner in which the parent protein is broken down, and 2) use DPP IV to degrade any peptides that happen to form. It is interesting to note that this same approach is being used to develop an enzyme-based therapy for celiac disease.[1]

Enzymes may be helpful in other ways for those with autism. Keeping the gut free of undigested material prevents putrefaction that may lead to pathogenic bacterial blooms and yeast problems. Gas and bloating may be minimized by using carbohydrase enzymes such as lactase and alpha-galactosidase. Some vegetables contain carbohydrates such as stachyose and raffinose that are difficult for humans to digest. The human gut lacks the enzymes to degrade carbohydrates that become a food source for gas-producing bacteria. Alpha-galactosidase enzyme supplements can make up for the deficiency and ease the bloating. Chronic diarrhea may also be helped through the addition of enzymes such as amylase and glucoamylase that degrade starchy foods.

Other enzymes, such as xylanase, may modify some plant polyphenolic compounds by removing certain sugar groups that are attached to these compounds within the plant cells. These "phenolic compounds" are sources of antioxidants and other nutritional substances and may play a role in modifying oxidative stress.[2] Removal of the sugar groups allows absorption of many polyphenolics and their subsequent metabolism by human cells.[3]

Enzymes are one of the safest dietary supplements available. No upper limit has been established for dosing of any food-grade enzyme. No amount of plant-based digestive enzyme has been found to cause toxicity or side effects. Dosing of enzymes is not based on body weight or age, as most of the ingested enzyme stays in the gut and is eliminated or broken down in the colon by microbial proteases. Enzymes are optimally given at the beginning of each meal to allow more contact time with the food in the stomach. Enzymes will not interfere with most medications, unless the medication is made of protein, carbohydrate, or triglyceride.

Well-controlled studies of enzyme use for the digestive problems associated with autism will eventually happen. The long history of safe use of enzymes in the food industry, however, should provide optimism and encouragement to try enzyme supplements without worry of significant side effects. It is paramount that the parents of those with autism find and develop a relationship with an enzyme company that truly understands the scientific basis of how enzymes work.

Enzymes are regulated as dietary supplements. This means that just about anyone can start a company selling enzymes and claim to be an "enzyme expert." Ninety-five percent of the enzyme supplement companies today have no science department or anyone on staff with actual hands-on experience in enzyme research. Enzymes are safe but the danger to the consumer is by using a product not correctly formulated for their specific dietary needs. It is strongly recommended that you contact a potential supplier of enzyme products and compare their staff and educational backgrounds. Time spent researching these companies will go a long way to helping you get the best enzyme supplement for your money.

HOW ENZYMES COMPLEMENT THERAPEUTIC DIETS

By Kristin Selby Gonzalez

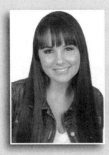

Kristin Selby Gonzalez

President and Chairman, Autism Hope Alliance
Autism Hope Alliance
18501 Murdock Circle Suite 303
Port Charlotte, FL 33983
www.autismhopealliance.org
www.kristinselbygonzalez.com
www.facebook.com/kristinselbygonzalez
www.facebook.com/autismhopealliance
www.twitter.com/KSelbyGonzalez
www.twitter.com/autismhopealli

Kristin Selby Gonzalez joined Enzymedica in 2008, serving as Director of Autism Education. As the company's primary link to the autism community, she has advised Enzymedica with respect to company policy and product formulation for children on the spectrum, and counseled directly with parents on the use of Enzymedica's products. She has given lectures worldwide, educating thousands throughout the years on different strategies to help children on the autism spectrum. In addition to her trainings and certifications, Kristin brings her own experience as a mother of a child on the spectrum. As of September 2012, Kristin leads Enzymedica's philanthropic work at Autism Hope Alliance where she is now serving as President/Chairman. Kristin has been working with her son for over nine years and has seen him progress from very withdrawn with no language to a playful and interactive boy who now speaks. She possesses an extraordinary body of knowledge and experience with both educational and biomedical interventions for autism, including enzyme therapy, dietary intervention, sensory integration, and play therapy. Kristin holds a Bachelor of Arts degree in Elementary Education and Theater Arts.

First, I think it is best to understand why it is so important for our children (no matter what age) to have proper digestion of their foods. Vitamins and nutrients can't be absorbed into the body and brain without enzymes. Many of our children are experiencing enzyme deficiencies. What does an enzyme deficiency look like? Well, there can be many symptoms to look for when trying to discern digestive sensitivities. Some of the behaviors and physical signs are: dark circles under the eyes, red cheeks, red ears, rashes, hyperactivity, lethargy, sweating, aggression, mood swings and/or sleep issues, bloating, gas, acid reflux, heart burn, constipation, diarrhea, particles of food in their stool and really the list goes on and on. We need to become better detectives in figuring out the causes of these signs and listen to what our bodies are trying to tell us.

Digestive enzymes are produced by our bodies, found in raw foods, and sold as nutritional supplements. Enzymes are the workers of the body and will never go wasted in the body. From the moment food enters the mouth, enzymes start to go to work. As we chew we begin to activate enzyme activity. As food travels throughout our digestive system there are enzymes assisting with breaking up the food all along the way. Visualize your digestive tract as somewhat of a conveyer belt. Imagine as the first bottle drops at a bottling factory there is a worker to oversee that it lands upright; then the bottle travels down to where the liquid will be added and there is a worker there overseeing that; the bottle still needs to be capped off . . . well, you can see where I am going with this. Enzymes work in a similar fashion as each one has a specific job and purpose.

As I mentioned previously, digestive enzymes are also found in raw food. It was Dr. Edward Howell, author of *Enzyme Nutrition*, who illustrated what would happen if someone were to pick an apple from a tree and leave it on the kitchen counter for two weeks. Some of us might say the apple would rot, and that would be correct in a sense. Mother Nature supplied that apple with enough enzymes to digest itself. So, it would only make sense that the fresher the apple, the more enzyme activity the apple would provide to help you digest it when you eat it.

Digestive enzymes are also found in a supplemental form that can be purchased at a health food store. A person would typically take this type of enzyme supplement with the first bite of food. Taking a digestive enzyme with a meal allows for the enzymes to aid proper digestion by breaking down foods into valuable nutrients for the body.

I know that digestive enzymes were a crucial piece for my son. Although, he was on a therapeutic diet, if he couldn't break up the foods then nothing would work properly in his body for him. It would also cause him much pain and discomfort every time he would eat.

Now, let's talk about therapeutic diets as I have often heard that some believe supplemental enzymes can replace a therapeutic diet. I wish that were true, but in most cases it just isn't. Supplemental enzymes and therapeutic diets are what I like to think of as the "dynamic duo," working synergistically in the body for optimal results. For the majority of those who have sensitivities, they should consider looking into a clean diet, a good digestive enzyme, a good probiotic, and a good omega fatty acid supplement. In my own son's case, even though I had him on the cleanest diet imaginable, I still needed to give him a good digestive enzyme to help break down food. My son was constipated and would only have a bowel movement every three days until we figured out how to help his body absorb the nutrients he was taking in by his food. Many other children have constipation for longer periods of time—sometimes dangerously so, including possible impaction and reabsorption of toxins. Anything that is not broken down by the gut can, in essence, putrefy and feed bad bugs that have pathological physiological effects and sometimes negative cognitive consequences. Also, the brain needs to receive nutrients. By giving my son a diet that his healing tummy could handle, appropriate for each level in the process, and combining this with the use of a good digestive enzyme, probiotic, and omega supplement, we have seen wonderful results.

What does this mean in terms of children with autism learning and functioning well? Imagine if you have tried to learn algebra while you had a headache or a stomach ache. It would be quite difficult. We focus so much of our time on different educational and other therapies that often we overlook the foundational importance of healing and sealing the gut. Other therapies are more successful when a child feels healthy and is free of pain. And when foods are broken down completely causing less irritation to the gut and resulting in fewer undigested substances entering the bloodstream, then fewer substances cause allergic-type reactions that affect the immune system and, consequently, the nervous system, thinking, and learning. Furthermore, I think that everybody would agree that everyone thinks and functions better when nutrients are absorbed to be utilized for the many cognitive and other processes of the body.

There are many different levels of digestive sensitivities for individuals on the autism spectrum. Some are truly allergic to specific foods, while others may show signs of intolerance to foods (an adverse reaction to a food not associated with an allergy and, therefore, not shown on an IgG allergy test). I recommend keeping a food diary, which can be very beneficial when trying to pinpoint food intolerances. When discovering which diet works best for an individual on the spectrum, it is crucial not to give up and keep searching until you find one that works. Sometimes taking it one step at a time and eliminating one food at a time can be easier for you and your child. This way you can really see how each food affects your child.

At the end of the day there is not one thing that works for every child—ultimately it takes trial and error to see what is best for each individual. We do know that no matter how healthfully you eat, if your digestive system isn't breaking down and absorbing the nutrients in your food, then the body can't function and operate to capacity. When the gastrointestinal system is operating properly, this benefits our immune system, our energy level, and our emotional and physical well-being. I think that the quote by Jean-Anthelme Brillant-Savarin (1755–1826) says it best: "Digestion, of all the bodily functions, is the one which exercises the greatest influence on the mental state of an individual." I also think my son says it best with the smile on his face after he eats and is not in pain. If you were to ask him why he takes his enzymes with his food he would tell you, "Because it helps my tummy feel better." And really at the end of the day isn't that what we all want for our children.

FLAVONOID FORMULATION FOR ALLERGY-LIKE SYMPTOMS AND BRAIN INFLAMMATION IN AUTISM

By Dr. Theoharis Theoharides and Shahrzad Asadi

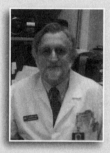

Theoharis C. Theoharides, PhD, MD
Shahrzad Asadi, PHARMD
Molecular Immunopharmacology and Drug Discovery Laboratory,
Department of Molecular Physiology and Pharmacology
Tufts University School of Medicine
136 Harrison Avenue
Boston, MA 02111
617-636-6866
Fax: 617-636-2456
www.mastcellmaster.com

Dr. Theoharis C. Theoharides, is the Director of the Molecular Immunopharmacology and Drug Discovery Laboratory as well as a professor of pharmacology, biochemistry, and internal medicine at Tufts University. He received all his degrees from Yale University. He has published over 300 research papers and three textbooks. Dr. Theoharides was the first to show that mast cells can be stimulated by non-allergic triggers, such as stress hormones, to secrete inflammatory mediators selectively leading to disruption of the gut-blood-brain barriers. He and his colleagues then showed that a brain/gut peptide, neurotensin, is elevated in the serum of autistic children and induces extracellular secretion of mitochondrial DNA that acts as an "auto-pathogen" inducing and auto-inflammation response. Based on his discoveries, Dr. Theoharides proposed the novel concept that mast cells play a critical role in brain inflammation and autism.

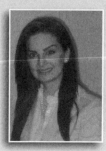

Shahrzad Asadi, PharmD, performs investigations in the Molecular Immunopharmacology and Drug Discovery Laboratory at Tufts University. She is currently working on the role of mast cells in stress-induced neuro-inflammatory diseases. She has been investigating the effect of corticotropin-releasing hormone (CRH) and the role of mitochondria on human mast cell release of molecules that could disrupt the blood-brain-barrier and contribute to the pathogenesis of autism.

Treatment for Autism Spectrum Disorders (ASD) has been elusive because of the absence of specific pathogenesis or biomarkers. In the majority of cases, the cause of ASD is unknown. Although some autism susceptibility genes have been identified, no single gene or group of genes can explain the disturbing rise in ASD from 2/100,000 children 20 years ago to 1/88 children today. Unfortunately, autism is still considered a psychiatric disease. As a result, research has mostly focused on the behavioral manifestations of autistic spectrum disorders instead of what led to them. We believe ASD derive from a perinatal/postnatal insult to the brain, leading to an "epineurologic" condition.

Gut-Blood-Brain Barrier Disruption, Mast Cells, and Brain Inflammation

We hypothesized that autism starts when the protective gut-blood and blood-brain barriers break down either during pregnancy or early postnatally. Barrier disruption allows neurotoxic molecules, such as propionic acid derived from gut bacteria, to reach the brain, ultimately resulting in inflammation and defective nerve processing. This premise is supported by the fact that many autistic patients have antibodies against brain proteins, which implies that immune cells reached the brain through a leaky blood-brain-barrier (BBB). Mast cell activation could be particularly critical during gestation, since mast cell-derived mediators might act epigenetically to alter the expression of autism susceptibility genes. Moreover, recent evidence indicates that there is increased number, spatial distribution, and activation of microglia, the innate brain immune cells, contributing to dysfunctional neuronal communication. Mast cells were recently considered as glial regulatory cells.

Allergic Symptomatology, Mast Cells, and Autism

The possible association between autism and mast cells was first investigated because many symptoms that characterize patients with autism are also present in patients with mastocytosis, a spectrum of disorders that involve proliferation and activation of mast cells in the skin (urticaria pigmentosa, UP) and other organs. Preliminary results indicate that the prevalence of autism in mastocytosis patients is about tenfold higher (1/10 children) than the general population. The *Mastocytosis Society, Inc.* together with the American Academy of Allergy, Asthma, and Immunology (AAAAI) recently produced a video, entitled "Mast Cell Activation Symptomatology" (www.tmsforacure.org), which highlights the fact that allergies may be only one aspect of mast cell activation.

The observation that most children with autism have either a family or personal history of immune or allergic disorders prompted the proposal that autism may be a "neuroimmune" disorder. There have been numerous papers that support this proposal. One study investigated infants born in California between 1995-1999 and reported that maternal asthma and allergies during the second trimester of pregnancy were correlated with more than double the elevated risk of autism in their children. In another study, 30 percent of autistic children had a family history of allergies as compared to 2.5 percent age-matched "neurologic controls." A more recent study reported that immune allergic response, represented by the frequency of atopic dermatitis, asthma, and rhinitis was increased in 70 percent of Asperger patients compared to 7 percent in age-matched healthy controls. In a National Survey of Children's Health, parents of autistic children reported symptoms of allergies more often than those of other children, with food allergies being the most prevalent complaint. Another study reported an increased prevalence of non-IgE mediated food allergy in the autism group compared to normal controls. It is also interesting that a recent study conducted in Germany reported an independent association between atopic eczema and Attention-Deficit Hyperactivity Disorder (ADHD), which has considerable phenotypic overlap with autism.

The link between allergic symptomotology and autism is also supported by the observation that in many cases, autistic symptoms worsen when a patient's "allergic" symptoms flare up. However, even in these symptomatic cases, "allergy" tests, such as skin prick or RAST, are often negative. These circumstances suggest a non-allergic trigger of mast cells. This possibility is now recognized by AAAAI as a new diagnosis, "mast cell activation disorder."

Environmental and Stress Mast Cell Triggers

Mast cells are critical for allergic reactions, but are also important in regulating immunity and inflammation. Mast cells are located close to blood vessels in both the gut and brain. Functional mast cell-neuron interactions occur in these locations and nerve endings increase both intestinal and brain permeability. This may help to explain the intestinal and neurologic complaints of ASD patients. Many substances originating in the environment, intestine, or brain can trigger mast cell secretion. These triggers include: bacterial, fungal, and viral antigens, as well as environmental toxins such as polychlorinated biphenyl (PCB) and mercury. We published that thimerosal can stimulate human mast cells to release pro-inflammatory molecules. A recent study also reported that children exposed to mold had cognitive dysfunction. The ability of viruses to trigger mast cell activation is also important for their possible contribution to autism pathogenesis. A number of rotaviruses have been isolated from asymptomatic neonates and could activate mast cells at that age.

Neuropeptides, such as neurotensin (NT) and corticotropin-releasing hormone (CRH), secreted under stress, stimulate mast cell release of vascular endothelial growth factor (VEGF). New evidence indicates that prematurity and stress experienced by the mothers during gestation increase the risk of children to develop autism. In fact, a recent paper reported that mothers who experienced stress during gestation had high

IgE levels in the cord blood and their children were more likely to be allergic to dust mites.

Once activated, mast cells secrete numerous vasoactive, neurosensitizing, and pro-inflammatory substances that are relevant to autism, including IL-6 and TNF. IL-6 can disrupt the gut-blood-brain barriers, as well as promote the development of Th17 cells which are critical for the development of autoimmune diseases.

Recent Evidence

We recently showed that NT was increased in the serum of young children with autistic disorder. This molecule, found also in the skin and the gut, activates not only mast cells, but also glial cells. Moreover, the highest concentration of NT receptors is in the Broca area of the brain, which regulates speech, known to be inexplicably lost in many children with ASD. We also showed that NT induces extracellular secretion of mitochondrial DNA (mtDNA), which was also increased in the serum of the same children that had high NT in their serum. Extracellular mtDNA acts as an "auto-pathogen" leading to auto-inflammation and can also increase IgE receptor expression in mast cells. Moreover, we showed that mitochondrial components can induce IgE receptor expression and augment allergic stimulation of human mast cells.

Why Use a Select Flavonoid Formulation?

Certain molecules have antioxidant actions. These include glutathione, resveratrol, and Pycnogol. However, certain flavonoids are more potent antioxidants, while also having the ability to inhibit activation of microglia, the brain innate immune cells, recently shown to be overactive in autism, and are also protective against neuronal mitochondrial damage.

Flavonoids are naturally occurring compounds mostly found in green plants and seeds. There are approximately 3,000 flavonoids. Whether taken as pills, tablets, or hard capsules, all flavonoids are difficult to absorb in powder form and are extensively metabolized to inactive ingredients in the liver. In fact, less than 10 percent of orally ingested flavonoids are absorbed.

Flavonoids are natural molecules found mostly in green plants and seeds. Unfortunately, our modern diet contains progressively fewer flavonoids and those that are consumed are difficult to absorb because they do not dissolve in water. Under these conditions, the average person cannot consume enough to make a positive health difference.

Quercetin, and its closely structurally related flavonoids rutin and luteolin, have potent antioxidant and anti-inflammatory actions. Quercetin and luteolin can also inhibit the release of histamine and prostaglandin D_2 (PGD_2), as well as the pro-inflammatory molecules IL-6, IL-8, and TNF from human cultured mast cells. Moreover, quercetin inhibits mast cell activation stimulated by IL-1, and mast cell-dependent stimulation of activated T cells involved in autoimmune diseases. Luteolin also inhibits IL-6 release from microglia cells, as well as IL-1-mediated release of IL-6 and IL-8 from astrocytes. Quercetin and luteolin also reversed acute stress-induced autistic-like behavior and the associated reduced brain glutathione levels in mice.

However, there are about 3,000 flavonoids in nature, and many impure flavonoids are sold under such names as "bioflavonoids," "citrus flavonoids," "soy flavonoids," or "Pycnogenol." Unfortunately, such preparations DO NOT specify either the source or the purity of the flavonoids. This problem is even worse given that many ASD patients could have reactions to the impurities, fillers, or dyes. Very few flavonoids are beneficial; many others such as morin have no anti-inflammatory activity, while Pycnogenol is weakly active (as compared to luteolin or quercetin), but could cause liver toxicity. As an additional consideration, the most common source of the flavonoid quercetin is fava beans, which can induce "hemolytic anemia" (destruction of all the blood cells) in those 15 percent of people of Mediterranean origin, such as Greeks, Italians, Jews, and North Africans, who lack the enzyme glucose-phosphate dehydrogenase (G_6PD). Another cheap source of querstetin is peanut shells, with the possible risk of anaphylactic reactions in those patients allergic to peanuts.

The selection of specific beneficial flavonoids, as well as the source, purity, and absorbability of the selected flavonoids is, therefore, of great importance. We searched for flavonoids that may block as many of the pathogenetic processes suspected to be involved in autism. It turns out that the natural flavone luteolin, purified from chamomile or artichoke, exhibits most of the designed benefits: 1) antioxidant, 2) anti-inflammatory, 3) mast cell inhibitor, 4) NT-induced mitochondrial secretion inhibitor, 5) microglial inhibitor, 6) BBB disruption protector, 7) neuroprotective, 8) mitochondrial protective, 9) metal chelator, and 10) thimerosal-induced inflammatory mediator release inhibitor. Luteolin also can reverse ASD behavior in mice and in humans.

Basic Description

NeuroProtek® (www.neuroprotek.com) is a unique dietary supplement formulation, with an exclusive patented combination of these flavonoids, selected to reduce oxidative stress and inflammation in both the gut and brain. The purpose of Neuro-Protek is to maximize the beneficial effects of flavonoids while overcoming absorption obstacles. NeuroProtek contains: luteolin, quercetin, and the quercetin glycoside rutin (>95 percent pure). To increase their absorbability, these flavonoids are formulated in microvesicles (liposomes) mixed in unprocessed olive kernel oil imported from

Greece, also providing the benefits of the Mediterranean diet. There are NO preservatives and NO dyes.

Preliminary Evidence of Benefit

Though to date, trials of NeuroProtek in ASD are limited, the results are very promising. In an open case report of thirty-seven children (ages 4-14) result derived from thirty-seven children with ASD, by the end of 4 months, there was a significant improvement in eye contact, communication skills, and social interactions. Four of these children (one boy and three girls), who had not been able to speak since regression at age 3 years, started using words and answering simple questions. Two of them (one boy, and one girl) are more fluent and attend regular middle school. NeuroProtek is not available in health food stores in order to keep the price affordable.

Formulation and Suggested Use

NeuroProtek is formulated in a soft gel capsules. The capsules must be taken with food in a dose of two capsules per 20 kg small (44 lb) weight per day. It may take 4-6 months before benefits are observed depending on the age, duration, and severity of symptoms. NeuroProtek does not require a prescription, but its use should be made known to the health providers responsible for ASD patients.

Safety

Quercetin and its related flavonoids rutin and luteolin are safe because they are purified from chamomile, to avoid the problems associated with fava beans and peanut shells mentioned above, and are highly pure (>95 percent). There are no side effects known; however, this formulation (as well as any flavonoids) must be used with caution with drugs that are heavily metabolized by the liver (e.g. antihistamines), as it may affect the resulting blood levels of such compounds. Nevertheless, parents and health providers should be aware of the fact that there could be unwanted interactions among drugs, dietary supplement, vitamins, and other treatment regimens that we reviewed recently.

The main metabolism of luteolin is by glucoronidation, methylation, and sulphation. Some ASD children appear to be sensitive to polyphenols, presenting symptoms of increased hyperactivity (http://www.allnaturaladvantage.com.au/Phenol%20Sensitivity.htm). Not all phenolic compounds carry the same potential risk. For instance, Pycnogenol from pine bark has 15 phenolic groups and naringin has 8, as compared to myrecetin's 6, quercetin's 5, and luteolin's 4. In response to concerns about "phenol sensitivity," NeuroProtek-LP (low phenol) has been developed and is available for such patients (www.neuroprotek.com).

Patents

Dr. Theoharides is the recipient of US patents No. 6,624,148; 6,689,748; 6,984,667; 7,115,278 and EPO 1365777, which cover methods and compositions of mast cell blockers in neuro-inflammatory conditions, US patent application No. 12/861,152 covering Auto-inflammatory compositions for treating brain inflammation (allowed), as well as US Patent applications 12/534,571 and 13/009,282 covering diagnosis and treatment of ASD. All patents have been assigned to Theta Biomedical Consulting and Development Co., Inc. (Brookline, MA, USA).

Trademark

The name NeuroProtek® has been trademarked in the USA with US registration No. 3225924 and has also been assigned to Theta Biomedical Consulting and Development Co., Inc. (Brookline, MA, USA).

Background live presentations:

http://www.mastcellmaster.com
http://www.autismedia.org/media3.html
http://www.youtube.com/watch?v=pNQsK9PQL3c&feature=related
http://www.youtube.com/watch?v=3QFa36TBtvA

GASTROINTESTINAL DISEASE: EMERGING CONSENSUS

By Dr. Arthur Krigsman

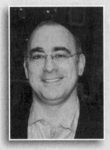

Arthur Krigsman, MD

148 Beach 9th Street
Far Rockaway, New York 11691
516-239-4123

Dr. Krigsman is a pediatrician and board-certified pediatric gastroentero-logist. He has extensive experience in the evaluation and treatment of gastrointestinal disease in children with autistic spectrum disorder and participates in the growing field of research designed to better understand GI disease in this group of children. He has presented his findings in peer-reviewed journals and has shared his experience at scientific and lay meetings, and at a congressional hearing dealing with autism and its possible causes.

The presence of chronic gastrointestinal (GI) symptoms in children with autism spectrum disorder (ASD) has been well established. Prospective reviews of the frequency of these chronic and often intense GI symptoms, based upon thoughtful questioning of the parents, reveal that they occur in as many as 70–80 percent of ASD children. The GI symptoms in these children are of a wide variety and include abdominal pain, diarrhea, constipation, abdominal distention, and growth failure ("failure to thrive"). In my experience with over 1400 such patients, I have often heard the parent state, "I can live with the autism, but I can't stand to see my child suffer with pain and severe constipation." Because the communicative and behavioral aspects of autism are the most obvious, and because the GI symptoms frequently begin during infancy (prior to the onset of the behavioral and cognitive problems), parents are often unaware of the impact of the GI problems on their child's health until years later.

Historically, when parents do finally bring these GI complaints to the attention of their general practitioner or pediatric gastroenterologist, their significance is often minimized or dismissed. There are many reasons for this, including lack of familiarity with the GI diseases frequently seen in ASD, uncertainty on the part of the physician about how to properly proceed in the evaluation of these diseases, and long-standing beliefs in the medical world that GI symptoms in the "mentally handicapped" are mysterious and poorly defined, similar to what is observed in many patients with mental retardation. Lastly, the political controversy and unending media misinformation swirling around the three scientists who were the first to describe bowel disease in ASD patients has given rise to doubts in some academic circles as to whether anything is really wrong at all with the bowels of these children.

Fortunately, the GI problems of children with ASD are now getting attention. First was a full-day conference jointly sponsored by NASPGHAN (North American Society for Pediatric Gastroenterology, Hepatology, and Nutrition), the American Academy of Pediatrics, and Autism Speaks. It was dedicated solely to further our understanding of the GI disease in these children. In addition, there are two consensus statements published in a January 4, 2010, supplement to the journal *Pediatrics,* offering guidance to clinicians as to how best evaluate gastrointestinal symptoms within the setting of ASD.

The two most important points to keep in mind are that (a) GI symptoms should be evaluated no differently in children with ASD than they would in neurotypical children, and (b) problem behaviors may be the sole manifestation of a gastrointestinal problem. Let us explore these two statements.

The presence of chronic (i.e., long-standing) GI symptoms demands medical evaluation. The fact that the child has autism is merely an interesting sidebar item. The clinical story typically begins with the parents' concern over the chronicity and intensity of their child's GI symptoms. It is this that brings them to the pediatrician or gastroenterologist. The symptoms typically consist of any, some, or all of the following:

- abdominal pain
- diarrhea (defined as unformed stool that does not hold its own shape but rather conforms to the shape of the container/nappy/diaper that it is in)
- constipation (defined as infrequent passage of stool of any consistency or passage of overly hard stools regardless of frequency)
- soft-stool constipation
- painful passage of unformed stool
- rectal prolapse
- failure to maintain normal growth
- regurgitation
- rumination
- abdominal distention
- food avoidance

An additional layer of complexity appears when there is an observed correlation between the intensity of the GI symptoms and the level of cognitive-behavioral dysfunction. Parents will often say that they can predict their child's behavior on any given day based on how their stool looks. In the non-ASD world of pediatric gastroenterology, the GI pathology responsible for these varying symptoms is often difficult to determine from the symptoms alone. The same holds true in the ASD patient group. In both cases, numerous underlying GI problems can cause these symptoms. In my experience with ASD children, the following diagnoses have been endoscopically confirmed and determined to be causing some or all of these symptoms:

- eosinophilic esophagitis (EoE)
- esophageal hypereosinophilia (EH)
- reflux esophagitis
- *Candida* esophagitis
- esophagitis of unknown origin
- Barrett's esophagus
- peptic gastritis
- eosinophilic gastritis
- lymphocytic gastritis
- autoimmune gastritis
- gastric ulcer
- gastropathy of unknown origin
- *Helicobacter pylori* gastritis
- peptic duodenitis
- duodenal ulcer
- white-spot (micro-erosive) duodenitis
- *H. pylori* duodenitis
- non-specific enteritis
- celiac disease
- non-specific colitis
- Crohn's disease

Of course, ASD children may suffer from the same common GI ailments as neurotypical children (e.g., constipation, reflux, transient stomach virus infections, etc.), so a GI complaint in an ASD child does not automatically suggest the presence of the above-mentioned diagnoses. It is certainly appropriate to undertake a trial of empiric therapy (that is, treatment of a suspected disorder without prior confirmation of the true diagnosis) for any of the common childhood GI problems (e.g., reflux, constipation, etc.).

However, if the symptoms prove resistant to conventional empiric therapies or if the suspected diagnosis is that of a chronic disorder that will require long-term treatment (i.e., inflammatory bowel disease), empiric therapy is inappropriate and contraindicated. The fact that most ASD children experience chronic GI symptoms, and that most ASD-GI-symptomatic children have demonstrable causal pathology of the types listed above, has led many to conclude that GI pathology occurs with increased frequency in ASD children when compared to neurotypical children. This is certainly the conclusion I have drawn in working with these children.

The approach to evaluating these chronic symptoms should be the same as those employed to diagnose and treat neurotypical children. Established diagnostic algorithms exist for all of the above-mentioned symptoms and include a careful taking of the history, physical examination, blood tests, stool tests, urine tests, abdominal imaging studies, nutritional assessment, and assessment of growth patterns. These tests should be designed to cover as broad a spectrum of potential diagnoses as possible, including metabolic diseases such as mitochondrial disorders. Needless to say, these tests are most useful when they provide strong evidence of a specific diagnosis. However, more often than not, even the most comprehensive non-invasive evaluation does not shed light on the cause of the symptoms in the ASD-GI patient. These are the cases that usually require direct visualization of the GI tract via endoscopy. Endoscopy not only provides direct visualization of the lining of the GI tract but also the ability to obtain a small sample of tissue (biopsy) for microscopic examination by a pathologist. The recent introduction of wireless capsule endoscopy (commonly referred to as the "pillcam")

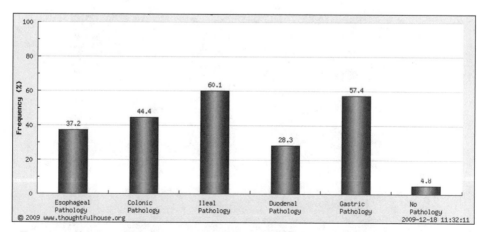

Frequency by Anatomic Location of Various GI Pathologies in ASD-GI Symptomatic Children Undergoing Endoscopy and Colonoscopy. Performed by Arthur Krigsman, MD. 2003-2009. Reported by Independent Pathologists (Mount Sinai Hospital, NY, Lenox Hill Hospital, NY, and CPL Labs, TX).

allows direct visualization of the small intestinal lining not accessible to more conventional endoscopy and has contributed greatly to our understanding of bowel disease in ASD children. ASD-GI patients who have undergone diagnostic endoscopy and biopsy frequently have more than one of the diagnoses listed above, and the precise order in which they need to be treated, as well as the nature of their relationship to each other, has to be further studied.

For the most part and for the sake of simplicity, the various diagnoses of the esophagus and stomach depicted above are also seen in the neurotypical population, but the ASD-associated enterocolitis (ASD-EC) present in the majority of ASD-GI patients, and well described in the medical literature, appears to be unique to ASD patients. (The exception to this appears to be a focal enhanced gastritis described only within the population of ASD-GI patients.) Because of this, established treatments for the esophageal and gastric (stomach) diagnoses exist, but the best treatment for the ASD-associated enterocolitis is unknown. It is uncertain whether treatment of non-specific enterocolitis may also treat some of the esophageal and gastric pathology. Much work needs to be done in this area. It does seem clear, though, that ASD-associated enterocolitis is, in many cases, a chronic disease. Because academic interest in the area of autism-associated bowel disease is increasing, it will be interesting to see the results of clinical trials aimed at determining the treatment outcomes of a variety of pharmaceutical and dietary interventions for autism-associated enterocolitis. Many researchers believe that

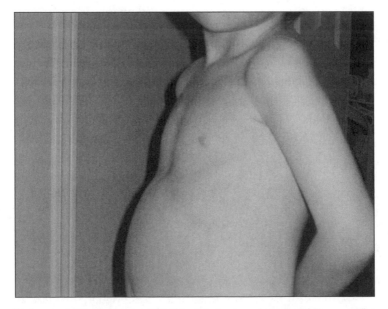

Abdominal Distension in a Child with Autism Associated Enterocolitis

these clinical trials should include established therapies for other inflammatory bowel diseases (IBDs) such as Crohn's disease and ulcerative colitis. The rationale for this is that preliminary data demonstrate an interesting overlap between the clinical presentation, laboratory findings, and endoscopic/histologic findings of autism-associated enterocolitis and IBDs. As in Crohn's disease, the symptom presentation of ASD-associated enterocolitis may consist of abdominal pain, diarrhea, abdominal distention, and growth retardation. Interestingly, constipation and difficulty in passing soft or unformed stools is a frequent presenting symptom in ASD-associated enterocolitis though this is not thought to be typical of the symptoms of Crohn's disease (though there are reports of just such presentation in Crohn's disease as well). Abdominal x-rays of ASD children presenting with chronic GI symptoms characteristically show fecal loading, meaning a colon loaded with stool. The colon in these patients does *not* typically appear distended on x-ray, thus providing reassurance that there is no obstruction. Obstruction would represent a medical emergency and requires urgent medical attention. In such cases, the patient is quite ill and toxic looking. The constipation most typical in ASD-GI children is best referred to as "soft stool constipation." This means that the child will go many days (often up to a week or more) without a bowel movement. During this period, the abdomen becomes progressively more distended. Parents often report that the progressive retention of stool correlates with progressive worsening in the child's *behavior* (e.g., "stimming," aggression, self-injurious behaviors, hyperactivity) and *cognition* (i.e., focus, processing, thought, and language, etc.). The stool that is finally produced after many days is semi-formed or unformed and is often produced only with great straining.

Other interesting overlaps in the clinical presentation of ASD-associated enterocolitis and Crohn's disease exist as well. Disturbance in growth patterns is often noted at presentation. Interestingly, even after all other gastrointestinal symptoms are resolved with the appropriate medications and diet, disturbances in growth patterns often persist. The deviation from normal growth can affect linear growth (height), weight, or both. Preliminary data indicate that this growth delay occurs despite adequate caloric intake and in the absence of any evidence of malabsorption. However, in some patients, there may indeed be a component of GI disease related malabsorption. There are reports of decreased bone mineralization in ASD children, independent of their being on any specific restrictive diet. In addition, reports of duodenal brush border enzyme deficiencies (not associated with known genetic defects) in ASD-GI patients further suggests a possible underlying mucosal inflammatory process that may contribute to growth retardation.

Overlap in laboratory testing between ASD-associated enterocolitis and IBD includes the finding of an elevated erythrocyte sedimentation rate, C-reactive protein, and platelet counts as well as the presence in the stool of lactoferrin, calprotectin, and lysozyme. The latter three stool markers are considered specific for the presence of intestinal inflammation. The relative frequency with which these markers of inflammation are present in ASD-associated enterocolitis as compared to IBD has not yet been determined. Perhaps most interesting in terms of laboratory overlap is the frequent presence of elevated IBD-specific serologic markers. These markers are serum antibodies to both bacterial and fungal gut flora that are statistically associated with the presence of IBD and are rarely found in the non-IBD population. It is important to point out that these markers are *not* considered to be a diagnostic test for IBD. They are most appropriately used when a clinician is trying to distinguish Crohn's disease from ulcerative colitis and when attempting to determine the likelihood of particularly aggressive forms of Crohn's disease. However, their frequent presence in ASD-GI children suggests that a similar mechanism of disease might be present there as well and provides potential avenues of further research.

In patients undergoing clinically indicated diagnostic endoscopy for the above symptoms, there is the frequent occurrence of a non-specific mucosal inflammation. The term "non-specific" indicates that the features seen under the microscope, though not normal, do not indicate the presence of a specific disease. It implies that the finding is not normal, but that many causes are possible. Though there are specific microscopic features of Crohn's disease that allow one to make a definitive diagnosis, it is not unusual for Crohn's disease patients to produce biopsies that are non-specific in nature. Such is the case with ASD-associated enterocolitis where the majority of the patients demonstrate non-specific findings upon biopsy. However, there are a number of ASD-GI children whose intestinal biopsies demonstrate the changes strongly suggestive of Crohn's disease.

These clinical, laboratory, and endoscopic/histologic overlaps provide strong preliminary support for clinical trials that investigate the efficacy of pharmaceuticals commonly used to treat IBDs. It is our hope that such clinical trials will be undertaken soon.

Moving on to the second of our statements made at the outset of this article, parents, physicians, and therapists must realize that difficult-to-treat ASD behaviors or behaviors that have not been responsive to standard behavioral interventions may be the *sole* manifestation of a GI diagnosis. This means that unprovoked aggression, violent behavior, and irritability may have an underlying GI cause, and this must be taken into consideration prior to the reflexive desire to begin a psychotropic drug such as risperidone (despite its FDA approval for the treatment of autism). Gastroesophageal reflux disease, gastritis/gastric ulcer, and constipation are just three examples of GI diagnoses that are known to cause such behavioral symptoms. In addition, poor focus and an inability to make significant academic or communicative progress despite intensive interventions may indicate the presence of a treatable bowel disease that, once treated, can significantly improve the child's degree of disability. The concept of behavioral problems as a symptom of GI disease was strongly supported in the consensus article published in the January 4, 2010, supplement of the journal *Pediatrics*.

The take-home messages are as follows:

1. Treatable GI disease is exceedingly common in ASD.
2. The signs and symptoms that alert one to the possible presence of GI disease are both conventional (e.g., diarrhea, abdominal pain, etc.) and ASD-specific (e.g., behaviors, aggression, poor response to therapies, etc.).
3. The approach to the GI evaluation of these signs and symptoms should be no different from a child without autism.
4. Parents and therapists who note such signs and symptoms must strongly advocate for the child regarding the need for a comprehensive GI evaluation.
5. Treatment of GI disease should follow established treatment protocols for the particular diagnosis.
6. GI diagnoses unique to ASD require further study to determine best treatment practices.
7. Empiric treatment for common, transient childhood conditions is appropriate but should be halted if the patient demonstrates non-responsiveness.
8. Empiric treatment for suspected chronic disease is inappropriate and contraindicated.

BIOME DEPLETION, HELMINTHS, AND AUTISM

By Judith Chinitz

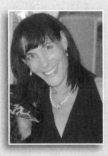

Judith Chinitz, MS, MS, CNC

New Star Nutritional Consulting
(914) 244-3646
www.newstarnutrition.com
judy@newstarnutrition.com

After her son's diagnosis with autism in 1996, Judith Chinitz has spent the last eighteen years searching for answers. After saving her son's life through diet, and seeing firsthand the healing power of food, Judy earned a second master's degree in nutrition. She is also a certified special education teacher. Judy is the author of *We Band of Mothers: Autism, My Son, and the Specific Carbohydrate Diet,* which also contains commentary by Dr. Sidney Baker. She also assisted Dr. Baker in founding Medigenesis (available at www.autism360.org), an Internet-based, interactive medical database. Currently, Judy is volunteering to help set up a new company that will be providing a helminth for biome reconstitution.

Autism, Immune Abnormalities, and Biome Depletion

In 1964, Dr. Bernard Rimland published his book, *Infantile Autism: The Syndrome and Its Implication for a Neural Theory of Behavior,* proving that autism was a physiological—as opposed to a psychological—condition. By the 1970s, researchers began to note immune system abnormalities in autistic children. In the 1980s, researchers such as Dr. Reed Warren, for example, demonstrated that those with autism had abnormal lymphocyte responsiveness (that is, their white blood cells don't respond normally to germs) and abnormal levels of various types of immune cells, including low levels of natural killer cells. (This means that children on the autism spectrum have a hard time fighting pathogens, like yeast, viruses, and bacteria.)

In 1998, Dr. Sudhir Gupta of the University of California, Irvine, published a paper in the *Journal of Neuroimmunology* entitled, "Th1- and Th2-like cytokines in CD4+ and CD8+ cells in autism." This paper states that the ". . . data suggest that an imbalance of Th1- and Th2-like cytokines in autism may play a role in the pathogenesis of autism."

To date, a few of the specific abnormalities found in individuals with autism include:

a. In an unstimulated state, individuals with autism have higher levels of proinflammatory cytokines (chemical messengers of the immune system) than control groups.

b. With stimulation of the immune system (i.e., with the introduction of pathogens), individuals with autism spectrum disorders (ASD) have markedly higher levels of proinflammatory cytokines than controls.

c. Specific proinflammatory cytokines that have been found to be high in people on the spectrum include tumor necrosis factor-α (TNF-α) in both the blood and the gut; interferon gamma (IFN-γ) in both the blood and the gut; and higher levels of IL-12 in the blood.

d. Individuals with ASD have lower levels of regulatory cytokines (those chemicals that turn off inflammation) like interleukin-10 (IL-10) than control groups.

e. Brain specimens from subjects with autism exhibit signs of ongoing inflammation and abnormalities in immune signaling and immune function.

These proinflammatory chemicals appear to affect not just how these individuals respond (or don't respond) to disease-causing microbes; they also affect the health of the body in general, the digestive system and the function of the brain itself.

Dr. Martha Herbert, an Assistant Professor of Neurology at Harvard Medical School, and a pediatric neurologist at the Massachusetts General Hospital in Boston, a leading figure in the research of autism, has stated repeatedly that the brain is downstream from the digestive system, meaning that if the latter is compromised, the former suffers. The lining of our digestive system comprises about seventy percent of the immune system. Our bodily systems are not separate entities, but all parts of one whole. If one part is compromised, the rest are affected.

Also evident from the medical literature is the finding that many individuals with ASD have abnormal gut microbiota. What does this mean? The human body contains trillions of microbes, far more than there are cells in our bodies. No one really knows exactly what the composition of these microbes should be. However, we do know that there should be something like 400–500 different types of bacteria living in our intestines. Multiple researchers have now demonstrated that individuals with ASDs have not only excessive amounts of bacteria living in their digestive systems, but also seemingly abnormal kinds as well. It's a chicken-and-egg scenario: abnormal gut microbiota leads to abnormal gut conditions compromising the immune system, but the reverse is also true. That is, abnormal immune functioning within the gastrointestinal tract will lead to abnormal microbiota.

In January of 2011, a paper was published in the *Proceedings of the National Academy of Science*, entitled, "Normal gut microbiota modulates brain development and behavior." The researchers found that mice raised in a germ free environment, devoid of normal gut microbes, had highly abnormal development when compared to normal peers. If normal microbes were introduced early enough in development, as adults the two groups were indistinguishable. However, introducing normal flora to an adult germ-free population did not remediate the developmental abnormalities. They conclude: "Our results suggest that the microbial colonization process initiates signaling mechanisms that affect neuronal circuits involved in motor control and anxiety behavior." Of course this study was done on mice, and animal models do not always translate into the same meaning for humans. However, these data are certainly compelling.

That our "old friends," the flora that live in and on us, are absolutely crucial to normal, healthy life, is accepted fact. That disturbances in this ecosystem early in life can affect the development of the immune and central nervous systems has now also become the focus of intensive research around the world. Our body is an ecosystem and our modern way of life has led to what Dr. William Parker, of Duke Medical School, calls a depleted biome.

The hygiene hypothesis, which was first proposed about twenty-five years ago, conjectures that we have become "too sterile." With the advent of germ theory a century ago (the recognition that many diseases arise from specific germs), we have concentrated our efforts on eradicating bacteria, yeasts, and more complex organisms called helminths, from our environment and ourselves. However, the fact is that many species of these organisms were normal parts of human flora for all of human history, and without our old friends, we have tipped our immune systems into a chronic state of imbalance.

So, where does this leave us? Many individuals with autism have abnormal gut biomes and abnormal immune functioning. How best to handle this is not yet known. Dr. Sidney Baker, one of the world's foremost authorities on autism, states that the practice of medicine is essentially deciding if the patient has too much of something or too little of something. Currently, many doctors focus on the "too much" and target the killing of the bad stuff — antibiotics for bad bacteria, antifungals for Candida, etc. And this helps . . . sometimes. Another line of thought, though, is to shift the immune system and gut back into normalcy by *adding* good flora and fauna (the "too little" side of the coin), rather than, or as well as, subtracting bad—especially when the lines between good and bad may be more blurred than originally thought.

Enter Helminths

The presence of helminths was natural and endemic for the evolving humanoid species up until seventy-five or so years ago. We lived on and with the soil, and thus our intestines were filled not only with bacteria and yeasts, but protozoa and other life forms too—including helminths. Helminths are a family of organisms that include nematodes (round-worm like hookworm and whipworm), trematodes (fluke) and cestodes (tapeworm).

In her book, *Riddled with Life: Friendly Worms, Ladybug Sex, and the Parasites That Make Us Who We Are*, Marlene Zuk writes, "What happens if we think of parasites not as enemies or friends, but as members of our family? We do not choose to have them, but our lives are unimaginable without them, and for better or worse, they have made us who we are."

With our current anti-germ way of thinking, many are immediately horrified when they first think about "infecting" themselves with such organisms. "Aren't these parasites? And aren't parasites bad?" is the typical first question from those learning about this form of therapy. Well, yes, they certainly can be. We are all very well aware of the health benefits of yogurt, with its live bacteria. Do you equate this with eating salmonella? Some helminths are good and some are bad. And like bacteria, some are meant to be in us. And like bacteria, the amount matters. An absence of good bacteria in the gut will seriously compromise the health of the individual. Research now suggests that an absence of helminths is a major factor in the development of many inflammatory disorders.

Perhaps most fascinating of all, several papers were published in 2010 pointing to the fact that the bacteria of our intestines seem to work synergistically with helminths. Dr. Joel Weinstock, a preeminent researcher of helminths' role in curing disease, who is now at Tufts University in Boston, recently looked at a mouse model of inflammatory bowel disease and found that helminthic infection actually positively altered the bacterial content of the gut. He concludes, "These data support the concept that helminth infection shifts the composition of intestinal bacteria." In fact, researchers at the University of Manchester in England found that a certain type of helminth is reliant upon the microflora of the intestine to reproduce. When the number of bacteria in the mice intestine were reduced, so were the number of helminth eggs: "Critical interactions between bacteria (microflora) and parasites (macrofauna) introduced a new dynamic to the intestinal niche . . ." It appears that mammals evolved carrying an entire complex, inter- and intra-dependent ecological system within them.

In 2007, Dr. Kevin Becker of the National Institutes of Health published an article in *Medical Hypotheses* entitled, "Autism, asthma, inflammation, and the hygiene hypothesis." Dr. Becker concludes, "Altered patterns of infant immune stimulation may hypersensitize the early immune system not toward allergic sensitivity and bronchial hypersensitivity but to inflammatory or cytokine responses affecting brain structure and function leading to autism. It is well documented that immune cytokines play an important role in normal brain development as well as pathological injury in early brain development. It is hypothesized that immune pathways altered by hygiene practices in western society may effect brain structure or function contributing to the development of autism."

In 2012, Dr. William Parker et. al. published the paper, "Is Autism a Member of a Family of Diseases Resulting from Genetic/Cultural Mismatches? Implications for Treatment and Prevention." Dr. Parker and his colleagues state, "Several lines of evidence support the view that autism is a typical member of a large family of immune-related, noninfectious, chronic diseases associated with postindustrial society. This family of diseases includes a wide range of inflammatory, allergic, and autoimmune diseases and results from consequences of genetic/culture mismatches which profoundly destabilize the immune system. Principle among these consequences is depletion of important components, particularly helminths, from the ecosystem of the human body, the human biome."

Marlene Zuk sums this all up beautifully: "Scientists are beginning to speculate that the absence of challenge to the immune system, which defends us against foreign intruders like bacteria and worm eggs, may have unanticipated repercussions. Like bored children, immune system cells may start working mischief, attacking the cells of the very body they inhabit or initiating an elaborate assault on an innocuous pollen grain or mote of dust. Having evolved with parasites, could we suffer when they are gone?"

As the evidence continues to pile up, the answer to her question appears to be a more and more emphatic YES. Dr. Parker states in his 2011 paper, "Reconstitution of the human biome as the most reasonable solution for epidemics of allergic and autoimmune diseases," that "A wide range of hyperimmune-associated diseases plague postindustrial society, with a prevalence and impact that is staggering. Strong evidence points towards a loss of helminths from the ecosystem of the human body (the human biome) as the most important factor in this epidemic."

Research thus far has shown that certain helminths raise levels of regulatory cytokines (those chemicals that turn off inflammation) and they lower levels of inflammatory cytokines, including TNF-α. That is, helminths may do exactly what is needed to improve the immunological functioning of individuals on the autism spectrum. There have now been several clinical studies done on individuals with asthma, allergy, multiple sclerosis (MS), and inflammatory bowel disease. Results have varied depending on the disease and the type of helminth tested and of course may have been affected by the length of the trial and the dosages used. However, multiple trials have now demonstrated significant positive effects of helminths on inflammatory bowel disease and multiple sclerosis. At the time of writing, there are multiple trials not yet completed, including a very small one on adults with autism. Anecdotally, many people have now benefitted enormously from therapeutic doses of parasites for diseases such as MS, inflammatory bowel diseases, asthma and allergy, Samter's triad, Sjögren's syndrome, and of course autism.

Over the last few years, more and more parents have begun to use a variety of helminths to treat their children with autism. Most have tried courses of TSO (Trichuris suis ova), which are porcine (pig) whipworm larvae. As these are not native to humans, they live for only two to three weeks in the human gut. Anecdotal reports have been astounding, to say the least. The children are showing global improvements, which are sometimes dramatic. The incidence of negative side effects is extremely low, and consists of nothing more than reports of increased hyperactivity, some agitation, and sleep disturbances, which go away over time (usually by week 10). Parents report improved digestive functioning, increased language and cognition, improved social skills, better mood and mood regulation, and more. The average amount of time it takes to begin to observe the changes is about twelve weeks. Some children, however, have certainly taken longer, even up to eighteen weeks. TSO is taken orally: small vials of saline solution containing the invisible ova are drunk every two to three weeks. However, TSO is so expensive at the moment that it is beyond the reach of many families, especially considering that it must be done continuously.

Several other human helminths are now also commercially available including whipworm (*Trichuris trichuria*) and hookworm (*Necator americanus*). Hookworm and whipworm cannot reproduce directly in their host. They live in the intestines and lay eggs, which are passed out in stool. Under certain specific environmental circumstances, the eggs then mature to an infective stage, at which point they can enter the host. (When we lived without modern plumbing and hygiene practices, stool would end up on soil or in water.) Thus, there is no danger of being "infested." If any adverse symptoms do occur, the worms can be destroyed with a dose or two of an anti-parasitic medication, such as Albendazole. There are potentially greater side effects with these two helminths, since they do take up residence in humans. Again, anecdotal reports have generally been good, especially in terms of hookworm alleviating allergy issues and TTO alleviating ulcerative colitis.

Hymenolepis diminuta cysticercoid (also known as rat tapeworm) is also now on the helminthic therapy horizon. Like TSO, these helminths are not native to humans (as cystoids, they have a slightly more complex life cycle, moving in development between rodents and grain beetles), and die in us in approximately 17 days. (Very preliminary anecdotal reports are excellent for IBD, allergy, and migraines, although at the time of writing this, no one has yet used them in autism.) There are no known side effects to date, and these, unlike TSO, TTO, and hookworm (which are class 2 organisms) are considered class 1 organisms by the CDC, meaning that they are not known to cause disease in healthy adults.

There are not yet any formal studies done on children with autism, and, as stated above, only one on adults with autism, which is ongoing. Those contemplating trying this therapy should be aware that it is untested, not approved yet by the FDA (although Coronado Biosciences is currently running phase 2 clinical trials on TSO in inflammatory bowel disease, in an attempt to get FDA approval) and that no one can guarantee safety 100 percent. (Then again, this is true for almost all therapies for autism, both accepted and alternative.)

There is far more we don't know than we do about the immunological causes of autism, the events that have triggered the abnormalities, and mostly the way to remediate the condition. We don't even know for sure if these abnormalities are the cause of autistic symptoms, and—if they are the culprit—exactly what mechanisms caused the developmental problems. Science is necessary, meaningful, and crucial—but it moves too slowly to help our children now. Helminthic therapy may seem radical to many, but in actuality, it is far safer than many pharmaceutical products. As Dr. Parker states in his paper on autism and biome depletion: ". . . the easiest way to evaluate the idea that autism is related to biome depletion is probably to conduct the experiment. Whether prophylactic biome reconstitution does or does not affect thte incidence of autism will answer all questions conclusively . . ." Another way to look at it is, as Dr. Herbert said at the Autism One Conference in May of 2008, "When faced with prolonged scientific uncertainty, use your best judgment."

INTESTINE, LEAKY GUT, AND AUTISM: IS IT REAL AND HOW TO FIX IT (INCLUDING WITH PROBIOTICS)

By Dr. Alessio Fasano

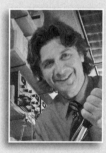

Alessio Fasano, MD

University of Maryland School of Medicine
Mucosal Biology Research Center and Center for Celiac Research
Health Science Facility II, Room S345
20 Penn Street
Baltimore, MD 21201
410-706-5501
Fax: 410-706-5508
afasano@mbrc.umaryland.edu

Dr. Fasano is Professor of Pediatrics, Medicine, and Physiology at the University of Maryland School of Medicine and is the Director of the Mucosal Biology Research center at the same institution. Dr. Fasano was born in Italy, where he completed his training as a pediatric gastroenterologist. In 1993, he was recruited at the University of Maryland and founded the Division of Pediatric Gastroenterology and Nutrition. In 1996, he established the Center for Celiac Research, a unique facility that offers state-of-the-art research, teaching, and clinical expertise for the diagnosis, treatment, and prevention of celiac disease. Dr. Fasano's research program encompasses both basic and clinical areas, including bacterial pathogenesis, intestinal pathophysiology, and prevention and treatment of both acute and chronic diarrheal diseases. In recent years, Dr. Fasano's research has focused on intercellular tight junctions (TJ) pathophysiology and its role in the pathogenesis of autoimmune diseases, with special emphasis on celiac disease. Dr. Fasano has published more than 170 peer-reviewed papers, and his research quality and creativity is further reflected in the filing of more than 160 patent applications, many of which are approved. He is an elected member of the American Society for Clinical Investigation. Because of his translational science, he has been awarded several prizes, including the 2005 Innovator of the Year Award, the 2006 Best Academic/Industry Collaboration Award, the 2006 Entepreneur of the Year Award, the 2007 America's Top Doctor's Award, and the 2009 Researcher of the Year Award. His research has been funded by the National Institutes of Health since 1995. Dr. Fasano has been a permanent member of the NIH study section, and continues to serve as an ad hoc reviewer.

The Intestine and ASD

The human intestine is a deceptively complex organ. It is lined by a single layer of cells exquisitely responsive to stimuli of innumerable variety, and is populated by a complex climax community of microbial partners, far more numerous than the cells of the intestine itself. Under normal circumstances, these intestinal cells form a tight, but selective barrier to "friends and foes": microbes and most environmental substances are held at bay, but nutrients from the essential to the trivial are absorbed efficiently. (1,2) Moreover, the tightness of the epithelial barrier is itself dynamic, though the mechanisms governing and effecting dynamic permeability are poorly understood. What is becoming increasingly clear is that a leaky gut is associated with a large number of local and systemic disorders, including autism spectrum disorders (ASDs). (3)

ASD and Diet

ASDs are heterogeneous neurodevelopmental disorders that affect approximately 1 percent of the general population. (4) It is generally agreed that there are multiple causes for ASD, with both genetic and environmental components involved. Gastrointestinal (GI) symptoms are frequently experienced by subjects with ASD, but their prevalence, nature, and therefore best treatments, remain elusive. (5,6) The most frequent GI symptoms experienced by subjects with ASD include constipation, gastroesophageal reflux, gastritis, intestinal inflammation (autistic enterocolitis), maldigestion, malabsorption, flatulence, abdominal pain or discomfort, lactose intolerance, enteric infections, etc. Of the almost fifty treatments proposed for ASD, seven (antifungal therapy, chelation, enzymes, GI treatments, intestinal parasite therapy, nutritional supplements, and dietary options for autism) are specifically focused to the GI tract, and they will be addressed in detail in other parts of this book. It is worthwhile to note that in a recent survey conducted by the Autism Research Institute involving more than 27,000 parents of autistic kids, avoidance of gluten (~9,000 cases) and/or casein (~7,000 cases) were the most frequent treatments implemented in their children, with a better : worse ratio of 30:1 and 32:1, respectively.

Intestine, Microbiome, and Leaky Gut

A possible unifying theory to "connect the dots" of all the factors mentioned above would link changes in gut microorganisms ecosystem with leaky gut, passage of digestion products of natural food, such as bread and cow's milk that would activate immune inflammatory cells that cause inflammation both in the intestine (autistic enterocolitis) and the brain (ASD). Alternative to the inflammatory hypothesis, it has been proposed that the defect in the intestinal barrier in ASD patients allows passage of neuroactive peptides of food origin into the blood and then into the cerebrospinal fluid, to interfere directly with the function of the central nervous system (CNS). No matter which of the two theories turns out to be correct, changes in intestinal microbiome and the consequent leaky gut seem to be the common denominators. Therefore, it would be logical to consider manipulation of the gut microbiome as the most effective intervention to treat ASD. Among the different strategies currently available to change the gut microbiome, the use of probiotics seems to be the most promising and feasible long-term intervention.

Definition of Probiotics

Probiotics are nonpathogenic bacteria that are claimed to have several beneficial effects related to their capability to either reduce the risk or treat a series of diseases. (7) Most probiotics are bacteria, which are small, single-celled organisms. Bacteria are categorized by scientists with genus, species, and strain names. For example, for the probiotic bacterium *Lactobacillus rhamnosus* GG, the genus is *Lactobacillus*, the species is *rhamnosus,* and the strain is GG. Most probiotic products contain bacteria from the genera *Lactobacillus* or *Bifidobacterium,* although other genera, including *Escherichia, Enterococcus, Bacillus,* and *Saccharomyces* (a yeast) have been marketed as probiotics. The requirements for a microbe to be considered a probiotic are simple. The microbe must be alive when administered, must be documented to have a health benefit, and must be administered at levels shown to confer the benefit. Probiotic products should be safe, effective, and should maintain their effectiveness and potency through the end of product shelf life.

Formulation of Probiotics

Once destined for commercial use, these bacteria are purified, grown in large numbers, concentrated to high doses, and preserved. They are provided in products in one of three basic ways: (8)

- as a culture concentrate added to a food at medium levels, with little or no opportunity for culture growth
- inoculated into a milk-based food (or dietary supplement) and allowed to grow to achieve high levels in a fermented food
- as concentrated and dried cells packaged as dietary supplements such as powders, capsules, or tablets, and delivered at a range of doses

Probiotic bacteria have a long history of association with dairy products. This is because some of the same bacteria that are associated with fermented dairy products also make their homes in different sites of the human body. Some of these microbes, therefore, can play a dual role in transforming milk into a diverse array of fermented dairy products (yogurt, cheese, kefir, etc.), and contributing to the important role of colonizing bacteria. Dairy products may provide a desirable "probiotic delivery vehicle" for several reasons. To date, however, there is little research on the impact of delivery vehicle and probiotic efficacy for any of the possible formats. This is an important area for future research.

The table below lists some commercial strains currently sold as probiotics. (9) Species are listed as reported by manufacturer, which may not reflect the most current taxonomy. Note that to be legitimately called a "probiotic," a strain must have undergone controlled evaluation for efficacy. The strains listed in this table may or may not have been adequately evaluated. The purpose of this table is to give the reader a sense of what is commercially available, not to provide recommendations for probiotic strain use.

Strain	Commercial products	Source
L. acidophilus NCFM *B. lactis* HN019 (DR10) *L. rhamnosus* HN001 (DR20)	Sold as ingredient	Danisco (Madison, WI)
Saccharomyces cerevisiae (boulardii)	Florastor	Biocodex (Creswell, OR)
B. infantis 35264	Align	Procter & Gamble (Mason, OH)
L. fermentum VRI003 (PCC)	Sold as ingredient	Probiomics (Eveleigh, Australia)
L. rhamnosus R0011 *L. acidophilus* R0052	Sold as ingredient	Institut Rosell (Montreal, Canada)
L. acidophilus LA5 *L. paracasei* CRL 431	Sold as ingredient	Chr. Hansen (Milwaukee, WI)
B. lactis Bb-12	Good Start Natural Cultures infant formula	Nestle (Glendale, CA) Chr. Hansen (Milwaukee, WI)
L. casei Shirota *B. breve* strain Yakult	Yakult	Yakult (Tokyo, Japan)
L. casei DN-114 001 ("L. casei Immunitas")	DanActive fermented milk	Danone (Paris, France)
B. animalis DN173 010 ("Bifidis regularis")	Activia yogurt	The Dannon Company (Tarrytown, NY)
L. reuteri RC-14 *L. rhamnosus* GR-1	Femdophilus	Chr. Hansens (Milwaukee, WI) Urex Biotech (London, Ontario, Canada) Jarrow Formulas (Los Angeles, CA)

Strain	Commercial products	Source
L. johnsonii Lj-1 (same as NCC533 and formerly *L. acidophilus* La-1)	LC1	Nestlé (Lausanne, Switzerland)
L. plantarum 299V	Sold as ingredient; Good Belly juice product	Probi AB (Lund, Sweden); NextFoods (Boulder, Colorado)
L. rhamnosus 271	Sold as ingredient	Probi AB (Lund, Sweden)
L. reuteri ATCC 55730 ("Protectis")	BioGaia Probiotic chewable tablets or drops	Biogaia (Stockholm, Sweden)
L. rhamnosus GG ("LGG")	Culturelle; Dannon Danimals	Valio Dairy (Helsinki, Finland) The Dannon Company (Tarrytown, NY)
L. rhamnosus LB21 *Lactococcus lactis* L1A	Sold as ingredient	Essum AB (Umeå, Sweden)
L. salivarius UCC118		University College (Cork, Ireland)
B. longum BB536	Sold as ingredient	Morinaga Milk Industry Co., Ltd. (Zama-City, Japan)
L. acidophilus LB	Sold as ingredient	Lacteol Laboratory (Houdan, France)
L. paracasei F19	Sold as ingredient	Medipharm (Des Moines, IA)
Lactobacillus paracasei 33 *Lactobacillus rhamnosus* GM-020 *Lactobacillus paracasei* GMNL-33	Sold as ingredient	GenMont Biotech (Taiwan)
L. plantarum OM	Sold as ingredient	Bio-Energy Systems, Inc. (Kalispell, MT)
Bacillus coagulans BC30	Sustenex, Digestive Advantage and sold as ingredient	Ganeden Biotech Inc. Cleveland, OH)
Streptococcus oralis KJ3 *Streptococcus uberis* KJ2 *Streptococcus rattus* JH145	ProBiora3 EvoraPlus	Oragenics Inc. (Alachua, FL)

Safety of Probiotics

Although the safety of traditional lactic starter bacteria has never been in question, the more recent use of intestinal isolates of bacteria delivered in high numbers to consumers with potentially compromised health has raised the question of safety. The safety of lactobacilli and bifidobacteria has been reviewed by qualified experts in the field. The general conclusion is that the pathogenic potential of lactobacilli and bifidobacteria is quite low. This is based on the prevalence of these microbes in fermented food, as normal colonizers of the human body, and the low level of infection attributed to them. However, reports of association of lactobacilli and bifidobacteria with human infection (commonly endocarditis) in patients with compromised health suggest that these microbes have rare opportunistic capability.

In many countries, the use of probiotics is not regulated by legislation comparable to that applied to drugs. Hence, the use of probiotics has become widespread despite the fact that their efficacy in clinical practice is not based on solid scientific evidence. For this reason, probiotics are often catalogued as "alternative" therapies.

Efficacy of Probiotics

While the initial use of probiotics was based on anecdotal reports of their beneficial effects, we have more recently witnessed a series of more rigorously designed clinical trials documenting the potential use of probiotics for the treatment of a variety of pediatric disorders, including enteric infectious diseases, allergic and atopic disorders, and intestinal inflammatory diseases. The two most studied probiotics are lactobacillus GG and bifidobacteria BB12, and there have been a large number of studies with these organisms in the pediatric population, with consistent good safety data (lack of side effects) but mixed efficacy. The inconsistent positive therapeutic results may be related to the fact that each probiotic organism has different effects, and therefore they cannot be used indiscriminately for each disease. Indeed, different conditions may be triggered by different microbiota composition and therefore may require different probiotics to be effectively treated. By performing more detailed studies to link gut microbiota composition to certain conditions, such as ASD, we will be able to decipher the host-microbe cross talk and, therefore, we will be able to customize probiotic treatment for specific conditions (i.e., personalized medicine). Another strategy that may complement the use of probiotics is the treatment with prebiotics. Prebiotics are nondigestible oligosaccharides (i.e., sugars), which pass through the intestine into the colon, where they are fermented by the colonizing bacteria. (7). The fermentation products, short-chain fatty acids, produce an acid milieu, which facilitates the proliferation of health-promoting bacteria.

Despite the fact that in a recent survey involving 539 primary pediatricians, 19 percent of them suggested the use of probiotics for the treatment of their ASD patients, (9) no well-designed studies have been conducted to justify their routine use in autism. Ideally, all treatments should be based on principles of evidence-based medicine proving the efficacy of treatment judged on the basis of the strength of evidence, including randomized, controlled clinical trials, which are at the peak, followed by cohort studies, case control studies, and then case reports.

Probiotics are available in the United States in foods, dietary supplements, and medical foods. There are no drugs approved for human use in the United States. In the past few years, the diversity of food products containing probiotics has expanded considerably. Not all products, even those claiming to be "probiotic," deliver adequate levels of probiotic microbes that have been documented to have health benefits. Nevertheless, probiotics represent very promising strategies and, therefore, it would be desirable to perform well-designed, multi-center studies to establish the microbiota of ASD patients in order to choose the proper probiotics to reestablish a healthy gut ecosystem able to decrease or completely ameliorate the clinical presentations of ASD.

IVIG: INTRAVENOUS IMMUNOGLOBULIN

By Dr. Michael Elice

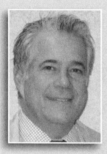

Michael Elice, MD

AIM Integrative Medicine
80 Crossways Park Drive
Woodbury, New York 11797
(516) 802-5028

Dr. Elice is a board-certified pediatrician and has been in practice for thirty years. Dr. Elice is a graduate of Syracuse University and the Chicago Medical School. He completed his pediatric residency at the North Shore University Hospital in Manhasset, New York. He has academic teaching positions and is on the staff of North Shore University Hospital and Schneider Children's Hospital. He is an associate professor of pediatrics at the New York University Medical School and the Albert Einstein School of Medicine. He is on the medical advisory board of the New York Families for Autistic Children (NYFAC) and is a member of the National Autism Association New York Metro Chapter. He has lectured at Defeat Autism Now! conferences around the country.

Autism spectrum disorders (ASDs) are currently defined as a syndrome of impaired social interaction, impaired communication skills, and restricted repertoire of activity and interests. The diagnoses contained within the spectrum range from attention deficit disorder (ADD), with hyperactivity (ADHD), obsessive compulsive disorder (OCD), tic disorders (such as Tourette's syndrome, aka TS), pervasive developmental disorder, not otherwise specified (PDD–NOS), and oppositional defiant disorder (ODD). These diagnoses are usually made prior to age three years, and have been on the rise over the past thirty years. The current statistics released by the Centers for Disease Control (CDC) and state health departments report the incidence of autism is 1:58 to 1:110 children, depending on geographic location, making autism spectrum disorders one of the greatest epidemics in pediatric medicine.

Intravenous immunoglobulin (IVIG) therapy has been used for common variable immunodeficiency syndrome (CVID), a disorder characterized by low levels of serum immunoglobulins and increased susceptibility to infections. The variability refers to the degree and type of immunoglobulin deficiency the patients had. Most individuals with CVID present first with recurrent bacterial infections. The underlying biomedical etiologies on children with autism have been under investigation. Genetic disorders possibly associated with epigenetic activity may lead to an increased incidence of multiple system disease in these children. Certain subsets of these children have a high incidence of immunological abnormalities and autoimmune disease. They also have markedly decreased serum immunoglobulin levels and impaired antibody responses. Based on the immunological abnormalities, a number of trials of IVIG have been utilized in autistic children. Gupta et al., in an open clinical trial, administered IVIG to ten children aged three to twelve years at four-week intervals for six months. Evaluations from the IV infusion nurse, physician, parents, and therapists showed clinical improvement in most of the patients. Younger patients showed greater improvement. Plioplys treated ten autistic children, ages four to seventeen years, with IVIG, four times every six weeks and found similar results. Delgiudice-Asch et al. administered IVIG monthly for six months to five autistic children. The sensory response Ritvo-Freeman scale showed a clinically meaningful response.

Based on this information, new research in autism spectrum disorders dictates the measurement of serum immunoglobulins, B and T cell lymphocyte levels, and anti-streptococcal antibodies. Patients who have received immunizations against polio, measles, diphtheria, tetanus, and strep pneumoniae may have low or absent antibody levels to one or more of these vaccines indicating a degree of immunodeficiency.

A subgroup of patients with OCD, ADD/ADHD, and tics or Tourette's syndrome has been identified who share a common clinical course characterized by dramatic symptom exacerbations following group A beta-hemolytic streptococcal (GABHS) infections. The term PANDAS has been applied to these patients, signifying Pediatric Autoimmune Neuropsychiatric Disorders Associated with Streptococcal Infections. The clinical symptoms are characterized by presence of the OCD and/or tic disorder, prepubertal onset of symptoms, intermittent exacerbations, neurological abnormalities such as motoric hyperactivity, adventitious movements, and the temporal association of the symptom exacerbations and GABHS infections.

In the 1980s, studies of childhood onset OCD and parallel investigations of rheumatic fever and its associated symptoms suggested a useful model of pathophysiology of these symptoms. It was thought that in certain children, susceptibility to genetic disorders possibly associated with epigenetic and transposon activity may lead to an increased incidence of multiple symptom disease in these children. Thus, certain strains of GABHS incite the production of antibodies that cross-react with central nervous system cellular components to cause inflammation of the basal ganglia in the brain resulting in these neuropsychiatric symptoms. Nearly 75 percent of these patients have symptoms of childhood onset OCD, worries about harm to self and others, violent images and behaviors, and ritualistic behaviors. These symptoms commence about four weeks prior to onset of the adventitious chorea-like movements, leading to the speculation that OCD might occur as a sequel of strep infections.

In a study by Swedo, et al. of fifty children meeting the PANDAS criteria, 40 percent met the DSM-IV (*Diagnostic and Statistical Manual of Mental Disorders, Fourth Edition*) criteria for ADHD, 18 percent ODD, 28 percent anxiety disorder. Exacerbations of OCD/tic symptoms were also accompanied by emotional lability and irritability, tactile/sensory defensiveness, motoric hyperactivity, messy handwriting, and symptoms of separation anxiety; a unique constellation of symptoms. The treatment for PANDAS is currently being studied including prophylactic antibiotics to prevent recurrent streptococcal infections and IVIG therapy. The children demonstrated dramatic improvements in OCD symptoms, anxiety, depression, emotional lability, and global functioning based on global change scores (41 percent). In contrast, placebo administration was associated with little or no change in overall symptoms severity. Side effects were limited to the duration of the procedure and included dizziness, nausea, and headache. In most cases, the discomfort occurred only during the first or second infusion and often persisted for twelve to twenty-four hours. Over 80 percent of patients who received IVIG remained much or very much improved at one-year follow-up, with their symptoms now in the subclinical range of severity. These results are particularly impressive in light of previous reports of the intractable nature of pediatric OCD and tic disorders. Long-term outcome studies in OCD have found less than one third of the patients with clinically meaningful symptom improvements.

In 2005 Boris, et al. published a study showing beneficial response of IVIG therapy in autistic children to whom 400 mg/kg IVIG was administered each month for six months. Baseline and monthly Aberrant Behavior Checklists were completed on each child in order to measure the child's response to IVIG. The participants' overall aberrant behaviors decreased substantially soon after receiving their first dose of IVIG. Total scores revealed decreases in hyperactivity, inappropriate speech, irritability, lethargy, and stereotypy (stimming, repetitive behaviors). This led to a reasonable rationale ratio to utilize IVIG therapy in children with autism.

The procedure of intravenous infusion of immunoglobulin is quite simple. The serum is sent to the doctor's office and remains frozen until the patient arrives, to ensure freshness. The volume to be infused is set up in a calibrated mechanical pump that begins the infusion at a slow rate to make sure the patient is tolerating the infusion. Depending on the volume to be infused, which is based on the weight of the patient, the procedure usually takes four to five hours.

Several days before the infusion, the patient receives information regarding premedication and hydration. Premedication might consist of oral ibuprofen and Benadryl at home or approximately one hour before arriving at the office. Sometimes it is necessary to administer IV Benadryl or Valium to relax the patient so that the IV catheter can be placed. This is a simple procedure, much like venipuncture to draw blood from a vein. The difference is that a catheter, a plastic extension of the needle, is threaded into the patient's vein and remains there for the duration of the procedure. The catheter allows a bit more flexibility of movement, so the patient may be more comfortable. In our office, the patient has the option of lying on an exam table with a comfortable backrest and pillow so they can sleep through the infusion or in a reclining chair so they can read or watch TV or a DVD of their choice. We encourage parents to bring these items for the comfort of the child.

A trained IV nurse is always present and will monitor vital signs; i.e., temperature, blood pressure, and pulse, as well as monitor the pump to be certain the infusion is proceeding efficiently. In the unlikely event that the patient demonstrates vital sign alterations or any other problem, the nurse will assess and report to the supervising physician. A crash cart for CPR/medications is always available. Thus far, we have never had any such incident.

Once the procedure is completed, the catheter is removed, instructions for at-home care are given, and the patient is discharged. There is a small possibility that the patient may develop fever, malaise, nausea, or headaches. These are rare and can be dealt with additional ibuprofen or Benadryl. The patient is instructed to make an appointment for the next monthly infusion. After the first infusion, seeing how simple it actually is, parents and children are very comfortable with the experience.

The treatment for common variable immunodeficiency characterized by low levels of serum immunoglobulins is similar to that of other disorders such as PANDAS. Intravenous immunoglobulin (IVIG) has led to improvement of symptoms. IVIG is a plasma product formed by taking antibodies from thousands of donors. The plasma undergoes processing for mixing, antibody removal, chemical treatment, and filtration to remove viruses, and then is freeze dried. This extensive processing dictates the high cost of the infusion, which is approximately $4,000 per child. This varies depending on the weight of the patient calculated based on 1 gram/kg of weight.

Intravenous immunoglobulin replacement combined with antibiotic therapy has greatly improved the outcomes of patients with PANDAS, CVID, and other autism spectrum disorders. The aim is to keep the patients free of infectious disease and to prevent the ensuing chronic inflammatory changes that may occur as a consequence of this immune system dysregulation. In our clinical practice, we have many children who have received IVIG. Based on anecdotal reports of parents, educators, and therapists, there have been improvements in focus and attention, and decreases in OCD/tic behaviors. In addition, these children—who are often sick with strep throats and other illnesses—have sustained longer intervals of health, compared to their previous history. Most recently, one of our patients visited Disney World, where he had been at least twenty times in his life. His older brother got strep throat and was treated with appropriate antibiotics. Forty-eight hours later, the patient became violent, started screaming, could not sleep, and was basically out of control. Within twenty-four hours of starting antibiotics, his behavior improved dramatically. Like "apples to oranges," said his father. This underscores the value to prophylactic antibiotics and IVIG which is the next step in treating this "autistic twelve-year-old male."

The results of these investigations, as well as clinical response noted in our practice, suggest that IVIG is highly beneficial to a subgroup of patients with tics and obsessive-compulsive symptoms. However, they do not provide support for routine use of immunomodulatory agents in OCD and tic disorders. IVIG is a potent immunological therapy. A NIH Consensus Statement asserted that the risks involved in the use of IVIG are minimal.

Other articles have confirmed their safety, after two decades of experience. Latov et al. reported that IVIG is used in the treatment of immunological diseases that affect the entire neuroaxis, including the brain, spinal cord, peripheral nerves, muscles, and neuromuscular junction. In prospective, controlled, double-blind clinical trials, IVIG was found to have proven efficacy in Guillain-Barré syndrome, chronic inflammatory demyelinating polyneuropathy, multifocal motor neuropathy, and dermatomyositis. It was found to probably be effective in myasthenia gravis and polymyositis, and possibly effective in several other neuroimmunological diseases. Further studies are needed to evaluate the use of IVIG for neuroimmunological diseases in which its efficacy is suspected but not proven and to elucidate its mechanisms of action.

Ongoing Results

The year 2010 was a successful one for intravenous gamma globulin therapy in our practice. We treated five patients age 7 to 15 years, all males. Their clinical presentation of ADHD, OCD and tics suggested the etiology of their behaviors was PANDAS. Laboratory values confirmed hypogammaglobulinemia (low IgG levels), elevated AntiStreptolysin O Antibodies (ASO) and elevated Anti DNAse B Antibodies. There was a past history of strep infections but none of the patients had recent strep illnesses according to the parents.

IVIG was administered monthly over the course of six months. The dosage was calculated in a range of 0.4 to 1.0 gram per kilogram of body weight. The rate of the infusion never exceeded 100gms. per hour. Some of the infusions lasted for 8 hours.

Premedication varied from patient to patient. Most were given Ibuprofen and Benadryl prior to arriving at our office. Depending on the individual, IV benadryl, toradol, solumedrol or valium was given to keep the patient calm and in some cases diminish the exacerbation of choreiform movements and tics. The tics varied from motoric behaviors to vocal/verbal sounds and repetitive speech. A physician or nurse was present with the family at all times. There were no adverse reactions observed other than an occasional complaint of headache.

Vital signs were assessed at regular intervals to insure stable blood pressure, pulse and temperature. None of the patients experienced any alterations in these modalities.

Parents completed the Aberrant Behavior Checklist (ABC) before the first infusion and after the sixth infusion. The total 'before' and 'after' scores were compared as a percent change and is reported below.

Patients

Patient #1—G.I. 7 year old male. Score change = behaviors actually increased 9%. However, the changes were noted in language since he progressed from non verbal to speaking, although inappropriately. Tantrums and adverse behaviors increased but were age appropriate since they occurred when he didn't get what he wanted where previously he didn't respond. He no longer required antibiotic prophylaxis for strep infections. He is now reading, writing and doing mathematics on an age appropriate level. He is more compliant and follows directions.

Patient #2—A.S. 12 year old male. Score change = 25% reduction in aberrant behaviors.

Most significant changes were decreases in aggression, temper outbursts and self-injury.

Recurrent body movements (chorea) involving shaking extremities and stereotypy diminished significantly. Attention, obedience and compliance with instructions improved. He was able to sit for longer periods of time and is showing more positive social reaction to others.

Patient #3—C.G. 15 year old male. Score change = 88% improvement

This was one of our more difficult cases. This fully developed teenager lost language and the ability to control motor and vocal tics to the extent that he couldn't sleep at night or sit still during the day. Between the fifth and sixth infusion, family noticed less hyperactivity and bizarre behavior. Choreiform movements diminished. Less staring blankly into space, repetitive speech and self-talk as use of language reemerged. Most significantly, he no longer has tantrums, stereotypical behaviors and restlessness. He doesn't cry or bang his head. Hand ticking and erratic mood changes have been reduced to a minimum. He is definitely more socially aware as expressive language reemerges.

Patient #4—C.D. 9 year old male. Score change = 38% improvement.

Most significant change in this child was in the diminishing of repetitive speech which was an obstacle to his progress in school. Choreiform movements, restlessness, stereotypy and bizarre behaviors all decreased. Hyperactivity, including running and jumping, distractibility and self-talking decreased as well. Social interaction with peers and adults and attention span increased.

Follow-up laboratory investigation showed normalization of IgG levels and the absence of ASO and AntiDNAseB antibodies.

Although the results of the ABC Checklists were not scored to assess true statistical significance, parent observation and reporting, physician observation and patient responses all support the effectiveness of IVIG treatments in these individuals. As the physician who examines them at regular monthly intervals, I can attest to these clinical improvements. As new double blind, placebo controlled studies are under way at the National Institute of Mental Health, it is still important to document evidence based observational improvements on a case by case basis.

MEDICAL CANNABIS AS A TREATMENT FOR SYMPTOMS ASSOCIATED WITH AUTISM SPECTRUM DISORDERS

By Nathan Coombs

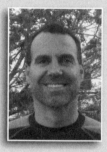

Nathan Coombs, MEd
contactus@asdconnection.com
asdconnection.com

Mr. Coombs is a respected educator. He possesses a Master's Degree in Special Education and has over 10 years of experience in this field. He is also co-owner of The Autism & Compassionate Care Connection, a medical marijuana collective that was created in 2010. It is his mission to help individuals with autism increase their self-awareness and quality of life through a scientific approach of cultivating high-quality strains of medical cannabis strategically targeted at alleviating their specific symptoms, through seamless administration methods of ingestion and inhalation. It is his deepest desire to offer individuals with autism and their families this holistic alternative to alleviating symptoms and behaviors associated with autism spectrum disorders.

Introduction

There is legitimate scientific rationale for the use of cannabis to benefit human physiology. There are also many fallacies of stigmatization regarding its medicinal efficacy. The historical political background relating to cannabis legislation in the United States has been quite tumultuous since the 1930s, although cannabis has been known to be used medicinally on a global scale for thousands of years. Fortunately, for patients who suffer from immunological and neurological conditions, the current socio-political landscape in the US is changing, with an enhanced awareness of cannabis as an effective medical treatment. Cannabis can now be obtained legally in 20 states for medicinal use. The use of this organic herb as an appropriate alternative or supplement for certain pharmaceutical drugs with severe side effects has been quite beneficial to many patients.

Socio-political background

Cannabis has been used to benefit health and human physiology for centuries globally. The historical use of marijuana has been dated back to ancient China, where it was administered for relief from gout, rheumatism, malaria, and constipation. Hua T'o, a famous Chinese surgeon, used cannabis for pain in surgery in the 2nd century A.D. According to ancient Roman writings, oil from the hemp seed was used for earaches and flatulence, and it was regularly prescribed for pain. In 1994, an archeological find in an Egyptian tomb dating back to the 3rd century A.D. showed evidence of a girl who died in childbirth with traces of hashish, apparently used for pain. William Brooke O'Shaughnessy, M.D., brought knowledge of cannabis to Europe from India in 1839, after observing its use there. Also, cannabis was commonly used in tinctures in the U.S. up until 1936.

In 1937, the Marijuana Tax Act was introduced by Harry Anslinger, a prohibition officer, banning cannabis. The American Medical Association (AMA) was one of the most vocal groups to oppose the bill. Hence, the AMA recognized the medical benefits of cannabis. In 1941, cannabis was withdrawn from the U.S. pharmaceutical market due to burdensome requirements of the law. Even to this day, the Food and Drug Administration's (FDA) procedural guidelines and protocols to start a cannabis research study are so rigorous and time-consuming that most researchers do not even attempt it. Notwithstanding, during the 1940s, government sponsored panels of medical experts continued to find cannabis harmless and potentially useful. In 1944, an expert panel from the New York Academy of Medicine concluded that cannabis was not addictive, did not lead to abuse of other drugs, and public hysteria was unfounded. Harry Anslinger denounced the report and destroyed as many copies as he could find. In 1970, the Controlled Substance Act was brought into law. This act gave the Drug Enforcement Agency (DEA) and the FDA full control to schedule substances or drugs.

There are currently five different levels of scheduling. Schedule I substances are those that have the following findings: the drug or other substances have a high potential for abuse; the drug or other substances have no currently accepted medical use in treatment in the United States; there is a lack of accepted safety for use of the drug or other substances under medical supervision. Heroin, LSD, and marijuana are some of the drugs classified as Schedule I. Schedule II substances are those that have the following findings: the drug or other substances have a high potential for abuse; the drug or other substances have currently accepted medical use in treatment in the United States or currently accepted medical use with severe restrictions; abuse of the drug or other substances may lead to severe psychological dependence. Cocaine, morphine, and oxycodone are some of the drugs classified as Schedule II. And so on.

In 1971, President Nixon appointed the Presidential Commission on Marijuana and Drug Abuse, which was led by Governor William Shaffer of Pennsylvania.

The commission unexpectedly recommended the repeal of the laws against the use of cannabis. President Nixon promptly disavowed their report. In 1982, another study done by the National Academy of Science came to similar conclusions and was ignored by President Ronald Reagan. In 1988, DEA administrative judge Francis Young ruled that the medical benefits of cannabis were clear beyond question and that it should be reclassified from a Schedule 1 drug to a Schedule 2 drug. Judge Young's recommendation was overruled by the DEA chief, John Lawn. In 1993, after continued lengthy federal litigation, the Federal Appeals Court upheld the DEA ban of cannabis. Triumphantly, in 1996, California voters approved the California Compassionate Use Act (Proposition 215). This exempted patients from prosecution for possessing or cultivating cannabis for medical use if they had a doctor's recommendation. Unfortunately, the passing of this piece of legislation prompted the federal government to threaten physicians with arrest. This action was blocked by a federal court decision, *Conant v. Walters,* which held that physicians were protected under the First Amendment in recommending cannabis. In 1997, the then-acting director of the Office of National Drug Control Policy, Barry McCaffrey, also known as the "Drug Czar," commissioned the national Institute of Medicine (IOM) to review the scientific evidence on the benefits of cannabis and drugs derived from it. The IOM reported that cannabinoids had potential therapeutic value, especially for nausea reduction, appetite stimulation, anxiety reduction, and pain relief. The report recommended further research and clinical trials, including the development of non-smoked delivery systems. In 2005, the US Supreme Court upheld the position of all cannabis use being illegal in its ruling regarding *Gonzalez v. Raich.* This ruling did not question the validity of state laws. Therefore, patients are still protected from prosecution under state—but not federal—law. Despite federal opposition, support for medical cannabis has grown steadily, and as of this writing, 20 states have legalized medical cannabis (or effectively decriminalized it).

Cannabis, for any use, is illegal under federal law. Even if you live in a state that has enacted legislation or passed a ballot initiative that recognizes the medical utility of cannabis, you are still subject to arrest by federal officials for possession or cultivation of cannabis. Again, the Controlled Substance Act classifies cannabis as a schedule 1 drug and defines it as a drug with no accepted medical value in treatment. Despite its long use as a medication, cannabis is classified as a new drug and legal access is only possible through the Investigational New Drug Application issued by the FDA.

Scientific rationale

"Cannabinoids" refers to a family of chemicals found in the cannabis plant. There are 86 cannabinoids found in nature. Of this total number, there are 60 cannabinoids found in the cannabis plant. The two main cannabinoids in the cannabis plant are THC (delta-9-tetrahydrocannabinol) and CBD (cannabidiol). THC is the main psychoactive ingredient in cannabis. Unlike THC, CBD lacks noticeable psychoactive effects. There is growing evidence that CBD has valuable medical properties. It works together with THC, bolstering its medicinal effects while moderating THC's psychoactivity. CBD has anti-inflammatory, anti-anxiety, anti-epileptic, sedative, and neuroprotective actions. Strains of marijuana high in CBD and low in THC make it possible to inhale or ingest high cannabinoid doses without affecting one's ability to operate normally.

Receptors are sites within the body that react to specific chemicals and produce specific reactions. Cannabinoid receptors in the brain affect the perception of pain, mood, hunger, and muscle control. Cannabinoid receptors in the extremities (i.e., arms and legs) and immune tissues (e.g., spleen, white blood cells, and lymphatic system) provide an anti-inflammatory effect when cannabis is inhaled or ingested, when THC and CBD attach to cannabinoid receptors throughout the body. Several areas of the brain (e.g., cerebral cortex, hypothalamus, brain stem, hippocampus, cerebellum, and amygdala) have high densities of these receptors, which helps explain the different psychoactive effects of the drug. The cerebral cortex controls memory and cognition; the hypothalamus governs appetite; and the brain stem controls basic functions, including arousal, the vomiting reflex, blood pressure, and heart rate (it also plays a role in pain sensation, muscle tone, and movement). The hippocampus is key to memory storage and recall. The cerebellum governs coordination and muscle control. The amygdala plays a role in emotions.

Our bodies produce endocannabinoids naturally. Endocannabinoids are substances produced from within the body, whereas cannabinoids are produced in nature. The functions of endocannabinoids play a role in regulating immunity, inflammation, neurotoxicity, trauma, blood pressure, body temperature, appetite, gastrointestinal functions, epilepsy, depression, stress, bone formation, and intraocular pressure. Endocannabinoids have a homeostatic function, signifying a role in restoring and maintaining balance. Endocannabinoids tend to fine tune biological responses upwards or downwards as needed within the range necessary to maintain healthy function.

Clinical endocannabinoid deficiency syndrome (CEDS) is a proposed contributor to autism spectrum disorder. It is associated with a range of illnesses, including irritable bowel syndrome, migraine, and fibromyalgia. CEDS could be responsible for these common conditions as well as many related ones. According to a literary review conducted by Ethan B. Russo, M.D., senior medical advisor for GW Pharmaceuticals, migraine, fibromyalgia, irritable bowel syndrome, and related conditions display common clinical, biochemical, and pathophysiological patterns that suggest an underlying clinical endocannabinoid deficiency that may be suitably treated with cannabinoid medicines.

It is speculated that cannabinoid deficiency affects 20–30 percent of the population and is a factor in many conditions associated with aging, such as arthritis, obesity, and autoimmune disorders. Anxiety, autism, attention-deficit/hyperactivity disorder, obsessive-compulsive disorder, depression, eating disorders, hyperactivity, stuttering, tics, and more have been linked to CEDS, although there is still no common explanation. Hence, the connection among all of these conditions may be CEDS since properly administered cannabinoids have helped so many patients with these conditions.

Regarding any comments about a lack of cannabis research, there are different reasons why this research would be disadvantageous for pharmaceutical companies. There is no patent on a plant that would thereby allow pharmaceutical companies to control the source or access. Furthermore, cannabis could be a cost-effective product placed in competition with already established, more expensive drugs, which would negatively affect profits of prescription drugs. There are no double-blind studies to date on cannabis: it currently costs approximately 800 million dollars to put a drug through testing for FDA approval! Pharmaceutical companies are not interested in developing an herbal medicine without the ability to control the source through a patent. As of yet, the cannabinoid products that have been developed, such as Marinol and Cesamet, which are synthetic, are not nearly as useful as whole herbal cannabis.

GW Pharmaceuticals in the United Kingdom has developed a whole plant derivative called Sativex, which contains equal parts of THC and CBD. It has been approved for treatment of multiple sclerosis in Canada and is available in 22 countries. Unfortunately, the US is not one of those countries. GW is planning further research on the use of CBD for arthritis, inflammatory bowl diseases, psychotic disorders, and epilepsy. Recent laboratory and animal studies have suggested that CBD could protect against the development of diabetes, certain types of cancer, rheumatoid arthritis, brain and nerve damage due to stroke, prion infections, and Huntington's disease.

Safety

Cannabis has a remarkable safety record. It has been used for thousands of years and by millions of people. A review published in the *British Journal of Psychiatry* in February 2001 said that there have never been reports of death directly due to acute cannabis use. THC has an extremely low toxicity and the amount that can enter the body through consumption of the cannabis plants poses no threat of death. Anecdotal evidence is often underestimated. It commands much less attention than it once did, yet it is a source of much of our knowledge of synthetic medicines as well as plant derivatives. Controlled experiments were not needed to recognize the therapeutic potential of drugs such as chloral hydrate, which has been used as a sedative. Furthermore, it was through anecdotal evidence that we learned of the usefulness of propranolol for angina and hypertension and of diazepam for status epileptucus, which is a state of continuous seizure activity. These drugs were originally approved by the FDA for other purposes.

Autism

There are no autism-specific medications. All medications to treat people with autism are used by physicians to treat other conditions, such as in the use of antiepileptic and psychotropic drugs. Some of the drugs that may be prescribed to people with autism include blood pressure medications, attention/hyperactivity medications, bipolar disorder medications, antidepressants with anti-anxiety properties, antipsychotic medications, and vitamins, minerals, and probiotics. Many of these drugs, with the exception of the vitamins, minerals, and probiotics, have potentially very harmful side effects. Cannabis, on the other hand, if determined to be an efficacious treatment for symptoms of autism, poses no harmful side effects when vaporized or ingested. Medical cannabis is not a cure for autism, but it is a viable treatment that helps alleviate some of the symptoms associated with autism without a whole host of severe side effects that are inherent in many pharmaceuticals. Medical cannabis treatment must be medically supervised by a doctor familiar with its properties.

Administration

Medical cannabis can be smoked, vaporized, and/or ingested. Vaporizing is recommended over smoking in order to avoid respiratory issues. Vaporizing may not be the most appropriate form of administration of cannabis for many individuals with autism due to insufficient ability to mindfully attend to inhaling and exhaling. Quite often, the most appropriate means of administration is through ingestion. Many of the edibles do not please the palate of most individuals—with or without autism—so it is recommendable that it be taken in a tasteless pill form, such as by placing in empty veggie caps that can be swallowed. For information about proper preparation, please consult with your dispensary.

Follow regulations appropriately

In order to obtain and use medical cannabis legally, first and foremost, you must obtain and/or use medical cannabis in a state where it is legal for medical use. It is important to consult with a neurologist regarding cannabis and for this neurologist to consult with a physician who can appropriately recommend cannabis and who also understands and has experience with autism. It is also advisable that you obtain a Medical Marijuana Card issued to you from your state's Board of Health. Even caregivers who administer cannabis need to have their own individual Medical Marijuana Card—not just the patient.

In closing

Medical cannabis can be a helpful and healthful tool in the toolbox when used with appropriate medical oversight for medically indicated conditions and while following applicable regulations.

METHYL-B$_{12}$: MYTH OR MASTERPIECE

By Dr. James Neubrander

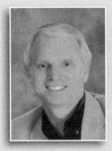

James A. Neubrander, MD, FAAEM

Road to Recovery Clinic
485A Route 1 South, Suite 320
Iselin, NJ 08830
(732) 726-1222
www.drneubrander.com

Dr. Neubrander trained in Pathology and Laboratory Medicine and is Board Certified in Environmental Medicine. He is the Medical Director of the Road to Recovery Clinic in Iselin, NJ. He serves on many scientific advisory boards dedicated to treating autism and neurodevelopmental disorders. He frequently lectures at National and International Conferences and Physician Training Courses. His lectures are scientific, evidence-based, and emphasize newer treatments or modifications of established protocols that appear to enhance clinical outcomes beyond the results previously reported. He is the coauthor of several peer-reviewed articles, has been interviewed and filmed for many documentaries and television spots, has been referenced in many books written about autism, nutrition, and environmental medicine, and has been quoted innumerable times by scientists, researchers, clinicians, and lay persons, most notably for methylcobalamin, hyperbaric oxygen, and heavy metal detoxification.

Since the mid nineties, I was one of a handful of physicians who had been using the only two available forms of vitamin B$_{12}$, cyano-B$_{12}$ and hydroxy-B$_{12}$, to treat children with autism. We used these forms of B$_{12}$ because the majority of children with autism had an abnormal elevation of the organic acid known as FIGLU (formimino-glutamic acid). Though we believed we saw minor improvements by using B$_{12}$, we never saw anything remarkable. In the eighties and nineties, the Japanese had been studying the methyl form of B$_{12}$ for many disorders, none of which were autism. It was not until the late '90s that the methyl form finally became available in the United States, though it was not commonly used. In March of 2002, I became the first physician in the world to ever use the methyl form of B$_{12}$ in a child with autism. Amazingly, the child showed many significant changes.

The second child I treated, who previously used three- to four-word utterances, began speaking in six- to eight-word sentences within two weeks. Not only was he now talking, he was also interacting with everyone. This included his shocked school bus driver whom he tried to kiss, and his even more shocked crossing guard whom he started hugging and talking to every day! Such social interactions, especially spontaneously initiated, were something that he never did prior to methyl-B$_{12}$. His parents jokingly said that things might have been better for them before they started the shots, because then they had a little peace and quiet in the house and not all his constant chatter!

Now, more than a million dose evaluations later, the single most predictable treatment I have seen to positively affect more than 90 percent of children on the spectrum is methyl-B$_{12}$ injections if done according to the protocols I have continued to improve upon over the lastnine years. Though shots are initially "feared" by most parents, they soon learn that the shots are painless, easy to administer, and give the greatest number of clinical responses when compared to oral, nasal, or transdermal routes of administration. Interestingly, prior to starting therapy, the majority of children who respond to methyl-B$_{12}$ injections have high normal to high levels of B$_{12}$ in their blood, rather than the low levels that would be expected. The reason for this appears to be what I call "B$_{12}$ diabetes." Just as blood sugar builds up in the plasma of a diabetic because it cannot get into the cell, B$_{12}$ builds up in the plasma and does not get into the cell, possibly due to a transcobalamin transporter problem.

Methyl-B$_{12}$ is *methylcobalamin*. Every time you see the word "cobalamin," you can substitute the word "B$_{12}$." In the late 1920s, when vitamins were first discovered, they were called "*vital amines.*" Eventually the words were combined to form what we know today as "vitamin." When B$_{12}$ was discovered, it was called the "cobalt vital amine" because a cobalt atom is found deep within the molecule. The name was later shortened to be called the "*cobalt* vit*amin,*" what we know today as "cobalamin." The cobalamins represent a *family* of cobalt containing vitamins. To better understand this, consider "cobalamin" to be the last name of a family, analogous to "the Smiths." The different types of B$_{12}$ are analogous to the first names of each family member that identifies them from each other. For the Smiths, there could be Jennifer, Ashley, Megan, Michael, Matthew, or Jeremy. For the Cobalamin family, the individual family members are named Methyl, Adenosyl, Hydroxy, Cyano, Glutathionyl, and Sulfito. They each have their own jobs and assignments to do. *The two senior family members of the cobalamin family are methyl-B$_{12}$ and adenosyl-B$_{12}$.* Only these two forms have "*coenzyme*" properties that allow them to *complete* special assignments with specific enzymes found in the body, especially in the brain and mitochondria when we are discussing clinical benefits for children with autism.

Methyl-B$_{12}$'s unique coenzyme activity unlocks the enzyme *methionine synthase*. Every time it is unlocked, methionine synthase transfers a methyl group to homocysteine allowing homocysteine to re-enter the methionine cycle. This reaction is vital for methyl groups to be passed from one molecule to the next, a process called *transmethyl-ation*. For children with autism, the results of transmethylation are *increased language, focus and attention, awareness, cognition, independence, socialization and interactive play, appropriate emotional responses, affection, eye contact, and improvements in gross and fine motor skills*.

The science behind why methyl-B_{12} works for autism is sound. *The [1]folate cycle, [2]methionine-homocysteine cycle, and [3]homocysteine-glutathione pathway are intricately interwoven in a delicate balance that exists to create and then pass along methyl groups, and to create* glutathione*, the body's most important intracellular antioxidant*. The folic acid cycle receives premethylated folic acid molecules from food, vitamins, or from a folic acid recycling process. *Premethylated folic acid* molecules are presented to the *MTHFR enzyme* to become *methylated folic acid*. Methylated folic acid donates its methyl group to "naked B_{12}" for it to become *methyl-B_{12}*. Methyl-B_{12}, in the presence of *methionine synthase*, passes its methyl group to *homocysteine* which then becomes methylated (or re-methylated) homocysteine, also known as *methionine*. Methionine, with the aid of a magnesium atom, then adds an adenosyl molecule to become S-adenosylmethione (*SAMe*), the "universal methyl donor." It is SAMe's job to transfer the methyl group (*transmethylation*) to many different types of molecules in the brain to produce the clinical results previously -described. Once the methyl group has been transferred, the remaining molecule, S-adenosylhomocysteine (*SAH*) still retains the adenosyl group. Unfortunately, SAH blocks further transmethylation until the adenosyl group is removed, a process that requires adequate zinc, the digestive enzyme "DPP-IV", and at times the removal of dairy products. Once SAH loses the adenosyl group, what is left is "naked" (or parent) *homocysteine*, devoid of methyl and adenosyl groups.

Depending on various factors, "parent homocysteine" will proceed one of two ways. [1]When oxidative stress is under control, homocysteine will enter the methionine-homocys-teine cycle just described. *[2]However, when oxidative stress is high, homocysteine will be shunted down the homocysteine-glutathione pathway to create glutathione, the body's pri-mary intracellular antioxidant*. Oxidative stress is a condition where "wild unpaired electrons" cause significant tissue and cellular damage before they find a mate. Anti-oxidants provide such mates.

Jill James, PhD, demonstrated that *children on the autism spectrum had lower values of active glutathione than controls*. Richard Deth, PhD, found that methionine synthase is critical for a special dopamine receptor and normal brain function. Dr. Deth also documented that *many substances damage or block methionine synthase activity*, including mercury, the infamous agent found in vaccines containing Thimerosal.

With this scientific background, one can begin to understand how the administra-tion of injectable methyl-B_{12} works for children with autism from each of the three pathways previously described. *In the ^{1}folate cycle, the MTHFR enzyme is frequently mutated.* This results in *low production of the methyl groups needed to make methyl-B$_{12}$.* By injecting methyl-B$_{12}$, we bypass the problem. *In the ^{2}methionine-homocysteine cycle*, the addition of methyl-B$_{12}$ allows *more methyl groups to first be donated to SAMe and subsequently passed along to the crucial molecules in the brain that will reduce autistic symptoms. In the ^{3}homocysteine-glutathione pathway, methyl-B$_{12}$ has been shown to help restore the critical balance between methylation and transsulfuration.*

Since March of 2002, I have treated thousands of children on the autism spectrum and have personally monitored over a million doses in my clinic. My research has included the clinical responsiveness to all forms of commercially available B$_{12}$: cyano-B$_{12}$, hydroxy-B$_{12}$, adenosyl-B$_{12}$, and methyl-B$_{12}$. It has investigated the clinical responsiveness from all routes of administration: oral, sublingual, transdermal, nasal, intravenous, intramuscular, suppository, and subcutaneous. It has evaluated the clinical responsiveness from shots varying from weekly to daily, from various stock concentrations, and from different pH values. It has evaluated the clinical responsiveness when B$_{12}$ has been used in combination which other agents, most commonly folinic acid, glutathione, and/or N-acetylcysteine. It has investigated the clinical benefit and side effect patterns when used concurrently with TMG, SAMe, methionine, NAC, glutathione, B$_6$, folic acid, folinic acid, 5-MTHF, DMG, ALA, etc. *In summary, from twelve years of intense clinical research I cannot emphasize enough how much the right protocol matters. Which protocol and methyl- B$_{12}$ product that is selected can make or break how effective the shots are for any given child.*

In my clinic, according to the protocols I have developed over the past twelve years, I consistently find that *the injectable form methyl-B$_{12}$ is far superior to any other route of administration* when one considers the percentage of children who respond, the intensity of each response, and how many responses each child exhibits.

Key factors necessary to achieve maximum effectiveness are beyond the scope of this chapter. They include, but are not limited to the pH and concentration of the stock solution, the mcg/kg of the dose used, the frequency of the injections, the route of administration, and if given subcutaneously, the site of the injections, the evaluation tools used by the parents to report their findings, and the presence of selected key supplements reaching predetermined dosage ranges prior to implementing higher doses of methyl-B$_{12}$ or prior to increasing the frequency of the injections. The *most common initiation protocol* I use is a dose of 65 mcg/kg drawn from a stock solution of 25 mg/mL given at a ten-degree angle into the adipose tissue of the buttocks once every three days. A local anesthetic cream can be locally applied at the site of the injection.

As previously stated, the primary categories of improvement include increased language, focus and attention, awareness, cognition, independence, socialization and interactive play, appropriate emotional responses, affection, eye contact, and improvements in gross and fine motor skills. In my clinic, the frequency for at least some of these responses is 94 percent. The average number of responses is thirty to fifty out of a possible total of 135. Though the intensity of response can be very strong at times, the majority of parents report mild, mild-to-moderate, or moderate improvements. The positive effects build over 2½ to 4 years. Should the shots be discontinued prior to that amount of time, many children will regress. After 2½ to 4 years, many children can be weaned off their shots. In my clinic, 70 percent of children do better on daily shots, but *only if certain key supplements are being taken at the recommended ranges* provided in the Supplement Review Program as shown on my website.

Compounding pharmacies must make the injections. Depending on the pharmacy used, *the shots usually range from $0.50 to $1.50 each.* In the past I always prescribed preservative-free methyl-B_{12} which is no longer available due to new safety regulations placed upon compounding pharmacies by the FDA and State Boards of Pharmacies in 2013. At this time it is too early to know whether or not these additional government regulations will result in increased costs to the parents now that compounding pharmacies are required to perform sterility and stability tests much more frequently than were required in the past. Unfortunately methyl-B_{12} products made by different pharmacies can vary significantly. I say this because over the years dozens of parents have come to my clinic stating that they had previously tried methyl-B_{12} from their compounding pharmacy using "the Neubrander protocol"and saw little to no response in their child's symptoms. When I started them on the shots I use, they were amazed that methyl-B_{12} really did work for their child and they wondered why. So did I. In June of 2012 I got my answer from a study I had performed by one of the leading biochemists in America who evaluated methyl-B_{12} products made by different pharmacies. Though we did not find issues with final concentrations of methyl-B_{12} or sterility, we did note that the pH values and balance between the active forms of B_{12} varied greatly. In addition, mass spectroscopy demonstrated impurities ranging from none to many depending on the sample being examined. From our preliminary study, we concluded that optimum clinical benefits are the composite result of the *concentration* and *purity* of methyl-B_{12}, the final *pH*, and the *process* by which it is made, something that can vary considerably among pharmacies. In addition, the evaluation process used by the parents is critical to determining if the child is or is not a methyl-B_{12}responder. The one I find to be the most effective was due to parents' input from which I created the *"Pegboard System."*

Best case anecdotal stories, including a section showing Recovered Kids, can be viewed in the video section of my website; www.drneubrander.com. One remarkable story is Caitlin's. Her mother was a speech pathologist who, while in training, refused to do a rotation to learn about autistic children because she wanted to have nothing to do with it. Unfortunately, when Caitlin was 2½ years old, Caitlin's mother was dev-astated when the doctor told her Caitlin was not just autistic, but severely so. Caitlin progressed very quickly from methyl-B$_{12}$ shots and fully recovered. Today, no one can tell she was ever autistic! *Unfortunately, best case scenarios are unusual.* The majority of patients show mild or moderate improvements which, as they follow my protocols for 2½ to 4 years, continue to improve. The April 2010 Okada Rat Study demonstrated that only the methyl form of the B$_{12}$ family showed significant benefits, and that regen-eration of transected nerves was possible when given in high doses.

Long-term use is safe as documented from pernicious anemia patients. *Serious side effects do not occur.* However, *nuisance side effects* are fairly *common*. The good news is that they usually pass within four to six months as the body adjusts to keep the good and delete the bad. Common side effects are *hyperactivity, stimming, and mouthing objects or biting.* Occasionally sleep is disturbed though more often it improves. Side effects belong in two categories: positive-negative vs. negative-negative, and tolerable vs. intolerable. A common positive-negative side effect for young children is pinching or tantruming, as they become much more aware of what they want and ask for it in perfectly good "autism-ese." When you do not understand, they get upset and tantrum or pinch to get your attention so you will do what they want you to do. Now that they are much more aware of what they want, they also get upset and tantrum when you tell them to do something they don't want to do.

In summary, every child on the autism spectrum deserves a clinical trial of inject-able methyl-B$_{12}$ because it has proven to be an effective treatment for the majority of children on the autism spectrum, *if done correctly.*

Cobalamin and methyl-B$_{12}$ references are hosted in the download section on my website at www.drneubrander.com.

14

TREATMENTS FOR MITOCHONDRIAL DISEASE AND DYSFUNCTION

By Dr. Richard E. Frye

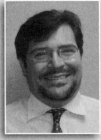

Richard E. Frye, MD, PhD

Arkansas Children's Hospital Research Institute
University of Arkansas for Medical Sciences
Slot 512-41B
Room R4041
13 Children's Way
Little Rock, AR 72202
Email: REFrye@uams.edu

Dr. Richard E. Frye received his MD and PhD in physiology and biophysics from Georgetown University. He completed his residency in pediatric at University of Miami and residency in child neurology at Children's Hospital Boston. Following residency Dr. Frye completed a clinical fellowship in behavioral neurology and learning disabilities at Children's Hospital Boston and a research fellowship in psychology at Boston University. Dr. Frye also completed a MS in biomedical science and biostatistics at Drexel University. Dr. Frye is board certified in General Pediatrics and in Neurology with Special Competency in Child Neurology. Dr. Frye has been funded to study brain structure function in individuals with neurodevelopmental disorders, mitochondrial dysfunction in autism and clinical trials for novel autism treatments. Dr. Frye is the Director of Autism Research at the Arkansas Children's Hospital Research Institute and the Director of the Autism Multispecialty Clinic at Arkansas Children's Hospital.

Recent studies suggest that autism spectrum disorder (ASD) may be associated with abnormal function of the mitochondria, at least in a subset of children. The mitochondrion is the powerhouse of the body's cells. It is primarily responsible for producing cellular energy although it is important for producing the building blocks of cell, such as amino acids, during development and also has an important role in regulating oxidative stress and cell health. Mitochondrial dysfunction can affect both energy and non-energy producing metabolic systems since many metabolic systems feed their final biochemical products into mitochondrial pathways and/or derive their biochemical substrates from mitochondrial pathways. Furthermore, dysfunctional mitochondria can create a high level of reactive oxygen species that can damage the mitochondria and other important cellular components.

Those affected by mitochondrial dysfunction manifest non-specific symptoms including developmental delay, loss of developmental milestones (i.e., regression), seizures, easy fatigability, gastrointestinal abnormalities, and immune dysfunction. In general, mitochondrial dysfunction affects body systems that have high energy demands such as the brain, gastrointestinal system and immune system. Some of the same body systems that are dysfunctional in mitochondrial disorders are also dysfunctional in ASD. Recently studies have suggested that approximately 5 percent of individuals with ASD have strictly defined mitochondrial disease while a larger number of individuals with ASD, possibly 30 percent or more, might have dysfunction of the mitochondrial that may or may not be considered mitochondrial disease.

Mitochondrial dysfunction is treated through four approaches: (1) precautions to prevent metabolic decompensation; (2) vitamin supplements to support mitochondrial function; (3) modification of the diet to optimize mitochondrial function; and (4) investigation and treatment of medical disorders associated with mitochondrial dysfunction. Although no drugs specific for mitochondrial disease are available, several companies are developing novel compounds for the treatment of mitochondrial disease.

Precautions

Individuals with mitochondrial dysfunction should avoid physiological stressors such as fasting, extreme cold or heat, sleep deprivation, dehydration, and illness. If an individual with mitochondrial dysfunction becomes sick, fever should be treated aggressively and good hydration should be maintained, potentially with intravenous hydration with carbohydrates if necessary. Certain drugs and environmental toxins which depress mitochondrial function should be avoided. For example, common toxins which inhibit mitochondrial function including heavy metals, insecticides, cigarette smoke, and monosodium glutamate. Common drugs that inhibit mitochondrial function include acetaminophen, non-steroidal anti-inflammatory drugs, alcohol, some antipsychotic, antidepressant, anticonvulsant, antidiabetic, antihyperlipidemic, antibiotic, and anesthetic drugs. Specific precautions are required for surgery and anesthesia.

Vitamin Supplementation

Vitamins may enhance mitochondrial enzyme function and may result in improved efficiency of energy generation. In addition, some vitamins serve as antioxidants, which may slow the progression of the mitochondrial dysfunction due to high amounts of reactive oxygen species. Standard supplementations for mitochondrial dysfunction include Co-enzyme Q10 (5-15mg/kg/day), L-carnitine (30-100mg/kg/day) and B vitamins.

Typical B vitamins include thiamine (50-100mg/day), riboflavin (100-400mg/day), nicotinamide (50-100mg/day), pyridoxine (200mg/day) and cyanocobalamin (5-1000 mcg/day). Certain forms of co-enzyme Q10, specifically ubiquinol, have better bioavailability than other forms of co-enzyme Q10, providing the same affect at 1/10th the dose. Acetyl-L-carnitine (250-1000mg/day) is a natural constituent of the inner mitochondrial membrane. Biotin (5-10mg/day) is an important cofactor for several mitochondrial enzymes, especially those that process fatty acids. Antioxidants useful for individuals with mitochondrial dysfunction include vitamins E (200-400 IU/day) and C (100-500 mg/day), alpha-lipoic acid (50-200 mg/day), and folic acid (1-10 mg/day).

Diet Modifications

Some patients respond to frequent meals high in complex carbohydrates. For some patients an overnight fast can be enough to destabilize mitochondrial function. Such patients can be treated with complex carbohydrates such as corn starch before bedtime while some can be awakened in the middle of the night for a snack while others may require a feeding tube to receive feeding overnight. Other patients respond to low carbohydrate diets such as the ketogenic diet. The ketogenic diet should be initiated and monitored by a practitioner familiar with the diet as it can exacerbate metabolic disorders by causing acidosis is certain cases. Some patients respond to medium chain triglyceride oil supplementation since these fats do not require carnitine to be transported into the mitochondria.

Associated Medical Disorders

Individuals with mitochondrial disease have high rates of nervous system, gastrointestinal, endocrine, growth, cardiac, vision, and immunological abnormalities. Thus, such organ systems should be screened for dysfunction. The common abnormalities associated with mitochondrial disease that are seen in children with autism are outlined below.

Nervous System

Seizures and subclinical electrical discharges are relatively common in mitochondrial disorders and in autism, so practitioners should have a high index of suspicion for epileptiform abnormalities and should consider an overnight electroencephalogram to screen for subclinical epileptiform abnormalities.

Cerebral folate deficiency has been reported in both mitochondrial disorders and ASD. This disorder can be treated with folinic acid so it should be strongly considered in individuals with mitochondrial dysfunction. The gold standard test for this disorder is a lumbar puncture to measure 5-methyltetrahydrofolate in the cerebrospinal fluid.

Certain neurotransmitters require proper mitochondrial function. For example, acetylcholine requires acetyl-CoA production from the mitochondrial and Y-aminobutyric acid neurons have high firing rates which require significant energy.

Gastrointestinal System

The function of muscles is particularly dependent on mitochondrial function. Thus, motility of the gastrointestinal system can be affected in individuals with mitochondrial disease, resulting in digestive problems, constipation, and gastroesophageal reflux.

Endocrine System

The thyroid is extremely important for regulating metabolic rate and brain development. Hypothyroidism is associated with mitochondrial disease. Adrenal function requires functional mitochondria. Mitochondrial dysfunction can result in abnormalities in stress hormones including cortisol.

Immune System

The immune system is highly dependent on mitochondrial function to defend the body against infectious agents. Immune function should be assessed in all children with mitochondrial disease.

History of Development

In 1962 two independent researchers linked dysfunctional mitochondria to medical disease. In the last thirty years, several dozen genetically-based mitochondrial disorders have been described—all of them rare. It is becoming increasingly recognized that mitochondrial dysfunction, as opposed to mitochondrial disease, may contribute to the development and progression of many common neurodegenerative diseases such as Parkinson's disease.

Although mitochondrial dysfunction in ASD has only recently been more widely recognized, the first biochemical evidence of mitochondrial dysfunction was reported over twenty years ago. Dr. Mary Coleman from Georgetown University described an elevation in serum lactic acid in a subset of children diagnosed with autism. Over the past five years, others have confirmed elevations in lactic acid, as well as abnormalities in other metabolic markers of mitochondrial dysfunction in children with ASD.

Success rate (including a "Best case" anecdote): In general, milder mitochondrial dysfunction responds better to treatment than more severe dysfunction and treatment initiated sooner in the course of the disorder will probably be more effective than treatment initiated after long standing mitochondrial dysfunction. However, the success rate of treatment is very variable for several reasons. First, the efficacy of mitochondrial treatment, even for well-known mitochondrial disorders, has not been well studied. Second, the mitochondrial dysfunction identified in ASD has not been well character- ized and treatment for mitochondrial dysfunction in ASD has not been well studied. Third, the benefit of treatment may not be obvious as treatment my simply prevent progression of symptoms rather than reverse symptoms. Fourth, any benefit from treatment may take several months to observe.

Risk and/or side-effects (including a "Worst case" anecdote): Most vitamins are well tolerated, even at high doses. Some children with ASD may have behavioral side- effects from some vitamin. Thus, it is important to start vitamins one at a time so that any side-effects can be linked to a particular vitamin. Pyridoxine has been suggested to result in peripheral neuropathy at high doses but in practice this is not reported. Chil- dren should be carefully monitored when the ketogenic diet is started as the diet can worsen the metabolic acidosis associated with mitochondrial dysfunction.

Contact information for developers/practitioners/clinics/etc.

MitoAction
www.mitoaction.org

The United Mitochondrial Disease Foundation
www.umdf.org

Autism Research Institute
www.autism.com

Autism Speaks
www.autismspeaks.org

15

NEUROFEEDBACK FOR THE AUTISM SPECTRUM

By Dr. Siegfried and Susan F. Othmer

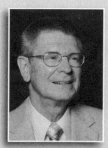

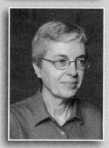

Siegfried Othmer, PhD
Susan F. Othmer

The EEG Institute
6400 Canoga Avenue
Suite 210
Woodland Hills, CA 91367
818-456-5975

Siegfried and Susan F. Othmer were attracted to the emerging field of neurofeedback in 1985 to help with the epilepsy of their son Brian. If Brian were diagnosed today, he would surely also be labeled Asperger's, so his may have been the very first case in which a child benefited for his Asperger's from having training with neurofeedback. Siegfried Othmer is a physicist with long experience in aerospace research until he was drawn into the field of neurofeedback. Susan Othmer studied physics and neurobiology at Cornell until her PhD research was derailed by her son's epilepsy. The Othmers have taught neurofeedback to thousands of professionals over the last 20 years in some 9 countries. The neurofeedback training instruments they either developed or inspired are used by more clinicians than any other. The Othmers have published research on neurofeedback in application to ADHD, mental retardation, addictions, chronic pain, and PTSD. Siegfried Othmer is co-author of the book *ADD: The Twenty-Hour Solution*. Siegfried Othmer is currently Chief Scientist at the EEG Institute in Los Angeles, CA. Susan Othmer is the Clinical Director. Their younger son Kurt is CEO of EEGInfo, a neurofeedback service organization for clinicians. Siegfried Othmer is also President of the Brian Othmer Foundation, under whose auspices neurofeedback services are being delivered worldwide to our veterans and active duty servicemen.

Neurofeedback is a highly promising emerging therapy for the autism spectrum. At issue here is a tool for the direct training of brain function, one that has already shown itself highly effective in addressing a wide range of "mental health" concerns. As has been the case for other therapies, its application to the autism spectrum has been complicated by the inherent complexity of the condition we confront. In the following, we recapitulate the development of neurofeedback for the autism spectrum and give some guidance to both therapists and parents with regard to the choices open to them.

Our own work with the autism spectrum using neurofeedback goes back some twenty-five years. In those early days of the field, the principal application of neuro-feedback was to Attention-Deficit Hyperactivity Disorder (ADHD), but the very same procedures were clearly also helpful for a variety of other issues. So it came naturally to want to try these methods also with children on the autism spectrum. These early attempts were just as likely to make things worse as they were to make things better, so we quickly placed a virtual fence around autism and decided we did not know enough to venture there. Some years later, a few practitioners in our network reported some good results with newer techniques, so the door was once again opened to working with the autism spectrum.

Neurofeedback procedures have proliferated in kind over the years, and with a broader set of clinical tools, it was also possible to match up to a broader set of clinical challenges in the autism spectrum. The point was being reached where one could rea-sonably expect worthwhile progress with nearly all autistic children. At the same time, scientific understanding of the issues was advancing to the point where the neurofeed-back work could now be understood in terms of an accepted model. Before going into more detail on the neurofeedback approach, it is helpful to have that model in mind.

Therapies for autism can be broadly lumped into approaches that address bio-medical issues that lie in the causal chain and methods that attempt to ameliorate the behavioral consequences. At first blush, neurofeedback fits into the latter category, and indeed neurofeedback practitioners tend to belong to the "mental health camp." But in truth, this assignment is not a good fit at all. By addressing behavior at the level of the brain itself we are in fact opening up an entirely new terrain that does not fit com-fortably either within the standard biomedical model or the standard mental health or behavioral model.

Looked at from the perspective of brain behavior, autisms' most obvious short-coming lies at the level of integration of function. Moreover, this deficit is not uni-form across functional domains, but rather afflicts particularly our emotional core that allows us to function in socially-connected ways. At the level of the brain, even our emotional functioning is organized by neural networks. We already know that there are developmental flaws in the structural connectivity of these networks. Beyond that, however, there are also deficits in the functional connectivity that operates on this flawed architecture. If we just survey the structural deficits in the white matter, we find no reason to believe that emotional networks should be selectively impacted. At the level of functional connectivity, they clearly are. This is where neurofeedback comes in. In this kind of training, we work to bring the neural network of emotional connectivity back online, among other things. We must necessarily operate within the limitations of what is available in terms of structural connectivity, but the good news is that emotional connectivity in the autistic child lies largely in the functional domain and is therefore clinically accessible to us. *EEG neurofeedback* allows us to do this efficiently. There is at present essentially no other comparable means to bring this about.

In addition to adopting the "brain perspective" on autism, it is helpful also to adopt the child's perspective for additional insights. What is the life experience of the autistic child who is not emotionally connected? We can gain insights into this by reflecting on other children who have severe attachment issues (often known by the term "Reactive Attachment Disorder"), for example, those who may have been raised in Chinese, Russian, or Romanian orphanages without the benefit of early nurturing. Such children live in extreme states of raw fear. We derive our sense of safety in the world from our early social relationships. In the absence of these comforting social bonds, the experience of life can be uncertain, capricious, and even threatening. The lack of assuredness in navigating one's world drives the nervous system toward heightened states of activation and arousal. The brain can never relax its vigilance because the child lacks the experience of a sense of safety. Even if the child presents as shut down, the internal state of that system is invariably one of high arousal—without apparent exception.

There is an even larger truth here. In the presence of various kinds of dysfunction, the brain will attempt to compensate by increasing activation generally. The effect may, however, be counterproductive. In any event, it imposes costs. We know very well what happens when we try to function in a highly agitated state. Brain function suffers. The larger principle at issue here is that problems in functional connectivity are not merely consequence. They are also the cause of yet further dysfunction. This is best visualized by reference once again to another affliction, namely Post-Traumatic Stress Disorder (PTSD).

In this condition, there may be nothing in the causal chain beyond the witnessing of a highly traumatizing event. Yet the lingering physiological consequences can devastate the rest of that person's life. In this case, we have no choice but to trace all these adverse consequences back to the original event, and all we have to work with is functional connectivity (which is demonstrably altered). There had been no physical injury, after all. Everything that occurred in that trauma experience lay in the functional domain at the outset. Very clearly, then, deficits in functional connectivity are quite sufficient to wreak all kinds of havoc with our physiology, and that is what also happens in the autistic spectrum.

The significance of this observation is that by addressing functional connectivity in autism directly, we are not only helping with the consequences of other biomedical deficits, we are also remediating an important element in the causal chain of dysfunction in its own right. This helps to make the case that neurofeedback should be an early intervention in the autistic spectrum. Given what we now know, we believe that it should be the very first thing undertaken by any family whose child is suspected of starting to exhibit autistic features. Families already involved in other therapies should consider folding neurofeedback in early as a high priority. But this is getting ahead of the story. Just what goes on in neurofeedback training, and how is it done?

Given the above model, it would be simple enough (at least in principle) to just characterize the deviations in functional connectivity and target those in training. The deviations are numerous, however, and one still needs a guiding principle to determine the appropriate order in which they should be addressed. And then one runs into the usual conundrum that some approaches help and others don't. So matters turn out not to be so simple at all. We have evolved a very different approach, one that starts with the observation already made above that the autistic child lives with an over-aroused nervous system, and that status does not do the child any favors.

In a kind of triage mentality, we find it most appropriate to move the child's brain out of emergency mode as the first order of business. "Calm the stressed and agitated nervous system" is the operative principle. This can be done relatively straightforwardly with essentially any autistic child, irrespective of level of functionality or of age. This strategy finds additional support in our work with servicemen coming back from Iraq and Afghanistan with PTSD and traumatic brain injury and in our work with children with severe attachment issues. All three of these classes of problems will be started with the very same neurofeedback approach because the initial objective is common to them all: to move the nervous system to a calmer and more controlled place. All three confirm for us that we are doing the right thing for each of them.

What actually happens in a session is as follows: The child sits in a large comfy chair in front of a large video screen. (Alternatively a young child may be held on a parent's lap or in a car seat.) Three electrodes are adroitly mounted on the child's scalp while the child is, hopefully, distracted by images on the screen. A skilled clinician can accomplish this task in about thirty seconds. The electrode leads are held out of the child's field of view. The images on the screen already relate to the "game" that the child will be watching for the feedback. This video game-like display encodes information derived from the child's EEG, so that the ebb and flow of game performance relates directly to a salient feature in the child's EEG. For example, the EEG variable may be reflected in the speed of a car or rocket or train. Other visual features in the image may be used as well to provide corroborative cues. Auditory feedback likewise encodes the information. And there is a tactile feedback module that also reflects the desired signal. So the child experiences immersive feedback in which the relevant information is corroborated with appeals to different sensory systems.

Functional improvements are observed almost immediately, simply by virtue of this change of state in which the nervous system functions. Of course one needs to do a number of sessions in order to get the brain to acquire new habits of functioning. All the while, additional functional improvements continue to surface while others continue to consolidate. What has been learned here is that the matrix of functional connectivity is itself a strong function of the state of arousal of the central nervous system. The greatest and swiftest payoff for our efforts therefore lies in first tending to the brain's emergency mode of function into which it has escalated.

One can often witness the effect on the child within the very first session. Understandably, the child most commonly starts out terrified of the novelty of neurofeedback and at minimum suspicious of the electrodes about to be attached to the scalp. But almost as soon as the training gets under way, one can often see a kind of tranquility settle on the child's face and a certain composure descend over his body. The child may even become completely still, and some have been observed to shift to a meditative pose—all quite uncharacteristic of the child who was brought in by the parents just hours earlier. The child's brain will have noticed that the information presented on the screen in some way actually mirrors its own activity. It cannot help but be intrigued to see its own activity mirrored back to it in this fashion, and so it becomes engaged in the process. Once the brain is thus entrained into the experience, then of course the child readily goes along for the journey. One can even think of this as guided meditation for the autistic brain. It clearly relishes the experience, and those dreaded electrodes are long forgotten by the child.

The immediate payoff for the child is that he is just more comfortable in his own skin. The secondary payoff is in terms of emotional relating. This follows from the fact that affect regulation is intimately coupled to arousal regulation. Regulating the one influences the other and vice versa. In fact, we have chosen to target our emotional circuitry as the most direct way of training arousal regulation, taking advantage of this relationship. A third critical payoff is that the brain is progressively much more stable. In general, the child will then go through life more on an even keel. More specifically, this training can be very helpful for children whose autistic presentation is further complicated by a seizure disorder. In fact, epilepsy was the first clinical indication for which efficacy of EEG feedback was proved in animal and human subject research, so the focus on seizure susceptibility is appropriate. The story is consistent throughout: Moving the child to better-regulated arousal states helps brain stability, and so does the re-normalization of connectivity relationships. Control of seizures then may open the door for enhanced cognitive function. We will have kindled a virtuous cycle in which every specific advance also promotes the overall objective of enhanced functionality.

Over time, the training process is repeated at various scalp sites in order to pursue other specific functional objectives, and in each case the training is shaped into its most productive course by the response of the child within session and across sessions. If everything goes as expected, the agenda gradually proliferates in terms of targeting and progresses on many fronts. Every feature of autistic behavioral presentation can be selectively targeted one after another. This is typically done in an order that emulates our original developmental sequence. Thus, for example, right-hemisphere function is addressed before left-hemisphere function. The first placement is always on the right parietal region, which leads to profound bodily calming and to bringing the child into body consciousness and into awareness of large-scale spatial relationships, i.e., of the relationship of self to the outside world. Right prefrontal training targets emotional connectivity directly. And interhemispheric placement is specifically helpful for the instabilities such as seizures. Eventually, left-side training may be introduced for more specific purposes.

Right-hemisphere training is quite commonly the key to the emergence of language because the right hemisphere is in charge of acquiring new skills. Language becomes a left-hemisphere function only once it becomes routinized. Moreover, the problem may not be language ability per se at all, but rather the very concept of communication itself. Once that concept is grasped, language may suddenly burst forth in fully formed sentences.

After a sufficient number of sessions to thoroughly establish the method for a particular child, it is often advisable to let parents take over the training at home, using a rented instrument, with ongoing remote supervision from the clinician. There is no obvious endpoint to the training, as the increasingly competent brain just continues to develop new competencies. Somehow our society needs to assure that every autistic child has the opportunity to expand his mental horizons with neurofeedback.

16

USING NUTRIGENOMICS TO OPTIMIZE SUPPLEMENT CHOICES

By Dr. Amy Yasko

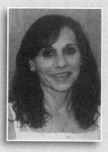

Amy Yasko, PhD, CTN, NHD, AMD HHP, FAAIM

Bethel, ME
207-824-8501
www.DrAmyYasko.com

Amy Yasko received her undergraduate degree in chemistry and fine arts from Colgate University and her PhD in the department of Microbiology, Immunology, Virology from Albany Medical College. Her postdoctoral work included fellowships in the Department of Pediatric Immunology and the Cancer Center at Strong Memorial Hospital, as well as the Department of Hematology at Yale Medical Center. Dr. Yasko was Director of Research at Kodak IBI as well as a principle/owner of several biotechnology companies including Biotix DNA and Oligos Etc., Inc. After receiving additional degrees as a traditional Naturopath and becoming a Fellow in Integrative Medicine, Dr. Yasko shifted her focus from biotechnology to natural medicine. With her knowledge in these various fields, she developed a protocol including a nutrigenomic test used to aid in addressing such complex conditions as autism, chronic fatigue syndrome, and other chronic neurological issues. Through the use of herbs and supplements and biochemistry testing to chart client progress, many who follow her protocol have improved and have even recovered. Dr. Yasko has spoken at conferences hosted by the NY Academy of Science, is listed in *Who's Who in Women*, has received the CASD Award for RNA research in autism, and has published numerous articles as well as chapters in books related to her more conventional work in biotechnology. At present she donates much of her time on her discussion group www.ch3nutrigenomics.com and offers advice and suggestions to the many who seek her help on their path to recovery.

I believe that autism is a *multifactorial condition,* meaning that a number of circumstances need to go awry simultaneously for autism to manifest. I often refer to my Princess Diana example…if the car wasn't speeding, if the paparazzi weren't chasing her, if they weren't in a narrow tunnel, if she had been wearing a seat belt…if you could eliminate any one of those factors then perhaps the end result would have been different. So too, I believe is the case with autism. I see and address autism as a multifactorial condition that stems from underlying genetic susceptibility combined with assaults from environmental toxins and infectious diseases. It has been shown in other instances that multifactorial diseases are caused by infections and environmental events occurring in *genetically susceptible individuals*. Basic parameters like age and gender, along with other genetic and environmental factors, play a role in the onset of these diseases. Infections combined with excessive environmental burdens only lead to disease if they occur in individuals with the *appropriate genetic susceptibility*. I believe this is the case in autism, and using this theory to approach autism has resulted in positive improvements.

Personalized Genetic Screening

One clear, definitive way to evaluate the genetic contribution of multifactorial conditions is to take advantage of new methodologies that allow for personalized genetic screening. Currently, tests are available to identify a number of underlying genetic changes in an individual's DNA.

The field of **nutrigenomics** is the study of how natural products and supplements can interact with particular genes to decrease the risk of diseases. By looking at changes in the DNA in these nutritional pathways, people are enabled to make supplement choices based on their particular genetics, rather than using the same support for every individual regardless of their unique needs. Knowledge of imbalances in nutritional genetic pathways makes it possible to utilize combinations of nutrients, foods, and natural ribonucleic acids to bypass mutations and restore proper pathway function.

The *methionine/folate pathway* is a central pathway in the body that is particularly amenable to nutrigenomic screening for genetic weaknesses. The result of decreased activity in this pathway causes a shortage of critical functional groups in the body called *methyl groups* that serve a variety of important functions.

Your Body's Editing Function

While the term may seem intimidating, a methyl group is actually just a group of small molecules, similar in size to the water molecule (H_2O). Water is a key to life, as are methyl groups critical for health and well-being. Methyl groups are simply "CH_3" groups; they contain 'H' like in water and a 'C' like in carbon or diamonds. However, these very basic molecules serve integral functions; they are moved around in the body to turn on or off genes.

One way to look at the function of methyl groups is that it is analogous to the editing function on your computer. If we think about your body like a computer then you have just one computer that you need to maintain over the course of your life. The longer you have that computer, the more outdated it will become. Over the course of a lifetime, many of the keys may become stuck or broken. You may drop the computer and damage its function or spill your coffee on it. However, the editing function of the computer remains intact and compensates for these broken keys, misspelled words, and sticky space bars due to accidents of wear and tear. In the absence of this editing function, assume that these "misspells" are accumulated in your body over the course of your life. If the editing function is impaired, then you have no way to get around these misspelled words and other issues that affect your ability to function. Over your lifetime you will accumulate so many misspelled words, missed keys, etc., that at a certain point it would be impossible to read a "document" amidst all of these mistakes. You can start to see why the proper functioning of the pathway that serves to edit your genes is so important. In addition to the editing of genes, this pathway also serves more direct roles in your body and is thus critical for proper function. While there are several particular sites in this pathway where blocks can occur as a result of genetic weaknesses, thankfully, supplementation with appropriate foods and nutrients can help to bypass these mutations to allow for restored function of this pathway.

The Role of the Methylation Cycle in Your Body

The methylation cycle is the ideal pathway to focus on for nutritional genetic analysis because the places where mutations occur is well defined and it is clear where supplements can be added to bypass these mutations. In addition to its editing role, the function of this pathway is essential for a number of critical reactions in the body. One very simplistic way to view methylation is that methyl groups serve as "traffic lights" for the genetic roadways in your body. Lack of proper traffic signaling can lead to a multitude of health problems. One consequence of genetic weaknesses (mutations) in this pathway that generates these "traffic lights" is an increased risk for a number of serious health conditions. Defects in methylation lay the appropriate groundwork for the further assault of environmental and infectious agents resulting in a wide range of conditions, including diabetes, cardiovascular disease, thyroid dysfunction, neurological inflammation, diabetes, chronic viral infection, neurotransmitter imbalances, atherosclerosis, cancer, aging, schizophrenia, decreased repair of tissue damage, improper immune function, neural tube defects, Down's syndrome, Multiple Sclerosis, Huntington's disease, Parkinson's disease, Alzheimer's disease, and autism.

- **Inflammation, bacterial and viral infection**
  When you have bacterial or viral infections in your system, the level of inflammation in your body is increased. This too relates back to this same *methylation cycle*. Increases in certain inflammatory mediators of the immune system due to infection such as IL6 and TNF alpha lead to decreases in methylation. Chronic inflammation would therefore exacerbate existing genetic mutations in this same

pathway. The inability to progress normally through the methylation pathway as a result of methylation cycle mutations combined with the impact of viral and bacterial infections further compromises the function of this critical system in the body.

- **New cells and the immune system**
  The building blocks for DNA and RNA require the methylation pathway. Without adequate DNA and RNA it is difficult for the body to synthesize new cells. New cell synthesis is needed to repair damaged cells, to maintain the lining of the gut, to make new blood cells as well as for your immune system that defends you against infection. T cells are a key aspect of your immune system and they require new DNA in order to respond to foreign invaders. T cell synthesis is necessary to respond to bacterial, parasitic and viral infection, as well as for other aspects of the proper functioning of the immune system. T cells are necessary for antibody producing cells in the body (B cells), as both T helpers and T suppressors are needed to appropriately regulate the antibody response.

- **Herpes, hepatitis, and other viruses**
  In addition, decreased levels of methylation can result in improper DNA regulation. DNA methylation is necessary to prevent the expression of viral genes that have been inserted into the body's DNA. Loss of methylation can lead to the expression of inserted viral genes such as herpes and hepatitis, among other viruses.

- **Sensory overload**
  Proper levels of methylation are also directly related to the body's ability to both myelinate nerves and to prune nerves. Myelin is a sheath that wraps around the nerve to insulate and facilitate proper nerve reaction. Without adequate methylation, the nerves cannot myelinate in the first place, or cannot remyelinate after insults such as viral infection or heavy metal toxicity. A secondary effect of a lack of methylation and hence decreased myelination is inadequate pruning of nerves. Pruning helps to prevent excessive wiring of unused neural connections and reduces the synaptic density. Without adequate pruning, the brain cell connections are misdirected and proliferate into dense, bunched thickets. When nerves grow in this unregulated fashion, it can cause confusion processing signals. *Synesthesia* occurs when the stimulation of one sense causes the involuntary reaction of other senses, basically sensory overload.

- **Serotonin, dopamine and ADD/ADHD**
  Methylation is also directly related to substances in your body that affect your mood and neurotransmitter levels of both serotonin and dopamine. Methylation

of intermediates in tryptophan metabolism can affect the levels of serotonin. Inter-mediates of the methylation pathway are also shared with the pathway involved in the actual synthesis of serotonin and dopamine. In addition to its direct role as a neurotransmitter, dopamine is involved in assuring your cell membranes are fluid and have mobility. This methylation of phospholipids in the cell membranes has been related to ADD/ADHD. Membrane fluidity is also important for a variety of functions including proper signaling of the immune system as well as protecting nerves from damage. A number of serious neurological conditions cite reduced membrane fluidity as part of the disease process including MS, ALS, and Alzheimer's disease. In addition, phospholipid methylation may be involved in modulation of NMDA (glutamate) receptors, acting to control excitotoxin damage.

Methylation as One Piece of a More Complex Puzzle

In general, single mutations or *biomarkers* are generally perceived as indicators for specific disease states. However, it is possible that for a number of health conditions, including autism, it may be necessary to look at the entire methylation pathway as a biomarker for underlying genetic susceptibility for a disease state. It may require expanding the view of a biomarker beyond the restriction of a mutation in a single gene to a mutation somewhere in an entire pathway of interconnected function.

This does not mean that every individual with mutations in this pathway will be autistic or will have one of the health conditions listed above. It may be a necessary but not a sufficient condition. Most health conditions in society today are multifactorial in nature. There are genetic components, infectious components, and environmental components. A certain threshold or body burden needs to be met for each of these factors in order for multifactorial disease to occur. However, part of what makes the methylation cycle so unique and so critical for our health is that mutations in this pathway have the capability to impair all three of these factors. This would suggest that if an individual has enough mutations or weaknesses in this pathway, it may be sufficient to cause multifactorial disease. Methylation cycle mutations can lead to chronic infectious diseases, increased environmental toxin burdens, and secondary effects on genetic expression.

By testing to look at mutations in the DNA for this methylation cycle, it is possible to draw a personalized map for each individual's imbalances, which may impact upon their health. Once the precise areas of genetic fragility have been identified, it is then possible to target appropriate nutritional supplementation of these pathways to optimize the functioning of these crucial biochemical processes. As seen in the diagram there are specific places in the cycle where support can be added. This support helps to bypass mutations in the pathway in a similar manner to the way you might take a

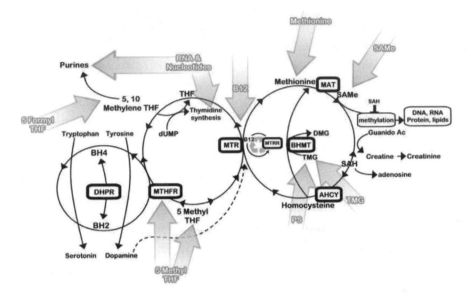

Methylation cycle indicating where supplements can be added to bypass mutations at specific points in the pathway. *Yasko, A. Pathways to Recovery. Bethel, Maine: Neurological Research Institute, 2009. Page 143.*

detour on a highway. We can look at a mutation in this pathway as analogous to a collision that has totally shut down traffic going in one direction on a highway. Support to bypass mutations in this pathway is like taking an alternate route to avoid the accident on the highway. Thus, the use of key nutrients or foods can aid in helping to bypass methylation cycle mutations and help restore function to this pathway.

The Newest Piece of the Puzzle: Genetic Susceptibility to *Helicobacter pylori*

As already discussed, genes can be turned on or off based on their degree of methylation. The ability of the CFTR gene (cystic fibrosis transmembrane conductance regulator) to function optimally appears to be regulated by methylation. Thus, lack of methylation cycle function may impair CFTR function, which can in turn lead to issues with appropriate mucus layer viscosity in the body. It has been observed that the number of individuals with autism testing positive for the bacterium *Helicobacter pylori* is much higher than would be expected. *Helicobacter pylori* (*H. pylori*) is a Gram-negative, spiral-shaped bacterium that lives in the mucus layer of the stomach and duodenum. Changes in the mucus layer environment may be a predisposing factor that accounts for this observed increase in *H. pylori*. This ulcer-causing gastric pathogen is able to colonize the harsh acidic environment of the human stomach. Although the stomach is protected from its own gastric juice by a thick layer of mucus that covers the stomach lining, *H. pylori* takes advantage of this protection by living in the mucus lining itself. In the mucus lining, *H. pylori* survives the stomach's acidic conditions by producing urease, an enzyme that catalyzes hydrolysis of urea into ammonia and bicarbonate. As strong bases, ammonia and bicarbonate produce a cloud of alkalinity around the bacterium, making it impossible for the body's normal defenses (such as T cells, natural killer cells, and other white blood cells) to get to it in the gastric mucus layer. Because *H. pylori* burrows into the mucus layer of the stomach and is very persistent there, it is difficult to get a positive test for it even when it is present. In addition, *H. pylori* can remain for long periods of time and is extremely difficult to eradicate. It appears that *H. pylori* may play a role in a number of the recognized pieces of the puzzle of autism. Many factors that have been identified as playing a role in autism are related to *H. pylori*, including problems with gluten and casein, breakdown of glutathione, excess stomach acid, and the high norepinephrine seen in ADD and ADHD. *H. pylori* affects neurotransmitters and brain neurochemistry. *H. pylori* infection increases the incidence of food allergy by facilitating the passage of intact proteins across the gastric epithelial barrier. *H. pylori* depletes secretin, which had previously been reported to have positive impacts in some cases of speech. Arginine makes urea to neutralize stomach acid, or, alternatively, makes intermediates (such as nitric oxide) that relax blood vessels. When *H. pylori* infection is present, it induces arginine to produce urea as opposed to nitric oxide because urea provides the alkalinity necessary for its survival. In this way, *H. pylori* depletes arginine through its overuse of the enzyme arginase. The depletion of arginine impacts the mitochondria, reducing mitochondrial energy production from glucose. When *H. pylori* infection is present, it changes the way important phospholipids are positioned in the cell membrane. Phospholipid orientation has been described as playing a role in ADD/ADHD as well as in immune system signaling. *H. pylori* also decreases levels of B_{12} in the body; decreases iron levels; increases ammonia and taurine; and can produce glaucoma in young individuals that resolves when the *H. pylori* is treated. *H. pylori* infection is not just an immediate acute infection. Rather, it is a long-term chronic problem that may take months or years to eradicate. Chronic *H. pylori* gastritis alters feeding behaviors, delays gastric emptying, alters gastric neuromuscular function, and impairs acetylcholine release; these effects can persist for months after the infection has been eradicated.

Taken together, the role of *H. pylori* in autism may be significant, and its ability to colonize the gut may be closely related to inadequate CFTR function, which in turn may be related to methylation cycle function.

The Bottom Line

It has been my experience that viruses, bacteria (including, but not limited to *H. pylori)*, toxic metals, and excitotoxins (like glutamate or MSG) also play a key role in the condition of autism. I do feel it is important to address these issues and to decrease the body's burden of metals and excitotoxins as well as to eliminate bacterial and viral issues in the body. Restoring healthy gut function is another critical area of focus on the path to recovery. However, if we begin with a knowledge of our nutrigenomic weaknesses, it makes it easier to address all of these aspects. While autism is a general term, there are multiple levels of severity, as well as a huge range of clinical presentations. Using nutrigenomic information takes into account that each child is an individual and needs to be seen as unique. This then allows for individualized supplement programs to target areas of weakness that customize support to address specific needs.

17

NUTRITIONAL SUPPLEMENTATION FOR AUTISM

By Larry Newman

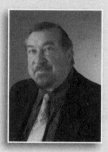

Larry Newman

Chief Operating Officer
Technical and Regulatory Affairs
Kirkman Group
6400 SW Rosewood St.
Lake Oswego, OR 97035
503-783-2704
lnewman@kirkmangroup.com

Larry Newman has been formulating nutraceuticals for autism and other developmental conditions for Kirkman Laboratories since 1999. As the chief operating officer for technical and regulatory affairs, he has worked with the leading physicians and clinicians in the special needs arena to develop science-based nutritional products that are utilized by patients with developmental disorders and special needs conditions.

Prior to his association with Kirkman, Larry ran the operations and technical departments of several large pharmaceutical, nutritional, and cosmetic companies, including IVC Industries, Hall Laboratories, Pharmavite Pharmaceutical, and Bergen Brunswig Laboratories. He is experienced in developing all product types including liquids, tablets, capsules, creams, lotions, and liquid pharmaceuticals.

Larry has a bachelor's degree from California State University and also attended USC school of pharmacy.

When we talk about cutting-edge therapies for autism spectrum disorders (ASDs), it is important to understand that no one type of therapy is effective for all persons with autism. Each individual has their own biochemical profile. What may be very effective for one autistic person may have no effect, little effect, or even a negative effect on another. The therapies we will be discussing here are those that have had a significant positive effect on an above average percentage of individuals over time.

A cutting-edge therapy is not purported to be a cure, but rather a treatment that consistently produces positive effects for those who try the therapy.

The most recent clinical work with autistic individuals indicates that a certain basic model with a defined set of priorities is the most logical way of implementing biomedical and nutritional interventions. This model allows parents or caregivers just getting started to set priorities and initiate a plan.

This chapter is mainly about how supplements will help the individual with autism. However, a discussion of the gut and diet establishes an essential foundation and is a necessary precursor to talking about supplementation. A properly functioning gut is better prepared to absorb nutrients and work in harmony with the immune and nervous systems, and an appropriate diet helps the gut and staves off detrimental immune and neurological effects.

Therapy #1—Clean up the Gastrointestinal Tract

It is well known and clinically documented that autistic individuals have a much greater incidence rate of gastrointestinal disorders than what is considered normal. A study done by Autism Speaks' Autism Treatment Network (ATN) reported that gastrointestinal (GI) symptoms occur in nearly half of children with ASD, and the prevalence increases as children get older. The results of this study were presented by ATN at the Pediatric Academic Societies annual meeting in Vancouver, British Columbia, Canada, on May 2, 2010. This study is extremely important in helping to set priorities in approaching autistic conditions. Patients with autism are medically ill, and addressing their gastrointestinal problems needs to be a first step.

In general, physicians have known for centuries that a well-functioning gastrointestinal tract and digestive system are crucial to good health. When digestion is working optimally, other organs and systems in the body have a better chance of working optimally as well. This is because the digestive system is responsible for processing the nutrients in our food, which in turn are used for growth, reproduction, development, tissue repair, healing, and organ function. In addition to providing fuel for the body through nutrition, the intestinal tract also plays an integral role in the functioning of the immune and nervous systems. The intestinal tract's relationship with neurological and cognitive function is often referred to as the gut-brain connection.

There are many distinct, recognizable signs of gastrointestinal disturbances, but as is often the case with autistic individuals who can't communicate, these are not always obvious to the parent or caregiver. Examples include the following:

- abdominal discomfort or cramping (often includes crying, screaming, or holding the abdomen)
- constipation or diarrhea
- indigestion, bloating, and gas

- inadequate digestion (the evidence of which is often seen in stools)
- inflammation
- yeast or bacterial overgrowth
- serious food sensitivities

When gastrointestinal disorders are suspected, a thorough examination by a gastroenterologist is called for. That examination may include an endoscopy and/or colonoscopy. Based on this exam, the physician has many options to help support whatever conditions are present. These options may include:

- prescription antifungals, antibiotics, or other drugs
- over-the-counter pharmaceuticals
- special diets including gluten-free/casein-free (GF/CF) or Specific Carbohydrate Diet™ (SCD™)
- probiotics to support good flora and crowd out undesirable organisms
- products that support tissue healing
- digestive enzymes to support proper food digestion

TRYING SPECIAL DIETS

Hidden sensitivities are often a contributing factor to GI problems. During a GI evaluation, the health professional may suspect a sensitivity to casein, gluten, soy, or complex carbohydrates as is the case with a majority of autistic individuals. If that is the case, a special diet would become an obvious intervention to try. Special diets can be very useful in alleviating GI symptoms as well as eliminating the cascade of other behavioral, neurological, and immunological symptoms. The most popular diet with the greatest success rate is undoubtedly the GF/CF diet. After following a strict GF/CF diet for a sufficient period of time (up to 6 months), if the desired results have not been seen, some practitioners recommend SCD. Please refer to the chapters in this book that explain these diets.

Therapy #2—Improving Nutritional Status

Following gastrointestinal evaluation and utilizing special diets if appropriate, improving nutritional status should become the next focus. This should be done by combining the proper healthful, nutritious foods with nutritional intervention using dietary supplements. Poor nutrition is very prevalent in autistic individuals for numerous reasons. A balanced diet is usually not the rule. This can happen for any (or all) of several reasons: (1) special diets such as GF/CF or SCD may be in place; (2) a person's tastes and attitudes can be such that their diet is very deficient in vitamins, minerals, or other necessary nutrients; or (3) a facet of biochemistry can be irregular, making the absorption of nutrients suboptimal.

The first step in improving nutritional status in an autistic patient is to do a thorough analysis of the patient's eating habits and supplement regimens. Physicians often turn this task over to a registered dietician or certified nutritionist who will lay out the person's typical diet and make recommendations for diet and supplementation.

Typical questions will include:

- What are the food groups consumed?
- How much in the way of protein sources, fruits, vegetables, carbohydrates, sugars, fiber, fats and oils are eaten daily?
- Are the foods consumed healthful?
- What nutrients do they provide?
- Are quantities consumed in the correct proportions?
- Is the method of cooking such that nutrients are not substantially depleted?
- What dietary supplements are also being taken?
- Given the food consumed and the additional supplements included, how does the regimen need to change to balance the person's nutritional status?

The diet must often change. But will it or can it? Often it is not possible because of the behavior or preferences of the individual. If the diet cannot improve sufficiently, then dietary supplements providing vitamins, minerals, essential fatty acids, fiber, and antioxidants need to be added. An individualized diet plus the addition of the required supplements will greatly improve nutritional status, and results and rewards will generally be very obvious as signs of poor nutrition diminish.

Poor nutrition can often be recognized by the following:

- vision issues
- unhealthy skin tone
- extreme tiredness or lack of energy
- lethargy
- behavioral issues
- failure to thrive
- frequent illness because of immune dysfunction

For those on a casein-/dairy-free diet, calcium supplementation is essential to ensure proper bone development and growth. In addition, a comprehensive vitamin and mineral supplement is essential when the diet is unbalanced and nutrients are deficient, which is often the case if all food groups including protein and carbohydrate sources and fruits and vegetables are not being consumed. Cod liver oil and omega-3 fatty acid supplements can help support good vision and healthy skin. Irregularities in biochemical pathways are often supported by B-6/magnesium supplements, folic or folinic acid, or sulfation aids (see below).

Certain nutrients are essential for proper support of the immune system. Zinc, vitamin A, vitamin C, vitamin D-3, vitamin E, and selenium are examples of nutrients that improve immune response. Suboptimal levels of these nutrients can sometimes lead to a weak immune system which can lead to frequent illnesses.

Proper absorption of nutrients as another factor in nutritional status

Often with autistic persons, even a balanced diet with the addition of the required dietary supplements fails to improve nutritional status to optimum levels because of a deficiency of pancreatic digestive enzymes or a lack of their proper secretion.

Digestive enzymes are those enzymes found in the body and secreted by the pancreas that function as biological catalysts to begin the breakdown of foods so that the important nutrients in the food can be properly absorbed and utilized. All food contains nutrients and potential nutritional value; however, until enzymes start the digestive process, the nutrients are "locked up" in the cellular structure and are not yet available to be absorbed by the body. For example, the fiber and vitamins in breakfast cereal provide no value until digestive enzymes start the digestion process and unlock the nutrients. Similarly, meat or fish do not deliver the protein necessary for growth and development until protease enzymes digest the protein.

When this type of enzyme insufficiency is taking place, adding oral digestive enzymes can make a dramatic, positive difference for an individual by improving digestion and absorption of nutrients. These enzymes can be administered as a prescription medication or as a dietary supplement. Some of the conditions that suggest digestive enzyme insufficiency include:

- malnutrition due to insufficient absorption of nutrients
- abnormal growth patterns
- vitamin and mineral deficiencies
- immune system impairment and frequent illness
- abnormal skin conditions
- gas, diarrhea, constipation, and/or foul smelling stools
- undigested food in the stool
- digestive tract discomfort (e.g., stomach, colon, or rectum)

Typically, a 3- to 4-week trial on a comprehensive multiple digestive enzyme will determine whether this intervention will be helpful.

Therapy #3—Use of Probiotics

Probiotics are defined scientifically as "living microorganisms that when ingested or locally applied in sufficient numbers can fill one or more specified, demonstrated functional or health benefits on the host." Probiotics have been called nature's "internal healers" because of their crucial role in the health and functioning of the intestinal tract. Probiotics are actually friendly (desirable and beneficial) bacteria that help keep the flora of the gastrointestinal tract within the correct balance of good and bad organisms.

One hundred trillion bacteria live in the human body, and of those, a healthy individual normally has a balance of about 85% good bacteria and 15% bad bacteria. When this ratio gets significantly out of balance, gastrointestinal problems arise. Individuals with autism are known to have imbalanced intestinal flora, with an excess of bad bacteria and a deficiency of good bacteria.

Supplementation of probiotics containing *Lactobacillus*, *Bifidobacterium* and other lactic acid bacteria strains are known to exert a profound positive influence in balancing intestinal flora. They are recognized to guard against intestinal inflammation, strengthening the immune barrier function of the intestines, and in helping to normalize intestinal permeability problems (aka "leaky gut"). They also produce antimicrobial substances, which are active against harmful bacteria, yeast, and viruses. By competing for intestinal nutrients and attachment sites, probiotic bacteria perform a crucial function in inhibiting the growth of harmful and potentially pathogenic bacteria.

Benefits of probiotics include:

- helping to regulate intestinal mobility, thereby normalizing bowel transit time
- producing lactic acid for reduction of colonic pH
- aiding digestion
- helping alleviate occasional diarrhea or constipation
- breaking down toxic byproducts of invading bad bacteria through a natural detoxification process
- increasing concentrations of healthy flora
- enhancing immune response
- decreasing infectious disease rates
- decreasing use of antibiotics
- decreasing serious allergic-type reactions

Results of using probiotics with individuals with autism having gastrointestinal and immune issues have been remarkably successful.

RESULTS OF THERAPIES 1, 2, AND 3

Gastrointestinal evaluation and support, a special diet (if required), and improving nutrition with use of digestive enzymes and probiotics should yield noticeable, favorable results for the person with autism within several weeks to several months. Once those improvements are noted and continuing support is established, there are other therapies that can be tried for numerous other symptoms the individual may exhibit.

Therapy #4—Improving Sleep Patterns

Individuals with autism suffer from sleep problems such as trouble falling asleep, periodic night waking, and nightmares. Parents of children on the autism spectrum have observed these problems to be more severe and/or frequent than those that occur in neurotypical children. These sleep problems can be all or in part due to underlying physiological conditions such as digestive discomforts; gastrointestinal pain from irritation, ulceration, reflux, or inflammation; or other causes of pain. Poor nutrition and metabolic issues can also contribute to poor sleep patterns.

Dietary supplements that have proven very useful in allowing autistic persons to maintain restful sleep include:

- melatonin
- magnesium
- L-Taurine
- 5-HTP
- GABA
- L-Threonine

All of these supplements are safe, usually without side effects, and should be tried one at a time for about a week in the order listed above. If one does not seem to help, stop and try the next one. Occasionally a combination of more than one is required. Getting restful sleep can greatly improve other symptoms of autism because the body is rested and operating efficiently.

Therapy #5—Improving Behaviors, Cognition, and Social Skills

Behavioral, learning, and social challenges are very common in autistic individuals. Because each person displays different behavioral traits and ultimately has a unique biochemical profile, it is sometimes challenging to find the right interventions.

Common behavioral and social challenges involve the following:

- speech delay or absence of speech
- inability to put words or sentences together
- learning disabilities
- social skill/communication challenges
- lack of eye contact or unable to focus eyes on an object
- aggressive behavior
- passive behavior
- depression
- anxiety
- tics or abnormal nerve responses

The list of supplements and interventions that have been used in dealing with these behavioral, learning, and social issues is long. The supplements that qualify for the cutting-edge label based on their frequent success rate are high B-6/magnesium supplements, dimethylglycine (DMG) or trimethylglycine (TMG), L-Taurine, omega-3 fatty acids, and cod liver oil. The Autism Research Institute publishes a list of nutritional supplements and drug products, listing their success rate as reported by responding parents. These rank amongst the top performers.

Omega-3 fatty acids are somewhat of an exception because they are good for all individuals with autism and will, without a doubt, improve overall health status long-term, so it is important to continue omega-3 supplementation even though short-term effects may not be noticeable.

Therapy #6—Improving Immune Function

The immune system is a complex and dynamic network of many soluble components including specialized cells, membranes, and a mini circulatory system separate from blood vessels. These entities all work together to protect us from infection by opportunistic microbes, bacteria, viruses, fungi, and parasites. The immune system also constantly scans our bodies for any signs of abnormal cell growth and keeps our bodies in check with regard to recognizing the differences between antigens and allergens. This is why a compromised immune system often leads to a shift in T cell types, which can lead to an individual developing more allergic-type reactions. Autistic individuals are almost always immunocompromised in some ways. Gastrointestinal issues often are immune related as are sensitivities to foods and allergens.

The signs of an immune problem are often quite easy to recognize over time. Persistence of the following conditions is key to suspecting immune deficiencies.

- frequent illness or illnesses of long duration
- continuous food allergies or an increased number of such allergies
- inadequate detoxification as indicated by laboratory testing
- low glutathione levels as indicated by laboratory testing
- impaired methylation pathway and inability to detoxify

Autistic individuals are especially prone to immune problems, and parents' observations conveyed to the physician are extremely important in helping the doctor recognize this problem because it is often hard to judge at an office visit.

There is a long list of nutritional supplements that support and strengthen the immune system. The most important of these include:

- zinc
- vitamin C
- vitamin D
- vitamin E
- selenium
- coenzyme Q-10
- reduced L-Glutathione (as prescribed by your physician)

You will recognize some of the above nutrients as being present in the multiple vitamin and mineral you may be using, but generally the multi will contain relatively low potencies. To better support a compromised immune system, additional supplementation of these immune-boosting nutrients is recommended. Increasing zinc to 50 mg. daily, vitamin C to 1000-3000 mg. daily, vitamin D-3 to 1000 IU or more daily, vitamin E to 200-400 IU daily, selenium up to 75 mcg. daily, and coenzyme Q-10 up to 100 mg. daily will be beneficial. As with the omega-3 supplements mentioned earlier, a regimen boosting immune response will be advantageous to all autistic individuals, so there is no reason not to use this proven therapy.

Therapy #7—Improving the Sulfation Pathway

The sulfation process is linked to an enzyme system known as phenol sulfotrans ferase (PST). Normally, PST is involved in a process called sulfoconjugation, whereby a group of potentially harmful chemicals known as phenols are attached to sulfate and thereby eliminated from the body. When there is a deficiency of sulfate in the bloodstream, phenolic compounds may build up in the body, and this in turn can interfere with neurotransmitter function. Sulfate deficiency and the resulting impairment of PST activity may explain some sensitivity reactions to a variety of phenol-containing foods, such as apples, grapes, chocolate, food colorings, and some herbs and spices.

Autistic individuals seem to have only about 20% of the normal level of sulfate in their bodies, the rest having been excreted excessively in the urine. In addition to the phenolic buildup described above, sulfate deficiency can contribute to other negative aspects of body chemistry including:

• preventing the detoxification of metals and other environmental toxins from the body
• inhibiting the release of pancreatic digestive enzymes, thereby hindering digestion
• limiting the activation of the hormone cholecystokinin (CCK), which plays a role in socialization
• contributing to a leaky gut because of an unhealthy ileum

Sulfation can often be regulated and improved by giving individuals Epsom salt baths once or twice daily. Dissolve some pharmaceutical grade Epsom salt (magnesium sulfate) in warm bath water. These baths have been remarkably helpful in autism. A topical Epsom salt preparation such as a cream or lotion can also be useful to improve sulfation, or a combination of the two may be convenient (such as using the cream in the morning and giving a bath at night). Oral sulfate such as glucosamine sulfate may be effective to some degree in certain individuals, but it is not purported to be as effective as the Epsom salt preparations or baths. Epsom salts are particularly helpful on days when an individual with autism has been swimming in a chlorinated pool.

Therapy #8—Improving the Methylation Pathway

Methylation is a series of very important biochemical reactions in the body that are responsible for overall good health. In individuals with autism, this process is very often lacking, making these individuals poor methylators. A properly functioning methylation pathway is necessary for the following:

• proper brain function
• healthy detoxification
• proper reproduction
• DNA protection
• a healthy, normal, non-premature aging process

There are many nutritional supplements that support proper methylation. Options should be discussed with the physician carefully because each autistic individual's needs are unique, and the protocol should be specifically tailored to their lab test results. Products used to support the methylation process include:

- methyl B-12 injections or other form of supplementation
- DMG or TMG
- folic or folinic acid
- vitamin B-6/magnesium
- SAMe (S-Adenosyl methionine)
- selenium
- zinc

Therapy #9—Detoxification

Substantial evidence is emerging linking a myriad of medical irregularities to negative environmental factors, including many conditions that are found in individuals diagnosed with autism and attention-deficit/hyperactivity disorder (ADHD). The frequency of many of these irregularities is increasing, which leads to further speculation that outside environmental factors are involved. Several recent clinical studies cited below certainly support this theory.

A recent study at Stanford School of Medicine on 192 sets of twins was conducted to evaluate the risk of autism posed by genetic factors and environmental factors. Surprisingly, this study indicated that environmental factors played a larger role than genetics (about 60% to 40%).

Clinical studies at three different research institutions (Mt. Sinai School of Medicine, University of California, and Columbia University) all revealed that children born to mothers with higher pesticide levels during pregnancy go on to experience lower IQ levels than those children born to mothers with lower values.

A study done by Phil Landrigan, MD, a pediatrician and public health expert at Mt. Sinai School of Medicine, reported that a study done in Canada on 1145 children revealed that children with high pesticide residues in their urine were twice as likely to be diagnosed with ADHD than those children with lower levels of urine pesticides.

Included in the list of environmental insults that can affect disease states are toxic chemicals, heavy metals, PCBs, and pesticides present in the products we use, the air we breathe, and the water we utilize and drink. Preservatives may also contribute. In April 2011, the EPA published a list of neurotoxicants that damage the nervous system and are linked to the continuing rise in learning, behavior, and developmental problems. Consumers need to be aware of potential product contaminations and select their food and consumable products carefully. The increasing utilization of organic diets indicates that this movement is gaining momentum.

These environmental pollutants can affect the body in numerous ways. Natural body defense mechanisms such as immune response can be bombarded with the insults, thereby becoming less effective because of the toxic load. The following conditions may be linked to continued exposure to environmental toxins:

- learning or speech difficulties
- social skills challenges
- aggressive behavior
- passive behavior
- poor immune response
- biochemical pathway issues

Certain nutrients are considered natural detoxifiers and can help mitigate exposures and enhance the body's natural detoxification process. Examples of such vitamins and minerals are zinc, vitamin C, vitamin E, vitamin D-3, and selenium. Other nutritional factors that can be helpful are L-Taurine, N-Acetyl cysteine, and reduced L-Glutathione.

In addition to the nutritional detoxifiers mentioned above, chelation using approved drugs can be very effective in detoxifying certain heavy metal contaminants, such as lead, mercury, arsenic, cadmium, antimony, and others deemed to be a health risk. On the Autism Research Institute's chart of effective therapies, chelation actually heads the list in its success rate. This would be a topic to discuss with the individual's physician, because regular medical monitoring, laboratory testing, and specific nutritional supplementation are usually recommended when chelating agents are used.

Conclusions

It is likely that some of these interventions will help all autistic individuals to some degree. The challenge to parents after receiving an autism diagnosis is finding out which of the specific therapies will help their child. A doctor trained and experienced in the physiological conditions underlying an autism diagnosis may help, especially in conjunction with a certified nutritionist. Many children, parents, and families have found positive rewards at the end of the process.

18

NEUROFIELD pEMF FOR THE TREATMENT OF AUTISM

By Dr. Nicholas Dogris

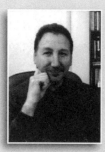

Nicholas Dogris, PhD

PO Box 426
Bishop, CA 93515
(760) 872-9153
nicholasdogris@verizon.net
www.NeuroField.com

Dr. Dogris has been in the mental health field since 1985. He is a California licensed psychologist and a board certified neurotherapist who practices in the Eastern Sierra mountain range. Dr. Dogris began working with EEG technology in 1987 while attending Humboldt State University. He was initially trained in neurotherapy by Margaret Ayers and would go on to develop treatment protocols for multiple neurofeedback systems. NeuroField, Inc. was opened and founded by Dr. Dogris and Brad Wiitala in 2008. Dr. Dogris is dedicated to the research and development of neurofeedback technologies and continues to practice in Bishop, California.

NeuroField was developed out of necessity. After all, most medical advances occur as a result of necessity. For me, my inspiration came from my son who was born anoxic and premature. I had been practicing neurofeedback for several years and knew from my experience that my son would need my help. However, in an effort to see if he would recover on his own, I waited until he was one and a half to begin treating him using neurotherapy methods. Injured from birth, my son had been making slow, poor progress. He walked at 18 months and had a vocabulary of two words at that time. He suffered from severe sensory integration problems that were primarily auditory and visual. He had low muscle tone and poor fine motor skills. We were working with some professionals on these issues and attempted to use Western methods to rehabilitate him, but things were not working out. I knew from my training in psychology that he was losing ground and that by the time I could treat him with standard neurotherapy methods, I would be playing catch up. So I started treatment when it was abundantly clear that his developmental delays were real and would impact him negatively. I chose a disentrainment method at first because it does not require the person to do anything except receive the treatment. Disentrainment is a painless method in which very low intensity electromagnetic waves are passed through the brain, which decouples the system and forces it to reorganize itself. After the brain is disrupted, it reorganizes itself within hours of the treatment, with the result being higher levels of functionality. This method worked for a period of time. My son's response to treatment using entrainment and disentrainment neurotherapy methods was good, but when he was roughly two and a half years old, he plateaued with regard to progress from treatment.

I became aware that if the brain does not have a history of good premorbid functioning (pre-injury functioning), then it would not know how to reorganize itself beyond a certain degree. After coming to this realization, it was obvious that we would have to show the brain how to reorganize itself. But how? My son was too young to engage in operant conditioning (learning-based) neurofeedback, which requires a specific level of understanding and cooperation by the person in order to obtain good clinical results.

Believing that more progress was possible, I began the process of searching the world for ways to heal him. My search led me through a wide variety of modalities. I would eventually arrive at the conclusion that I would have to do this myself. So, I searched, meditated, and prayed for help, and before I knew it, I had the idea that would eventually become NeuroField. I do not believe in accidents, and shortly after I developed the idea, I met Brad Wiitala; Brad had the engineering ability to bring NeuroField to life. By October 2007, we had the first prototype, and by April 2008, we had the first pulsed electromagnetic (pEMF) stimulation unit completed. It was not my intention to release NeuroField to the public but, rather, to use it for my son. However, while I was attending a conference, I showed it to a trusted colleague who told another colleague who told another and so on. Before I knew it, I was being asked to release the prototype to other professionals for the purpose of testing it. I agreed to do this and released ten systems to my beta testers. After several months of testing, it became clear that we had created something truly amazing and that I had the ethical responsibility to release it so others could benefit from this device.

NeuroField is an electromagnetic device that is capable of generating pulsed electromagnetic fields (pEMF) ranging from 0.31 to 300,000 Hz, with an output intensity ranging from 1-400 milligauss. To put it in perspective, NeuroField is 10,000,000 times weaker than the pulses given during an MRI. The EMF output of your computer and refrigerator is equivalent to the maximum stimulation intensity of NeuroField. In other words, the EMF is so low that it can be safely administered to the brain at slow and fast frequencies without causing tissue damage. At first, we did not know if this low intensity pEMF could even affect the brain. After all, transcranial magnetic stimulation (TMS), which also uses EMF to disrupt the brain, is 10,000,000 times stronger than NeuroField and is approved as a safe and effective method for the treatment of depression by the FDA as of 2008. How could such a low intensity EMF pulse impact the brain and/or the body in a positive way? What we would eventually learn is that NeuroField's low intensity pEMF is copied or mimicked by the brain. pEMF traverses the skull effortlessly and passes through the entire brain at low or high intensity. As the pEMF passes through the brain, the brain creates a dominant frequency of whatever frequency it "sees." In essence, the brain can be made to mimic whatever frequency you introduce to it between 1-1000 Hz. This is not a new breakthrough as neurologists have been doing this with light stimulation devices in hospitals for decades in order to diagnose seizures and epilepsy. The difference is that with NeuroField we were doing it with pEMF and could affect any region of the brain that we selected as needing therapy. The question then (and now) is one of how to determine which brain regions to stimulate and which pEMF frequencies do you use?

For the past six years, we have been researching that very question. Our research has revealed three major observations regarding NeuroField pEMF technology. The first observation is that the brain will mimic or copy low intensity pEMF frequency. The second observation is that pEMF causes inflammation reduction anywhere in the body. The third observation is that pEMF causes capillary dilation, which increases blood flow in the region where the stimulation is being given. It was these observations that lead us to develop several procedures in which quantitative electroencephalogram (QEEG) analysis, NeuroField pEMF stimulation, and 19-channel, operant conditioning, norm-referenced neurofeedback are combined to rehabilitate the brain. Using a program called Neuroguide, a 19-channel EEG can be obtained to analyze the brain cortically and subcortically. Neuroguide uses norm-referenced data to analyze the EEG and generates a report—very much like a blood test—that shows you how and where the brain is deregulated. The clinician then utilizes QEEG data and matches this data to the presenting problems of the person in order create a treatment plan. Using the NeuroField system, pEMF is then given to the person so as to assist the brain in regulating or balancing itself. The NeuroField community has been testing these procedures for several years, and the results suggest that they are valid and reliable methods that can assist a person in their recovery.

The NeuroField system is being tested on a wide variety of issues such as autism, Asperger's syndrome, pervasive developmental disorder, attention-deficit/hyperactivity disorder, depression, anxiety, traumatic brain injury, and Parkinson's disease. This writer has treated over 50 children with autism, and clinicians in the NeuroField community combined have treated over 200 children with autism. The QEEG, norm-referenced data that the NeuroField community has obtained over the years shows some consistent findings in children with autism. We have identified two subtypes of autism, with the first being the alpha-deficient type and the second being the theta-excessive type. The alpha-deficient type appears to have significantly reduced alpha activity in the central, parietal, and occipital lobes. They also have decreased delta activity in the parietal lobes. Lastly, they appear to have increased high beta activity in the sensory motor strip. The combination of reduced alpha and delta wave activity combined with high beta in the sensory motor strip creates a state in which the person is a sensory "raw nerve" and is easily overwhelmed by any form of sensory stimuli. In other words, the brain is unable to slow down or take in the external information at a rate that a person can tolerate without getting overwhelmed. In my opinion, people with autism are easily overstimulated and overwhelmed by external stimuli and engage in self-stimulation behaviors to slow down the rapid amount of information that they do experience. Once the alpha deficiency is resolved, sensory stimuli are tolerated much better, allowing the person to function in environments in which auditory and visual stimuli had been overwhelming previously. The theta excessive type has excessive theta activity that is widespread throughout the brain along with excessive high beta in the sensory motor strip. People with this profile usually have seizures and are also sensory sensitive. Treatment focuses on reducing the delta and theta activity, which reduces the amount of seizure activity that the person experiences. Once this is achieved, high beta activity is slowly reduced so as to stabilize the sensory issues and reduce the raw "nerve effect" associated with the brain processing information too quickly. Notably, both subtypes have gastrointestinal and metabolic issues that limit the body's ability to absorb food and eliminate toxins. Another part of the NeuroField treatment focuses on giving pEMF stimulation directly to the gut in an effort to assist with elimination and absorption issues. At first, treatment was given once a week, but as time went on it became clear that intensive, daily treatment had a much better and longer lasting effect on the brain and the body. The following are some case studies that demonstrate the effectiveness of NeuroField.

Case Study 1. A little girl, four years of age and diagnosed with autism, was brought in by her mother after her symptoms had resulted in her having no success in school. She was nonverbal when we began treatment. Her QEEG showed her to be in the alpha-deficient subtype, with alpha being greater than three standard deviations below the norm and high beta being greater than three standard deviations above the norm. She was a sensory "raw nerve" and could not tolerate loud noises or rooms of people talking all at once. She was given NeuroField pEMF over a period of four years, with treatment occurring once a week. During that time, she also engaged in applied behavior analysis (ABA) treatment and special education classes in school. Within the first year of treatment, she began talking. This began with verbal babbling and progressed in a consistent pattern to fluent language development. She emerged from the autistic state (i.e., no speech, no eye contact, completely internalized) in roughly two years. Her ability to understand where she ended and others began steadily improved as treatment progressed. In time, she was able to be in school without the need for an aide. Her ability to follow directions improved to the point where she could carry out multiple directions and stay on task. Her QEEG improved steadily over time with alpha amplitude increasing to the normative range. As alpha improved, she improved.

Case Study 2. A little boy, eight years of age, was brought in by his parents as he was nonverbal and not responding to a wide variety of interventions. He was identified as the alpha-deficient subtype. He participated in multiple intensive treatments in which he received two treatments per day for two weeks at a time. Since beginning treatment, he has participated in intensive treatment every other month since 2012. His parents report continued improvement after each set of intensive treatments. His alpha level continues to increase, which is usually followed by better eye contact, increased verbalizations, and the use of "I" statements. During one of his intensives, his ability to respond to questions emerged. After being asked how he felt, this little boy made direct eye contact and said, "I'm fine." When asked how he felt, he said, "I feel good." His progress has also been observed by his teachers and aides who report continued improvement.

Case Study 3. An 11-year-old male who was diagnosed with autism and seizure disorder was identified as the theta-excessive subtype. He participated in one treatment a week for 14 months. The frequency of his seizures decreased from 2-3 times per week to *maybe* once a month. His ability to communicate and make eye contact improved dramatically to the point where he did not require an aide in school. It was also discovered that his gastrointestinal problems greatly contributed to his seizure activity and that once those issues were corrected, his response to NeuroField pEMF was greatly improved.

NeuroField continues to evolve and improve. Continued research and development of this modality is ongoing in the NeuroField community. The technology shows promise as a standalone and adjunct treatment for children, adolescents, and adults diagnosed with autism.

TRANSCRANIAL MAGNETIC STIMULATION FOR THE TREATMENT OF AUTISM

By Dr. Joshua M. Baruth, Dr. Estate Sokhadze,
Dr. Ayman El-Baz, Dr. Lonnie Sears, and
Dr. Manuel F. Casanova

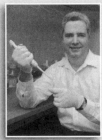

Joshua M. Baruth, PhD[1,4]
Estate Sokhadze, PhD[1]
Ayman El-Baz, PhD[2]
Lonnie Sears, PhD[3]
Manuel F. Casanova, PhD[1,4]

Affiliations:

[1]Department of Psychiatry and Behavioral Sciences, University of
Louisville School of Medicine, Louisville, KY 40202
[2]Department of Bioengineering, University of Louisville J.B. Speed
School of Engineering, Louisville, KY 40208
[3]Department of Pediatrics, University of Louisville School of Medicine, Louisville, KY
40202
[4]Department of Anatomical Sciences and Neurobiology, University of Louisville School of
Medicine, Louisville, KY 40202

Dr. Manuel Casanova did his basic training at the University of Puerto Rico and continued his specialty training at the Johns Hopkins University and the National Institutes of Mental Health. He is a board certified neurologist with specialty training in both neuropathology and psychiatry. At present Dr. Casanova serves as the Vice Chair for Research within the Department of psychiatry at the University of Louisville. He is also the Gottfried and Gisela Kolb Endowed Chair in Psychiatry for the same institution. Dr. Casanova was a founding member of the National Alliance for Autism Research (now merged with Autism Speaks) and the Autism Tissue Program. He chaired for several years the Developmental Brain Disorders Study section of the National Institute of Health. He serves as an editor for five different journals. Dr. Casanova is the recipient of many recognitions, including an EUREKA award from the NIMH for innovative research in regards to autism. In 2010 he was a plenary speaker at the World Organization of Autism Congress in Monterrey Mexico. His CV shows 191 refereed articles, 49 books chapters, 3 edited books, and close to 300 congress presentations.

Transcranial magnetic stimulation (TMS) allows scientists to stimulate the brain noninvasively in alert, awake patients. The first TMS device that could stimulate focal regions of the brain was developed in Sheffield, England by A. T. Barker and colleagues in 1985 (Barker et al., 1985). TMS operates based on Faraday's law of electromagnetic induction (1831) which describes the process by which electrical energy is converted into magnetic fields and vice versa. The TMS apparatus achieves the induction of a magnetic field by using a power supply to charge capacitors which are then discharged through the TMS coil, and this creates a magnetic field pulse. The principle of electromagnetic induction proposes that a changing magnetic field induces the flow of electric current in a nearby conductor—in this case the neurons below the stimulation site. Typically TMS coils are designed to produce magnetic fields in the range of 1 tesla (T) which is powerful enough to cause neuronal depolarization. The focal point of stimulation is about 1 cm^2 in area, and maximal induction is proposed at 90 degrees to the magnetic field (see George & Belmaker, 2007).

TMS can be administered in a single-pulse manner where single or paired pulses are delivered non-rhythmically and not more than once every few seconds or repetitively (rTMS) where pulses are delivered at specific frequencies in trains with precise inter-train intervals (ITI). Generally, single-pulse TMS is used for physiological research or diagnostic purposes while rTMS is used to alter the excitability and function of targeted areas of cortex. rTMS can be divided into low-frequency rTMS (≤1Hz) and high-frequency rTMS (>1Hz), which categorically affect cortical excitability in different ways. Studies have shown that low-frequency or "slow" rTMS (≤1Hz) increases inhibition of stimulated cortex (e.g., Maeda et al., 2000), whereas high-frequency rTMS (>1Hz) increases excitability of stimulated cortex (e.g., Pascual-Leone et al., 1994). It has been proposed that the effect of "slow" rTMS arises from increases in the activation of inhibitory circuits (Pascual-Leone et al., 2000). Long-term potentiation may be a model for understanding the mechanisms of high frequency rTMS, whereas long-term depotentiation (whereby synaptic weights are "reset" to baseline levels) may be proposed as the most relevant model for understanding the inhibitory effect of low-frequency rTMS (Hoffmann & Cavus, 2002).

rTMS is a simple outpatient procedure lasting approximately 30 minutes. Patients are seated in a comfortable, reclining chair and are fitted with a swim cap to outline the TMS coil position and aid in its placement for each session. Before the procedure begins the "motor threshold" is determined in each patient. "motor threshold" is the intensity of the pulse delivered over the motor cortex that produces a noticeable motor response. Sensors are applied to the hand muscle (i.e., the first dorsal interosseous) opposite the site of stimulation and motor responses are monitored with physiological monitoring tools on a computer. The output of the machine is gradually increased by 5 percent until a 50μV deflection on the monitor (i.e., electromyograph) or a visible twitch of the muscle is observed. Once the patient's "motor threshold" is determined the coil is moved to the site of stimulation (e.g., the prefrontal cortex) and the pulse intensity is adjusted relative to the patient's "motor threshold". Common dosing schedules include one to two visits per week, and typically patients are welcome to read a book or magazine during the procedure (Fig. 1).

TMS is generally regarded as safe without lasting side effects. Reported side effects include a mild, transient tension-type headache on the day of stimulation and mild discomfort due to the sound of the pulses; earplugs are recommended especially at higher frequencies of stimulation. Given the modulatory effect of rTMS on cortical excitability, there is a very small risk of inducing a seizure (see Wasserman et al., 1996). Given this risk, participants with epilepsy or a family history of epilepsy are generally excluded of rTMS studies, and as a safety precaution, some rTMS studies adjust the stimulation intensity below the participant's "motor threshold" (e.g., 90 percent of motor threshold). rTMS is generally considered safe for use in pediatric populations, as no significant adverse effects or seizures have been reported (see Quintana, 2005 for review).

rTMS has been applied to a wide variety of psychiatric (e.g., ADHD, depression) and neurological disorders (e.g., Parkinson's Disease) in adult populations and more recently rTMS has been applied in child and adolescent populations (see Croarkin et al. 2011). A number of studies report an improvement in mood after repeated frontal lobe stimulation in both depressed adults (e.g., George et al., 2010) and adolescents (Wall et al., 2011), and it has been reported that rTMS may improve symptoms of Attention Deficit Hyperactivity Disorder (ADHD) (e.g., Bloch et al., 2010). Furthermore, it has been found that rTMS may improve certain symptoms associated with anxiety disorders, like Post Traumatic Stress Disorder (PTSD) and Obsessive-Compulsive Disorder (OCD) (see George & Belmaker, 2007). In Parkinson's disease (PD) most studies have shown beneficial effects of rTMS on clinical symptoms (Wu et al., 2008).

Within the context of autism spectrum disorders (ASD) rTMS has unique applications as a treatment modality. ASD

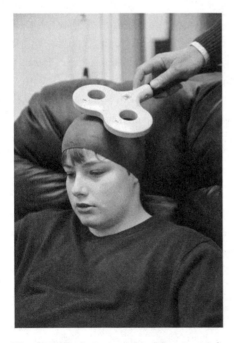

Figure 1 Patient receiving Transcranial Magnetic Stimulation Treatment

is associated with disturbances in social interaction and communication, restricted and stereotyped behavioral patterns, and frequently abnormal reactions to the sensory environment (American Psychiatric Association, 2000; Charman, 2008). It has been suggested that a wide range of deficits in autism might be understood by an increase in the ratio of cortical excitation to cortical inhibition (Rubenstein & Merzenich, 2003) and increases in local cortical connectivity accompanied by deficiencies in long-range connectivity (Rippon et al., 2007). Locally overconnected neural networks may explain the superior ability of autistic children in isolated tasks (e.g., visual discrimination), while, at the same time, deficiencies in long-range connectivity may explain other features of the disorder (e.g., lack of social reciprocity). An increased ratio of cortical excitation to inhibition and higher-than-normal cortical "noise" may explain the strong aversive reactions to auditory, tactile, and visual stimuli frequently recorded in autistic individuals as well as a higher incidence of epilepsy (Gillberg & Billstedt, 2000).

One possible explanation for higher-than-normal cortical noise and abnormal neural connectivity in ASD is the recent finding of minicolumnar abnormalities. Minicolumns are considered the basic anatomical and physiological unit of the cerebral cortex (Mountcastle, 2003), and contain pyramidal cells that extend the cortical width surrounded by a neuropil space consisting of several species of GABAergic, inhibitory interneurons (i.e. double-bouquet, basket, and chandelier cells) (Casanova, 2007). The double-bouquet cells impose a strong vertically directed stream of inhibition (Mountcastle, 2003) surrounding the minicolumnar core. The narrow vertical distribution of the double bouquet cells is so specific and restricted that it creates a narrow vertical cylinder of inhibition running geometrically perpendicular to the surface of the brain (Mountcastle, 1997; Douglas & Martin, 2004). Our preliminary studies indicate that minicolumns are reduced in size and increased in number in the autistic brain, especially the prefrontal cortex (Casanova et al., 2002ab, 2006ab). More specifically, minicolumns in the brains of autistic patients are narrower and contain less peripheral, neuropil space (Casanova, 2006ab). The lack of a "buffer zone" normally afforded by lateral inhibition and appropriate neuropil space may adversely affect the functional distinctiveness of minicolumnar activation and could result in isolated islands of coordinated excitatory activity (i.e., possible seizure foci); this autonomous cortical activity may hinder the binding of associated cortical areas, arguably promoting focus on particulars as opposed to general features. In addition the effect of loss of surround inhibition may result in an increase in the ratio of cortical excitation to inhibition and signal/sensory amplification which may impair functioning, raise physiological stress, and adversely affect social interaction in patients with ASD.

We hypothesize that contrary to other inhibitory cells (i.e., basket and chandelier), whose projections keep no constant relation to the surface of the cortex, the geometrically exact orientation of double-bouquet cells and their location at the periphery of the minicolumn (inhibitory surround) makes them the appropriate candidate for induction by a magnetic field applied parallel to cortex (Fig 2). Over a course of treatment "slow" rTMS may restore the balance between cortical excitation and cortical inhibition and lead to improved long-range cortical connectivity.

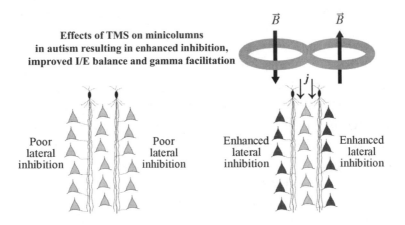

Figure 2 Magnetic field applied parallel cortex enhances surround inhibition on periphery of minicolumn

Thus far we have focused on clinical, behavioral, and neuroimaging outcome measures, in order to access the effectiveness of rTMS treatment in ASD. One neuroimaging modality that has unique applications to ASD research is electroencephalography (EEG). EEG is the non-invasive measurement of the summation of postsynaptic currents via scalp electrodes; the oscillatory frequency ranges of the postsynaptic currents can be divided into delta (0-4Hz), theta (4-8Hz), alpha (8-12Hz), beta (12-30Hz) and gamma (30-80Hz) frequencies. It is well known that the generation of normal gamma oscillations directly depends on the integrity of networks of inhibitory interneurons within cortical minicolumns (Whittington et al., 2000). Additionally the synchronization of cortical activity over wide-ranging cortical regions in the gamma range as been linked to the connectivity or "coherence" of assemblies of neurons working on the same object (percept, idea, cognition) (Brown et al., 2005).

In one of our previous investigations (Sokhadze et al., 2009b) we measured the EEG gamma band in 12 children with ASD and 12 controls during a visual attention task, and then measured the EEG gamma band in the ASD group after 6 sessions of "slow" rTMS to the prefrontal cortex. We hypothesized that the ASD group would have excess gamma band activity due a lack of cortical inhibition and treatment with "slow" rTMS would help restore inhibitory tone (i.e., reduce excess gamma band activity). We also analyzed clinical and behavioral questionnaires assessing changes in symptoms associated with ASD after rTMS treatment. The visual attention task employed Kanizsa, illusory figures which have been shown to readily produce gamma oscillations during visual tasks (Fig. 3). Subjects are instructed to press a button when they see the target Kanizsa square and ignore all other stimuli: Kanizsa stimuli consist of inducer disks of a shape feature and either constitute an illusory figure (square, triangle) or not (colinearity feature); in non-impaired individuals gamma activity has been found to increase during the presentation of target visual stimuli compared to non-target stimuli.

We found that the power of gamma oscillations was higher in the ASD group and had an earlier onset compared to controls—especially in response to non-target illusory figures over the prefrontal cortex (Fig. 4). Additionally there was less of a difference in gamma power between target and non-target stimuli in the ASD group particularly over lateral frontal and parietal recording sites. After six sessions of "slow" rTMS applied to the left prefrontal cortex the power of gamma oscillations to non-target Kanizsa figures dramatically decreased at frontal and parietal sites on the same side of stimulation, and there was more of a difference between gamma responses to target and non-target stimuli. According to clinical and behavioral evaluations the ASD group showed a significant improvement on the repetitive behavior scale (RBS), which assesses repetitive and restricted behavior patterns associated with ASD (e.g., stereotyped, self-injurious, compulsive, and restricted range) (Bodfish et al., 1999).

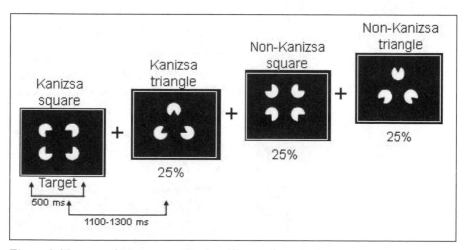

Figure 3 Target and Non-target Kanizsa illusory figures

In a more recent investigation with more participants (Baruth et al., 2010a) we investigated gamma band activity in 25 subjects with ASD and 20 age-matched controls using Kanizsa illusory figures and assessed the effects of 12 sessions of bilateral "slow" rTMS applied to the prefrontal cortices in 16 of the ASD participants. In individuals with ASD gamma activity was not discriminative of stimulus type, whereas in controls early gamma power differences between target and non-target stimuli were highly significant. Following rTMS individuals with ASD showed significant improvement in discriminatory gamma activity between relevant and irrelevant visual stimuli, and there was also a significant reduction in irritability and repetitive behavior as a result of rTMS (Fig 5 & 6).

In another investigation our laboratory analyzed gamma coherence before and after 12 sessions of "slow" rTMS in 14 subjects with ASD. Analysis at 4 sites of EEG over frontal and parietal sites revealed significantly lower coherence in the ASD group before rTMS while after rTMS there was a significant improvement pointing to an increase in global cortical connectivity.

We have also been interested in investigating event-related potentials (ERP) abnormalities in ASD: ERPs provide a neurobiological measure of perceptual and cognitive processing and represent scalp-recorded, transient changes in the electrical activity of the brain in relation to the onset of a stimulus. In a previous paper (Sokhadze, et al. 2009a) we investigated ERPs in a three-stimuli, visual task of selective attention in 11 high-functioning children and young adults with autism spectrum disorder (ASD) and 11 age-matched, typically developing control subjects. Patients with ASD showed significantly amplified and prolonged cortical responses to irrelevant, visual stimuli compared to controls; these results were recently confirmed in a following study assessing ERP responses in 15 subjects with ASD and 15 controls in a similar task using illusory figures (Baruth et al., 2010b).

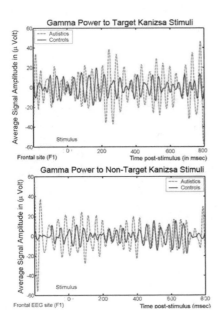

Figure 4 Gamma power is higher in ASD group compared to controls especially to non-target stimuli

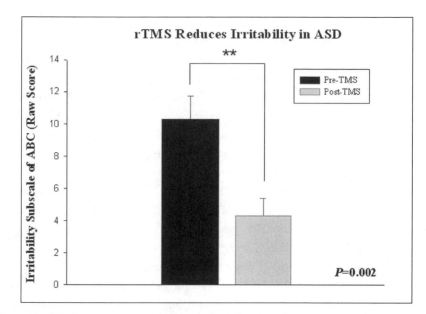

Figure 5 rTMS treatment resulted in a significant reduction in irritability in ASD (Baruth et al., 2010a).

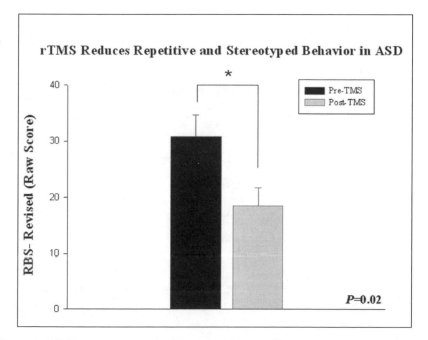

Figure 6 rTMS treatment resulted in a significant reduction in repetitive and stereotyped behavior in ASD (Baruth et al., 2010a).

In a follow-up investigation (Sokhadze, et al. 2010a) we assessed the effects of 6 sessions of "slow" rTMS stimulation applied to the left prefrontal cortex on performance in a three-stimuli, visual task of selective attention, as well as clinical and behavioral questionnaires in 13 individuals with ASD. Low-frequency rTMS minimized early cortical responses to irrelevant stimuli in this task and increased responses to relevant stimuli indicating improved selectivity and better stimulus differentiation. Additionally, there was a significant reduction in the percentage of errors in motor responses to target stimuli, and in agreement with our previous results (Baruth et al., 2010a; Sokhadze et al., 2009b), we found a significant reduction in repetitive behavior according to the RBS. Furthermore, these results were recently confirmed in 25 subjects with ASD following 12 sessions of bilateral "slow" rTMS by finding significantly improved ERP indices of selective attention, reduced motor response errors, and reductions in both repetitive behavior and irritability (Casanova et al., 2012) (Fig. 7).

Additionally, we investigated executive functioning in 14 individuals with ASD and 14 age- and IQ- matched controls by evaluating error monitoring and correction (Sokhadze et al., 2010b). The ASD group showed significant evidence of compromised error detection, evaluation, and correction which may underlie a general impairment in self-monitoring related to behavioral and/or social disturbances in ASD. We then evaluated the effects of 12 sessions of bilateral "slow" rTMS on error monitoring and correction. The active rTMS group showed significant improvement in error detection and correction compared to a randomized, non-active rTMS group (Sokhadze et al.,

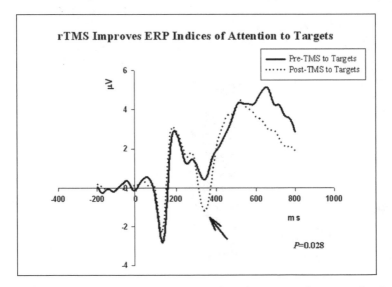

Figure 7 ERP indices of attention were significantly improved as a result of rTMS treatment

2012); this may point to improved executive functioning and behavioral performance in ASD as a result of rTMS.

We recently extended our results by including an analysis of outcome measures following 18 sessions of low-frequency (1Hz) rTMS applied bilaterally over the prefrontal cortex (Sokhadze et al., 2013). Treatment sessions were once-per-week at 90% of motor threshold (~200 pulses/per session) in 27 individuals with ASD. Results were compared to a wait-list group comprised of 25 age-, gender-, and IQ-matched controls with ASD, who did not receive TMS but were tested twice within 2 months. Following 18 sessions participants showed decreased irritability and hyperactivity as well as decreased stereotypic and compulsive behaviors compared to the wait-list group. Furthermore, the TMS group showed reduced cortical reactivity to non-target distractor stimuli and increased reactivity to targets using an ERP task of selective attention. Participants in the TMS group also had significantly improved reaction times to target stimuli and improvement in error monitoring function compared to the wait-list group. These results replicate our prior studies using a shorter rTMS course and extend our results to include 18 sessions.

Our findings of excessive gamma oscillations and ERP responses in visual tasks are in agreement with other studies noting that neural systems in the brains of autistic patients are often inappropriately activated (e.g., Belmonte & Yurgelin-Todd, 2003); this may be due to a disruption in the ratio between cortical excitation and inhibition (Casanova et al., 2002ab; Casanova, 2006ab; Rubenstein and Merzenich, 2003). In autism, increased cortical activity made evident by gamma and ERP responses indicate that activity induced by perceptual processes starts earlier and continues longer, because the neural networks subserving cognitive processes involved in combining information processing are not functioning normally. A reduction in the ability to decrease these cortical responses may reflect inhibitory deficits, and may result in the brain of autistic patients being over-activated. Abnormally large cortical responses to sensory stimuli (i.e. signal/sensory amplification) may play an important role in the manifestation of symptoms of ASD (e.g., sensory hypersensitivity, impaired social interaction). Enhanced and weakly differentiated responses to both target and non-target stimuli in sensory specific cortical areas (e.g., visual cortex at occipital EEG sites) and low functional connectivity supports the hypothesis of abnormal regional activation patterns (local over-processing vs. global under-processing).

Overall, our preliminary findings show promising results for TMS as a treatment modality targeting core symptoms of ASD. Treatment with "slow" rTMS decreased excess gamma activity and amplified ERP responses in ASD patients during visual tasks and improved the signal differentiation between processing relevant and irrelevant stimuli (Baruth et al., 2010a; Sokhadze et al., 2009b; Sokhadze et al., 2010; Casanova et al., 2012; Sokhadze et al., 2013); there was also a significant reduction in the percentage of errors in motor responses to target stimuli (Sokhadze, et al. 2010; Casanova et al., 2012; Sokhadze et al., 2013), and rTMS was associated with a significant improvement in indices of error detection and correction (Sokhadze et al., 2012; Sokhadze et al., 2013). Additionally "slow" rTMS dramatically improved the coordinated activity or coherence between different regions of the brain and significantly improved repetitive and restricted behavior patterns associated with ASD (Baruth et al., 2010a; Sokhadze et al., 2009b; Sokhadze, et al., 2010a; Casanova et al., 2012; Sokhadze et al., 2013). Our results suggest that low-frequency rTMS has the potential to become an important therapeutic tool in ASD treatment and may play an important role in improving the quality of life of many with the disorder.

THE ROLE OF THE MICROBIOME/BIOME AND CYSTEINE DEFICIENCY IN AUTISM SPECTRUM DISORDER

By Dr. James Jeffrey Bradstreet

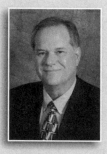

James Jeffrey Bradstreet, MD, MD(H), FAAFP

104 Colony Park Drive, Suite 600
Cumming, GA 30040-2793
470-253-7445
DrBradstreet@aol.com

Dr. James Jeffrey Bradstreet, received his medical degree from the University of South Florida in Tampa and his residency training at Wilford Hall USAF Medical Center in Texas. He is widely published on the various aspects of autism-related biology and comorbidities and is a member of the American Academy of Toxicology as well as a Fellow of the American Academy of Family Physicians. Dr. Bradstreet is an adjunct professor of pediatrics at Southwest College of Naturopathic Medicine in Tempe, Arizona, and is licensed in Georgia, Florida, California, and Arizona. Both his son and stepson have autism spectrum disorders and have experienced significant recovery as a result of intensive biomedical interventions. Dr. Bradstreet's interests include the interactions between the immune system and the brain, stem cell therapies, and the relationship of vitamin D to macrophage activation and viral pathogens. Using new techniques, he has been able to see significant progress for some of the most challenging cases. Please visit www.drbradstreet.org.

A utism spectrum disorders (ASD) are complex developmental abnormalities defined on the basis of the severity of symptoms in three domains: language, socialization and stereotypical behaviors. Although it is recognized that various chromosomal, mitochondrial and metabolic disorders can present with autistic features, the biological aspects of this disorder are not generally considered in the evaluation and diagnosis of the condition. Over the last 3 decades we have seen accumulating evidence of immune dysregulation in ASD. Although the nature of the immune aberrations is somewhat elusive and inconsistent, the general pattern indicates an imbalance resulting in proinflammatory and autoimmune conditions. This was recently reviewed by Careaga, et al.[1] as well as Gupta, et al.[2] These effects are present in the gut and the brain of a significant subset of ASD affected individuals.[3] As early as 1982, Weizman, et al., found abnormal cell-mediated immune responses to brain proteins in 13 of 17 ASD children tested.[4] Chez and colleagues noted extremely high cerebral spinal fluid to plasma ratios of TNF-alpha (a powerful inflammatory mediator), even in immunologically treated cases of ASD.[5] Researchers at Johns Hopkins also found persistent neuroinflammatory changes at the time of autopsy even into the 4th decade of life.[6] The implication of these inflammatory changes persisting despite either steroids or intravenous immunoglobulin therapies cannot be understated. Some force is driving the ongoing central inflammatory response in ASD. It is tempting to speculate that a persistent neurotropic pathogen (e.g., virus, atypical bacteria, etc.) is present in the central nervous system (CNS), but after several decades none has been identified with any consistency. However, in 2004, working with molecular virologists at Coombs Women's Hospital in Dublin, Ireland, Bradstreet, et al., reported the first three cases of measles virus F gene in the spinal fluid of ASD children with concurrent gastrointestinal inflammation.[7] That same year they reported MV F-gene was present in the cerebral spinal fluid (CSF) from 19 of 28 (68%) cases and in only one of 37 (3%) controls (RR = 25.12; 3.57-176.48, p<0.00001).[8] The three original cases are part of this cohort as well, so to date only 19 cases have been positively identified and reported. Even with the detection of the MV gene in the CSF, the actual cause and effect relationship between viral genome and autistic symptoms is hotly debated.[9]

In the absence of consensus on a central nervous system pathogen, others have focused on the role of the gut's complex ecosystem, the intestinal microbiome, as a potential source for immune activation and toxins capable of influencing the brain's development. This is an appealing theory that fits at least some of the clinical and laboratory observations. In 2000, Sandler et al., observed that 8 of 10 (80%) of children with ASD, regardless of intestinal symptoms, significantly improved after treatment with vancomycin.[10] The speculation was that this was related to *Clostridia* colonization, overgrowth or infection in the intestinal tract of these children. However, in this study, the researchers did not attempt to identify specific organisms that may be responding to the vancomycin. Dr. Sydney Finegold (who was a part of the vancomycin study) and colleagues recently applied pyrosequencing DNA detection techniques to evaluate the bacteria present in the feces of children with ASD.[11] This is a highly specific and sensitive method, and the results support the potential explanations why vancomycin could have been effective. At the same time, this study points us away from clostridial species to other anaerobic bacteria. One of the predominate organisms vastly overrepresented in the ASD group (as well as in their siblings) is the *Desulfovibrio* species. This becomes intriguing because of its potential relationship to the observations of cysteine deficiency in ASD. *Desulfovibrio* will compete with the host organism (a child with autism) for cysteine. So this provides at least one potential mechanism for the observed deficiency of cysteine in ASD.[12]

While it is easy to see how brain inflammation could lead to autistic features, it is more challenging to comprehend the microbiome-gut-brain connection in both creating and maintaining this ongoing CNS inflammatory response.

In the late 1990s, I had observed cysteine deficiency on amino acid testing of children with ASD. The availability of cysteine is considered to be the rate limiting step in the body's ability to manufacture intracellular glutathione. It would be hard to overemphasize the role of glutathione to human health. It is the main intracellular antioxidant and has been known for decades to protect neurons from oxidative stress.[13] In addition to more recent observations in autism, glutathione deficiency has long been known to be associated with a variety of disorders, including Parkinsonism,[14] schizophrenia,[15] ADHD,[16] HIV,[17] inflammatory bowel disease[18] and premature aging.[19] While working on research with Professor S. Jill James from the University of Arkansas for Medical Sciences, I observed dramatically lower cysteine and glutathione, as well as corresponding increases in oxidative markers in the ASD population.[20] With that study, we also found increased frequencies of genetic vulnerabilities to oxidation and glutathione metabolism.

Let's examine another critical part of this intestinal-immune puzzle. This part also relates to the vital role of cysteine. Defensins are produced by Paneth cells and are an inducible, yet nonspecific, antimicrobial defense mechanism, regulating the gut microbiome.[21] Thus defensins might be considered the extracellular counterpart of glutathione. They, too, are cysteine-dependent peptides critical to host immune function and protection.[22] It's likely, although at this time still speculative, that the type and magnitude of cysteine deficiency observed in ASD creates a relative defensin deficiency just as it creates a glutathione deficiency. This would be especially relevant to the local intestinal mucosal environment where *Desulfovibrio*, as a dominate organism, would be most locally competing for cysteine resources. In ulcerative colitis we see sulfur-reducing bacteria implicated in causation.[23]

So far we have the following overlapping observations: CNS inflammation, an abnormally skewed microbiome capable of competing with the body for valuable cysteine resources, low cysteine in the blood of ASD children, evidence of oxidative stress, potential responses to antibiotics capable of reducing anaerobic bacteria like *Desulfovibrio*, and suspected defensin deficiency. But is this enough to explain the catastrophic developmental changes we label "autism"?

Over the past several decades, both children and their mothers have been exposed to increasingly powerful broad-spectrum antibiotics. This is an unprecedented factor in human development since there is growing acceptance that humans coevolved with their microbiome.[24] Undoubtedly, this has radically altered the gut microbiome in a way that predisposes to inflammatory bowel disease.[25] At the same time, cultural changes as humans left the farm and gathered in cities have resulted in what is now referred to by Dr. William Parker of Duke University as "biome depletion."[26] Simply stated, biome depletion recognizes the regulatory roll of helminthic species (worms). Rather than being the yucky and the presumed evil bloodsuckers envisioned by most of us, there is abundant evidence that certain helminths are mutualistic symbionts. In an excellent review on this subject, McKay states the following:

> There is unequivocal evidence that parasites influence the immune activity of their hosts, and many of the classical examples of this are drawn from assessment of helminth infections of their mammalian hosts. Thus, helminth infections can impact on the induction or course of other diseases that the host might be subjected to. Epidemiological studies demonstrate that world regions with high rates of helminth infections consistently have reduced incidences of autoimmune and other allergic/inflammatory-type conditions.[27]

Elliott and colleagues at the University of Iowa had this to say about our dependent relationship with worms:

> Immune-mediated diseases (e.g., inflammatory bowel disease, asthma, multiple sclerosis, and autoimmune diabetes) are increasing in prevalence and emerge as populations adopt meticulously hygienic lifestyles. This change in lifestyles precludes exposure to helminths (parasitic worms). Loss of natural helminth exposure removes a previously universal Th2 and regulatory immune biasing imparted by these organisms. Helminths protect animals from developing immune-mediated diseases (colitis, reactive airway disease, encephalitis, and diabetes). Clinical trials show that exposure to helminths can reduce disease activity in patients with ulcerative colitis or Crohn's disease.[28]

Mount Sinai School of Medicine has an ongoing trial of helminthic therapy for autism. No results are available at this time. The study is investigating *Tricuris suis* ova (TSO: pig whipworm eggs). As with any monotherapy for a complex disorder like autism, it is doubtful it will produce dramatic results in language and stereotypical symptoms over a short course. TSO does show impressive results in refractory inflammatory bowel disease,[29] but there we are not dealing with complex CNS/developmental abnormalities. When applied to existing respiratory allergies, TSO had no measurable benefit on nasal allergy symptoms in a recent controlled study.[30] It has been observed that there is a mutually exclusive relationship between *Schistosoma* infection and multiple sclerosis, implying a protective effective of helminthic colonization.[31] And while helminths have been shown to have a protective effect by preventing the induction of experimental encephalomyelitis,[32] it is unknown if it can reverse the course of established brain inflammation as observed in ASD.

It is reasonable—even likely—that the regulatory role of both the biome and the microbiome needs to be first established in the maternal environment prior to pregnancy.[33,34] These data point to very early immune programming of the brain's future developmental response. They also establish a link between maternal immune dysregulation and ASD. It may also be that the same microbiome/biome effects that disrupt the maternal immune system are passed along environmentally to her offspring. As will be described in detail later, the ecosystem of the gut is set very early in life.

This brings up the issue of artificially changing the intestinal ecosystem. The logic seems to follow that if the nature of the gut flora is the problem, why not just change them with different—presumably healthier—bacteria (probiotics)? This was discussed briefly by Garvey,[35] but no systematic investigation has been published. Despite this, numerous clinicians and parents undertake the use of bacteria supplementation.[36] My experience provides a mixture of results from the use of probiotic supplements. Some children are immediately benefitted by probiotics: demonstrating improved bowel function, decreased hyperactivity, increased eye contact, and better attention. The dose and type of probiotic tolerated seems highly variable. Some children do well, but only with small doses (in bacterial terms this is 1-10 billion bacteria per day). Other children are helped, but only by massive doses (upwards of 450 billion per day). There is support in the pediatric literature for high-dose *Lactobacillus* in ulcerative colitis (UC).[37,38] VSL-3® has been tested in adults with proven efficacy for UC in this older population as well.[39] However, evidence is lacking for VSL-3® efficacy in Crohn's disease, which is a different type of inflammatory bowel disease.[40]

The nature of the inflammatory bowel disease in autism is immunologically distinct from both UC and Crohn's disease.[41] So, this creates the need for specifically testing the ASD population for the efficacy of any proposed probiotic. At this point, any large scale scientifically rigorous study of probiotics in ASD is unlikely to be financially feasible. Despite this obstacle, clinicians can reasonably try probiotics in population on an N of 1 study model. In essence, each child's baseline serves as his or her own control point for observations. The probiotic can be started initially at low doses and subsequently increased to tolerance. It is especially helpful to use biomarkers of gut inflammation wherever possible. For a review of these biomarkers and the clinical application of them to autism interventions, please see Bradstreet, et al.[42]

Recently, another form of microbiome modification has been proposed for autism: fecal transfer or transplantation (Finegold, et al. ibid 11). This presents some daunting challenges. There is growing evidence the immune system programs itself to accept a specific microbiome very early in life.[43] Within days of birth, the gut of all infants is colonized by the child's mother and specific environment and diet. Various factors, including the route of delivery, formula versus breast and in various combinations, influence the composition of the child's gut microbiome.[44] Once established, the microbiome drives nutrient digestion and absorption, further determining the composition of the intestinal ecosystem.[45]

There is evidence this ecosystem becomes stable by 1 year of life, and even after antibiotics it tends to return to the immunologically programmed microbiome within a few months.[46]

When and how this microbiome became disrupted in autism is poorly understood. As mentioned earlier, vancomycin resulted in temporary improvement of autistic symptoms, but after a few months the children relapsed, implying a return to the old microbiome. In some cases, microbiome disruption caused by antibiotics is potentially life-threatening, as with *Clostridium difficile* colitis. Some cases are refractory to treatment with *C. difficile* specific antibiotics. In these cases the new harmful microbiome becomes established and the host lacks the ability to revert to the earlier ecosystem. Various factors contribute to this: 1) the chronic form of colitis is debilitating and creates nutritional deficiencies; 2) the inflammatory response alters local bacterial regulatory factors; and 3) the *C. difficle* biochemically defend their ecological niche.

In these entrenched, chronic cases, doctors have resorted successfully to fecal bacteriotherapy (FB), also known as fecal transfer or transplantation.[47] This has been successful in pediatric cases as well.[48] Naturally, there is going to be significant consumer resistance to this therapy for many obvious reasons. I have had the pleasure of discussing the early use of fecal bacteriotherapy with Professor Emeritus Tore Midtvedt, MD, PhD, from Karolinska University in Sweden. In the early 1950s, he was asked to help a Norwegian community plagued with chronic infectious diarrhea that had resisted all efforts of the local physicians to eradicate the infections. With a great deal of effort, they identified an ideal donor and were able to instill the feces into the infected individuals using enemas. This early experience was complicated by the challenges of finding a suitable donor. The difficulty of donor screening and identification has escalated in an age of antibiotics and occult viruses like HIV and the newly discovered retrovirus, XMRV (xenotropic murine leukemia virus-related virus). Despite these challenges, FB research continues at several institutions.

Fecal bacteriotherapy can be accomplished in a variety of ways.[49] The simplest technique would be swallowing oral time-delayed capsules. This is envisioned but to my knowledge not available to consumers at this time. The high-end recent research has used colonoscopies to deliver the fecal transplant to the cecum (first portion of the large bowel). Both nasogastric tubes and retention enemas have also been used to deliver the new microbiome. Most of the protocols involve pretreating the gut with some antibiotic (like vancomycin) or antibiotic combinations. Since there have been few clinical trials published, the best methods are not yet established, and no one has yet to publish the application of this therapy to treat the microbiome of ASD. Given the link between bowel flora and at least some of the behaviors observed in autism as well as its potential benefit on the immune dysregulation observed in ASD I suspect we will see more discussions and potential clinical trials with FB and ASD.

Now we face the challenge of linking these observations into a logical disease model to guide both our diagnostic evaluations and therapeutic efforts. The data points out the following potential problems leading to and then likely maintaining the autistic state.

1. Disruption of the maternal ecosystem.
2. Altered microbiome with flora which tend to disrupt her immune balance and that of her offspring, including antibodies directed against the fetal brain.
3. Further complicated by biome (helminthic) depletion such that the pregnant woman is unable to counter the autoimmune/proinflammatory influences of her microbiome.
4. The early-life establishment of an undesirable microbiome for her offspring.
5. Cysteine depletion created at least in part by sulfur-reducing intestinal bacteria overgrowth.
6. Cysteine-dependent defensin deficiency that alters the microbiome and permits greater numbers of potentially pathogenic organisms (presumed).
7. Glutathione deficiency and increased intracellular oxidative stress in all organs. The brain is especially sensitive to glutathione deficiency.
8. This combination of antecedents opens the door to brain inflammation and altered development (perhaps as early as intrauterine development).

Intervening in this process must start early in life—ideally prior to conception—with properly conditioning the maternal biome/microbiome. That will be no small challenge in its own right—given the resistance to change noted in the gut ecosystem. For existing cases of autism, early and appropriate restoration of the gut flora could offer significant benefits. In clinical observations, we have seen efforts to benefit the microbiome proving successful—if only temporarily so. Improved diagnostic methods of detecting microbiome disruption (e.g., pyrosequencing) may become clinically available soon and assist the clinician in therapeutic interventions. Multiple means are available in our efforts to alter the intestinal ecosystem. Although not previously discussed, dietary changes may offer significant advantages during the attempts to alter the gut environment. Anecdotal observations support interventions ranging from gluten and casein elimination to even more restrictive and challenging diets, such as the Specific Carbohydrate Diet™. All of these dietary changes would be expected to modify the immune and microbiome responses of the child. Novel microbiome therapies like fecal bacteriotherapy loom in the future even as biome therapy with TSO is being investigated. Probiotics are readily available, but dosing and strain selection is still incompletely understood. Methods to address brain inflammation are being discussed, and some have proposed nature provided anti-inflammatories to address this need.[50]

In conclusion, the complex interactions of maternal and child immune and intestinal environments seem to play a major role in the development of ASD and, therefore, are important targets for therapeutic interventions.

EFFECTS OF AMBIENT PRISM LENSES AND VISUAL-MOTOR TRAINING ON HEART RATE VARIABILITY AND BEHAVIORAL OUTCOMES IN AUTISM

By Dr. Brynn Dombroski, Dr. Melvin Kaplan,
Dr. Barbara Kotsamanidis-Burg, Dr. Stephen M. Edelson,
Marie K. Hensley, Dr. Estate M. Sokhadze, and
Dr. Manuel F. Casanova

Department of Psychiatry & Behavioral Sciences, University of Louisville, Louisville, KY,
Center for Visual Management, Terrytown, NY, and Autism Research Institute,
San Diego, CA.

Brynn Dombroski, PhD

Brynn Dombroski, PhD, is the center director of Learning Rx. She is a graduate of the Department of Anatomical Sciences & Neurobiology at the University of Louisville School of Medicine. She did her dissertation under Dr. Casanova's mentorship. Dr. Dombroski participated at the each stage of the study when she was a graduate student and PhD candidate at the University of Louisville. She is a specialist in behavioral treatment methods in autism, ADHD, and other developmental disorders.

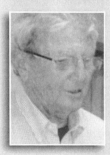

Melvin Kaplan, OD

Melvin Kaplan, OD, is Director of the Center for Visual Management in Terrytown, New York. He is a qualified Doctor of Optometry, and has previously worked as a clinical instructor of behavioral sciences at New York Medical College. He has published a significant body of research on ambient lenses and their role in the rehabilitation of individuals who display dysfunction in learning or emotion, and those with autistic spectrum disorders.

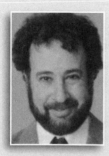

Stephen M. Edelson, PhD

Stephen M. Edelson, PhD, is the director of the Autism Research Institute and has been active in the field of autism for over 30 years. Dr. Edelson has conducted research in a variety of areas comprising behavior, sensory issues, and cognition; he has published peer-reviewed research articles with many notables in the autism field, including Drs. Bernard Rimland, Ivar Lovaas, Temple Grandin, and Margaret Bauman. Dr. Edelson is the consulting editor for the research journal *Focus on Autism and Other Developmental Disabilities.* He is a participant on the Panel of Professional Advisors for the Autism Society of America (ASA). He is a former ASA Board member and a past president of the Autism Society of Oregon.

Marie K. Hensley

Marie is a graduate student of Bioengineering pursuing Master's degree in Bioengineering at the Speed School of Engineering at the University of Louisville. She was actively involved in HRV and other data processing and analysis.

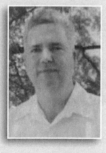

Manuel F. Casanova, MD

Manuel F. Casanova, MD, is a professor in the Department of Psychiatry and Behavioral Sciences and Kolb Endowed Chair in Psychiatry. Dr. Casanova has had over twenty years of experience in the neurosciences and is well published in a multitude of postmortem techniques including neuronal morphometry, neurochemistry, and autoradiography. Although trained in the classical methods of neurology and neuropathology, his interest has gradually shifted towards the study of abnormalities of cortical circuitry. His most recent studies have investigated the presence of abnormalities of minicolumnar organization and lateralization in the brains of patients who exhibit language disturbances, including autism, Asperger's syndrome, and dyslexia. He is internationally known for his work in autism.

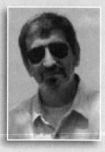

Tato Sokhadze, PhD

Estate (Tato) Sokhadze, PhD, is Associate Professor at the Department of Psychiatry & Behavioral Sciences at the University of Louisville. This study was conducted at the laboratory that he is directing. His research is focused on alternative and complementary methods of treatment of neurodevelopmental disorders (rTMS, neurofeedback, etc.).

Introduction

We rely on our sense of vision to gather information about our surroundings, read directions, recognize familiar faces, and numerous other activities. Vision can be classified into two main types. The first, focal, is conscious and allows us to see objects in high-resolution color. At the doctor's office it is focal vision that is tested and given a score, sometimes resulting in the prescription of corrective lenses for near- or farsightedness. The other type of vision is known as ambient vision, which is largely non-conscious and is used in spatial orientation and depth perception. Unlike focal vision, which is restricted to two degrees of visual field, ambient vision involves the entire visual field and integrates with other sensory systems to determine one's position in space. Deficits in this ambient vision system could clearly cause confusion, disorientation, and stress. In fact, such deficits have been linked to autism spectrum disorder (ASD), attention deficit hyperactivity disorder (ADHD), and other developmental disorders by previous studies.

Autism spectrum disorder is a pervasive developmental disorder of childhood characterized by deficits in social interaction, language, and stereotyped behaviors along with a restricted range of interest. It is further marked by an innate inability to perceive and respond to social and emotional signals in a typical manner. This is due to the functional disconnectedness of networks important for specific aspects of social cognition and behavioral control. The underlying neural deficits are related to developmental abnormalities of functional disconnectivity of the associative frontal cortical areas with posterior neocortical areas which leads to abnormal global processing in autism and contributes to an inability to integrate incoming individual parts and perceive them as a whole. According to several recent theories, sensory processing abnormalities may play an important role in impairments of perception, cognition, and behavior in individuals with autism. Among these sensory abnormalities visual distortion may contribute to such typical symptoms of autism as relying on peripheral vision, strabismus, and manifestation of stereotypic behaviors.

Also frequently observed in ASD is an imbalance between the two branches of the autonomic nervous system (ANS), specifically, increased sympathetic tone and decreased parasympathetic tone. Several types of autonomic dysfunctions have been reported in autism, including increased basal sympathetic tone, as well as reduced baseline parasympathetic activity in association with increased baseline sympathetic tone (Ming et al., 2011; Porges, 2001). The sympathetic nervous system is activated during times of stress, increasing heart rate and blood pressure while slowing digestion. Activation of the parasympathetic nervous system has the opposite effect, decreasing heart rate and blood pressure and allowing for normal digestion. Thus, deviations from typical ANS function, as seen in ASD, can result in gastrointestinal or cardiovascular symptoms. As Heart Rate (HR) is determined by sympathetic and parasympathetic signals, we chose to use Heart Rate Variability (HRV) as a useful indicator of autonomic balance. Heart rate variability (HRV) measures are widely used in psychopathology research for assessment of phasic and tonic cardiac autonomic control. Reduced HRV, specifically the attenuated power of high frequency (HF) component of the HRV (often referred to as Respiratory Sinus Arrhythmia) along with high power of low frequency (LF) component of HRV is an indicator of limited psychophysiological flexibility. Several studies have shown that typical children suppressed the HF in HRV more than autistic children, and autistic children have unusually small deceleratory HR phasic responses to stimuli. Therefore, analysis of the HRV, the HF and phasic HR responses associated with dynamic parasympathetic activity, may provide very important information regarding the autonomic dysfunctions in autism. Studies have demonstrated several manifestations of abnormal sympathetic functions in measures other than HRV. For example, Skin Conductance Response (SCR) studies in autistic children have shown a lack of the normal SCR habituation to the same stimulus over time (Toichi & Kamio, 2003). It is often reported that the autistic group had a higher baseline Skin Conductance Level (SCL). It has been reported that children with autism had blunted autonomic responses to social stimuli. Furthermore, our own pilot studies also support excessive but less differentiated SCR to affective sounds, visual, and audio-visual stimuli. Since SCL is controlled solely by the sympathetic inputs (Boucsein, 2012), above effects indicate high sympathetic tone and low selectivity in autism.

Therefore, the main objective of the study described in the following chapter was to evaluate the effects of improving ambient vision, through the use of prism lenses, on HRV and overall autonomic function in children with autism. To test the effectiveness of prism lenses in improving autonomic balance, a protocol was set in place which involved visual-motor exercises while wearing prism lenses. Then during each visit to the office, the patient's HR was recorded while he or she watched selected emotional scenes from the Disney movie, "The Lion King." Participants were evaluated at baseline, and post-6 months long visuo-motor training and wearing ambient lenses using following questionnaires: Aberrant Behavior Checklist (ABC), Achenbach's Child Behavioral Checklist (ASEBA), and Repetitive Behavior Scale – R (RBS-R).

Methods

Participants

Fourteen out of 24 children enrolled in the study completed whole course of ambient lenses treatment and visuo-motor training, along with baseline and post-treatment assessments. Mean age of participants was 13.1 years (SD = 3.37 yrs), range varied within 8-19 years, and 4 of them were girls. All participants had autism spectrum disorder

(ASD) diagnosis made according to the DSM-IV-TR (APA, 2000) and further ascertained with the Autism Diagnostic Interview—Revised (ADI-R) (Le Couteur, Lord, & Rutter, 2003). They also had a medical evaluation by a developmental pediatrician. All subjects have normal hearing based on past hearing screens. All autistic participants were high-functioning persons with ASD with full scale IQ > 80 assessed using the Wechsler Intelligence Scale for Children (WISC-IV; Wechsler, 2004). Four out of 14 participants had diagnosis of Asperger's Disorder. Study participants were recruited c/o advertisement posted at local autism advocacy organizations (e.g., Louisville Chapter of FEAT) and some were recruited from existing pool of children with ASD seeking treatment.

Determining each subject's prism lenses prescription

Dr. Kaplan from the Center for Visual Management (Terrytown, NY) visited University of Louisville twice and on-site observed each patient's head tilt, body posture, facial expressions, and breathing during visual pursuits, ball catching, and watching TV to determine which base direction of ambient lenses should be prescribed for each patient (Figure 1ab). Prism lenses were manufactured at the optic center in the state of New York following Dr. Kaplan's prescription to each participant.

Daily vision exercises

At the beginning of each month, each study participant along with prescribed lenses received a packet of visuo-motor exercises program that were to be done for Week 1, Week 2, Week 3, and Week 4. Each week's exercises were designed to build neurosensory and neuromuscular skills from one week to the next. A description of the materials, lenses, setup, procedure, observations and time expected to be spent on each exercise were all included in the instructions. Additionally, graduate research students filmed a demonstration of each procedure in the lab and transferred the video demonstrations onto DVDs that were disseminated to each study participant. The prescription prism lenses, the dysruptive lenses and the red/green lenses were all provided by the Center for Visual Management. The materials needed involved a combination of household items and a few items that were relatively inexpensive to buy or build on your own, such as a balance board and a chalk board. At the end of each month, patients came into the lab at the University of Louisville for a post-assessment evaluation and video recording of selected procedures chosen by the Center for Visual Management. The graduate researcher instructed the patient on which exercises to demonstrate in the lab and evaluated the patient's performance as either "efficient," "satisfactory," or "needs improvement," and wrote additional notes in regards to the patient's posture, breathing, or other involuntary movements to be

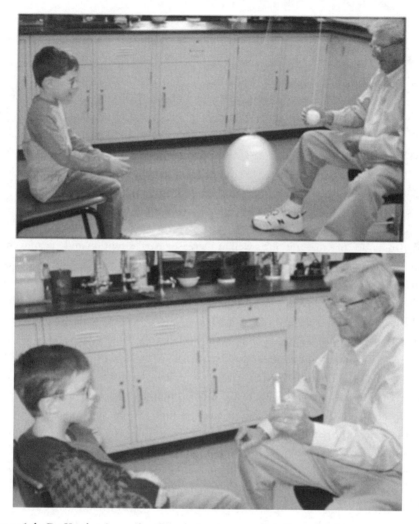

Figure 1ab. Dr Kaplan is conducting evaluations to prescribe prism lenses.

reviewed by the Center for Visual Management. The video recordings were mailed to the Center for Visual Management for oversight in determining each patient's progress throughout the study.

<u>Month 1:</u> The purpose behind the exercises assigned for month 1 was to disrupt and reintegrate the visual system. Observational changes could be seen in the patient's stress level, ease or difficulty in reorganizing visual perception and balance to the each base direction, level of comfort or discomfort in completing the exercise, sustained visual attention, awareness of double vision, visual tracking, hand-eye coordination, smooth or uncoordinated movements, visual convergence, proper posture, as well as improved

perception of distance and speed. In addition to wearing prescription prism lenses, disruptive lenses and/or red/green lenses as described, some of the equipment used in these exercises included a balance board, a trampoline and a yoga mat.

Month 2: The visuo-motor exercises assigned for the second month utilized a visual-vestibular technique to enhance body schema and self-awareness, develop visual-vestibular integration, coordinate balance and visual attention to self, and engage binocular fusion. Additionally, patients practiced sustaining visual feedback to a focal target, while increasing ambient awareness and reorganizing current visual perceptual patterns and visual fields which may have been previously compressed prior to wearing prism lenses and visuo-motor therapy. Additional equipment used in some of these exercises included a full length mirror, a "Star" chart, and a chalkboard.

Month 3: The purpose of this month's exercises was to engage bilateral movements and visual-auditory integration as well as increase visual attention and eye movement skills including tracking and coordination. Other objectives included the introduction of fixation jumps to expand the visual eye field while incorporating proprioception of body movement and auditory input to reorganize the patient's current visual perceptual patterns as well as promote smooth tracking and breathing skills. New equipment introduced during this month's exercises included a metronome, bongos, a checkerboard, a circle and square chart, and a Hart chart.

Month 4: During month 4 exercises, patients were asked to read before and after visuo-motor therapy and trainers were instructed to observe differences in speed, reading fluency and comprehension as well as changes in breathing and posture, including whether or not the patient appeared relaxed or tense. The primary goal of this month's exercises was to integrate two visual tracts, both focal and ambient vision while also creating depth perception, increasing smooth eye movements, and increasing visual attention and tracking ability. Additional equipment during this month's exercises included a pie tin, a slinky on a dowel, two matchbox cars or tennis balls, and bubble blowing solution with a wand.

Month 5: A constant theme throughout visuo-motor therapy is to increase visual attention, eye movements and tracking ability. For this month's exercises, several previously learned procedures were repeated, but now combined with other procedures to create depth perception, increase smooth eye movements, develop visual-vestibular integration and increase visual processing ability. Much of the same equipment was reused during this month's exercises; however, a walking rail was added to incorporate balance and depth perception with an exercise that was previous done standing or sitting in a stationary position.

Month 6: The final month's exercises for this study highlighted the fusion of vision and auditory integration with controlled breathing, increased proprioceptive input, visual attention, convergence skills and depth perception. This study concluded with the integration of visual-verbal sequences in which the patient was directed to name items such as animals or fruits in alphabetical order or simply count or recite the alphabet while bunting the ball. The ability to provide a correct verbal response while visually attending to and physically making contact with the ball is the direct result of cortical reorganization of the vision system. The patients in this study were successful in integrating their visual, auditory and proprioceptive systems through the daily use of prescription prism lenses in combination with visuo-motor exercises for a period of six months (Figure 2ab). A more detailed explanation of the types of vision lenses, visuomotor exercises and equipment used in this study can be found in Dr. Kaplan's previously published book, *Seeing Through New Eyes* (Kaplan, 2006).

Psychophysiological reactivity tests

Our interest was also in evaluating the effects of corrective ambient prism lenses on autonomic nervous system activity, as well as contributing to the understanding of abnormal autonomic reactivity mechanisms present in autism. The study used emotionally arousing video excerpts taken from the classic Disney film "Lion King." Each episode (high and low emotional context block) was 2 minutes long, while totally 4 episodes were used, thus making the period of watching video up to 10 minutes. The order of movie episodes were counterbalanced across all subjects. HR was monitored and collected during the session and later analyzed block by block. Physiological activity was recorded using C-2 J&J Engineering Inc. (Poulsbo, WA) real-time physiological monitor with USE-2 Physiodata software. Analysis of HRV was enhanced using Kubios HRV software (Helsinki, Finland). The test was conducted twice, at the baseline (before treatment) and after completion of prism lenses treatment course.

Measures of interest were overall HR, low frequency (LF) power, high frequency (HF) power, and the ratio of the two (LF/HF). Mean HR, the standard deviation of the HR (SDHR), power and percentage of high frequency (HF), low frequency (LF), very low frequency (VLF) HRV components, and the ratio of the LF over the HF (LF/HF ratio) of HRV were calculated using Kubios software (Finland). LF power is indicative of sympathetic nervous system activity, while HF power is indicative of parasympathetic nervous system activity, in particular *n. vagus* effects on cardiac chronotropic functions. Our hope was that wearing prism lenses and performing the visuo-motor exercises would enhance the patient's ambient vision, thus reducing the confusion and stress caused by deficits in this type of vision. Expected outcomes were a decrease in HR, increase in high frequency (HF) power and decrease in low frequency (LF) power, indicative of enhanced parasympathetic nervous system activity and/or decreased sympathetic activity, and a decreased LF/HF ratio, which is considered as an indirect cardiac autonomic balance index. Lower LF/HF ratio of HRV is considered as an indication of better cardiac autonomic balance and improved psychophysiological flexibility in autism.

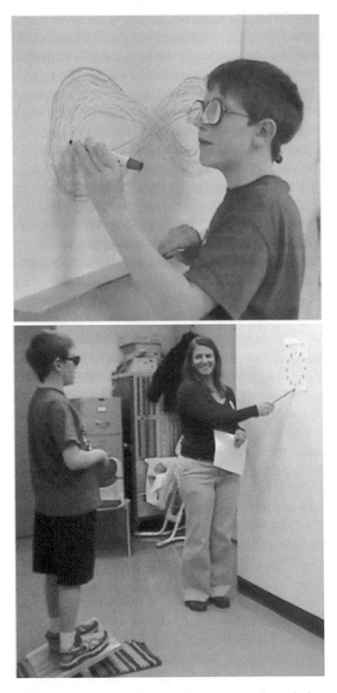

Figure 2ab. Child with autism is performing visuo-motor tasks with disruptive prism lenses during midterm assessment in the lab.

Results

Behavioral ratings results

Empirical behavioral data outcomes was reported using the Autism Behavior Checklist (ABC) and Repetitive Behavior Scale (RBS) (Figures 3-4). In the ABC, three out of five scaled scores were reduced. In particular, scores tended to be decreased in Lethargy (t = 2.09; df = 13, p = 0.058) and Inappropriate Speech (t = 2.06, df = 13, p = 0.06) while significantly decreased in Hyperactivity (t = 2.39; df = 13, p = 0.034) compared to baseline scores. According to the Repetitive Behavior Scale (RBS), three out of six subscale scores were significantly different. These subscale scores included: Stereotypic Behavior (t = 3.47; df = 11, p = 0.01), Compulsive Behavior (t = 3.49; dr = 11, p = 0.01) and overall Total Score (t = 2.70; df = 11, p = 0.031) compared to baseline scores. Achenbach's ASEBA (Figure 5) showed significant decrease on Rule-Breaking Behavior (mean = -1.54, t = 2.60, df = 11, p = 0.026) and ADHD symptom scores (mean = -3.34, t = 2.56, df = 11, p = 0.029).

Heart Rate Variability results

Post treatment it was observed a significant decrease in average heart rate among the participants from the baseline 94.6 ± 2.99 beats/min to post-sessions 89.6 ± 3.65 beats/min, with paired-sample t-test showing significant change (t = -2.52, df = 13, p = 0.025). There was a decrease in LF power from 60.2 ± 2.81 power units to 48.6 ± 3.57 units (t = -2.38, df = 13, p = 0.033) and an increase in the percentage of HF power from 24.8 ± 2.16 percent to 37.6 ± 4.61 percent (t = 2.42, df = 13, p = 0.03). VLF component of HRV (another measure of sympathetic activity) tended to decrease from 37.8 percent down to 29.7 percent but the change was not statistically significant (t = -1.69, df = 13, p = 0.11) (Figure 6). Lastly, the LF/HF power ratio decreased from 1.70 ± 0.22 to 1.06 ± 0.13 (t = -2.52, df = 13, p = 0.025).

The above results are very encouraging in that they support the hypotheses that ambient prism lenses in combination with therapy vision exercises had the desired effect on HRV variables reflecting improved autonomic balance in children with ASD. First, the decrease in average heart rate suggests the participants were in a more relaxed state with corrective prism lenses than without. Second, the decrease in LF power and the increase in HF power were changes in the desired direction toward improved autonomic balance. This is also seen in the decreased LF/HF power ratio. These results are in favor with increased parasympathetic and decreased sympathetic tone, a significant improvement from ANS activity in autism. Behavioral measures also reflect improvements in hyperactivity, ADHD symptoms and repetitive behaviors.

Changes of Repetitive Behavior Sub-Scales Scores Post-Prism Treatment
Compulsive Behavior Rating and Total Score of Repetitive Behavior Scale Decreased

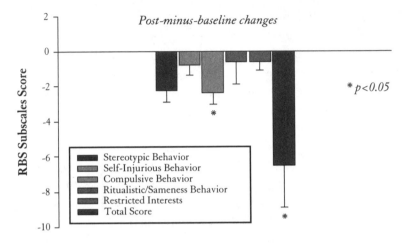

Figure 3. Outcomes of Repetitive Behavioral Scale questionnaires (RBS-R) showing decreased Compulsive Behaviors Score and Total Score post prism lenses treatment.

Aberrant Behavior Checklist Scores Changes Post Prism Lenses Treatment in 14 Children With Autism Spectrum Disorder
6 months long course of wearing ambient lenses and visuo-motor exercises

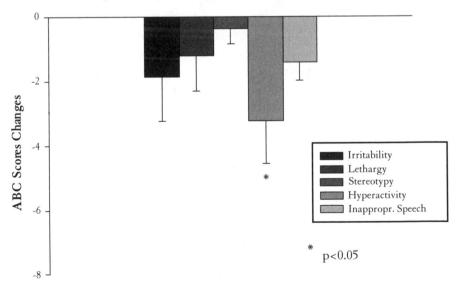

Figure 4. Outcomes of Aberrant Behavior Checklist questionnaires (ABC) showing decreased Hyperactivity score post prism lenses treatment.

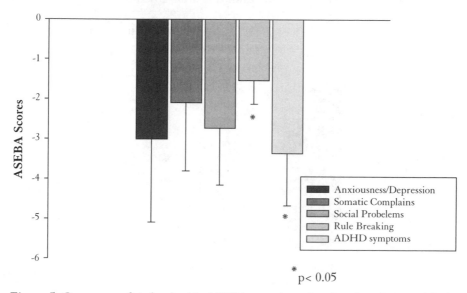

Achenbach's ASEBA Scores Changes Post-Prism Lenses
Treatment in 12 Children with Autism Spectrum Disorder

Figure 5. Outcomes of Achenbach's ASEBA questionnaire showing decreased Rule
Breaking and ADHD symptom scores post prism lenses treatment.

Summary

Children diagnosed with autism spectrum disorder (ASD) are characterized by impairments in communication, social interaction, and repetitive behavior. Ambient vision deficiency is a common comorbid condition in autism that negatively affects peripheral vision, attention, hand-eye coordination, balance, and gross motor movement. Ambient vision is necessary for control of anatomical movement involved in spatial orientation and proprioception. Dysfunction of this system impairs the ability to process environmental cues used to control gait, posture, movement, and speech. Loss of spatial orientation negatively affects the vestibular system, which leads to the development of adaptive responses that are consistent with the behavioral symptoms observed in autism. In this study, fourteen autistic children (mean age 13.1) were recruited, evaluated, and individually prescribed corrective ambient prism lenses. Next, a six-month daily vision therapy protocol was implemented in an attempt to ameliorate ambient vision deficiencies and abate autistic behaviors. Patients were instructed to wear the corrective ambient lenses all day, except when vision therapy procedures instructed otherwise. Daily vision therapy procedures included exercises that required the patients to wear disruptive prism lenses and occasionally red/green lenses. The combination of the lenses and tasks were used to address problems involved in balance, visual organization, and

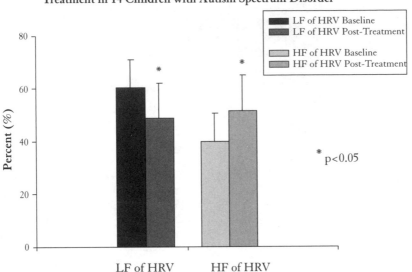

Figure 6. Low frequency (LF) and High frequency (HF) components of HRV showed post prism lenses and visuo-motor training exercises changes indicative of decreased sympathetic and increased parasympathetic cardiac activity. Proportion of the LF component of HRV decreased, while proportion of HF of HRV increased indicating improved cardiac autonomic balance during exposure to emotional video clips from "Lion King" movie.

depth perception. Empirical behavioral data was reported using the Autism Behavior Checklist (ABC), Repetitive Behavior Scale (RBS), and Achenbach (ASEBA) question-naires. Autonomic reactivity recordings at the baseline and post-treatment included Heart Rate (HR) and Heart Rate Variability (HRV), which were taken while the subject was watching scenes from the classic Disney film, "The Lion King," to evoke emotional responses. Results of this study showed that corrective ambient prism lenses combined with daily vision therapy both reduced autistic behaviors (according to ABC, ASEBA, and RBS rating scores) and enhanced autonomic cardiac balance during exposure to emotional stimuli in autism. Prism lenses address an important issue of ambient vision in ASD and possibly other developmental disorders as well. Our study with prism lenses and HR suggests improved ambient vision has a positive impact on autonomic function and behavior rating in children with autism, with the potential to ameliorate autistic behaviors and improve communication. We look forward to the future of prism lenses and their use in treating developmental disorders such as autism.

STEM CELLS AND AUTISM

By Dr. James Jeffrey Bradstreet

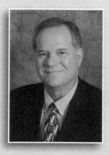

James Jeffrey Bradstreet, MD, MD(H), FAAFP

104 Colony Park Drive, Suite 600
Cumming, GA 30040-2793
470-253-7445
DrBradstreet@aol.com

Dr. James Jeffrey Bradstreet received his medical degree from the University of South Florida in Tampa and his residency training at Wilford Hall USAF Medical Center in Texas. He is widely published on the various aspects of autism-related biology and comorbidities and is a member of the American Academy of Toxicology as well as a Fellow of the American Academy of Family Physicians. Dr. Bradstreet is an adjunct professor of pediatrics at Southwest College of Naturopathic Medicine in Tempe, Arizona, and is licensed in Georgia, Florida, California, and Arizona. Both his son and stepson have autism spectrum disorders and have experienced significant recovery as a result of intensive biomedical interventions. Dr. Bradstreet's interests include the interactions between the immune system and the brain, stem cell therapies, and the relationship of vitamin D to macrophage activation and viral pathogens. Using new techniques, he has been able to see significant progress for some of the most challenging cases. Please visit www.drbradstreet.org.

Stem cells remain an unproven but enticing therapeutic option for autism spectrum disorders (ASDs) and other conditions. Regardless of your view of the science or lack thereof, stem cell therapies are being widely practiced around the world. I began writing this chapter about stem cells and autism for *Autism Science Digest* one year ago.[1] With what I have since learned, looking back at what I wrote then reinforces that my thinking about stem cell therapies was reasonable. In addition, the past year's first-hand journey with these therapies has brought forth some important new observations. Stem cells were a therapeutic option I felt was worth trying for my own sports-related injuries and for my stepson's autism. Although my choices don't validate stem cell therapies, receiving them personally has given me a real-world perspective.

The most significant change in my thinking related to stem cell therapy has to do with specific cell choices. Although this is a complex, controversial, and challenging topic, a discussion about cell choices is important for evaluating what is currently happening in many places outside the US. We also need to consider how effective this therapy might be for autism. I will be frank in this discussion, but at the same time, I hope I don't come across as insensitive to anyone's beliefs or ethics. I have great respect for human life and have dedicated my career to helping people enjoy a high quality of life. After years of studying stem cells, I believe they hold great promise as healers of what would otherwise be considered untreatable disorders.

Types of Stem Cells

Let's rewind our discussion back to the point where we learn about what a stem cell is, and then, let's explore what types of stem cells are being researched and used. First, stem cells must possess *both* the capacity to reproduce themselves and the potential to change into specialized cells. As an example, a neuronal stem cell must be able to make other stem cells and then ultimately turn into a neuron (brain cell) itself.[2]

There are five types of stem cells: embryonic stem cells, fetal stem cells, adult stem cells, induced pluripotent stem cells, and designer stem cells, each of which is defined in the paragraphs that follow.

Embryonic stem cells (ESCs): ESCs are derived from the very early stage of the growing embryo (around 50-150 cell stage) (see Figure 1). These cells are pluripotent (the most potent apart from a fertilized egg); however, of all the stem cell types, these are the most difficult to regulate and control. They show particular promise in spinal cord injury and retinal degeneration.

ESCs are the byproduct of infertility treatments and result when a greater number of fertilized eggs (turned embryos) are created than can be used by the mother. If the unused embryos are donated for medical use or research, they can be used in special studies. Because each of these cells is capable of producing a human being, they are ethically complex and controversial. Their use, therefore, is highly regulated. Few countries allow therapies with ESCs apart from legally regulated medical research, and many countries won't permit research on ESCs in any form. There are a few ongoing US studies using ESCs in spinal cord injuries and other serious disorders, but because there isn't a large supply of these earliest human stem cells at this time, they are not in significant

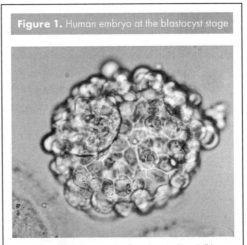

Figure 1. Human embryo at the blastocyst stage

Source: http://archive.eurostemcell.org/images/StemCell/
Human-blastocyst.gif

use in medical therapies anywhere in the world. For the purposes of this article, we can leave ESCs out of our remaining discussion since they are not, to my knowledge, being used by any clinic in any country to treat autism.

Fetal stem cells (FSCs): As the blastocyst grows in the womb, it creates three distinct germinal layers, which will ultimately become different structures in the fetus. FSCs can be derived from any of these three germ layers (ectoderm, mesoderm, or endoderm). Because FSCs are already committed to one of the three semi-specialized cell lines, they have less potential than the pluripotent (undifferentiated) ESCs. FSCs are, however, more potent than adult stem cells.

Adult stem cells (ASCs):[3] ASCs, by definition, must express several particular surface antigens and (absent lab manipulation) are less potent than other stem cells. There are many types of ASCs, but in practice we are limited at this time to mesenchymal stem cells (MSCs) from adipose tissue, bone marrow, or the umbilical cord (Wharton's jelly-derived MSCs, also known as WJMSCs). Umbilical cord blood has hematopoietic-related (blood-related) stem cells, but these do not have neuroprogenitor or MSC potential without laboratory manipulation.

Induced pluripotent stem cells (iPSCs): Somewhere between the native MSCs and the next type of stem cell (designer stem cells) lies the laboratory induction of specific stem cell types but without genetic (designer) manipulations. These cells come from adult cells, but they are induced with chemical signals to convert to specific cell types such as neuronal cells. These adult MSCs also can be converted into pluripotent cells just as though they were embryonic stem cells (see Figure 2).

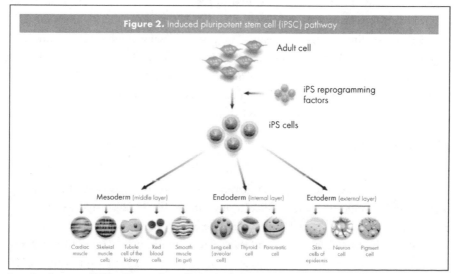

Figure 2. Induced pluripotent stem cell (iPSC) pathway

Adult cell

iPS reprogramming factors

iPS cells

Mesoderm (middle layer)

Endoderm (internal layer)

Ectoderm (external layer)

Cardiac muscle / Skeletal muscle cells / Tubule cell of the kidney / Red blood cells / Smooth muscle (in gut)

Lung cell (alveolar cell) / Thyroid cell / Pancreatic cell

Skin cells of epidermis / Neuron cell / Pigment cell

Source: http://www.sigmaaldrich.com/life-science/stem-cell-biology/ipsc.html

Designer stem cells: These are specialized stem cells created via biochemical manipulation of some other cell (generally an ASC or WJMSC). Biotechnology companies are hoping to cash in in a big way on these types of cells since they have the potential to be patented.[4] Already being used in research, I think we will see the vast majority of future research geared toward this type of cell—not because it is necessarily better—but because it is vastly more profitable. Presently, however, designer stem cells are not on the market.

Use of Fetal Stem Cells

FSCs are derived from elective abortions, generally those performed prior to 12 weeks gestation. FSCs derived at older gestational ages (after 12 to 16 weeks) express a more adult pattern of cell surface antigens and are more rapidly rejected by the new host. This makes them less suited for clinical treatments.

Obviously, use of FSCs raises some critical questions, including questions about how stem cell clinics get access to these cells and about legality, ethics, and safety. In many countries, there are no specific laws governing the unmodified use of fetal stem cell transplants for medical applications apart from the rules already on the books regarding human blood or organ donation and use. By *unmodified*, I mean that the cells have not been treated chemically to alter their characteristics. Thus, in the same way that doctors can transplant a cornea to correct a vision impairment, they can, in theory, transplant FSCs to treat anything agreed upon by patient and doctor. In actuality, however, it is far more complicated than that in most countries. To my knowledge, fetal tissue use in the US is limited to research conducted by universities and biotechnology companies. More specifically, this means that FSCs are not being used in US medical clinics to treat patients. The research being conducted on natural (as opposed to enhanced) FSCs is limited not just in the US but also in Canada, the United Kingdom and other member countries of the European Union, Australia, New Zealand, and South Africa. To date, I have not been able to find any specific information about Japan's use of fetal tissues in medical clinics.

FDA Guidelines

In 2006, the US Food and Drug Administration (FDA) issued updated and revised guidelines for stem cell therapies. Unfortunately, the revisions only further confused many people's understanding of the FDA's intent. In the 2006 update, the FDA extended its authority to medical practice previously regulated exclusively by state medical boards and hospital ethics and therapeutics committees. The FDA did this by expanding its authority under sections 351 and 361 of the Public Health Safety (PHS) Act. More specifically, the update added a discussion of the FDA's authority to regulate stem cells when they are used for something other than their *normal* function. Not surprisingly, a debate immediately ensued as to what defines the normal function of a stem cell. Discussion then quickly progressed to the currently heated debate about reimplanting stem cells derived from self-donation (i.e., harvesting one's own bone marrow or fat) and the controversy of transplantation from donors. (Regarding the latter, there is agreement that transplantation of stem cells from donors must meet the transplantation criteria of section 361 of the PHS Act, just as with any other organ or blood donation).[5]

While there is clear agreement that the FDA has no authority over the individual practice of medicine by doctors, in the 2006 update, the FDA seemed to say that it has control over what doctors do with stem cells. That statement represents a completely new area of federal authority over the practice of medicine. Up until that point, US doctors had been exclusively regulated by state medical boards (and were also subject to the legal authority of agencies such as the Drug Enforcement Administration). Unfortunately, however, as the example of stem cells illustrates, medical practices have advanced faster than state and national legislatures' capacity to pass regulatory guidance.

To this day, it remains unclear whether a stem cell that has not been manipulated biologically and which retains its natural properties is further subject to the jurisdiction of the FDA for its intended medical application. With this continued lack of clarity, issues surrounding the use of FSCs have gotten more and more complicated. Many years ago, through a process of complex and lengthy litigation against the agency, the FDA lost its ability to regulate the off-label use of medicines by doctors and consumers. An outcome is that, in general, the FDA does not regulate surgical procedures or guidelines but does regulate surgical hardware such as artificial joints. In my mind, this victory allowing off-label use to be at the discretion of the physician remains a cornerstone of healthcare freedom. The FDA does restrict the manufacturers of medicines and other products from *promoting* their products for off-label use. But stem cells are human cells or tissues, not medicines; only when they are manipulated should the FDA consider them a biological agent and have jurisdiction over their use. At any rate, because the FDA's jurisdictional reach remains blurry, many doctors have elected to pursue stem cell therapies in foreign (offshore) jurisdictions with more straightforward regulatory environments.

We will talk more about these issues in a bit, but for now, I want to continue discussing FSCs. In the US, the topic is presently a non-issue. There are no guidelines for donation or sale of aborted fetal tissue, and I can only imagine the uproar that "selling" aborted fetuses would create. Nonetheless, fetal stem cell research and therapies are a reality in other countries, including Russia, Ukraine, and China. I happen to know a good deal about FSC-related work in Ukraine (though I know less about FSCs in Russia and China). Ukraine gained its independence from the Soviet Union when the latter dissolved in 1991. Shortly after that, EmCell started as a public-private joint venture in Kiev, based on the pioneering work of Professor A.I. Smikodub from the National Medical University of Ukraine. The team created by Professor Smikodub was the first to describe and publish outcomes from treatments using FSCs for a range of disorders, including AIDS (HIV infection), types 1 and 2 diabetes mellitus, aplastic anemia, psoriasis, rheumatoid arthritis, degenerative diseases of the nervous system, Crohn's disease, ulcerative colitis, bowel cancer, and several other disorders. While this group's work is largely unknown, unrecognized, and even ignored in the US (perhaps due to its publication in Russian and Ukraine languages), the group's pioneering role is undeniable.[6]

Smikodub and colleagues started their work in the late 1980s even prior to the dissolution of the Soviet Union, and they have more combined therapeutic stem cell experience than any center in the world. Reportedly, over 7000 patients have received FSCs at EmCell in Kiev, with no reported infections or significant complications. Although EmCell's track record of no side effects offers room for optimism, randomized controlled trials are lacking as are English translations of EmCell's pioneering work (a gap that I am working on rectifying). Over the next few years, I anticipate that more objective data will emerge from the work at EmCell.

What May Stem Cells Offer for the Treatment of Autism?

Autism is a complex developmental neurological disorder that appears to manifest as immunological dysregulation of special neuroimmune cells (glia), with resultant disruption of brain organization.[7] On the surface, disruption of brain organization would seem to imply that the condition is irreparable. However, new evidence indicates that, at least in some cases, the immune disruption may be inhibitory as opposed to destructive, leaving room for hope that the effects may be reversible.[8]

That being said, let us revisit the previous discussions pertaining to fetal and mesenchymal stem cells. FSCs are the substance of human life—all that you are today comes from your FSCs. MSCs are the biological force behind repair and immune regulation. MSCs produce the chemistry to induce repair in recipient organ systems and to regulate the host's immune system.[9]

The human brain—particularly the developing human brain—is the most complex structure in nature. With its numerous dendritic connections and exceptional processing speed, the human brain rivals the best supercomputers. Repairing such an intricate organ is a daunting and overwhelmingly difficult task, which is why many consider autism to be incurable. By natural design, however, the purpose of stem cells in the brain is regulation, healing, and repair.[10] Biologically, therefore, stem cells appear to be better suited to heal the brain than any other current therapy.

No matter how challenging the task of repairing the brain may appear to be, case reports have built an argument for supporting the reversibility of autism using immunological interventions.[11,12] Additionally, another totally different approach, applied behavior analysis (ABA), has also achieved documented reversals of IQ loss and behavioral abnormalities in up to 50% of children with autism.[13] Regardless of what happens in the brain as a result of ABA, its success at least speaks to the fact that a large subset of children has reparable brain syndromes. This is not the place to elaborate on the potential biochemical and neurotransmitter changes resulting from ABA, but I would speculate that it increases acetylcholine and reduces dopamine and that this combination reduces oxidative stress and inflammation.

Cerebral palsy (CP), like autism, is also considered an incurable brain syndrome. CP is thought to be the result of perinatal hypoxic injury to the brain,[14] and until recently, there was no effective therapy. Some impressive news reports[15] about an autologous (self-donated) umbilical stem cell therapy study at Duke University (not yet published) as well as the first published case reports from two children treated in Thailand[16] both document this type of FSC treatment. Both children in the latter study showed rapid improvement in gross motor scores with no apparent side effects. The responses seemed to occur too rapidly to be due to actual neurological reconstitution from engrafting of the umbilical stem cells. Instead, the therapeutic results are more likely due to the production of cell mediators by the stem cells and the change in neurological dysregulation that followed.

Intravenous immunoglobulin (IVIG) therapy represents another relevant example of how a therapeutic treatment can modify immune responses. In the mid-1990s, Professor Sudhir Gupta from the University of California-Irvine published a case series of children with autism whom he treated with human IVIG.[17] Some of the children responded dramatically, quickly, and positively to the intervention. Professor Gupta has continued to use this therapy for children with autism as have I. Sometimes it is amazing how rapidly IVIG helps alleviate the symptoms of autism. In at least this subset of rapid responders, it has been theorized that IVIG removes an immunological inhibitor. As with the umbilical stem cell therapy results in Thailand, the restoration of function with IVIG occurs too rapidly to be due to neuronal regeneration and synaptic development.

In other children with autism and fragile X syndrome, the use of antiinflammatories such as steroids,[18] spironolactone,[19] pioglitazone,[12] and minocycline[20] has also resulted in rapid improvements. In a single case report, an older individual not formally diagnosed with autism but clearly on the autism spectrum responded rapidly to the anti-TNF-alpha drug entanercept (Enbrel®).[21] TNF-alpha is a powerful mediator of inflammation and a target for many specific anti-inflammatory medications.

Returning the focus to the stem cell discussion, stem cells offer a potentially self-renewing source of immunological regulation to the body and brain. They also offer a wide array of biochemically mediated cell signals to induce repair. In autism, many body systems could benefit from this process of healing signals from stem cells. The potential options and benefits are numerous, as illustrated by a few examples:

- In autism, it has been postulated that the blood-brain barrier (endothelium) does not function normally[22] and that autoantibodies to the endovasculature are commonly found.[23] As shown in Figure 3, the blood-brain barrier defines the environmental separation between the brain and the rest of the body. If the blood-brain barrier is chronically inflamed, abnormal function of the brain would be expected. Stem cells may, more properly than medications, regulate the immune system in the brain and provide a stable, more functional environment.
- Chronic inflammatory changes are noted in the intestinal tract of a significant subset of children with autism.[24] Other forms of inflammatory bowel disease have been responsive to stem cell therapies.[25]
- Similar to cerebral palsy but on a lesser scale, many children with autism demonstrate motor dysregulation and dyspraxia.[26] This includes abnormal proprioception, abnormal gross and fine motor control, and cross-extensor reflex abnormalities. Early positive observations demonstrated by stem cell interventions for treating CP suggest that motor planning issues in patients with autism may respond in a similar manner.
- Lastly and hopefully, stem cells may provide repair and replacement neurons over a long period of time to restore deficient function.[27] Although this remains an uncertainty, preclinical observations in animals suggest that, in theory, it is at least a potential outcome.[28]

Anecdotal Observations of Stem Cells in Autism

I maintain a blog where I strive to discuss a wide variety of health issues. Autism and stem cells, however, seem to take up most of our discussions. Through this forum, I have been attempting to follow the stem cell therapy outcomes (three of which I include below) from patients in my practice. (I have several more, but space does not suffice to include them.) The three following patients were all treated at EmCell, which uses fetal stem cells. Generally, the outcomes were about the same in each case. Behavioral changes seem to occur first and are often dramatic. Language is more challenging, although most children are experiencing some gains in both receptive and expressive language.

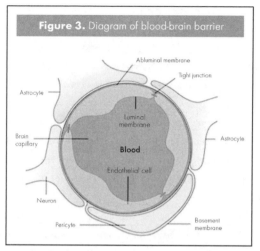

Figure 3. Diagram of blood-brain barrier

Source: http://media.tumblr.com/tumblr_lk7odmeeCu1qc9f5v.jpg

A mom from Canada sent me this post about her two boys and their responses to stem cells:

Dr. Bradstreet, I am so glad you are in Kiev learning about what EmCell is all about. I went to EmCell July 2011. I have to say our experience was very good. Our kids 7 and 8 with autism are getting better every day. K could not be in school full-time before we went to EmCell, now he goes to school full-time and is doing well. K can also read now, he talks in full sentences, asks questions and answers questions. It is just amazing how much our lives have changed since we went to EmCell. J and K are much happier. I think their quality of life is much better. It is nice to be able to chat with our kid now.

These parents from Dubai posted the following account to the blog:

Our 7-year-old boy has been going through major changes since the stem cell treatment at the end of November (EmCell). Within three weeks he added and retained seven words to his vocabulary, which is quite a feat considering he has only spoken and retained seven words in as many years. Because of his verbal dyspraxia, he has spoken more words over the years, but would lose them immediately. We have also realized that he no longer pronounces the end sound of a word first, which was a constant prior to the therapy. He is blending multiple sounds moving towards proper pronunciation, something he greatly struggled with. In fact, the first multiple sound word he added was in the taxi ride home from the airport after returning from Kiev. He saw the petrol station with a car wash and suddenly pointed and said "wash."

The last week or so his verbal growth has reached a plateau for the time being but major changes are still ongoing as he is obviously very displaced within himself, but in a positive sense. Lots of sensations going on in his mouth, his distended belly is now flat and almost defined, and has three regular [bowel] movements a day. He seems to have found a new store of energy as he is more hyper than usual and we have a lot more stim running, but this has always been the norm when he goes through growth spurts and another confirmation that a lot of change is going on inside his little body.

His teacher and therapists all comment on the changes, not just verbally, but also on his attention and willingness to participate in activities, even when he obviously cannot be bothered. There is an obvious correlation between the decline of his listening and participation skills when he is experiencing major changes within himself, but within a week or so he is back on form plus some.

Parental observations are anecdotal and not equal to rigorous scientific investigations, but they are important to document at this early stage of therapeutic application. This next parent account is particularly detailed and seemingly objective. The account pertains to a girl who had been largely static with language and other developments over the past year. The girl was 4 years old at the time of treatment.

We just hit the three-month mark and I wanted to touch down and let you know how she is doing these days after EmCell therapies. She's actually doing pretty good! Our ABA supervisor sent me an e-mail with some changes they've noted in the past 3 months. I didn't tell them about the stem cell treatment so I think their observations are pretty unbiased. We've also noticed that her PANDAS symptoms seem to be almost completely gone since the stem cell [therapy]. Anyway, here are some changes we've noted in the past 3 months. Most of these are new changes that her therapists have brought up so I feel good knowing that I'm not "imagining" anything.

1. *Significant decrease in rigidity, decreased obsessive-compulsive behaviors, and anxiety.*
2. *Increase in the following: attending, language comprehension, motor imitation skills, visual discrimination, and understanding of concepts.*
3. *Increase in her ability to tolerate changes and is more easily directed/redirected.*

4. *She understands the power of language and team has seen an increase in communicative intent and understands the back and forth of language.*

5. *She looks forward to her ABA sessions and has developed positive relationships with the therapists.*

6. *She is showing interest in other children and seems to want to play but doesn't know how to initiate (previously uninterested in other kids).*

7. *She is interacting more with her brother.*

8. *She's showing much more affection to family and friends.*

9. *She's dropped vanco [vancomycin], zithro [azithromycin], and nystatin completely and cut clonidine and omeprazole doses in half with no regression.*

10. *Increase in verbal attempts, but still very lacking in expressive language changes.*

Recently, I have had several patients treated at clinics other than EmCell. One clinic (located in the Dominican Republic) uses a combination of bone marrow MSCs and adipose-derived MSCs. MSCs are highly counter-regulatory to the immune system,[29] downregulating inflammation and promoting healing. However, there is an intrinsic problem with adipose-derived MSC therapy. Because the adipose tissue is surgically removed from the patient using liposuction, the process creates a wound. Stem cells naturally seek out areas of damage; as a result, they would be expected to return to the wound site. In an attempt to minimize that problem, the clinic banks the cells for 7 to 10 days before reinfusing the stem cells. Because it is doubtful that even 10 days are adequate to heal the surgery site, it is difficult to know what proportion of the stem cells later make it to the sites where we would want them to go to address symptoms associated with autism. Despite this shortcoming, these patients have reported some positive gains, including reduced self-stimulatory behaviors, improved mood in some cases, and decreased gut issues in one child. So far, in the procedure involving bone marrow and adipose-derived MSCs in combination, these patients haven't reported any language gains or other changes.

Several other children who are my patients were treated at a Panamanian center that apparently uses pooled or expanded umbilical stem cells. A paper published by this group suggests that indeed they are using expanded cord blood rather than WJ-related mesenchymal stem cells.[30] These expanded stem cells are adult-type and, depending on the techniques used, they would be expected to express HLA type II surface antigens.[31] What this means is that their longevity in the body is most likely going to be short due to their rejection by the recipient's immune system. This type of cell (while present) is anti inflammatory; in the children with ASDs treated at the Panama clinic, this has sometimes equated to short-term gains, but no sustained benefits have been observed. I am aware of one child with CP who, at age 3, was treated at the Panama clinic and showed very significant improvement in spasticity and motor control. This effect has been sustained for greater than 6 months.

Cell Choices: MSCs

Before concluding, I want to return the discussion to adult MSCs. Mesenchymal stem cells are derived from the fetal mesodermal layer. They are hardy and plentiful in both bone marrow and fat. Beyond their ability to create bone, connective tissue, cartilage, and adipose, they are strongly anti-inflammatory. In the laboratory, MSCs can also be biologically transformed to become other cell lines, including neuronal. For this reason, I expect that in the future these types of cells will be the resource for a variety of designer stem cells.[32] In autism, without further transformation, MSCs would be expected to have a peripheral anti-inflammatory effect, with the potential to heal the gut and quiet autoimmune reactions. It would be doubtful that they would directly convert to neurons and more likely that they would signal repair in the brain with their intrinsic cellular chemistry.[33]

Potential Risks

We must also ask if there are any significant potential risks associated with using stem cell therapies for the treatment of autism. This is a complex area because of the various protocols, multiple cell sources, and different cell types presented in the medical literature. First, it is helpful to note that we are not dealing with the more complicated

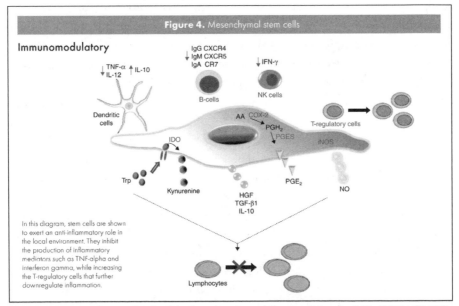

Figure 4. Mesenchymal stem cells

Immunomodulatory

IgG CXCR4
↓ IgM CXCR5
IgA CR7

↓ IFN-γ

↓ TNF-α ↑ IL-10
↓ IL-12

B-cells

NK cells

Dendritic cells

AA COX-2
→ PGH₂
↓ PGES

T-regulatory cells

IDO

iNOS

Trp

Kynurenine

PGE₂

NO

HGF
TGF-β1
IL-10

In this diagram, stem cells are shown to exert an anti-inflammatory role in the local environment. They inhibit the production of inflammatory mediators such as TNF-alpha and interferon gamma, while increasing the T-regulatory cells that further downregulate inflammation.

Lymphocytes

Source: Iyer SS, Rojas M. Anti-inflammatory effects of mesenchymal stem cells: novel concept for future therapies. *Expert Opin Biol Ther.* 2008 May;8(5):569-81.

graft versus host type of reactions. For example, unlike bone marrow transplants after chemotherapy for leukemia, where rejection is a potential issue, a person with autism has an intact immune system to prevent graft versus host reactions.

Although increased cancer risk for patients treated with both self-donated (autologous) and donor (allogeneic) stem cells has been suggested to be a potential issue by some authors,[34] the doctors at EmCell claim that no cancers have thus far been reported after treatments involving up to 20 years of follow-up. In fact, EmCell doctors have clinical observations indicating just the opposite, namely a reduction in cancer-related issues after stem cell therapy. The cancer risks appear to be limited to patients with prior chemotherapy for lymphoma and leukemia or in stem cells derived from induced pluripotent cells.[35] Most of the long-term observations related to cancer are in populations where ongoing anti-rejection drugs are being given, and in that population, a significant increase in cancer risk is observed. The issues that are associated with those scenarios don't apply to treating children with autism. In theory, ESCs would seem to have the greatest risk of cancer, although so little work has been done with these cells that it is hard to evaluate. One child who appeared to have ESCs injected into his spine for an unusual and fatal genetic disease developed benign tumors within the spinal canal that required decompression surgery.[36] While some protocols for ASD and CP utilize the injection of stem cells into the spine, I strongly encourage patients NOT to allow this procedure.

Infection transmission from contamination of the stem cell source is also a risk. A recent evaluation of cord blood samples by the American Association of Blood Banks showed that vaginal delivery significantly increased the risk of bacterial contamination of the cord (logical) and that the rate of bacterial contamination was at least 4 percent.[37] By using blood donation standards for any form of allogeneic transplantation, a recent review placed the risk of finding a contaminated specimen at the time of screening at about 0.5 percent but estimated post-screening contamination at close to zero for all the agents tested using modern screening techniques.[38] This type of conclusion raises the concern that not all infectious agents can be practically screened for, though current screening techniques encompass all major and common disorders. Freedom from contamination, therefore, depends largely on the quality of the screening technique and the pedigree (source documentation) of the stem cells. Consumers should ask for and expect certification of the sample's bacteriological (especially cord blood) and viral testing. Consumers should also know where the material to be transplanted was sourced and what recordkeeping is maintained by the transplantation facility.

Beyond this, I am additionally concerned that cultured (amplified) stem cells grown in the lab could test clean from the source but then subsequently be subject to additional laboratory contamination. I know with certainty that there is a potential for all labs to be subject to cell culture contamination; this is attested to by the recent recalls of flu vaccine in New York.[39] In my review of the medical literature, apart from umbilical cord blood testing, I could find no published reports estimating contamination of lab-grown stem cells.

Conclusion

Where does all of this leave us? If I put on my hat as a father of a child and stepchild with autism (yes, I have two boys in my life with autism), I am left with this sense: if the risks are reasonable and the finances allow it, I want to try everything that has the potential to improve my boys' health. As a physician, I have read hundreds of research papers on stem cells and their potential to heal as well as their unknown potential to do harm. All of the available choices have challenges. Self-donated umbilical stem cells would be first on my list for use with autism, but as of yet I have no experience with any child with autism receiving their own umbilical stem cells. Next, I would select fetal stem cells because of their potency. If considering autologous stem cells, the potential flaw associated with using autologous cells is the source of the cells: they are from a child with autism who is known to be genetically susceptible. In other words, whatever autism is, the stem cells of the autistic child did not prevent the autism from happening in the first place. That might mean that autologous stem cells lack the therapeutic capacity to heal the existing autistic state, yet this question still remains to be answered. Finally, another option is donated umbilical stem cells, which are potent, but as discussed, their survivability is most likely short. In the end, when weighing all these considerations, the complex decision of whether or not to use stem cells can only be made by us as parents.

THE THYROID-AUTISM CONNECTION: THE ROLE OF ENDOCRINE DISRUPTORS

by Dr. Raphael Kellman

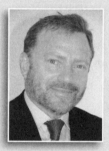

Raphael Kellman, MD

Dr. Raphael Kellman is a graduate of Albert Einstein College of Medicine. He is an internist and a pioneer in holistic medicine. Dr. Kellman is the author of two books, *Gut Reactions* and *Matrix Healing*. He has practiced in New York City since 1995. Dr. Kellman treats many children with autism and neurodevelopmental disorders. For more information, please see www.kellmanmd.com.

Hypothyroidism and autism are today strongly associated with the increasing burden of environmental toxicity. Both the brain and the thyroid are very susceptible to environmental toxins. Is there a connection between hypothyroidism and autism? The latest studies point to endocrine-disrupting chemicals (EDCs) as likely major causative or contributory factors in any such connection. This chapter lays out the details.

HAVE ASDs BECOME EPIDEMIC IN THE U.S.?

An article in *Environmental Health Perspectives* in 2006 noted that since the early 1990s alone, reported cases of autism spectrum disorders (ASDs) have increased tenfold. And in March 2012, the Centers for Disease Control and Prevention (CDC) announced an estimate of 1 in 88 US eight year olds (as of 2008) as having an autism spectrum disorder. Autism is the fastest growing developmental disability in the US, affecting more children than cancer, diabetes, and AIDS combined.

HAS THYROID DISEASE BECOME EPIDEMIC IN THE U.S.?

Thyroid disease is the most common endocrine disorder (defined as a problem affecting the hormone glands) in the US. An estimate based on statistics gathered by the American Association of Clinical Endocrinologists (AACE) indicates that approximately 27 million Americans—as much as 7-8% of the population—have some form of thyroid disorder. (According to this estimate, roughly half of these cases remain undiagnosed.)

Approximately eight out of ten thyroid disease cases (80%) are hypothyroid conditions (low or underactive thyroid), with the other two out of ten (20%) being hyperthyroid conditions (high or overactive thyroid). Women constitute about 80% of Americans with thyroid disease, and women are five times more likely than men to develop hypothyroidism.

Thyroid *autoimmune* disease (as distinct from thyroid disease) is the most common autoimmune disease in the US.[1] Because only one-third of those with thyroid autoimmune disease are diagnosed, the actual number may be 72 million Americans.[2]

HOW THE THYROID WORKS

The function of the thyroid is very important to overall health. Thyroid hormone is responsible for the energy production and metabolism of every cell in the body, including the brain. It is a critical hormone for brain development. Thyroid-stimulating hormone (TSH) is produced in the brain by the pituitary, which stimulates the thyroid to produce hormones such as T4 (thyroxine) and T3 (triiodothyronine). When a sufficient amount of hormone is produced by the thyroid, then the T4 and T3, in a feedback loop, tell the pituitary to stop producing TSH (or to slow it down). When there is a low amount of thyroid hormone (TH) in the blood, T4 and T3 tell the pituitary to start producing more TSH. The thyroid is very vulnerable to environmental toxins.

EVIDENCE SUPPORTING A THYROID-AUTISM CONNECTION

A number of strands of evidence support a link between hypothyroidism and autism, including research on brain development, gluten sensitivity, methylation defects, and mitochondrial dysfunction.

The Crucial Role of Thyroid Hormone in Brain Development

Thyroid hormone is essential for brain development during a period beginning *in utero* and extending through the first 2 to 3 years of life. Deficiencies in thyroid hormone during this crucial period can have significant behavioral and cognitive effects; many of the same symptoms are also associated with ASD.

Normally, thyroid hormone regulates neuronal proliferation, migration, and differentiation in discrete regions of the brain during definitive time periods. Thyroid hormone also normally regulates development of cholinergic and dopaminergic neurons in the brain.

Gluten Sensitivity

Celiac disease and gluten sensitivity are factors known to contribute to autism. Gluten antigen, similar to an antigen in the thyroid, also can provoke autoimmune thyroid disease.[3] Numerous studies confirm the strong link between gluten intolerance and autoimmune hypothyroidism.[4,5] In a 2000 study,[4] for example, researchers observed an association between untreated celiac disease, gluten intake, and autoimmune disorders. They reported, "We believe that undiagnosed celiac disease can cause other disorders by switching on some as yet unknown immunological mechanism. Untreated celiac patients produce organ-specific autoantibodies."

One of the most effective therapies for ASDs and PDD is a gluten-free (GF) diet. A gluten-free diet also can help heal an underlying thyroid disorder, as noted by the authors of the 2000 study just mentioned,[4] who observed that the organ-specific antibodies "disappeared after 3 to 6 months on a gluten-free diet." This may be one of the reasons why the GF diet is so effective in children with autism.

Methylation Defects

Hypothyroidism can contribute to methylation defects. T4 and T3 are tyrosine-based hormones that are primarily responsible for regulation of metabolism. T4 regulates the conversion of riboflavin to FAD (flavin adenine dinucleotide). Composed of riboflavin 5'-phosphate and adenosine 5'-phosphate, FAD serves as an electron carrier by being alternately oxidized (FAD) and reduced (FAeH2). It is important in electron transport in the mitochondria.[6]

With hypothyroidism, conversion of riboflavin to FAD and MTHFR (methylenetetrahydrofolate reductase) is impaired.[6] *MTHFR* is the name of a gene that produces an enzyme, also called methylenetetrahydrofolate reductase. In an individual with a genetic mutation that inhibits production of this enzyme, the mutation can lead to hyperhomocysteinemia, a condition in which elevated levels of an enzyme called homocysteine are found in blood plasma. When the body is deficient in MTHFR, its ability to absorb folate (vitamin B9 and folic acid, for instance) is inhibited. Folic acid and B9 are both essential to the development and health of the fetus. Genetic variation in the MTHFR gene also increases susceptibility to acute leukemia, colon cancer, neural tube defects, and occlusive vascular disease. Mutations in this gene are associated with MTHFR deficiency.

Mitochondrial Dysfunction

Hypothyroidism can cause mitochondrial dysfunction, and mitochondrial dysfunction, in turn, has been found to be associated with autism. A 2010 study by researchers at the University of California found that cumulative damage and oxidative stress in the mitochondria could influence the onset and severity of autism.[7] This study observed that mitochondrial dysfunction in autistic children appeared to decrease NADH (nicotinamide adenine dinucleotide) and increase oxidative stress. NADH, which is an activated form of the B vitamin niacin, behaves as a coenzyme that helps in energy extraction. It also enhances the immune system, fights disease, and repairs damage caused by the disease.[7] The researchers also observed over-replication or deletion of mitochondrial DNA in these children: "Whether the mitochondrial dysfunction in children with autism is primary or secondary to an as yet unknown event," remarked the researchers, "remains the subject of future work; however mitochondrial dysfunction could greatly amplify and propagate brain dysfunction, such as that found in autism."[7]

An earlier paper, published in 2003, found that hypothyroidism alters mitochondrial morphology and induces release of apoptogenic proteins.[8] We know that TH deficiency can lead to extensive apoptosis (programmed cell death) and that adequate levels of TH maintain mitochondrial architecture and inhibit release of apoptogenic molecules to prevent excess apoptosis during cerebellar development. A review article published in the *Journal of Molecular Endocrinology* in 2001 on TH action in mitochondria discussed, among other things, TH regulation of mitochondrial activity as a link between metabolism and development.[9]

BRAIN DEVELOPMENT: FURTHER CONSIDERATIONS

Before and after birth, thyroid hormone development is characterized by three distinct phases.

Phase I. The fetus is dependent on maternal TH during the first trimester of pregnancy. Fetal synthesis of TH takes place after the first trimester. Also during the first trimester, neurons which will develop into the forebrain proliferate, migrate, and differentiate—TH orchestrates all this activity.

Phase II. During the second phase, the fetus produces its own TH, which then chiefly orchestrates development. Maternal TH still plays a role. Neurons which develop into the cerebellum proliferate, migrate, and differentiate. The forebrain matures. Synapses are formed.

Phase III. After birth, the infant's TH, acting figuratively as a time clock, stimulates and subsequently terminates brain cell proliferation, migration, and differentiation. Thyroid hormones orchestrate these events at the precise time with the precise dose and in the correct sequence.[10,11]

Maternal thyroxine (T4) plays a pivotal role in fetal brain development. Iodine is necessary for TH production,[12] and iodine deficiency is related to low levels of T4, a condition known as hypothyroxinemia. Where maternal T4 levels are low normal (0-10th percentile) and maternal iodine is deficient from early gestation to birth, there is an increased risk of neurodevelopmental delay in the offspring.[13] The main developmental delays resulting from mild hypothyroxinemia are lower performance in gross and fine motor coordination and poorer performance in socialization. An increase in the incidence of autism is also associated with increased iodine deficiency.

According to Grandjean and Landrigan,[14] "The blood-brain barrier, which protects the adult brain from many toxic chemicals, is not completely formed until about 6 months after birth." These same authors further point out that "The human brain continues to develop postnatally, and the period of heightened vulnerability therefore extends over many months, through infancy and into early childhood. Although most neurons have been formed by the time of birth, growth of glial cells and myelination of axons continues for several years."[14] The symptoms of low thyroid function in the fetus and newborn are similar to the symptoms associated with ASD and ADHD.[15] These include:

- general developmental delays
- cognitive dysfunction
- hyperactivity
- attention disorders
- speech delays
- hypotonia/fine motor dysfunction
- repetitive behavior
- social and communication dysfunction

ENDOCRINE-DISRUPTING CHEMICALS (EDCS), AUTISM, AND THE THYROID

According to the Environmental Protection Agency (EPA), an EDC is an exogenous agent that interferes with synthesis, secretion, transport, metabolism, binding action, or elimination of natural bloodborne hormones that are present in the body and responsible for homeostasis, reproduction, and developmental processes. These chemicals disrupt the body's communication network in three main ways:

1. They block or mimic hormone messages.
2. They scramble the signals in these messages.
3. By "sowing misinformation," they fool the endocrine system into accepting new (but incorrect) instructions.

In cancer, one can say "the dose makes the poison," meaning that the duration or concentration of exposure to a toxic substance is mainly responsible for development of the illness. EDCs play by different rules. Here, one can say, "the timing makes the poison." Thyroid hormones secreted at the right time and in the right dose orchestrate the process of neurological development. In other words, neurological development is like a chemical ballet, dependent on the right hormone message being sent and received at precisely the right time and in the right amount. This ballet opens windows of vulnerability. If exposure to an EDC occurs at one of these vulnerable moments, abnormalities can result. During this critical period, even low doses of EDCs, which may have little effect on adults, can have devastating effects on the unborn, neonate, and child.

Many of the endocrine-disrupting chemicals that are associated with autism also cause thyroid disease. Further, many of the chemicals that contribute to autism mediate their effects through adverse action on the thyroid. Toxins with endocrine-disrupting effects include PCBs, dioxins, perchlorate, phthalates, PBDEs, lead, mercury, cadmium, insecticides, and bisphenol-A.[16] The neurodevelopmental effects of thyroid disruption by EDCs may include learning disabilities, behavioral problems, fine motor dysfunction, poor response to stress, attention problems and hyperactivity, language and speech deficits, and social development deficits.[10,11] Other effects on neurodevelopment in infants and children include visual-spatial deficits, visual and motor delays, decreased social and perceptual abilities, and decreased auditory discriminating abilities.[17]

Thyroid-disrupting chemicals operate through multiple mechanisms. Moreover, the different effects of endocrine disruptors on the thyroid can create cumulative and/or synergistic effects,[18] and different toxins can cause multiple "hits" at different points in the thyroid hormone signaling system (see Table 1).

As shown in Table 1, there are a large number of EDCs exerting a wide variety of effects on the thyroid. Several EDCs warrant a more detailed look.

Table 1. Effects of EDCs on the thyroid	
Endocrine-disrupting chemicals	**Effects on thyroid hormone signaling system**
Chlorinated pesticides, mercury, PBDEs, PCBs, dioxins/TCDD	Direct toxic effect on thyroid gland
Amitrole, benzophenone, Mancozeb	Blocked production of thyroid hormone
Bisphenol A (BPA), dioxins, flame retardants, PCBs, phthalates	Binding to thyroid receptor
Flame retardants, PCBs, pentachlorophenol, phthalates	Competitive binding to thyroid transport protein (TTR)
DDT, PCBs	Effects on TSH receptor
Bromates, perchlorates, phthalates, thyocinates	Blocked iodide uptake
Cadmium, C red dye #3, HCB, lead, mercury, octylmethoxycinnamate, PBDEs, PCBs	Inhibiting of deiodinases
Acetochlor, PBDEs, PCBs	Enhanced hepatic metabolism

Bisphenol A (BPA)

BPA is a monomer of polycarbonate plastics, which inhibits thyroid hormone receptor-mediated transcription by acting as an antagonist. In transient gene expression experiments, BPA suppressed transcriptional activity stimulated by thyroid hormone (T3) in a dose-dependent manner.[19]

Dioxins

Widespread, persistent, and highly toxic, dioxins are produced through industrial burning processes and production of herbicides. TCDD is the dioxin prototype and the most toxic. A single dose of TCDD in rats dose-dependently decreased T4 and free T4 and increased TSH.[20] In offspring of rats, a single dose of TCDD to the dam during gestation correlated to decreased T4, caused a twofold increase in TSH, and caused hyperplasia of the thyroid gland.[21] In humans, a large study of Vietnam veterans detected a significant increase in TSH in the group with the highest TCDD levels.[22]

In a 1993 study,[23] both PCBs and dioxins were found in high levels in breast milk and were associated with hypothyroidism in both mothers and newborns. This study also found inhibition of enzyme 5-deiodinase, decreased conversion of T4 to T3, and decreased nuclear T-3 receptor occupancy. In the pituitary gland, decreased nuclear T-3 occupancy stimulated TSH secretion.

PBDEs

Polybrominated diphenyl ether is used as a flame retardant in plastics, paints, electrical equipment and synthetic textiles. A report published in *Toxicological Sciences* in 2001 found that in rats that were weaning, a commercial PBDE mixture (DE-7) decreased levels of TH and induced activity of hepatic enzymes UDPGT. High doses of DE-7 caused histopathological changes.

PCBs

Polychlorinated biphenyls (PCBs) are synthetic environmental toxins with a striking structural resemblance to active thyroid hormones. Boas and colleagues describe the effects of PCBs as follows:[24]

> *There is substantial evidence that polychlorinated biphenyls, dioxins and furans cause hypothyroidism in exposed animals, and that environmentally occurring doses affect human thyroid homeostasis. Thyroid disruption may be caused by a variety of mechanisms as different chemicals interfere with the hypothalamic-pituitary-thyroid axis at different levels. Growth and development in fetal life and childhood is highly dependent on normal levels of TH (thyroid hormone). Normal levels of THs are crucial for the development of the central nervous system. This critical phase may be vulnerable to even subtle effects of synthetic chemicals. Such developmental deficiencies may not be identifiable until late in life.*

There is a negative correlation between maternal total T3 and PCBs, as well as with three pesticides (p-'-DDE, cis-nonachlor, hexachlorobenzene) and inorganic mercury at low levels of exposure. PCBs have a positive correlation to fetal TSH[25] and TSH levels in children.[26] As noted above, PCBs also interfere with the hypothalamic-pituitary-thyroid (HPT) axis by producing a subnormal response of the pituitary to TRH stimulation.[27] In adults, adolescents and children from areas highly exposed to PCBs, PCB levels correlate negatively to TH levels.[28]

In studies of breast milk, there is a positive association between PCB levels in breast milk and TSH levels in infants.[29] In Taiwan, a 1988 study of women (N=1,971) who consumed cooking oil contaminated with PCBs and furans during pregnancy found that all of the children studied (n=128) with *in utero* exposure exhibited subsequent impairments in mental and motor abilities, behavioral problems, and hyperactivity–attention deficits.[30]

Perchlorates

A report issued by the CDC in 2006 stated that American women, particularly those with low iodine intake, may have reduced thyroid function due to perchlorate exposure. According to the Environmental Working Group: "[An] analysis of the CDC data found that for more than 2 million iodine-deficient women nationwide, exposure to perchlorate in drinking water and the food supply, at levels equal to or lower than proposed national and state standards, could lower thyroid hormone levels to the extent that they would require medical treatment to avoid developmental damage to their babies."[31]

Phthalates

A 1998-2002 study conducted with children born at Mt. Sinai Hospital evaluated the relationship between phthalate and BPA exposure in mothers whose urine was collected during the third trimester of pregnancy and neurodevelopmental disorders in their children when they reached ages 7-9. Increased exposure to phthalates was associated with greater social deficits, including poorer social cognition, social communication, and social awareness. The investigators postulated that the mechanism of action related to phthalates' thyroid-disrupting effects.[32]

Prenatal phthalate exposure is associated with childhood behavior and executive function. In children evaluated at ages 4-9 for behavioral issues and executive function, phthalate levels correlated with poor executive function and decreased ability to control impulses, make a transition between situations, modulate emotional responses, initiate tasks, retain information for task completion, and set goals.[33]

The Insecticide-ASD-Thyroid Connection

Just as EDCs have myriad effects on the thyroid, so do they have numerous effects on development and developmental disorders such as autism.

In a study by Roberts and colleagues,[34] maternal residence near agricultural pesticide applications during key periods of gestation was shown to be associated with the development of ASD in children. In this study, ASD risk increased with the poundage of organochlorine pesticides applied and decreased with distance from the field sites. According to the researchers, the two pesticides (dicofol and endosufan) that pregnant women were exposed to during key periods of gestation do not primarily target the brain. Rather, they are endocrine disruptors that target thyroid and estrogen hormone signaling, which secondarily affect the brain. As the researchers put it, "Generally speaking the brain has not been highlighted as the primary target organ for the toxicity of either dicofol or endosulfan. The latter compound has been noted to have estrogen effects as well as effects on the thyroid gland which may be relevant to concerns about the role of the fetal hormonal milieu in ASD pathogenesis."

Organochlorine Pesticides

Organochlorine pesticides have a number of neurodevelopmental effects, including decreased psychomotor function and decreased mental function (such as depressed memory, attention, and verbal skills). Again, thyroid disruption is thought to be the mechanism of action.[35-37]

SIMILARITY OF CEREBRAL CORTICAL ARCHITECTURE IN AUTISM AND HYPOTHYROIDISM

Many of the studies just cited provide substantial evidence that thyroid disease and autism are intricately connected. An article by Roman published in 2007 [38] discusses the cerebral cortical architecture in the two types of disorders:

> *Experimental animal models have shown that transient intrauterine deficits of T hormones result in permanent alteration of cerebral cortical architecture reminiscent of those observed in brains of patients with autism... Both in autism and hypothyroidism, there is faulty differentiation of neurons, particularly Purkinje cells...*

Roman also notes that "Transient and limited T hormone deficiency *in utero* may cause the morphological brain lesions of autism." Discussing hypothyroxinemia, Roman observes that "hypothyroxinemia may have begun in a percentage of children with autism as early as the first trimester *in utero*. This may be caused by subbiochemical maternal hypothyroidism that either preceded pregnancy or developed subsequently due to the excessive need of TH and/or to a decrease in available iodine." To quote Roman one final time, "The current surge of autism could be related to transient maternal hypothyroxinemia resulting from dietary and/or environmental exposure to anti-thyroid agents."

As indicated by Roman,[38] decreased TH *in utero* causes alterations of cerebral cortical architecture by affecting neuronal migration reminiscent of the alterations observed in the brains of patients with autism. Although the etiology of autism is multifactorial, hypothyroidism *at any point during neurodevelopment* clearly can be a central cause of autism (emphasis added). Therefore, treating hypothyroidism should play a vital role in the treatment of autism.

MISSING THE THYROID DIAGNOSIS IN ASD?

Given that thyroid disease is likely a significant contributing cause of autism, why do routine blood tests then frequently miss the diagnosis? Why are so many children with autism not diagnosed with hypothyroidism? The answer to these questions has to do with the fact that the thyroid signaling system is controlled on two levels: the central HPT axis and control on a local and peripheral cellular level.

The HPT axis: The first level is the central HPT axis (the second level will be discussed hereafter). Routine blood tests frequently fail to detect abnormalities in the HPT axis for a variety of reasons, including that the general population range for TSH is significantly broader than the individual range. Because everyone has a unique set point for TSH, for many individuals even a slight deviation can have profound effects.

The main reason why hypothyroidism is missed in ASD is that the routine tests for TSH, T3, and T4 frequently miss the diagnosis. Only with the TRH (thyrotropin-releasing hormone) stimulation test can we pick up this problem in a large percentage of these children. Everyone has their own set point of TSH, and with routine tests we can't know if one is out of their set point. The TRH stimulation test will frequently detect an underactive thyroid and whether someone is past their set point (which is missed by routine tests).

A landmark study published in 2007 confirmed that routine TSH thyroid tests frequently fail to detect hypothyroidism. Some investigators have noticed, however, that depressed patients with normal TSH can have an exaggerated response to TRH.[39] When patients with normal TSH and TH but suggestive clinical symptoms of hypo-thyroidism were evaluated with a more sensitive TRH test, the researchers concluded: "An exaggerated TRH response indeed occurs in many subjects with normal biochemistry... Even though the TRH test is seldom used in clinical practice at present, a larger prospective study is in order. Until then, physicians may once again need access to TRH for diagnostic use."[40]

Another noteworthy 2007 study was conducted with 87 female patients with infertility but no other symptoms of hypothyroidism. One subgroup included 39 women with ovulation disorders and polycystic ovary syndrome (PCOS), while a second group (n=48) consisted of women with normal ovulation. The study found that although TH was normal and TSH was in the normal range of 1.72 to 1.87, the TRH test produced abnormal results in 13.8% of all women, and in 20% of women with ovulation disorders or PCOS. These abnormalities were only detected by the TRH test. The researchers concluded with the recommendation that TRH stimulation testing be performed in women suffering from ovulation disorders, even in the presence of normal basal TSH levels.[41]

Local control: In addition to the HPT axis that controls thyroid hormone production, there is also control on a local and peripheral cellular level. This is mediated in part by the deiodinase enzymes (see next section). These enzymes are essential control points of cellular thyroid activity which determine intracellular activation and deactivation of thyroid hormones. Even when the more sensitive TRH test is normal, the thyroid hormone signaling system can be underactive due to changes in the local control of thyroid hormones. These changes can elude accurate evaluation of thyroid testing, including the TRH test, because the blood test can come out apparently normal or with subtle inexplicable abnormalities.

Remember that even at subclinical and subbiochemical levels, hypothyroidism can adversely affect critical target organs and systems, including the developing brain, the adult brain (observed in depression studies), and the cardiovascular system. (Among angina patients who underwent cardiac catheterization, those with TSH levels above 2.1 were more likely to have multiple vessel disease.)[42] Thus, it is vital to receive an accurate diagnosis of hypothyroidism.

LOCAL CONTROL: ROLE OF THE DEIODINASE ENZYMES

The deiodinase enzymes include Type 1 deiodinase (D1) and type 2 deiodinase (D2), which increase cellular thyroid activity by converting inactive T4 to the active T3. Type 3 deiodinase (D3) reduces cellular thyroid activity by converting T4 to the anti-thyroid reverse T3.[43] The activity of each deiodinase enzyme type changes in response to differing physiologic conditions. Moreover, local control of intracellular T4 and T3 levels results in different tissue levels of T4 and T3 under different conditions. Because the deiodinases determine *cellular* thyroid levels and not *serum* thyroid levels, serum thyroid levels may not necessarily predict thyroid tissue levels under a variety of physiologic conditions.

Although D1 converts T4 to T3, D1 is not a significant determinant of pituitary T4 to T3 conversion, which is controlled by D2. D1 (but not D2) is suppressed and downregulated in response to physiologic and emotional stress, inflammation, autoimmune disease, exposure to toxins, and chronic illness. This state is known as "sick euthyroid syndrome."[44] (Interestingly, tumor necrosis factor or TNF, a potent inflammatory mediator known to play an important role in inflammation associated with autism, is also a mediator in sick euthyroid syndrome.) Under these conditions, TSH levels are usually normal because D2 bound in the pituitary is not downregulated and therefore is a poor indicator of tissue thyroid levels.

As should by now be apparent, a complete definition of thyroid status requires more than the measurement of serum concentrations of thyroid hormones. For some tissues, the intracellular T3 concentration may only partly reflect concentration in the serum. Recognition that intracellular T3 concentrations in each tissue may be subject to local regulation, and an understanding of the importance of this process in the regulation of TSH production, should permit a better appreciation of the limitations of the measurements of serum thyroid hormones and TSH levels.

In children with autism, stress and inflammation may cause reverse T3 (RT3) to be high. RT3 blocks D1 and T4 to T3 conversion, blocks T3 from binding to receptors, and blocks the T3 effect. As the pituitary does not contain D3, and D3 is responsible for RT3 production, the pituitary will have normal levels of T3, and the TSH can be normal. Nonetheless, because children with autism are stressed emotionally and physiologically and are in an inflammatory state, they are likely to have low cellular thyroid hormone levels (that is, an underactive thyroid). However, because their blood tests may be normal, their low cellular TH levels frequently are overlooked. Only with a comprehensive understanding of how various environmental toxins can affect local control, and how physiological conditions such as stress and inflammation can alter thyroid control, can one correctly "read" thyroid blood tests.

OTHER BIOMARKERS OF HYPOTHYROIDISM

Several other biomarkers can signal the presence of hypothyroidism even with normal TSH and serum T4 and T3. In children with autism, one cannot rely on routine thyroid blood tests to determine if they have low T3 in peripheral cells, including the brain.

The first set of markers includes TNF, IL-1, IL-6, CRP, and other inflammatory markers; because these decrease D1 activity and reduce tissue T3 levels, if they are high, one should consider hypothyroidism.

Secondly, autoimmune disorders (including autism, which is associated with autoimmune antibodies) should raise a red flag for tissue hypothyroidism, even with normal serum TSH, T4, and T3.[45] In autoimmune conditions, there is a decrease in T4 to T3 conversion in the tissues, but in the pituitary the inflammatory cytokines will increase the activity of D2, suppressing TSH production.

Thirdly, high cortisol levels also downregulate D1 and increase D3 activity in peripheral tissues, while stimulating D2 in the pituitary. This will lead to a decrease in TSH yet low levels of T3 in peripheral cells.

EDCS, THYROID RECEPTOR RESISTANCE, AND ATYPICAL THYROID BLOOD RESULTS

EDCs may interfere with thyroid hormone signaling in a variety of ways. Some environmental chemicals alter TH signaling by selectively interfering with subsets of TH receptors. The consequences for brain development, then, may be a mosaic of effects on the nervous system. This is because different thyroid receptors mediate different actions of TH during development.[46] To make matters more confusing, many toxins cause thyroid signaling dysfunction by binding to receptors, leaving thyroid hormone levels and TSH normal in the serum. Toxins can also affect the thyroid hormone signaling system at multiple sites. Both yield blood test results that are difficult to interpret.

A number of endocrine-disrupting chemicals cause a decrease in serum and total and free T4 without a concomitant increase in TSH. One example is Aroclor 1254, which causes a significant decrease in serum T4 (total and free) but does not affect serum TSH or T3 levels.[47] BPA can also render thyroid blood tests difficult to interpret. BPA can selectively bind to thyroid receptors in the pituitary, leading to elevated serum

T4 and either normal or slightly elevated TSH.[47] In this scenario, all other thyroid parameters will be normal. BPA selectively antagonizes the TR beta receptor in the pituitary, which blocks T4 uptake by the pituitary. Low levels of T3 will result, causing the pituitary to produce and release higher levels of TSH and high T4 in the thyroid.

Certain dioxins can also produce high TSH levels and high levels of total T4. Because there are structural similarities between some dioxins and T4, the dioxins might interfere with transport of T4 into the cell, the conversion of T4 into T3, or binding of T3 to its nuclear receptor. In the pituitary, decreased nuclear T3 receptor occupancy will stimulate TSH secretion. This causes the thyroid to produce high levels of T4.

In a 2010 paper in *Hormones*,[47] Zoeller advises: "Because of the complex nature of the regulation of thyroid function and TH action, the consequences of EDC exposure are also likely to be complex and our ability to understand these effects as well as to screen for potential EDCs must consider this complexity." Importantly, Zoeller adds:

> *Animal studies are revealing both the complexity of the thyroid system and the complexity of the ways in which EDCs may interfere with TH signaling...The current clinical strategy of evaluating thyroid disease (i.e., measure blood levels of hormones, antibodies and proteins) is not sufficient to identify EDC actions on thyroid hormone signaling that may well be associated with disease in the human population.*

MY FINDINGS

Nearly three-quarters of children with autism have an underactive thyroid. Many children who are being treated for hypothyroidism are either on the wrong dose or not on the appropriate balance of T3 and T4. Treatment with thyroid hormones helps children with autism achieve improvements in:

- language
- cognition
- hyperactivity
- motor function
- sociability
- gastrointestinal function

SUMMARY

Research indicates that thyroid dysfunction due to endocrine-disrupting toxins likely plays a role, perhaps a significant one, in autism. Through the use of the more sensitive thyroid test (the TRH stimulation test), and with an understanding of local control of thyroid signaling, I have found that approximately seven out of every ten children with ASD have an underactive thyroid. Yet many children with autism remain undiagnosed and untreated for their hypothyroidism. Treatment with properly balanced thyroid hormones and a dose guided by the TRH test can help many of these children experience significant improvement. Some make a complete recovery.

HYPERBARIC OXYGEN THERAPY—LET'S PUT THE PRESSURE ON AUTISM FOR RECOVERY

By Dr. James Neubrander

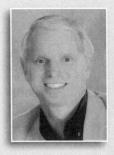

James A. Neubrander, MD, FAAEM

Road to Recovery Clinic
485A Route 1 South, Suite 320
Iselin, NJ 08830
(732) 726-1222
www.drneubrander.com

Dr. Neubrander trained in pathology and laboratory medicine and is board certified in Environmental Medicine. He is the Medical Director of the Road to Recovery Clinic in Iselin, NJ. He serves on many scientific advisory boards dedicated to treating autism and neurodevelopmental disorders. He frequently lectures at National and International Conferences and Physician Training Courses. His lectures are scientific, evidence-based, and emphasize newer treatments or modifications of established protocols that appear to enhance clinical outcomes beyond the results previously reported. He is the coauthor of several peer-reviewed articles, has been interviewed and filmed for many documentaries and television spots, has been referenced in many books written about autism, nutrition, and environmental medicine, and has been quoted innumerable times by scientists, researchers, clinicians, and lay persons, most notably for methylcobalamin, hyperbaric oxygen, and heavy metal detoxification.

Hyperbaric therapy, also known as hyperbaric oxygen (HBO) or hyperbaric oxygen therapy (HBOT), is a specialized therapy applying an increase in atmospheric pressure, with or without a concurrent increase in oxygen concentration, to incorporate more oxygen *onto* the red cells (very little increases are possible) and to dissolve more oxygen *into* body water: plasma, lymph, cerebrospinal fluid, interstitial fluid, etc. (significant increases are possible). This is accomplished by using specialized chambers, either *multiplace,* which treats many patients simultaneously, or *monoplace* in which only one person can be treated at a time.

Hyperbaric therapy is *classically defined* as the inhalation of 100 percent oxygen at greater than one atmosphere absolute (ATA) in a pressurized chamber. This definition is now *popularly defined* as the inhalation of varying degrees of oxygen at greater than one atmosphere absolute (ATA) in a pressurized chamber and referred to by the autism community as "HBOT."

Treatment pressures and oxygen concentrations are *always compared against values at sea level* where the pressure is one atmosphere and oxygen concentration is 21 percent. The basic principle of the gas laws states that the behavior of a gas is defined by the pressure, volume, temperature, solubility characteristics, and diffusion properties. In simple terms, the greater the pressure and/or the greater the oxygen concentration breathed, the more oxygen molecules that will be dissolved into the plasma. It is important to know that three factors are varied to achieve treatment protocols and clinical results for children with autism: a) how much pressure is applied, most commonly varying from 1.3 to 1.75 atmospheres; b) how strong the oxygen concentration is, most commonly varying from 24 percent to 100 percent; and c) how long the treatment session lasts, most commonly 1 hour to 1.5 hours per "dive" (the common term for a treatment). *Hyperbaric therapy is truly drug therapy* because too much is toxic, too little is ineffective, and the amount of time between dosing affects both its toxicity and effectiveness profiles.

Approved indications for HBO therapy do not include autism. They are intracranial abscess; anemia from severe blood loss; burns; carbon monoxide poisoning; compartment syndrome; decompression sickness (DCS); embolisms; gas gangrene; infections (refractory); injuries (crush, radiation); ischemia (acute and severe); wound healing, including skin flaps and grafts that are compromised. *Unapproved conditions* for HBO are many–autism being one. Each condition has shown HBO to be an effective adjunctive therapy as documented in published studies. Unfortunately, insurance companies rarely reimburse for these unapproved therapies.

The first known record for the use of hyperbaric therapy was in 320 BC, when *Alexander the Great* used a chamber that was submersed under water. In 1500, *Leonardo da Vinci* drew sketches of diving vessels but did not pursue the concept. In 1772, *Karl W. Scheele* discovered oxygen independently from *Joseph Priestly,* an amateur English chemist who in 1775 also discovered oxygen independently from Karl W. Scheele. Therefore, *Scheele and Priestley are both given credit* for its discovery. Priestly named it "dephlogisticated air." It was later renamed "oxygen" by *Antoine Lavoisier*.

In 1783, the French physician *Caillens* was the first doctor reported to use oxygen therapy as a remedy. In the mid-to late 1800s, the first severe problems with decompression sickness were seen in coal miners and caisson workers, many of whom died. In 1878, *Paul Bert* published *Barometric Pressure: Researches in Experimental Physiology,* describing caisson's disease and the bubble theory of decompression sickness (DCS) and oxygen toxicity. In 1889, *Moir* developed the first recompression chamber to treat DCS. In 1899, *Lorraine-Smith* described pulmonary oxygen toxicity. In 1921, *Cunningham* from Kansas City, Missouri built a 10-foot by 88-foot chamber that used compressed air to treat hypoxic states, hypertension, syphilis, cancer, and diabetes. This resulted in a successful challenge by the AMA in the 1930s. In 1928, *Henry Timken* from Cleveland, Ohio, built a six-story, seventy-two-room hyperbaric hotel, but the 1929 stock market crash caused the hotel to fail. Between the 1930s and 1940s, *Behnke* established oxygen tolerance limits for divers, which remain the basis for the oxygen recompression treatment tables still used today.

The recent history of hyperbaric medicine begins with *Boerema, the father of modern hyperbaric medicine.* In the late fifties, he filmed pigs, whose red cells had been removed, living with pure oxygen under hyperbaric conditions while only their plasma remained. This phenomenon was published in 1960 in *Life Without Blood.* In 1967, the *Undersea Medical Society (UMS)* was formed and considers itself to be the guardian of hyperbaric medicine. In 1977, *Davis and Hunt* published the first Hyperbaric Oxygen Therapy textbook.

The era of hyperbaric medicine for autism began in 2002 when *Heuser* published positive SPECT scan results from a four-year-old child with autism who had undergone HBO therapy. In 2005, though not directly related to autism, *Stoller* documented positive neurocognitive changes from hyperbaric oxygen therapy in a case of fetal alcohol syndrome sixteen years post injury.

The above two studies became the foundation upon which clinicians treating autism, at that time believed to be an untreatable "hard-wired" disorder, hypothesized that HBO may help their patients. In 2005, in an unpublished study, *Buckley and Kartzinel* described positive SPECT scan results and clinical findings after using low-pressure, low-oxygen concentrations in autistic children. From 2006–2009, *Rossignol* published several studies regarding HBO and autism. Included was the first double-blind placebo-controlled study from six centers (one of which was Neubrander's) that documented low-pressure, low-oxygen concentrations to be an effective treatment for autism. In 2007, at a Think Tank in California, *Neubrander* reported increased clinical responsiveness from a one-month *diagnostic protocol* he specifically designed for children with autism. In 2009, *Thatcher and Neubrander* published a paper which demonstrated, by quantitative EEG (qEEG) technique, the phase reset phenomenon that occurs in children with autism. Their study demonstrated that children with autism had a significantly *shortened* period of time for neuronal recruitment (*phase shift*) followed by a significantly *increased* amount of time necessary to process the information that was gathered (*phase lock*). Also in 2009, at a Think Tank in Chicago, *Neubrander* presented his preliminary findings demonstrating that his low pressure, low oxygen concentration "diagnostic protocol" and the standard high pressure, 100 percent oxygen protocols both began to correct the phase shift and phase lock abnormalities. The neuronal recruitment period was lengthened and the excessive processing time was decreased. However, at the same Think Tank, *Granpeesheh and Bradstreet* shared the findings of their double-blind, placebo-controlled study. Their study showed low-pressure, low-oxygen concentrations, similar to the ones used in the Rossignol study, to not be clinically significant. Those of us involved in the Rossignol study strongly disagree with their findings. It is my opinion that their study design was doomed to failure because its negative conclusion was based on children finishing 80 treatment hours over a 15 week period and not based on a uniform and specified number of treatment hours *per day* over a specified number of *consecutive weeks.* In their study some families could come in twice a week and do more hours on those days until they reached their 80 hour treatment total while other families could come in every day but only do one hour per day until they reached their 80 hour treatment total. This is analogous to saying "food doesn't work consistently to quench hunger" if one group of children would eat a lot of food but only twice a week while another group of children would eat less food but eat it every day. It is obvious that these two different groups of children would look and feel totally different after eating their 80 meals! In addition to my critique of their study, their findings do not reflect my clinical experience after closely monitoring over 800 children and 100,000 treatment hours for children with autism using the *specific protocols* I have designed for this important subset of the population.

When it comes to the use of hyperbaric oxygen for children with autism, parents don't really care much about definitions, history, philosophy, or our scientific debates. What they want is enough preliminary science to support its use and demonstrate its safety. Though *they prefer* double-blind, placebo-controlled, crossover studies, what *they require* is strong anecdotal evidence by other parents who have children just like theirs who face the same challenges that they face every day. *Their main concern is not whether* science has "dotted all its I's and crossed all its Ts" beyond a shadow of a doubt, *but rather* there be a treatment that has the potential of helping their child now, not at some distant point in the future. *Nor is their main concern whether or not* their doctor will support them, *but rather* have they attempted to do all they believe they could and should be doing before their child's window of opportunity permanently closes. *Contrary to the popular wisdom of an old paradigm,* parents who seek my colleagues' and my treatments are well-studied, well-read, and usually college-educated. They are definitely not a bunch of gullible, ill-informed lemmings, following charlatan Pied-Piper physicians who are just out to fleece them because they are desperate.

I could share *hundreds of stories of children who responded positively* to HBOT from my clinic. Should you be interested, you can see *videos of parents* talking about what HBOT did for their child at *www.drneubrander.com*. Though exceptions do occur, as a general rule, most children respond only mildly or mild-to-moderately within the first forty-hour treatment "set." However, HBO therapy, if continued intermittently for several cycles, is one of the most powerful treatments I have to induce language, increase awareness and cognition, and allow more normal socialization and emotional responses. As *an example of "a best-case scenario,"* consider two boys from different families who came to my clinic August 2007. One boy was eight years old and the other boy was eleven years old. Both boys spoke with only two or three word utterances, had little socialization, and engaged in parallel play with minimal to no interaction with peers. Thirty days later, both boys were speaking in six- to nine-word sentences, with adjectives, adverbs, prepositions, pronouns, and conjunctions. In addition, not only would they now participate in interactive play, they would initiate it with other children. *However, best-case examples do not paint the real picture* that most parents will experience if they try HBOT for their child. *The most common examples* I see in my clinic are initially reported by parents to *show mild or mild-to-moderate changes,* not moderate to significant ones. *The top twenty improvements* most commonly seen include positive changes in the areas of *language, eye contact, self-awareness, general awareness, independence, emotional responses, and gastrointestinal regulation.*

Success does not occur in a vacuum. In my experience, in order to increase the benefit-to-cost ratio, *pre-treatment with adjunctive therapies is required.* Those I use to accomplish this goal, prior to initiating HBO, require six to twelve weeks of *methyl-B$_{12}$ injections and key supplements.*

You ask, *"What are the risks?"* The worst-case scenario occurred in Florida late in the spring of 2009 when an *old* monoplace chamber ignited and fatally burned a child and his grandmother. In general, HBOT therapy, as done in the United States using up-to-date chambers that are not homemade, boasts an incredible safety record, with only this one incident having occurred in the last forty years. This includes chambers used in clinics and at home. When parents follow strict safety guidelines and receive prerequisite medical and technical training courses, like the ones we require at our clinic, contrary to what some organizations tell their patients and post on the Internet using scare tactics, portable HBOT chambers can be safely used in the home setting. This allows a valuable treatment to be ongoing rather than intermittent, and a treatment that becomes less expensive rather than more expensive over time for those who own their own chambers.

So, what are the real risks? *Barotrauma,* which occurs in 2 percent of individuals, is usually minor and analogous to "mildly spraining the eardrums." The risk of *seizures,* what parents worry about the most, increases by 0.01 percent to 0.03 percent. *Perforated eardrums* can occur when chamber operators pressurize or depressurize too quickly prior to the ears being able to "clear": The take-home message is that HBOT is as safe as flying in an airplane, when safety procedures are carefully followed.

There are many clinics in the country that will offer HBOT to children with autism. Hospitals will not offer this service because they are only allowed to use HBOT for the approved indications shown above. Private clinics do not have these restrictions, and are therefore more than willing to treat children with autism. Such clinics are not difficult to find by conducting a Google search. It is important to note that protocols from different clinics vary significantly. The variations include: 1) the pressures used, which vary all the way from 1.1 to 2.8 ATA; 2) whether oxygen is delivered by an oxygen concentrator or 100 percent pure oxygen or no oxygen at all; 3) the time used per session, commonly varying between sixty to ninety minutes; 4) the number of sessions used per day varying between one and two; 5) the time between sessions varying between two and twelve hours; 6) the frequency of treatments varying from once to twice per day; 7) and the number of treatment hours per treatment "set," most commonly forty hours but as high as ninety hours. Parents rightfully ask, *"What protocol or clinic is the best for my child?" The answer is, "No one knows."* Opinions abound. Clinicians do not agree. Unfortunately, the research needed to document that HBOT is a valuable treatment for children on the autism spectrum will require hundreds of thousands of dollars and no less than ten to fifteen years to complete and then to replicate prior to becoming an accepted practice that is reimbursable by insurance companies. Once that fact has been established, to determine which protocols are the most effective will require additional hundreds of thousands of dollars and an additional ten to fifteen years. Knowing that, *the last question parents must ask themselves is, "How old will my child be by then and what do I want to do in the meantime?"*

Therefore, parents wishing to investigate this treatment option for their children must be diligent in their research. They need to understand that the treatment is expensive and comes with no guarantees. If they want to do HBO, they need to look for a clinic that produces quality care, a clinic that has treated many children with autism, and a clinic that believes children with autism not only can be helped, but deserve to be helped *today*.

HBO references are hosted in the download section on Dr. Neubrander's website at www.drneubrander.com.

CEREBRAL FOLATE DEFICIENCY IN AUTISM SPECTRUM DISORDERS

By Dr. Richard E. Frye and
Dr. Daniel A. Rossignol

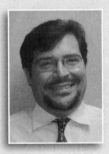

Richard E. Frye, MD, PhD

Arkansas Children's Hospital Research Institute
University of Arkansas for Medical Sciences
Slot 512-41B
Room R4041
13 Children's Way
Little Rock, AR 72202
Email: REFrye@uams.edu

Dr. Richard E. Frye received his MD and PhD in physiology and biophysics from Georgetown University. He completed his residency in pediatrics at University of Miami and residency in child neurology at Children's Hospital Boston. Following residency Dr. Frye completed a clinical fellowship in behavioral neurology and learning disabilities at Children's Hospital Boston and a research fellowship in psychology at Boston University. Dr. Frye also completed a MS in biomedical science and biostatistics at Drexel University. Dr. Frye is board certified in General Pediatrics and in Neurology with Special Competency in Child Neurology. Dr. Frye has been funded to study brain structure function in individuals with neurodevelopmental disorders, mitochondrial dysfunction in autism and clinical trials for novel autism treatments. Dr. Frye is the Director of Autism Research at the Arkansas Children's Hospital Research Institute and the Director of the Autism Multispecialty Clinic at Arkansas Children's Hospital.

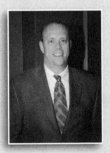

Daniel A. Rossignol, MD, FAAFP

Rossignol Medical Center
3800 West Eau Gallie Blvd.
Melbourne, FL 32934, USA

Dr. Daniel A. Rossignol received his MD at the Medical College of Virginia and completed his residency in family medicine at the University of Virginia. Coming from an academic background, Dr. Rossignol searched the medical literature looking for a solution after both of his children were diagnosed with autism. He has made it his mission to research and publish in autism. In the last six years, he has had twenty-three publications and three book chapters concerning autism and related conditions. Dr. Rossignol is a fellow of the American Academy of Family Physicians (FAAFP) and is president of the Medical Academy of Pediatric Special Needs (MAPS).

The importance of folate

Folate (vitamin B9) is a water-soluble B vitamin that is essential for numerous physiological systems of the body. Folate derives its name from the Latin word *folium*, which means leaf, to signify that the main natural source of this vitamin is from leafy vegetables. However, in the modern western diet, the main source of folate is from folate-fortified foods.

Some foods are fortified with folic acid, the inactive oxidized form of the folate compounds. The main active form of folate in the body is 5-methyltetrahydrofolate (5-MTHF). Folic acid is converted to dihydrofolate and then to tetrahydrofolate (THF) by the enzyme dihydrofolate reductase. This reaction, which requires niacin (vitamin B3), can be inhibited by certain medications. In addition, polymorphisms in the dihydrofolate reductase gene have been associated with autism. 5-MTHF is also converted to THF by the enzyme methylenetetrahydrofolate reductase (MTHFR). 5-MTHF is then converted back to THF through a cobalamin (vitamin B12) dependent enzyme called methionine synthase, a process that recycles methionine from homocysteine.

Folate is important for the de *novo* synthesis of purine and pyrimidine nucleic acids that are the molecules from which DNA and RNA are produced. DNA stores the genetic code and needs to be duplicated when a cell divides and replicates. Thus, folate is extremely important during cell replication, especially prior to birth during the development of the embryo and fetus. It is also essential during early life when cells are growing quickly. Folate deficiencies are related to errors in properly copying DNA during cell division and can increase chromosomal fragility.

The folate cycle interacts with the methionine cycle as well as the tetrahydrobiopterin production and salvage pathways. Deficiencies in folates can lead to abnormalities in these pathways. The methionine cycle is essential for the methylation of DNA, a process that is important in controlling gene expression. Tetrahydrobiopterin is essential for the production of nitric oxide, a substance critical for the regulation of blood flow, and for the production of the monoamine neurotransmitters, including dopamine, serotonin, and norepinephrine. Tetrahydrobiopterin is produced *de novo* using the precursor purine guanosine triphosphate, a substance that requires THF to be produced. Reactive oxygen species and the reactions which produce monoamine neurotransmitters result in an oxidation of tetrahydrobiopterin. One of the salvage pathways for reducing pterins in order to recycle tetrahydrobiopterin requires conversion of 5-MTHF to THF.

Several disorders have been linked to folate deficiency. For example, since blood cells need to be constantly replenished, a lack of folate commonly leads to anemia, an insufficiency of red blood cells. Folate deficiency during pregnancy can lead to fetal neural tube defects such as spina bifida.

Cerebral folate deficiency: A recently described neurodevelopmental disorder

One decade ago, Ramaekers and colleagues[1] described a new neurodevelopmental disorder called cerebral folate deficiency (CFD). They described five patients with normal neurodevelopment until four to six months of life. During the second half of the first year of life, these patients demonstrated developmental regression and progressively developed neurological symptoms, including irritability, cognitive slowing, unsteadiness, incoordination, cerebral palsy-like symptoms, visual loss, and seizures. Patients also demonstrated acquired microcephaly. 5-MTHF was found to be normal in the serum and red blood cells but was low in the cerebrospinal fluid. This new disorder was named CFD to describe the lack of folate specifically in the central nervous system.

Cerebral folate transporters

To understand CFD, it is necessary to understand that the central nervous system (CNS) is a protected area of the body. The blood-brain barrier highly regulates the entry of substances into the CNS. The active form of folate (5-MTHF) enters the CNS through one of two specialized blood-brain barrier transporters. The primary carrier uses a specialized folate receptor known as folate receptor α (FRα). Through this system, 5-MTHF binds to FRα, which is located on the apical side (blood vessel side) of epithelial cells of the choroid plexus. FRα then transports 5-MTHF to the other side of the cell where it is released into the CNS. This transport process requires energy in the form of an adenosine-5'-triphosphate (ATP) dependent mechanism. FRα is then recycled back to the apical side of the cell to pick up more 5-MTHF.

A secondary carrier of folate through the blood-brain barrier is the reduced folate carrier (RFC). The RFC has a lower affinity for folic acid and 5-MTHF than the FRα system but has a higher affinity for 5-formyltetrahydrofolate, also known as folinic acid or leucovorin. The RFC is also responsible for transporting 5-MTHF into neurons once it has entered the CNS.

If blood concentrations of folate are high enough, folate may also diffuse across the blood-brain barrier without a carrier.

Causes of cerebral folate deficiency

Ramaekers' group[1] examined the gene that encodes FRα to investigate whether or not genetic mutations accounted for dysfunction in the transport of 5-MTHF into the CNS but could not identify any such mutations. In 2004, Ramaekers and Blau[2] expanded their case series to 20 patients, none of whom were found to have a mutation in the FRα gene. However, these researchers did find non-functional FRα receptors in the patients' cerebrospinal fluid, leading to the hypothesis that some type of molecule, potentially an autoantibody, might be irreversibly binding to the FRα protein, causing it to become dysfunctional for binding folate. In 2005, Ramaekers and colleagues[3] identified high-affinity blocking autoantibodies against FRα in the serum of 25 of 28 children with CFD. These autoantibodies were not found in age-matched control subjects. More recently, Molloy and colleagues[4] described an additional blocking FRα autoantibody (termed a "binding" antibody).

In 2006, CFD was linked to mitochondrial disease in a case report of a child with an incomplete form of Kearns-Sayre syndrome.[5] Further case reports and case series later expanded the association between CFD and mitochondrial disorders to include complex I deficiency,[6] Alpers' disease,[7] and complex IV overactivity,[8] as well as a wide variety of mitochondrial disorders in both children and adults.[9] In most of these cases, the autoantibodies to FRα were not found, suggesting that it was the lack of ATP availability secondary to mitochondrial dysfunction that resulted in the impaired transportation of 5-MTHF into the CNS.

Cerebral folate deficiency and autism spectrum disorders

Seven of the 20 children portrayed in the second case series describing CFD were reported to have an autism spectrum disorder (ASD),[2] while five of the 28 patients first described to have the FRα autoantibody were found to have low-functioning autism with neurological features.[3] Further case reports[8,10] and case series[11,12,13] have expanded the description of CFD in children with idiopathic autism. Interestingly, Rett syndrome, a disorder considered to be a part of the diagnostic group of pervasive developmental disorders, has also been reported to have reduced 5-MTHF levels in the cerebrospinal fluid.[14,15]

Recently, Frye et al.[16] reported that 60 percent and 44 percent of 93 children with ASD were positive for the blocking and binding FRα autoantibody, respectively. This high rate of FRα autoantibody positivity was confirmed by Ramaekers et al.[17] who compared 75 ASD children to 30 non-autistic controls with developmental delay. The blocking FRα autoantibody was positive in 47 percent of children with ASD but only 3 percent of the control children. Overall, these reports suggest that early-onset low-functioning autism with neurological deficits may be characteristic of some children with CFD but that a wider group of children with idiopathic ASD may also be at risk for CFD and/or central folate abnormalities.

It should be noted that only some children with ASD who have CFD have been reported to possess FRα autoantibodies.[3,12] Because these reports of children with idiopathic ASD and Rett syndrome include children with and without the FRα autoantibody, this suggests that factors other than the FRα autoantibody might be important for the development of CFD in these children. Although not specifically investigated, it is possible that many children with CFD and idiopathic ASD or Rett syndrome who do not have the FRα autoantibody may have mitochondrial disease. Indeed, as previously noted, mitochondrial disease appears to be associated with CFD[5-9] and there appears to be an increased prevalence of mitochondrial disease in children with idiopathic ASD as compared to the general population.[18,19] At least one case series has linked children with mitochondrial disease and regressive-type ASD to CFD.[9] Interestingly, Rett syndrome has also been linked to mitochondrial abnormalities in both an animal model[20] and a case report.[21] To a lesser extent, children with idiopathic ASD might also manifest dysfunction of the mitochondria without necessarily fulfilling the criteria for strictly defined mitochondrial disease.[19] Thus, it is possible that mitochondrial dysfunction could contribute to the development of CFD in children with idiopathic ASD.

Diagnosing cerebral folate deficiency

Table 1 outlines the signs, symptoms and conditions associated with CFD. It is important to consider CFD in children with Rett syndrome or mitochondrial disease with or without ASD features. A combination of the neurological symptoms outlined in Table 1 that are not explained by a specific neurological condition should also prompt consideration of CFD. It is clear that CFD can present with atypical features. Thus, it is important to keep a high index-of-suspicion for this disorder in unexplained neurodevelopmental symptoms.

Table 1. When to Suspect Cerebral Folate Deficiency

- Low-functioning autism
- Mitochondrial disease or dysfunction
- Rett syndrome
- Epilepsy or seizures
- Abnormal electroencephalogram: subclinical electrical discharges or slowing
- Ataxia
- Microcephaly
- Dyskinesia: choreoathetosis, ballismus
- Pyramidal tract abnormalities
- Irritability
- Insomnia
- Delayed myelination
- Frontotemporal atrophy

Table 2 outlines the diagnostic workup for CFD. As shown in the table, it is important to begin by ruling out systemic deficiencies in folate or cobalamin that might cause symptoms similar to CFD (Step 1). Next, it is essential to test for FRα autoantibodies (Step 2).

If the FRα binding autoantibodies are discovered, it is important to investigate the function of other organs that use the FRα receptor for folate uptake to ensure that the antibodies are not the result of a more general autoimmune process (Step 3). It should be noted that because the reported relationship between FRα autoantibodies and cerebrospinal fluid levels of 5-MTHF is nonlinear, some individuals with FRα autoantibodies have normal levels of cerebrospinal fluid 5-MTHF.[13] If FRα autoantibodies are not found, it is possible that an underlying mitochondrial disorder might be resulting in secondary CFD. Thus, if CFD is still suspected despite negative FRα autoantibodies, screening for mitochondrial disorders using established guidelines[19] is recommended (Step 4). If the FRα autoantibody is detected or a mitochondrial disorder is diagnosed, a lumbar puncture may be required to confirm the diagnosis of CFD (Step 5).

A thorough workup should also measure levels of tetrahydrobiopterin because folate is essential in the production of this cofactor. As noted previously, deficits in tetrahydrobiopterin can lead to reduced production of the monoamine neurotransmitters. Interestingly, abnormalities in monoamine neurotransmitter metabolites have been reported in CFD[2,22] and may improve with folinic acid treatment. Neurotransmitter

---

Table 2. Diagnostic Workup for Cerebral Folate Deficiency

1) Rule-out systemic folate and cobalamin deficiency
   a) Serum folic acid level
   b) Serum cobalamin level
2) Test for FRα folate receptor autoantibodies
3) If FRα autoantibodies are positive:
   a) Test for dysfunction in other organs
      i) Thyroid function tests
      ii) Renal function tests
   b) Test for inflammatory disease
      i) Erythrocyte sedimentation rate
      ii) C-reactive protein
      iii) Antinuclear antibody
4) If FRα autoantibodies are negative or there are symptoms of mitochondrial disorders:[18]
   a) Test for mitochondrial markers[19]
      i) Fasting serum lactate, pyruvate, quantitative amino acids, ammonia, metabolic panel, liver function tests, creatine kinase, acyl-carnitine panel, carnitine panel, and CoQ10 level
      ii) Fasting urine organic acids

5)   If FRα autoantibodies are positive or mitochondrial markers are positive:
   a)   Consider lumbar puncture to confirm cerebral folate deficiency
   b)   Test cerebrospinal fluid for
      i)   5-MTHF
      ii)   Tetrahydrobiopterin
      iii) Neurotransmitters
      iv)   Neopterin
      v)   IgG index

metabolites in the cerebrospinal fluid should, therefore, also be measured during the lumbar puncture. Finally, because inflammatory conditions have been associated with CFD,[7] it is important to measure cerebrospinal fluid neopterin, a measure of inflammation, and an IgG index, a measure of intrathecal antibody production.

Unfortunately, a lumbar puncture is an invasive procedure that requires a specialist with significant experience to perform. For example, at many children's hospitals, an experienced neuroradiologist performs non-emergent lumbar punctures under general anesthesia with fluoroscopy guidance. In many cases, parents will not elect for their child to undergo such an invasive procedure and, in other cases, experienced personnel may not be readily available. Under these circumstances, empirical treatment with folinic acid or 5-MTHF can be a prudent option (see *Treatment of cerebral folate deficiency*). If empirical treatment is pursued, the patient should be closely monitored for behavioral and/or cognitive changes and side effects.

Treatment of cerebral folate deficiency

Treatments for CFD are outlined in Table 3. The first treatment used for CFD was folinic acid. This therapy, which has an excellent safety profile, has been shown to normalize cerebrospinal fluid levels of 5-MTHF in children with autism and CFD.[12] Reports have suggested that treatment with folinic acid has led to full control of epilepsy and resolution of brainstem, thalamus, basal ganglia, and white matter demyelination in a child with complex I deficiency,[6] resolution of neurotransmitter abnormalities,[2] and improvements in seizures, attention, motor skills, neurological abnormalities, verbalizations, preservative behavior, restricted interests, and social interaction in some children with autism.[3,10,11,12]

Recently, Frye et al.[16] reported that ASD children who were positive for at least one of the FRα autoantibodies demonstrated an improvement with 2 mg/kg/day of folinic acid treatment in two divided doses (maximum 50 mg daily) for an average of four months. Parents rated the intervention responses using a modified Clinical Global

Impression-Improvement subscale. These ratings were compared to a control group of ASD children who were awaiting test results but did not change any treatment over the same follow-up period. Children treated with folinic acid, as compared to the control group, demonstrated significant improvements in verbal communication, receptive and expressive language, attention, and stereotypical behavior with very few adverse effects.

Although typical doses of folinic acid range from 0.5-1 mg/kg/day in two divided doses with a maximum of 50 mg/day, some case reports have used doses as high as 4 mg/kg/day, especially in individuals with mitochondrial disorders. Therefore, some children may need higher levels of folinic acid. As described above, folinic acid enters the CNS through an alternative folate carrier known as the reduced folate carrier. Once it enters the CNS, folinic acid can particulate in the reactions that use THF. In these processes, folinic acid is converted to 5-MTHF, a step that requires cobalamin to be recycled to THF. Thus, it is essential that adequate levels of cobalamin be available when treating with folinic acid. As folic acid (the inactive, oxidized form of folate) can compete for the binding site on FRα, it is probably wise to discontinue the use of folic acid-containing supplements.

Interestingly, the human folate receptor cross-reacts with folate receptors contained in human, bovine (cow), and goat milk. In 2008, Ramaekers and colleagues[13] demonstrated that a cow's milk-free diet significantly reduced the level of FRα auto-antibodies and that re-exposure to milk significantly increased FRα autoantibodies. Furthermore, some of the children with autism were found to have marked or partial improvements in attention, communication, and stereotyped movements when placed on a milk-free diet. Interestingly, this provides compelling evidence that supports parental reports of improvements with a casein-free diet in some children with autism and supports previous studies suggesting gastrointestinal tract immune activation in children with autism.

Table 3. Treatments for Cerebral Folate Deficiency

- Discontinue drugs that can interfere with folate metabolism
- Start folinic acid at dose of 0.5 mg/kg/day in two divided doses and increase to 1-2mg/kg/day in two divided doses (maximum 50 mg/day)
- Consider cobalamin supplementation (vitamin B12)
- Stop folic acid supplementation
- Start a cow's-milk-free diet
- Monitor for changes in cognition and behavior
- Monitor adverse effects

Potential association of the cerebral folate antibody with birth defects

Several studies provide interesting and compelling evidence for a relationship between folate receptor autoantibodies and neural tube defects (NTDs). In 2004, for example, Rothenberg and colleagues[23] demonstrated that women from the United States with a current or previous baby with NTDs were more likely to have autoantibodies to the human placental folate receptor. In a larger study, Cabrera and colleagues[24] found that mid-gestation levels of both IgM and IgG autoantibodies to the human folate receptor collected from US women were associated with pregnancies complicated by NTDs. More recently, a study of Norwegian women by Bovies and colleagues[25] suggested that mid-gestation autoantibodies were specifically related to NTDs but not to oral facial clefts. Although another rather large study from Ireland (using previously frozen specimens not necessarily collected during pregnancy) did not find any difference between mothers who had a previous pregnancy with NTDs as compared with those without an affected pregnancy,[26] the prevalence of autoantibodies to FRα was very high in this population (approaching 35 percent), and the findings need duplication in populations where the prevalence is lower. Because these studies reflect important methodological differences (including whether or not autoantibodies were measured during pregnancy) as well as differences in national policies regarding dietary folate supplementation, further research is needed to define whether or not a relationship between folate receptor autoantibodies and NTDs truly exists.

Unanswered questions:

It is important to understand that because CFD has only been reported in case reports and case series, there may be a much wider variation in the symptoms associated with CFD. For example, children who do not have neurological symptoms or seizures will rarely undergo a lumbar puncture to look for CFD. This is especially true in autism, where there are diverse opinions regarding the disorder's medical basis. It is possible that many more children with ASD than are currently recognized may suffer from CFD, a treatable condition.

FROM PRECONCEPTION TO INFANCY: ENVIRONMENTAL AND NUTRITIONAL STRATEGIES FOR LOWERING THE RISK OF AUTISM

By Dr. David Berger

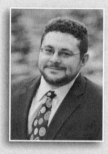

David Berger, MD, FAAP

Dr. David Berger is a board certified pediatrician who specializes in holistic pediatric primary care; nutritional and detoxification therapies for autism, ADHD, and related disorders; and immune dysregulation, such as allergies, asthma, and autoimmune disorders. Dr. Berger graduated from the Medical College of Pennsylvania in 1994. He has been in private practice since 1997, and in 2005 he opened Wholistic Pediatrics in Tampa, Florida. He has been an advanced practitioner of the philosophy formerly known as Defeat Autism Now! since 1999. In 2010, Dr. Berger was appointed to the position of assistant professor at the University of South Florida College of Nursing. Most recently, Dr. Berger became the vice president of the Medical Academy of Pediatric Special Needs. Please see www.medmaps.org and www.wholisticpeds.com.

INTRODUCTION

Autism spectrum disorders (ASDs) represent a cluster of neurobehavioral-developmental conditions characterized by varied levels of impairment in communication, behaviors, social interactions, and sensory integration. To date, no single medical hypothesis has adequately explained the increasing prevalence of ASDs as well as the wide range and intensity of symptoms. There is a growing belief in the medical world that ASDs have both genetic and environmental triggers, and there is growing interest in how the environment (both internal and external to the body) interacts with the genetic code as well as the various body organs to produce symptoms of ASDs.

At a glance, it is obvious that ASDs cannot have a purely genetic cause. There are multiple documented cases of identical twins where one child is severely affected by autism, while the other twin is neurotypical and indistinguishable from his or her peers. I have seen identical twins where one child received multiple courses of antibiotics while the other did not, and the antibiotic-exposed child (but not the unexposed twin) is now on the autism spectrum. I have also seen identical twins where one child received vaccines in accordance with the recommended schedule and subsequently developed signs of being on the autism spectrum, while the other twin did not receive early infant vaccines at 2 or 4 months of age due to illness at time of check-up and remained unaffected by autism. On the other hand, genetics play some role. It is well known that there is an increased prevalence not only of ASDs but also of allergies, asthma, and autoimmune and hyperinflammatory conditions in children for whom there is a family history of such conditions. Families with such histories may be particularly interested in strategies to prevent these conditions in their future children.

The purpose of this review article is to explore how environmental exposures and nutritional factors may play a role in the development of ASDs in children. This implies that there are also certain precautions and steps that may be taken to minimize the risk of having a child who develops an ASD (and other chronic/disabling medical conditions). These measures include avoidance of environmental exposures and implementation of nutritional testing and optimized nutrition. Since I began using these strategies 10 years ago with families, to the best of my knowledge, not a single child born into my medical practice has gone on to develop an ASD. Furthermore, of the more than 500 patients who joined my practice at birth, none have developed diabetes, just one has developed asthma, and only one family (of 3 children) has developed recurring ear infections.

Some of the recommendations listed below are not specific to and may have never been studied in relation to ASD. However, strategies intended to decrease antibiotic exposure, *Candida* development, and the incidence of allergies, asthma, and autoimmune diseases likely are relevant to lowering the incidence of autism as are strategies to increase cognitive development and optimize nutrition.

PRECONCEPTION AND PREGNANCY

Many families of ASD children have asked me throughout the years if there are things that they could do even prior to conception to decrease the likelihood of having another child develop an ASD. Few formal studies have looked into this issue, and with so many different variables in play, it would be very difficult to perform good research on this. Nonetheless, the approach I have taken over the past 10 years seems to be successful.

To the best of my knowledge, I have not had any subsequent siblings develop an ASD, although the incidence in siblings has otherwise been documented to be high (about 1 in 6)[1] when compared with 1 in 88 for the general population.[2] Most of the concepts that I take into account when evaluating and treating a woman prior to conception are similar for women who are pregnant. Factors that I consider both preconceptionally and prenatally are summarized in Table 1 and described in greater detail in the rest of the article.

Genetic Factors

Although there are genetic abnormalities that have been associated with ASD, no genes have been identified that are present in even close to a majority of children with ASD (and most of these gene tests are not commercially available). For example, the abnormal gene sequence found between the cadherin 9 and 10 protein on chromosome 5, which was widely reported in 2009, was only present in 15% of children with ASD.[3] Fragile X is present in about 2% of children with autism.[4,5] While this incidence of fragile X in ASD children is significantly higher than the 1 in 4000 males who carry the full fragile X mutation and the 1 in 1000-2000 who carry the premutations,[6] it still represents a very small percentage of children with autism.

Genes involved with methylation and transsulfuration (see Figure 1), the pathway that breaks down homocysteine and produces glutathione, may contribute to autism. Genes code for various enzymes, and these genes and enzymes often have the same name. Cystathionine β-synthase (CBS) is the enzyme that metabolizes homocysteine to cystathione, and methionine synthase (MS) is the enzyme that converts homocysteine back to methionine. CBS and MS genes may play a role in the abnormal biochemistry that can be observed in ASD, although most labs do not run these tests.

Table 1.
Preconceptional and prenatal considerations in autism prevention

Concept	Examples
Genetics	Genetic mutations Methylation/transsulfuration pathway Maternal single nucleotide polymorphisms (SNPs)
Cellular environment	Maternal nutrition Toxic exposures (i.e., bisphenol A)
Nutrition-related	Celiac disease Gluten and casein opioid peptides Maternal allergies
Intestinal flora	Candida Clostridia
Heavy metals	Mercury (thimerosal, amalgams, and environmental) Lead
Thyroid health	Hypothyroidism Thyroid autoantibodies
Nutrients	Vitamin D Iron Folate Calcium Omega-3 fatty acids

MTHFR (methylenetetrahydrofolate reductase), the enzyme that converts 5,10-methylenetetrahydrofolate to 5-methyltetrahydrofolate (a substrate in the homocysteine-to-methionine methylation reaction), is commercially available at most labs. As abnormal nucleotide sequences have been associated with fetal miscarriage[7,8] and cardiovascular disease,[9,10] MTHFR has become a particularly useful test.

The biochemical abnormalities that can occur due to these atypical genes may be at least partially overcome with the use of methylcobalamin (M-B12) and activated folate (folinic acid or L-methylfolate).[11] Supporting the methylation/transsulfuration pathway with proper B vitamin supplementation may be particularly important for a mother of a child with ASD as parents of children with autism have often been found to have similar abnormal biochemical markers to those of the children.[12] Interestingly, one study found that mothers of children with autism were less likely than those of typically developing children to report having taken prenatal vitamins during the 3 months before pregnancy or the first month of pregnancy.[13] Significant interaction effects were observed for maternal MTHFR 677 TT, CBS rs234715 GT + TT, and child COMT 472 AA genotypes. Children were 4.5 times more likely to be diagnosed with autism if their mothers had the homozygous MTHFR C677T single nucleotide polymorphism (SNP) (SNPs are DNA sequence variations) and 7 times more likely with the COMT SNP.[13] Because of the greater risk for autism when mothers did not report taking prenatal vitamins, the authors suggest that the B vitamin component of prenatal vitamins may protect against fetal brain development deficits.

Although vitamins for pregnancy are referred to as "prenatal," for an optimal pregnancy I propose the use of "preconceptional" vitamins, a product still under development. While waiting for a preconceptional product to become available, I suggest that women start taking prenatal vitamins prior to getting pregnant to ensure that adequate nutrition is provided from the moment of conception. A recently identified concern about multivitamins, in general, however, is the possibility that chromium, an essential mineral, could be present in its carcinogenic chromium VI (hexavalent chromium) form.[15] Unfortunately, most manufacturers do not test for the different forms of chromium to make sure that the hexavalent form is not present. I would, therefore, ask the manufacturer if they are testing for and rejecting hexavalent chromium and only use companies that do this.

Epigenetics and the Cellular Environment

An emerging hypothesis for potential causes of ASDs is related to epigenetics. An epigenetic trait is a stably heritable phenotype resulting from changes in a chromosome without alterations in the DNA sequence.[16] The environment within the cell can affect the way that genes are expressed. An example of this is found in Prader-Willi and

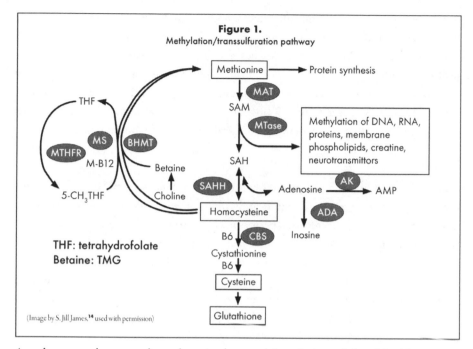

Figure 1.
Methylation/transsulfuration pathway

THF: tetrahydrofolate
Betaine: TMG

(Image by S. Jill James,[14] used with permission)

Angelman syndromes, where there is abnormal imprinting of the ubiquitin protein ligase E3A (UBE3A) gene.[17] In fragile X syndrome, the epigenetic effects result in a CGG-repeat expansion that triggers hypermethylation and silencing of the FMR1 gene.[18] I expect that in coming years, research will reveal specific alterations in the cellular environment that lead to these epigenetic changes. Ultimately, epigenetics may be the map that explains how the body and its environment interact in a manner that prevents or causes disease. While this is being figured out, we already know enough to minimize toxic exposures and enhance maternal nutrition to give cells an optimal environment in which to develop and reproduce.

Nutritional Issues

Certain laboratory tests that can be run on a woman preconceptionally or during pregnancy may be helpful in providing the information needed to support an optimal fetal environment. I often run a celiac panel because untreated celiac disease can cause nutritional deficiency.[19] And, although not well studied in humans, mammalian studies have suggested that celiac disease could increase intestinal permeability (leaky gut), which could, in turn, permit gluten-based opioid peptides and other toxins to gain access to the maternal bloodstream[20,21] and, thus, the fetus. In addition to testing for celiac disease, I often also test for the presence of opioid peptides derived from gluten and casein. Just as we would not want to have morphine or other pharmacological opiates present during fetal development, I presume that opioids derived from foods containing these two proteins could also have a negative effect on the developing fetus.

Circulating maternally derived antibodies may have a negative impact on the future health of children. The intake of foods that a woman is allergic to during pregnancy may increase the risk of allergy in the offspring.[22] Taking this into account, performing maternal IgE and IgG antibody testing for various foods and avoiding those foods during pregnancy may bring an immunological advantage to the child later in life.

Candida

As many families who have explored biomedical treatments for ASD have discovered, controlling *Candida* (yeast) can significantly reduce many of the symptoms of autism. Unfortunately, most of the research performed by gastroenterologists has yet to support these clinical findings. Nonetheless, especially for women who have a significant history of frequent antibiotic exposure or recurring yeast infections, I test for the presence of *Candida* species using stool microscopic evaluations and cultures as well as the urine Organic Acids Test. If the woman is not pregnant, I often treat with systemic antifungal medications (fluconazole, ketoconazole, itraconazole, or terbinafine), probiotics, and dietary control (low-carbohydrate diet or Specific Carbohydrate Diet™).

I do not use most systemic antifungal therapies during the first two trimesters of a pregnancy. However, the oral form of the antifungal medications nystatin and amphotericin B are not absorbed into the bloodstream, meaning that both can be considered safe to use orally at any point during pregnancy. Systemic amphotericin B is the antifungal medication that has been most studied during pregnancy. It is in the FDA's pregnancy risk category B (the second safest category but only recommended for use during pregnancy when the benefit outweighs the risk), and there have been no reports of fetal abnormalities from its use, even when administered intravenously.[23] Fluconazole is the most studied azole antifungal medication during pregnancy; abnormal fetal development has been seen at high doses (> 400 mg/day) but not at lower doses (150 mg).[24] Because herbs that are used to treat *Candida* have not been studied, in general, I avoid these during pregnancy.

Clostridia

Multiple species of clostridia bacteria have been implicated in contributing to symptoms of ASD. Elevated levels of a measurable clostridia metabolite, HPHPA, have been found in some individuals with autism and schizophrenia; use of a treatment appropriate for eliminating clostridia (vancomycin) reduced HPHPA levels and simultaneously improved symptoms.[25] Treatments for clostridia that are safe to use during pregnancy include *Saccharomyces boulardii* and certain strains of lactobacillus. Vancomycin oral capsules are a FDA risk category B pregnancy medication.

Environmental Exposures

Bisphenol A (BPA) has received wide media attention due to the concern about it being a hormone disruptor. Most baby bottles that are now produced are BPA free, and some states are banning its use in all baby feeding containers. BPA is used in many different products to harden plastics. It also can be found in or on tin can linings, dental sealants, and cash register receipts. It is believed that BPA is an estrogen hormone disruptor, and there is mounting evidence that exposure during pregnancy may lead to negative outcomes. Prenatal BPA exposure has been linked to aggression in 2 year olds[26] as well as anxiety, depression, and poor emotional control in girls.[27] Avoidance of BPA-containing products is the best strategy to minimize the impact of BPA on a fetus or young child.

There are many other substances that women and young children are exposed to that are raising concerns. For years, Dr. Stuart Freedenfeld of Stockton, New Jersey, has taught us about these chemicals and how they can negatively impact health. He points out that phthalates are used in various plastic products to give them flexibility and durability. Phthalates are also used in various medications as coatings for capsules as well as to stabilize and suspend certain liquid medications. There are concerns that phthalates may disrupt hormone and energy metabolism. Flame retardants in children's clothing and furniture contain antimony (a toxic metal) as well as polybrominated diphenyl ethers (PBDEs) that are similar in structure and toxicity to PCBs and dioxin. These substances can concentrate in dust, and children can either ingest or inhale them. We are exposed to pesticides both through our food supply as well as on the lawns and parks where our children play. These pesticides damage energy production, interfere with enzyme activity, and can interfere with methylation, sulfation, and digestive enzyme function. These are but a few of the thousands of chemicals that people are exposed to that have never been adequately tested, especially when people are exposed to them in combination. Dr. Freedenfeld talks in more detail about daily exposures in the home, such as cleaning products, and environment at his website www.stocktonfp.com.

Heavy metals such as mercury and lead are well established to be toxic to fetuses and young children, and all efforts should be made to minimize exposure in these populations.[28,29] Although there is no consensus on what defines increased heavy metal exposure or toxicity, I recommend that a woman consider performing a single dose chelation challenge with baseline urine metal testing *prior to getting pregnant* to determine if heavy metals are present. If there is a significant increase in heavy metals following this single dose, I would recommend that she consider chelation therapy with the agent that brought about the increased metal excretion. Chelation therapy should *not* be used during pregnancy, however.

Vaccines that contain thimerosal (a mercury compound), such as certain flu shots, should not be given to pregnant women. Consumption of fish that have significant mercury levels should also be avoided. (A list of the mercury levels in commercial fish and shellfish is available at the US Food and Drug Administration website.[30]) Women found to have high levels of mercury and who have amalgam (50% mercury) fillings should consider having the fillings replaced (except during pregnancy), but this should only be done by a dentist who is knowledgeable and experienced in safe removal procedures. Improper amalgam removal can lead to increased mercury exposure. Living in close proximity to coal-fired power plants also can increase exposure to mercury. An increased incidence of autism has been associated with communities that have high levels of mercury-releasing coal plants[31,32] (see Figure 2).

Hypothyroidism

Testing for hypothyroidism is one of several other tests that I perform before and during pregnancy, with correction of the abnormality if present. Hypothyroidism is a known cause of developmental delay in children,[33] and thyroid hormone is also a growth factor for fetuses and young children.[34] The prevalence of hypothyroidism in pregnant women has been estimated at 5%, and thyroid autoantibodies can be seen in 12% of pregnant women.[35] My personal observation is that the actual percentages are

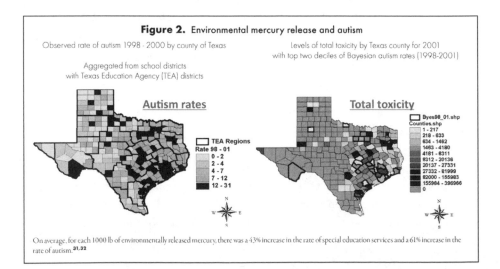

Figure 2. Environmental mercury release and autism

Observed rate of autism 1998 - 2000 by county of Texas

Aggregated from school districts with Texas Education Agency (TEA) districts

Levels of total toxicity by Texas county for 2001 with top two deciles of Bayesian autism rates (1998-2001)

Autism rates

TEA Regions
Rate 98 - 01
0 - 2
2 - 4
4 - 7
7 - 12
12 - 31

Total toxicity

Byes98_01.shp
Counties.shp
1 - 217
218 - 633
634 - 1462
1463 - 4180
4181 - 8311
8312 - 20136
20137 - 27331
27332 - 81999
82000 - 155983
155984 - 396966
0

On average, for each 1000 lb of environmentally released mercury, there was a 43% increase in the rate of special education services and a 61% increase in the rate of autism.[31,32]

higher. Women with true hypothyroidism and those with positive antibodies (especially those with consistently low basal body temperatures under 97°F) should receive consideration for thyroid hormone supplementation and be closely monitored during both pregnancy and lactation.

Vitamin D

Vitamin D has long been established to be essential for bone health, and emerging evidence is showing its importance for proper immune development. Children born to women who are low in vitamin D have an increased incidence of allergies and severity of asthma[36] and a greater incidence of type I diabetes.[37] The Vitamin D Council has hypothesized that vitamin D deficiency may be contributing to the increased incidence of autism.[38] Most recently, in *Pediatrics*, Whitehouse et al. demonstrated a link between maternal vitamin D insufficiency during pregnancy and offspring language impairment at 5 and 10 years of age. In the study, women with 25-hydroxyvitamin D levels under 18 ng/ml were twice as likely to have a child with language impairment when compared with those above 33 ng/ml. The Vitamin D Council recommends that pregnant women get their level of 25-hydroxyvitamin D (the storage form of vitamin D, also called calcidiol) above 50 ng/ml and suggests a dose of 5000 IU of vitamin D3 a day for pregnant women who cannot get their level checked.[39]

Iron

Iron is an essential mineral not only for the production of hemoglobin, but it also may affect a person's cognitive function. While a low hemoglobin level (anemia) is one indicator that a patient may be iron-deficient, a low blood ferritin level (<30 ng/ml) is a better early indicator of low iron stores.[40] Iron deficiency without anemia has been associated with autism,[41] attention-deficit/hyperactivity disorder (ADHD),[42] and lower math scores in children.[43] Correcting non-anemic iron deficiency has been shown to correct verbal learning and memory[44] as well as symptoms of ADHD.[45]

During pregnancy, a hemoglobin level under 10.5-11.0 g/dl (depending on trimester) is considered anemia. When I document that a woman has a low ferritin level, I try to correct the level to above 50 ng/ml.[40] During pregnancy, 40 mg of elemental iron per day is usually sufficient to prevent iron deficiency,[46] and doses of between 60-120 mg are recommended if there is already iron deficiency present.[40] Some forms of iron can cause intestinal discomfort and constipation, especially during pregnancy. I find that iron in the ferrous bisglycinate chelate form is best tolerated by the GI tract and has very good absorption. Iron absorption can be enhanced if taken at the same time as vitamin C but should be taken away from thyroid hormone supplementation. I have also found that using a cast iron skillet for pan frying and sautéing can increase food's iron content.

Folate

Folate is known to be essential for fetal brain development. Folate deficiency has been associated with spina bifida and other neural tube defects. All pregnant women should get a minimum of 400 mcg of folic acid daily. However, because women who have the abnormal *MTHFR* gene sequence may not be able to efficiently complete the conversion of folic acid to methylfolate, they may have issues if taking only folic acid. In such cases, I recommend that women not take folic acid but rather L-methylfolate or folinic acid or possibly a combination of both. These two forms bypass the faulty MTHFR enzyme and provide the fetus with activated folate.

Another potential complication of faulty folic acid metabolism is cerebral folate deficiency (CFD) and the presence of cerebral folate receptor antibodies. CFD has been associated with low-functioning autism, mitochondrial disease or dysfunction, Rett syndrome, epilepsy or seizures, and an abnormal electroencephalogram.[47] While this disorder is not something that I routinely check for in all preconception or pregnant women, testing for the presence of folate receptor 1 antibodies may be indicated if there is a significant family history of any of the above conditions. If CFD is identified, folic acid should be stopped and high doses of activated folate (i.e., folinic acid or L-methylfolate) taken, working up to 25 mg twice a day.[47]

ADDITIONAL CONSIDERATIONS DURING PREGNANCY

Beyond folate, iron, and vitamin D, there are two additional nutrients (calcium and omega-3 fatty acids) that I focus on with pregnant women to ensure that there are no deficiencies.

Calcium

Adequate calcium intake is essential for bone growth and long-term health. A pregnant woman should take between 1000-1200 mg daily. If a woman is avoiding dairy, this may be difficult to accomplish through the diet, and calcium supplementation may be needed. As lead has recently been found to be present in some calcium supplements, it is essential to use supplements from manufacturers who are testing for lead and rejecting calcium raw materials that have increased amounts of lead. (This means verifying that the manufacturer is screening for lead in the raw material or in each batch produced.) When taking calcium supplements, I suggest that women also take magnesium in a 2:1 ratio of calcium to magnesium.

Omega-3 Fatty Acids

Omega-3 fatty acids are essential for brain and cardiovascular development and growth. The DHA form of omega-3 fatty acid (available in certain sea algae and other marine sources but not plant-based sources of omega-3 fatty acids) is the one that is best utilized by the developing brain. It is recommended that pregnant and lactating women take at least 300 mg per day of DHA,[48] and some studies have suggested that significantly higher doses may be even more beneficial. Children of mothers who took 3.3 grams of combined EPA and DHA during pregnancy demonstrated greater hand-eye coordination,[49] and children of mothers who took about 2 grams of combined EPA/DHA (as 2 teaspoons of cod liver oil) had increased mental processing.[50] Fish oil supplementation during pregnancy has also been associated with lower potential for allergies and possibly other immune-mediated diseases.[51,52]

BIRTH AND POSTNATAL CONSIDERATIONS

An increased prevalence of autism has been identified in children born by both emergency and elective cesarean section (C-section).[53] It is logical to suspect that when an emergency C-section is performed due to fetal distress, this stress could be related to a lack of blood flow to the fetal brain that could lead to brain injury with resulting autism symptoms. Because the prevalence of autism is also higher with elective C-sections, however, all efforts should be made to avoid C-sections whenever possible. Although many women are told that they need to have a C-section if they had a previous C-section, the American Congress of Obstetricians and Gynecologists (ACOG) recently declared, "Attempting a vaginal birth after cesarean (VBAC) is a safe and appropriate choice for most women who have had a prior cesarean delivery, including for some women who have had two previous cesareans."[54]

I instruct parents that a baby is not considered past due until after 42 weeks. There is no reason to artificially rush the delivery of a baby before the baby and placenta indicate that it is time for delivery. If there is any concern, an ultrasound can be performed to ensure that the baby is healthy and not under stress. Induction of pregnancy itself may have a negative role on a child's development. In one study, there was almost a 2-fold increase in ADHD diagnosis in children born to mothers who were induced.[55]

Some families express concern about exposing their newborn to the antibiotic ointment that is placed in newborns' eyes soon after delivery. This is used specifically to prevent neonatal infection from sexually transmitted diseases (STDs) such as chlamydia and gonorrhea that can be contracted during passage through the birth canal. Therefore, this has to do with the STD status of the mother. (It should be remembered that these STDs can be asymptomatic or missed on vaginal screening.) While I am not overly concerned about a topical one-time exposure to an antibiotic (using a route that would not have an effect on the baby's intestinal flora), it is the case that the ointment may cause chemical irritation or interfere with the initial eye contact and bonding that happens when the mother is first holding the baby. Parents should evaluate the pros and cons and decide what they think is best for their baby.

Vitamin K is routinely administered by intramuscular injection soon after birth. This is done to prevent a rare newborn condition called hemolytic disease (a condition where the baby's blood cannot clot and the baby has a hemorrhage). The injected form does not contain thimerosal. Deficiency in vitamin K can cause the hemorrhagic condition in about 1 in 10,000 births, and the bleeding can occur up to 12 weeks after birth. For families who have concerns about the injected form of vitamin K, there are protocols available for its oral use from the Canadian Pediatric Society,[56] the Pediatric Society of New Zealand,[57] and the Australian government.[58]

Babies are routinely given the first dose of hepatitis B vaccine on the first or second day of life. I discuss vaccines at greater length below. Many parents question why they should give a newborn a hepatitis vaccine at birth if the mother tests negative for the virus during pregnancy and babies do not engage in activities that would spread hepatitis B. While the administration of the vaccine along with hepatitis B immunoglobulin may be effective in preventing the acquisition of hepatitis B in babies born to infected mothers, all pregnant women should have been tested for hepatitis B, meaning that their infection status should be known at the time of delivery. If the mother is not infected with hepatitis B, I see little benefit to vaccinating a baby for this at birth.

After birth, I advocate for discharging mother and baby from the hospital as soon as possible. Hospitals are known to harbor higher levels of certain infections (such as *Candida*, methicillin-resistant *Staphylococcus aureus* [MRSA], and clostridia) than most of the outside world, including most people's homes.

INFANCY

Breastfeeding

The importance of breastfeeding is now universally accepted. The American Academy of Pediatrics (AAP) recommends that babies be breastfed for at least the first year of life, and longer if desired by the mother and baby.[59] Babies who are breastfed have been suggested to have higher IQs and cognitive development[60,61] and a lower incidence of type 1 diabetes,[62] allergies (when compared with cow's milk and soy formulas),[63] asthma,[64] and ear infections.[65] Babies who receive cow's milk-based formula may have increased intestinal permeability (leaky gut) when compared with babies who receive breast milk,[66] especially if they were born prematurely.[67] Although some families express concern about feeding any form of milk to their babies due to the casein content, the amino acid composition of human milk is different from that of cow's milk.[68] For these and other reasons, I encourage adherence to the AAP breastfeeding recommendations.[59]

Babies who are breastfed are provided antibodies through the milk to fight off infection within hours of a mother being exposed to a virus or bacteria. This can protect the baby against a host of different pathogens that could otherwise lead to the baby being exposed to antibiotics. Another advantage of breastfeeding is that a mother who continues to optimize her nutrition (as already discussed with regard to pregnancy) provides the nutrients to her baby through the breast milk.

Introduction of Solid Foods

Infants who are fed solid foods too early are prone to developing food allergies. In general, the American College of Allergy, Asthma, and Immunology recommends that solid foods not be introduced until 6 months of age, with dairy products introduced at 12 months, eggs at 24 months, and peanuts, tree nuts, fish, and seafood not introduced until at least 36 months of age.[69] For younger siblings of children on the autism spectrum, I also recommend waiting at least until 1 year of age before introducing gluten. When foods are finally introduced, only small amounts should be offered for the first few days, and one new food should be introduced every 4 days to watch for negative reactions.

Vaccines

Much controversy surrounds the potential connection between vaccines and ASD. I find it interesting that pediatricians routinely tell parents that to prevent an undesirable immune reaction (allergies) they should wait six months to introduce a foreign substance (food) to their baby and advise parents to give foods one at a time to watch for reactions, yet recommend that vaccines be given starting at birth (hepatitis B) and continuing with another 21 antigens given simultaneously at 2 months of age: diphtheria, tetanus, pertussis, 3 strains of polio, 13 strains of pneumococcus, *Haemophilus influenzae* type b (HiB), and rotavirus. This displays a significant disconnect between pediatricians' feeding and vaccine advice.

In my pediatric practice, I follow the true meaning of informed consent, explaining vaccine benefits, risks, and alternatives to families so that they are fully and meaningfully informed when making their decision. Ultimately, parents have both the right and responsibility to make medical decisions and decide what is best for their child. They can choose to give vaccines according to the recommended Centers for Disease Control and Prevention (CDC) schedule, or they can split vaccines, delay them, or not give any at all. The AAP recommends that pediatricians listen carefully and respectfully to parents' concerns about vaccines, convey respect for continued refusals that follow adequate discussion,[70] and not discharge families who refuse vaccination from their pediatric practice. Notwithstanding these recommendations, almost 40% of pediatricians said they would not provide care to a family that refused all vaccines, and 28% said they would not provide care to a family that refused some vaccines.[71]

Although thimerosal is a known neurotoxin with no natural biological role, concerns about vaccines go beyond the mercury in vaccines. With the exception of flu shots and tetanus vaccine (DT has trace thimerosal and tetanus toxoid may have the full 25 mcg of mercury), thimerosal was removed from most vaccines in the early 2000s, yet the prevalence of autism has continued to climb. One possible explanation is that exposure to injected antigens from vaccines can cause undesirable immunological effects with or without the presence of mercury. The diseases that children are vaccinated against (with the exception of tetanus and hepatitis B) are not contracted in the natural world through injection but through the respiratory tract or the gastrointestinal (GI) tract, and, therefore, the immune system's first line of defense, which sets in motion the rest of the natural immune response, is bypassed. Both of these systems (respiratory and GI) have specific white blood cells and antibodies residing on their surface that serve as a first line of defense against invading organisms. The injection of vaccines prompts an artificial immune response. Abnormal shifts in white blood cells following vaccination were suggested to be the reason why children who were given the DTwP vaccine (note that this had a different form of pertussis antigen than the current vaccine and did contain thimerosal) at 2 months of age were significantly more likely to develop asthma than children who did not start receiving this vaccine until 4 or 6 months of age.[72] The authors of this study hypothesized that the vaccinations can be viewed as promoters of asthma development, perhaps by stimulating a Th2-type immune response and shifting the cytokine balance.[73] They also note that at birth the newborn immune system has a limited ability to produce Th1 cytokines, but levels increase over the next 6 months.[74]

More research is warranted to examine possible subtypes of autism relative to vaccine exposure and vaccinated versus unvaccinated children. Nonetheless, existing medical literature makes it clear that a role between autism and vaccines is biologically plausible. To cite a few examples:

- Some children with ASD have been found to have mitochondrial dysfunction.[75] In the case of Hannah Poling, the United States Court of Federal Claims decided that there was enough evidence to show that vaccines may have aggravated her mitochondrial disorder and triggered problems consistent with autistic-like behavior.[76] Some people even argue that vaccines can be the trigger for secondary mitochondrial issues.[77]

- Vaccines are documented to have the potential to induce autoimmune diseases,[78,79] and although rare, MMR vaccine has recently been associated with immune thrombocytopenic purpura.[80] As a subset of children with ASD has documented autoimmunity against the brain,[81-83] it is plausible that vaccines could induce auto-immunity against the brain with resulting symptoms consistent with autism.

- Large epidemiologic studies have been published that found statistically significant evidence to suggest that boys in the United States who were vaccinated with the triple series hepatitis B vaccine during the time period in which vaccines were manufactured with thimerosal were more susceptible to developmental disability than were unvaccinated boys.[84] In addition, a study based on vaccine records suggests that US male neonates vaccinated with the hepatitis B vaccine prior to 1999 had a threefold higher risk for parental report of autism diagnosis when compared with boys not vaccinated as neonates during that same time period.[85]

CONCLUSION

There is considerable interest in developing strategies to try and prevent autism, especially for families who are at higher risk by having one child on the spectrum already. In this article, I reviewed a variety of possible strategies that can be considered beginning at the time of preconception and beyond. These include supporting the methylation/transsulfuration pathway with proper B vitamin supplementation; avoiding or minimizing toxic exposures (including BPA and heavy metals); enhancing maternal nutrition (including supplementation, as appropriate, with vitamin D, iron, folate, calcium, and omega-3 fatty acids); assessing maternal food allergies and intolerances; screening for maternal hypothyroidism; controlling maternal fungal and bacterial infections; breastfeeding newborns and introducing solid foods with care; and carefully weighing the pros and cons of postnatal interventions including vaccines. Further study is warranted to examine the issues raised in this review article so that we can determine if the prevalence of autism can be reduced by correcting imbalances and insults that can occur preconceptionally, during pregnancy, and during early childhood.

TETRAHYDROBIOPTERIN METABOLISM IN AUTISM SPECTRUM DISORDER

By Dr. Richard E. Frye

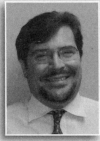

Richard E. Frye, MD, PhD

Arkansas Children's Hospital Research Institute
University of Arkansas for Medical Sciences
Slot 512-41B
Room R4041
13 Children's Way
Little Rock, AR 72202
Email: REFrye@uams.edu

Dr. Richard E. Frye received his MD and PhD in physiology and biophysics from Georgetown University. He completed his residency in pediatrics at University of Miami and residency in child neurology at Children's Hospital Boston. Following residency Dr. Frye completed a clinical fellowship in behavioral neurology and learning disabilities at Children's Hospital Boston and a research fellowship in psychology at Boston University. Dr. Frye also completed a MS in biomedical science and biostatistics at Drexel University. Dr. Frye is board certified in General Pediatrics and in Neurology with Special Competency in Child Neurology. Dr. Frye has been funded to study brain structure function in individuals with neurodevelopmental disorders, mitochondrial dysfunction in autism, and clinical trials for novel autism treatments. Dr. Frye is the Director of Autism Research at the Arkansas Children's Hospital Research Institute and the Director of the Autism Multispecialty Clinic at Arkansas Children's Hospital.

Tetrahydrobiopterin (BH_4) is a naturally occurring substance that is an essential cofactor for several metabolic pathways, including those responsible for the production of monoamine neurotransmitters, tyrosine, and nitric oxide as well as the breakdown of phenylalanine. Abnormalities in all of these metabolic pathways have been reported in individuals with autism spectrum disorder (ASD). In addition, deficiencies in central nervous system BH_4 concentration have been reported in individuals with ASD. Over the past twenty-five years, a limited number of clinical trials have reported encouraging results with BH_4 treatment for children with ASD.[1]

General role of tetrahydrobiopterin in metabolic systems

BH_4 is a naturally occurring pterin with a heterocyclic pteridine structure.[1] Biologically important pterins include BH_4, biopterin and neopterin, but BH_4 is the only biologically active pterin. BH_4 is synthesized *de novo* from the purine Guanosine-5'-triphosphate (GTP). BH_4 is a cofactor for several enzymatic reactions. Three aromatic amino acid hydroxylases, phenylalanine-4-hydroxylase, tyrosine-3-hydroxylase, and tryptophan-5-hydroxylase, use BH_4 as a cofactor in the production of monoamine neurotransmitters. These enzymes catalyze the conversion of phenylalanine, tyrosine, and tryptophan to tyrosine, L-dopa, and 5-hydroxytryptophan, respectively. These products of the hydroxylase enzymes are further converted into neurotransmitters: L-dopa is converted into dopamine, which is further converted into norepinephrine; 5-hydroxytryptophan is converted into serotonin. In this process, BH_4 is converted into 7,8-dihydrobiopterin, which can be recycled to BH_4 through a salvage pathway catalyzed by dihydropteridine reductase or dihydrofolate reductase, folate independent and folate dependent pathways respectively. BH_4 is essential in the production of nitric oxide, an important second messenger molecule used primarily for communication in vascular and neural tissues. In this reaction, nitric oxide synthase uses L-arginine and oxygen to produce L-citrulline and nitric oxide. Normally BH_4 is recycled locally during this reaction. However, in the context of low BH_4 levels, this reaction becomes uncoupled resulting in a consumption of BH_4 and the production of a peroxynitrite, a toxic reactive nitrogen species, instead of nitric oxide.

Abnormalities in BH_4 synthesis or recycling cause specific neurological syndromes. Type IV phenylketonuria (PKU), also known as hyperphenylalaninemia, is characterized by elevated phenylalanine levels in the blood at birth and represents the minority of PKU cases. Severe intellectual disability can result if phenylalanine levels are not reduced early in life. BH_4 appears to be effective for treating this type of PKU. BH_4 deficiency can also result in dopamine-responsive dystonia, a neurological disorder that demonstrates a wide range of symptoms and ages of presentations that is characterized by dystonia with diurnal variation.

Tetrahydrobiopterin deficiency in autism spectrum disorder

The concentration of BH_4 in the cerebrospinal fluid (CSF) has been reported to be 42 percent lower in children with ASD as compared to neurotypical children. A central BH_4 deficiency appears to be prominent in ASD children younger than seven years old. This younger group also demonstrated a reduction in total pterins and biopterin, essentially indicating that the deficit in BH_4 was not due to a synthesis or recycling deficit but a problem with the general availability of pterins.[2]

There is evidence that metabolic pathways that consume and recycle BH_4 are dysfunctional in children with ASD.[3] First, inflammation and immune system overactivation has been reported in ASD. Nitric oxide, which is a key mediator of inflammation and immune system response, is produced by a BH_4-dependent reaction. Thus, BH_4 could be depleted by this immune system overactivation and excessive inflammation through an excessive production of nitric oxide. Second, folate-dependent BH_4 recycling using dihydrofolate reductase may be reduced in ASD as several abnormalities in folate metabolism are found in individuals with ASD. Third, since BH_4 can act as a superoxide radical scavenger, it may be depleted in the setting of high oxidative stress states, such as those seen in children with ASD. Lastly, in the setting of low levels of BH_4 nitric oxide synthase becomes uncoupled, resulting in the production of a toxic reactive nitrogen species and BH_4 is not recycled. This depletes BH_4 in two ways as BH_4 is used up in the reaction and may act as an antioxidant to reduce oxidative stress caused by the reactive nitrogen species produced. A recent clinical study suggests that this BH_4-related abnormality in nitric oxide metabolism may be one of the major predictors of response to BH_4 supplementation in children with ASD.

Clinical trials of tetrahydrobiopterin for autism spectrum disorder

The first case studies of BH_4 treatment in children with ASD were conducted by Japanese researchers almost three decades ago[4]. Two boys with ASD, one seven-year-old and one five-year-old, were treated with 1-2.5 mg/kg/day of BH_4.[5] The seven-year-old showed marked improvement in hyperactivity, mood lability, and stereotypic behaviors; both boys showed moderate improvement in general autistic symptoms. Over a six-year period, from 1985 to 1990, four Japanese researchers treated over 300 mildly to severely affected autistic children in five open-label studies and one double-blind placebo controlled study.[4-12] Response was measured as the percentage of children who demonstrated moderate or marked global improvement. Treatment with oral BH_4 at a dose of 1–3 mg/kg/day over 4–24 weeks resulted in a response rate of 41 percent to 64 percent. Two additional clinical studies, one double-blind placebo controlled crossover and one open-label, were conducted by Swedish researchers using an oral BH_4 dose of 3 to 6 mg/kg/day.[13,14] More recently, an open-label biomarkers study and a double-blind placebo controlled study in the United States using much higher doses of BH_4 (20 mg/kg/day in one daily dose) has provided further support for improvement in ASD symptoms with BH_4 supplementation.[15,16]

Only a few clinical trials have examined the biological basis of BH_4 supplementation. Two Swedish clinical trials and one clinical trial from the United States measured CSF BH_4 concentrations. Fernell et al[14], Danfors et al[13] and Frye et al[15] treated children with CSF BH_4 concentrations of less than 12, 30 and 30 nM/L respectively. Danfors et al[13] found a borderline significant correlation between CSF BH_4 concentration before treatment and improvement in social interactions on the CARS (Childhood Autism Rating Scale) with BH_4 treatment. While Fernell et al[14] demonstrated that CSF BH_4 concentration increased by an average of 63 percent with treatment, the study did not correlate initial or final CSF BH_4 concentration with behavioral variables. Frye et al[15] did not find a correlation between CSF BH_4 concentration and improvement in behavioral or cognition.

Fernell et al[14] examined functional CNS changes with treatment. Using positron emission tomography, BH_4 treatment was shown to decrease the baseline elevation in D_2 receptor binding found in children with ASD. The authors suggested that BH_4 treatment resulted in a normalization of dopamine metabolism in children with ASD.

Frye et al[15] examined biomarkers of monoamine neurotransmitter, pterin, nitric oxide and redox metabolism as well as immune activation in ASD children treated with BH_4 in an open-label fashion. They found that baseline nitric oxide metabolism was highly predictive of whether and to what extent the participants responded to BH_4 treatment and that the responders to BH_4 supplementation demonstrated a greater increase in the reduced-to-oxidized pterin ratio, a key parameter which controls nitric oxide synthase uncoupling, as compared to non-responders.

Sapropterin

Daiichi Asubio Pharma was the first to develop a synthetic BH_4 for clinical use called Biopten Granules 2.5% (sapropterin) which was approved in Japan in 1992. BioMarin developed Kuvan® (sapropterin dihydrochloride) which is a synthetic preparation of the dihydrochloride salt of naturally occurring tetrahydrobiopterin (6R-BH_4 or BH_4). Kuvan® has the same active ingredient as Biopten and is approved by the Food and Drug Administration of the United States of America for BH_4-responsive PKU.[1]

Safety of Sapropterin

More than a decade of market experience with Biopten in Japan has established that it is generally safe.[1] Clinical trials have exposed more than 1100 human participants to sapropterin formulations at various dosages mostly ranging from 5–20 mg/kg/day. Kuvan® appears to be well-tolerated in healthy volunteers, in subjects with PKU, and in subjects with hypertension. The reported adverse effects in studies on children with ASD include sleep disruption, excitement, hyperkinesias, aggression, urinary frequency, gastroesophageal reflux, and loose stools. However, these adverse effects are reported in a minority of patients and sapropterin is usually well-tolerated in children with ASD.[1]

Potential for Sapropterin as a novel therapy in autism

Clinical trials suggest that treatment with BH_4 results in improvement in autism symptomatology in some children with ASD. Many of the clinical trials have used different doses of BH_4 ranging from 1–20 mg/kg/day, so the exact dose is not known. In addition, the exact biological mechanism of action of BH_4 in children with ASD is not clear. Children with ASD clearly have abnormalities in many biological systems that use BH_4 —this may be a reason why it might be an effective treatment for ASD. One particularly positive characteristic of BH_4 is that it appears to be safe without serious adverse effects.

OBSERVING THE AUTISM BRAIN WITH REAL-TIME IMAGING: THE ROLE OF TRANSCRANIAL ULTRASOUND (TUS) IN AUTISM, WITH IMPLICATIONS FOR THE BRAIN-IMMUNE SYSTEM LINK IN AUTISM AND AN EXPLORATION OF INTERVENTIONS

By Dr. James Jeffrey Bradstreet

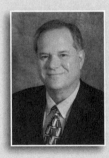

James Jeffrey Bradstreet, MD, MD(H), FAAFP

Director of the Brain Treatment Center of Atlanta
Adjunct Professor, Western University of Health Sciences, CA
104 Colony Park Drive, Suite 600
Cumming, GA 30040-2793
470-253-7445
DrBradstreet@aol.com

Dr. James Jeffrey Bradstreet, received his medical degree from the University of South Florida in Tampa and his residency training at Wilford Hall USAF Medical Center in Texas. He is widely published on the various aspects of autism-related biology and comorbidities and is a member of the American Academy of Toxicology as well as a Fellow of the American Academy of Family Physicians. Dr. Bradstreet is an adjunct professor of pediatrics at Southwest College of Naturopathic Medicine in Tempe, Arizona, and is licensed in Georgia, Florida, California, and Arizona. Both his son and stepson have autism spectrum disorders and have experienced significant recovery as a result of intensive biomedical interventions. Dr. Bradstreet's interests include the interactions between the immune system and the brain, stem cell therapies, and the relationship of vitamin D to macrophage activation and viral pathogens. Using new techniques, he has been able to see significant progress for some of the most challenging cases. Please visit www.drbradstreet.org.

First, a confession. I am quite obsessed with understanding the function of the autism brain and what regulates it. Chances are very good you are, too, since you are reading this chapter. By the time this reaches the publisher, my son with autism will leave his teenage years behind and turn 20, while my stepson with autism will reach 13 years of age. Those two boys shape my daily mindset about this disorder and drive my passion for answers.

The number of those of us who are personally affected by loving someone with autism (parents, siblings, grandparents, and close family members) is growing daily. Autism has exceeded affecting 1 percent of children in many nations, and there is no apparent lessening of the growth in prevalence of this tragic disruption of normal childhood development.

As I write this chapter, it is late December, and on Christmas Eve I received my early present from *Frontiers in Human Neuroscience:* my original research on transcranial ultrasound has been accepted (Bradstreet et al., 2014). The topic of this research was inspired and co-authored with Professors Ruggiero and Pacini from the University of Florence in Italy. Prof. Dr. Marco Ruggiero has become a dear friend and colleague over the past few years as our efforts to help children with autism has synergized thanks to a special protein related to immune regulation, GcMAF (Gc macrophage activating factor), which is a form of VDBP (vitamin D binding protein).

Marco and I had shared several telephone discussions about autism, but we finally met in Frankfurt, Germany, in early 2013. During a conference on various novel technologies, he presented his observations of real-time brain imaging via transcranial ultrasonography. If you have had a baby in the last 35 years, then you are already familiar with ultrasound, which is the technology doctors use to image the baby inside the womb. Ruggiero pioneered a new methodology using a linear probe to view the brain in real-time: TUS. It was amazing to observe the dynamic living brain as it changed with each heartbeat. TUS gives us unprecedented insight into certain aspects of the autism brain and its surrounding structures: the meninges.

Ruggiero first published his observations with his team from the University of Florence ("Firenze" for my Italian friends) in 2012 in *Medical Hypothesis.* Subsequently, the TUS anatomical observations were accepted by the *Italian Journal of Anatomy and Embryology* in 2013 (Figure 1).

The bright white image under the temporal muscle is the cranium. The subarachnoid space is visualized as a small gap under the meninges and bordered by the cerebral cortex (brain).

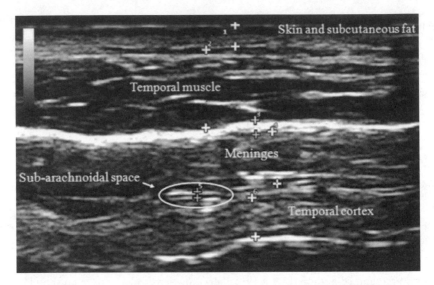

Figure 1 Italian Journal of Anatomy and Embryology: *Volume 188 (3), 2013.*

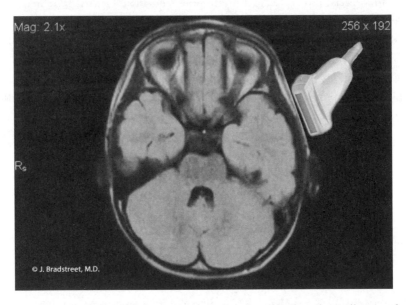

Figure 2 The relationship of the cortex and the ultrasound probe is illustrated with the superimposition of a scaled image of the linear probe and its relationship to the temporal boney window used to look inside the skull at the brain.

At Ruggiero's urging, I obtained a Sonosite ultrasound machine attributable to the kindness of a grant from the Newport Brain Research Laboratory. After obtaining ethical approval and registration with the NIH website (www.clinicaltrials.gov), we proceeded to look at the brains of children with autism and their neurotypical siblings. Ultrasound of the brain is considered safe when used at the frequencies and durations noted in our study and on the clinical trials website. What we found was remarkable. Before I tell that story, however, we need a little bit more background.

For several years, the UC Davis MIND Institute has been performing serial MRI brain imaging studies on the siblings of children diagnosed with autism. In the summer of 2013, they published their findings electronically in the esteemed journal *Brain*. Ruggiero and I were very excited about their observations because they were very consistent with our own early findings.

To help you understand, I am excerpting a figure from that paper (Shen et al., 2013) in order to illustrate their findings. The paper is in open access on the publisher's website, and I encourage you to download the entire study.

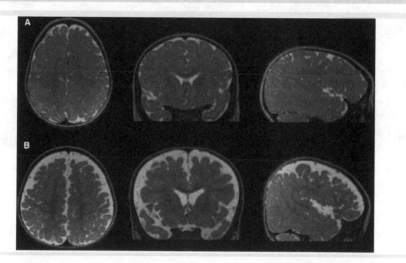

Brain and fluid volume in infants with ASD   Brain 2013: 136; 2825–2835 | 2829

Figure 3 (This is Figure 2 from Shen et al., 2013, and it demonstrated a remarkable amount of fluid excess [white signal] around the brain of Child B, but not that of Child A. Child A will not go onto to develop autism, but Child B will. Both have older siblings diagnosed with autism.)

We quickly realized the TUS methodology could image this fluid easily in a mere few moments of time. The findings were dramatic. Neurotypical siblings had no excess of fluid, while all (to date) of their autistic siblings had increased fluid between the arachnoid membrane and the surface of the brain. To properly categorize the observations, we created a criteria whereby we would measure the distance between the arachnoid membrane and the pia (covering of the brain) at the gyral summits. Now what are gyral summits? If you look at the image from the Shen 2013 paper, you will see folds in the brain, and the summits are where the brain comes very close to the skull. You will notice Child A has all gyral summits in very close proximity to the skull, indicating the subarachnoid cerebral spinal fluid is squeezed out of the space and the arachnoid and pia are nearly in contact with each other. In all of our observations of neurotypical siblings, the distance remaining for fluid to occupy between the brain and the meninges was less than 0.05 cm and often below our ability to measure it with ultrasound.

In contrast to this, importantly, with the entire autism associated population *that space was larger.* In this next image, the difference between these fraternal twins is obvious. [Note: the images above from Shen et al., (2013), use an imaging process that makes the EAF look white. In contrast, the TUS image of EAF is dark or black].

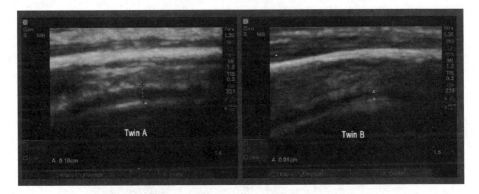

Figure 4 This is Figure 13 from Bradstreet et al., 2014. *Twin A with autism demonstrates a significantly increased extra-axial fluid space (EAF) [in the range of 0.11 - 0.16 cm measured at various locations -Sonosite zoom view]. In contrast with his autistic brother, neurotypical Twin B has an obvious narrowing of the EAF at the gyral summit (0.01cm) Sonosite zoom view. Twin A appears to have a somewhat thicker temporal bone; despite this, the image quality is very good. Both images are of the Broca-associated expressive language area of the left frontal cortex.*

In Figure 4, it is apparent that there is a lack of compression of the subarachnoid space – EAF in the autistic twin. Normally, the arachnoid membrane compresses due to the gyral summit of the brain squeezing it against the inside of the skull. As the arachnoid structures compress, there is a corresponding loss of volume in the subarachnoid – EAF space. In Twin A, the hydrostatic pressure of the EAF is sufficient to resist the natural compression effect of the gyral summit approaching the inside of the skull. In contrast, the EAF space of the neurotypical twin is observed to compress to a mere thin film of remaining fluid: this is typical of non-autistic subjects regardless of age, and we have observed narrowing of the summit EAF in apparently healthy children as young as 6 months of age.

So what does this extra fluid mean, and, more importantly, what do we do about it?

To answer that critical question, we need to look at the growing body of evidence encompassing the observations of immune dysregulation in many – perhaps most – individuals with autism. For this discussion, let's reference the work of Gesundheit et al. from 2013. In a review paper titled *Immunological and autoimmune considerations of Autism Spectrum Disorders,* the authors (a virtual who's who of immune research in autism) created a model of maternal immune interaction with the child during development in the womb (Figure 5).

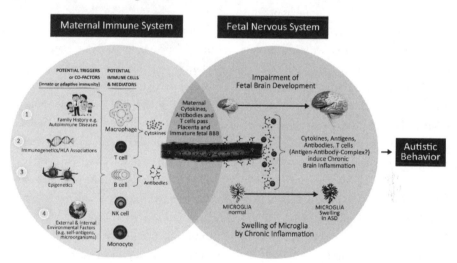

Figure 5 J Autoimmun. *2013 Aug;44:1-7. doi: 10.1016/j.jaut.2013.05.005. Epub 2013 Jul 15. Review.*

In this diagram of the *in utero* interactions of the maternal immune system with the fetal brain, chemical immune messengers (cytokines and antibodies) pass through the placenta and readily cross the poorly formed fetal blood–brain barrier. The net effect is microglial (residential immune cells of the brain) activation and disruption of brain function and development. With all respect for the authors' efforts, missing from the diagram are the postnatal environmental factors (toxins, infections, vaccines, gut microbiome, etc.) on the developing brain of the infant after birth. Without a complex review of the literature, let me propose here that there is an abundance of data supporting the postnatal environment in at the least the further progression of autism-related symptoms. I recently co-authored an article reviewing the epigenetic (biological influences unrelated to mutations of genes) factors influencing the development of the autism phenotype (expression of autism symptoms) (Siniscalco et al., 2013). A more complete discussion of those issues can be found in that open-access article.

Professor Theoharides from Tufts University has published numerous articles describing the potential role of mast cells in autism. Mast cells are derived from bone marrow stem cells which express CD34 surface markers. They are distinct from macrophages and microglial cells in their immune regulatory roles but have related embryogenesis linked to hematopoietic stem cells. Microglial cells are derived from macrophages that migrate out of the blood system into the brain during fetal development. They are responsible for coordination of neuronal migration and regulate the final structural development of the brain, and, as such, it is hard to underestimate their potential role in the development of autism.

What most people, including most physicians, don't know about both microglial cells and macrophages is that they exist in three primary functionally different states. What this means is that a microglial cell/macrophage can only be defined by its form and function. The primary states are: amoeboid, ramified, and activated. Amoeboid microglial cells are capable of migrating throughout the central nervous system. They are responsible for repair and development of the brain. Ramified microglial cells are resting and exist in the healthy state as caretaker cells for neurons that assist in the protection from oxidative stress and environmental toxins. Activated microglial cells have two states: phagocytic and non-phagocytic. The phagocytic state signifies responding to damage and death of neurons and actively removing cell debris. It has been theorized that it is the activated microglial which contribute to developmental abnormalities and symptoms seen in autism.

Mast cells interact and communicate with microglial cells and macrophages in a number of complex and incompletely understood ways. Mast cells in the meninges are now felt to result in increased risk of migraine. Equally, there is evidence of mast cell dysregulation in autism as proposed by Theoharides and colleagues. At this point, we speculate that mast cells, macrophages, and microglial cells are communicating in the meninges and the brain via immune chemical messengers and that the consequence of this immune conversation is the opening of the endovascular tight junctions in the brain blood vessels and the meninges. These effects would help explain the persistence of increased fluid surrounding the autism brain (Shen et al., 2103 and Bradstreet et al., 2014), and the remarkable sensitivity they experience to environmental influences, particularly gut-immune-brain factors.

Now, what can be done about this after the development of autism symptoms? Unpublished laboratory observations from the University of Florence research team on the vitamin D binding protein subtype known as GcMAF (MAF stands for macrophage activating factor) may give us some answers if these observations can be translated to both animal and human models. Those researchers found the vitamin D-related protein converted activated microglial cells to the ramified resting state as opposed to activating them. This is a very encouraging observation. So, rather than the misunderstood misnomer of MAF (implying it causes inflammation), it is actually a microglial and macrophage regulatory and counter-inflammatory factor.

Recently, at the Second World Conference on GcMAF, physicians from the United States, Turkey, Italy, Jordan, and Dubai presented their own observations and videos of how autistic children respond to GcMAF. It was an impressive and touching event; the conference was held on the first anniversary of the publication of my observations regarding GcMAF and autism (Bradstreet et al., 2012), and it was good to see this work bear fruit for the benefit of children. The worldwide positive cumulative experience of GcMAF in autism is over 4000 children at present, and none of the physicians report any significant adverse effects.

Theoharides and his colleagues (2012) have also found that luteolin (a natural anti-oxidant and anti-inflammatory found in celery, broccoli, green pepper, parsley, thyme, chamomile tea, carrots, olive oil, peppermint, rosemary, navel oranges, oregano, and more) has beneficial effects on behaviors of children with autism. In the laboratory, luteolin has dramatic effects insofar as stabilizing mast cells so they hold onto their immune chemistry and don't release it unnecessarily. The ease at which autism- related mast cells release their immune regulators is a presumed principle component of the brain-immune axis of dysfunction (Theoharides et al., 2007, and Conti et al., 2013).

I recently participated in a review paper of stem cells as an autism intervention (Siniscalco et al., 2013). In that article we wrote: "The development of molecular and regenerative interventions is progressing rapidly, and medicine holds great expectations for stem cell therapies. Cells could be designed to target the observed molecular mechanisms of ASDs, that is, abnormal neurotransmitter regulation, activated microglia, mitochondrial dysfunction, blood-brain barrier disruptions, and chronic intestinal inflammation. Presently, the paracrine, secretome, and immunomodulatory effects of stem cells would appear to be the likely mechanisms of application for ASD therapeutics." In addition, I would now add, "and potentially target abnormal meningeal immune dysregulation."

In summary, autism is a complex disorder with various epigenetic influences that likely has its roots in an early (within the womb) priming immune process related to maternal-fetal interactions. The presence of increased fluid around the brain observed by Shen et al. (2013) and which we also have observed persists as measured using transcranial ultrasonography, implying that the immune mechanism remains active long after birth of the at-risk infant. The treatment of this fluid will require carefully designed studies to understand; however, TUS is one rapid, safe, and cost-effective method of screening for this condition and its possible responsiveness to immunological therapies. GcMAF, luteolin, and, perhaps, stem cells, offer potential areas of future research.

CHLORINE DIOXIDE'S ROLE IN HEALING AUTISM

By Kerri Rivera

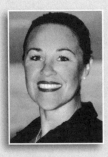

Kerri Rivera

Kerri Rivera is mom to two sons, with 13-year-old Patrick currently recovering from autism. In 2005, at the request of Dr. Bernard Rimland, Kerri translated what was formerly known as the Defeat Autism Now! protocol to Spanish so that it could be applied throughout Latin America, and she was trained as a Defeat Autism Now! clinician. Since then, Kerri has worked one-on-one with families throughout the world to help them improve the lives of their children on the autism spectrum. As of November 2013, her protocol was being utilized in over 57 countries, and since the addition of CD (chlorine dioxide) to her biomedical protocol, 110 children have lost their autism diagnosis.

An international lecturer, Kerri is the biomedical consultant for Curando El Autismo (Latin America) and Venciendo el Autismo (Venezuela) and the Liaison to Mexico for AutismOne. Kerri holds a diploma in homeopathy. Her book *Healing the Symptoms Known as Autism* details her protocol and includes many testimonials from families using the protocol as well as from families of recovered children. For more information about this book, please visit www.CDAutism.org.

*I*t is astounding to note that over one hundred children who were once considered on the autism spectrum dropped so many ATEC score points in such a relatively brief amount of time as to be considered off the spectrum—just by using an inexpensive item that is able to be utilized safely. Parents worldwide have reported their children's amazing results with joy, having renewed hope after having tried many other modalities. This item is called chlorine dioxide (CD).

Why would CD help autism? Autism is pathogenic in origin. Let me say that again because it is a completely different way to understand this problem we label "autism."

Autism is pathogenic. It is connected with the presence of bacteria, yeast (*Candida*), heavy metals, viruses, and parasites. In fact, parasites accumulate, propagate, and excrete bacteria, viruses, and yeast. Parasites build biofilm (extracellular polymeric substances) nests that harbor layers of heavy metals and other toxins, and they drill holes in the intestines,[1,2] while eating nutrients intended for our children and excreting chemicals (malondialdehyde, ammonia, histamine, formaldehyde, and morphine) into our children's bodies.[3]

What is chlorine dioxide?

Chlorine dioxide is an inexpensive, broad spectrum, gentle, anti-pathogenic oxidizer. A few years ago, I started using it with my own child in a synergistic combination with healthful diet and a parasite remediation protocol, after which I shared my experience with other parents. As of November 2013, over 100 children on the CD protocol had lost their autism diagnosis (i.e., as defined as having an ATEC [Autism Treatment Evaluation Checklist] score of 10 and below), and thousands more have made documentable improvements. The CD protocol brings HOPE for RECOVERY!

Technically defined, chlorine dioxide (ClO_2) is a gas produced by combining two liquids: sodium chlorite ($NaClO_2$) and a weak acid, most commonly citric acid ($C_6H_8O_7$) or hydrochloric acid (HCl). The addition of the acid to sodium chlorite brings the combined pH level to under 5, which destabilizes the sodium chlorite and causes the release of chlorine dioxide—an oxidizer with an oxidation potential of 0.95V.

Chlorine dioxide is an antibacterial, antiviral, and antifungal. CD is patented, among other things, for use as an antiseptic, for treatment of burns, and to stimulate the immune system.[3] In addition to patents, there are many products in the US marketplace, approved by the FDA that contain chlorine dioxide in their ingredients.[3] Furthermore, the FDA has approved the use of chlorine dioxide for disinfecting fruits and vegetables, and requires it in all meat-packing plants.[4]

Why chlorine dioxide for autism?

Children with autism nearly always have the following in common, all of which contribute to the behavioral issues that lead to their diagnosis:

- Viruses
- Bacteria
- Yeast (*Candida*)
- Parasites
- Heavy metals
- Inflammation
- Food allergies

A multitude of scientific studies exist linking underlying pathology to an autism diagnosis. In fact, there are various references citing some of these studies in the other chapters of this book. A PubMed search will yield many more; so with this in mind, I will only mention a few here.

Ekiel and coworkers[5] more frequently isolated strains of *Clostridium* species and enterococci, but rarely lactobacilli, from stool samples of autistic children when compared with healthy children. In addition, they noted quantitative differences in staphylococci, *Candida* species, and *Clostridium perfringens*. In a separate study, researchers found significantly higher levels (P<0.05) of DA (a marker of invasive candidiasis) in the urine of autistic children before and after probiotic supplementation.[6]

Bradstreet and colleagues[7] found most individuals with autism have substantially higher nagalase levels than the expected healthy ranges. Nagalase promotes immune suppression by inactivating macrophages,[8] and is recognized as an enzyme produced by cancer cells and viruses. One of the functions of nagalase is to get the virus into the cell while also decreasing the body's immune reaction to the virus. This provides evidence not only for viral prevalence in the bodies of children with autism, but immune dysfunction as well, hindering the body's ability to defend itself against these invaders.

A separate study published in *Pediatric Health* found that there is evidence that chronic infections and the immune reactions associated with them may contribute to causing autism spectrum disorders. These infections include *Babesia, Bartonella, Borrelia burgdorferi, Ehrlichia, Human herpesvirus-6, Chlamydia pneumoniae,* and *Mycoplasma*.[9] In my personal work within the autism community, my colleagues and I have seen these afflictions repeatedly on an international scale as evidenced by various objective laboratory tests.

The same pathogens, parasites, heavy metals, and inflammation that lead to an autism diagnosis are eliminated by chlorine dioxide. It has also been used for decades to eliminate biofilms in industry.[10] Chlorine dioxide is able to penetrate the biofilm matrix and destroy the pathogens coexisting inside,[11] thus allowing the body to pass biofilm in stool. (Many parents who are using the protocol with their children have provided photo documentation.)

As of this writing, 110 children have recovered from the symptoms known as autism through the use of chlorine dioxide as a part of a larger biomedical protocol that targets the excesses related to autism rather than the deficiencies. Pathogens eat nutrients. For example, parasites eat vitamin B12 and iron and then excrete bacteria, viruses, and *Candida*. **It is important to note that an excess of pathogens causes the deficiencies that my colleagues and I see in autistic children, and supplementing those deficiencies actually feeds the pathogen that is causing them. By targeting the excess of pathogens rather than attempting to supplement the deficiencies they cause, the children are making much greater progress.**

The protocol

The protocol responsible for healing these 110 children and counting, as well as the improvements seen by thousands more, is a series of seven steps, each one building on the previous. The first step is the diet, which should be gluten, dairy, soy, sugar, and chemical free. Removing foods that promote inflammation, allergies, and mucous is critical to healing autism.

We then add low, frequent doses of CD as our second step toward killing pathogens, oxidizing toxins in the body, neutralizing heavy metals, and reducing inflammation. CD is dosed orally, in baths, and in enemas. Ninety-five percent of children's ATEC scores reported back to us have dropped an average of 20 points after three months on the protocol. There is a significant reduction in undesireable behaviors, with an increase in desirable behaviors in speech, eye contact, socialization, affection, and other skills. My colleagues and I are seeing improvements at every age—from infant to adult—which shatters the belief that there's no hope if children don't recover by a young age.

The third step is the Kalcker parasite protocol, a 12-18 month protocol that focuses on the elimination of intestinal parasites. Parents add the parasite protocol after their child reaches their individualized full dosage of CD. Kalckler's parasite protocol consists of nonsystemic herbs and medications that can be purchased over the counter. The protocol is designed to target parasites around the full moon phase, when they are known to move to the gut to mate. The most commonly eliminated parasites are roundworms, such as *Ascaris lumbricoides*, tapeworms, flukes, and what we believe are a newly discovered species of helminth, the rope worm.[12]

Adding the Kalcker parasite protocol reduces behaviors and symptoms associated with an autism diagnosis, such as bruxism (teeth grinding), constipation, diar-

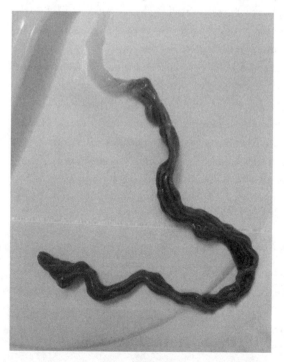

rhea, aggression, self-injurious behavior, butt and nose picking, and night waking. **It is vital to do CD in conjunction with the parasite protocol** because as parasites die they release more toxins into the body that CD targets. The available CD will oxidize the toxins released by the parasites along with other pathogens that form part of the parasite environment.

The following photos are representative of thousands more that have been received, depicting dead helminthes eliminated during the full moon phase of the Kalcker protocol.

The first three steps of the protocol are mandatory. What my colleagues and I have observed is that **after the pathogen load of the body has been lessened, other treatments become more successful**. For example, parents can consider adding specific supplements to support speech, mild chelators, hard chamber hyperbaric oxygen, or the relatively new immune system GcMAF (Gc protein-derived macrophage-activating factor). Each intervention needs to be considered on an individual basis in conjunction with CD and the ongoing parasite protocol. When the steps are applied in the correct order, then significant gains are seen in individuals with autism.

I would be remiss if I did not mention that this protocol is controversial. The FDA, even though they have approved patents for multiple products using chlorine dioxide, has come out against "MMS," Jim Humble's original name for dilute chlorine dioxide in aqueous solution. It is inexpensive, unpatentable, and it works. For these reasons, it will never be a moneymaker for the industry. Because of the FDA's warnings, it is difficult for many doctors in the US to recommend CD. Therefore, the final critical piece to this protocol is the support group "book clubs" that parents have formed online to help each other on Facebook and CDAutism.org.

This protocol works!

As of November 2013, this protocol had spread to more than 5000 families in 57 countries. Upon review of quarterly ATEC scores submitted by the parents of 163 children (ages 2–17) who had been on the protocol for over one year, my colleagues and I calculated that over 94% had shown a reduction in their ATEC scores.

I would like to share a few excerpts from testimonials submitted to us by parents who are using this protocol for their children on the spectrum.

> *Prior to starting CD, we had tried almost every autism biomedical protocol. We saw several DAN! and GI specialists and numerous other practitioners. We spent tens of thousands of dollars on consults, supplements, diets, medicine and medical procedures not covered by insurance. My daughter either had no response or negative ones, and she continued to get worse. She developed extreme self-injurious behaviors that progressed to the point of her needing to be restrained several times a day in an attempt to prevent her from pinching or biting herself until she drew blood. Her body was covered with bruises and cuts. She would also pull out big clumps of her hair. She would be up for hours screaming in the night with these behaviors. She was severely malnourished despite the fact that two registered dieticians had deemed her daily caloric intake adequate. She was 14 years old and weighed a little over 70 pounds. I honestly did not think that CD would be any different than anything else we had ever tried but figured things could not get much worse.*

Since starting CD her self-injurious behaviors are almost entirely gone. She went from having to be restrained almost daily to once in the last 5 months. Her former multiple daily 45-minute self-injurious tantrums are now a few minutes of crying or protest and happen once a week if at all. We have noticed gains in language and cognition (20 point drop in her ATEC score). After years of fluctuating between loose stools and constipation, she is now regular and has gained almost 10 pounds. She sleeps through the night and we are able to take her places that we would have never dared to before. If my daughter can make gains this drastic in 5 months at age 14, I can't wait to see what the future holds.

****

I, too, am so thankful for Kerri and her whole "crew." Thanks to Kerri for bringing CD to all of our kids on the spectrum worldwide. My Natalie is now OFF of her former roller-coaster ride of prescription anti-fungals, OFF of her former roller-coaster ride of prescription antibiotics, OFF of prescription antiviral, OFF of prescription low-dose naltrexone, etc. Her belly distention has disappeared, she's gained weight, she's gained height and she's now almost 103 days seizure free. She still has a ways to go toward more improvements, but she's happily climbing up from bottom of the trenches; she's climbing up from what seemed like the very bottom of the abyss that vaccine injury/injuries had placed her in. Thank you Kerri, Andreas Kalcker, Jim Humble and all of the moderators on the supportive websites!!!

****

My family and I are very grateful to Kerri Rivera for making available the CD protocol to treat autism which has recovered myself and made a huge difference to thousands of kids and families all over the world. CD can recover even a teenager like me whom others had given up on. Of all the bio-medical interventions, CD cost the least and made the biggest difference. Muchas Gracias por salvar mi vida Kerri.

****

The book *Healing the Symptoms Known as Autism* outlines the aforementioned protocol and contains hundreds of testimonials similar to the ones above, chronicling a myriad of improvements seen in children and adults on the spectrum and beyond.

REPETITIVE TRANSCRANIAL MAGNETIC STIMULATION AND MAGNETIC RESONANT THERAPY™ FOR AUTISM

By Dr. James Jeffrey Bradstreet

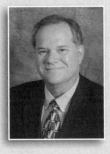

James Jeffrey Bradstreet, MD, MD(H), FAAFP

Director of the Brain Treatment Center of Atlanta
Adjunct Professor, Western University of Health Sciences, CA
104 Colony Park Drive, Suite 600
Cumming, GA 30040-2793
470-253-7445
DrBradstreet@aol.com

Dr. James Jeffrey Bradstreet, received his medical degree from the University of South Florida in Tampa and his residency training at Wilford Hall USAF Medical Center in Texas. He is widely published on the various aspects of autism-related biology and comorbidities and is a member of the American Academy of Toxicology as well as a Fellow of the American Academy of Family Physicians. Dr. Bradstreet is an adjunct professor of pediatrics at Southwest College of Naturopathic Medicine in Tempe, Arizona, and is licensed in Georgia, Florida, California, and Arizona. Both his son and stepson have autism spectrum disorders and have experienced significant recovery as a result of intensive biomedical interventions. Dr. Bradstreet's interests include the interactions between the immune system and the brain, stem cell therapies, and the relationship of vitamin D to macrophage activation and viral pathogens. Using new techniques, he has been able to see significant progress for some of the most challenging cases. Please visit www.drbradstreet.org.

Regardless of your opinion about what factors contribute to the development of autism, novel methods to overcome its symptoms are urgently needed. Our existing therapies—behavioral, speech, occupational, sensory integration, biomedical, and others—simply are leaving too many children with significant residual deficits. Having now observed over 50 cases of autism treated via transcranial magnetic stimulation, it is clear many of them respond in a positive and vigorous way to the therapy.

Over my last 16 years of working with and researching autism, I've been troubled by the difference in responsiveness to therapies demonstrated by individuals on the spectrum. Some children turn the corner quickly and return to normal development by the use of biomedical and/or behavioral interventions. Yet others remain much as they were prior to therapies despite everyone's best efforts.

In my efforts to understand why some children stay disconnected, I started exploring brain electrical harmonics and ways of retraining the brain with modalities like EEG (electroencephalogram) neurofeedback. Beginning in 2001, I studied with Professor Joel Lubar, one of the grandfathers of quantitative EEG analysis (QEEG) and neurofeedback, especially for symptoms related to attention-deficit/hyperactivity disorder (ADHD) (Lubar et al., 1995). That led me to Roberto Pascual-Marqui, PhD, the developer of low resolution electromagnetic tomography (LORETA). Roberto created a mathematical formula for localizing the source of any EEG signal within the 3-D space of the brain (Pascual-Marqui et al., 1994).

I then made the trek to Canada to visit Drs. Mike and Lynda Thompson at the ADD Centre outside of Toronto. Mike was passionate about the QEEG process and using it to guide the retraining of the brain, and he was convinced it could be applied to autism as it had been for ADHD-related issues. Lynda was the practical holistic therapist, who worked to integrate the entire picture for the ADHD children (Thompson and Thompson, 1998). She, too, was optimistic about autism. You can learn more about their work at their website: www.addcentre.com.

At a CME class in 2001, I met Professor John Hughes from the University of Illinois College of Medicine at Chicago. Hughes wrote the best clinical textbook on EEG I have studied. He is one of the most senior EEG researchers, with over 600 published articles and several books on the subject. Over several years, I studied extensively with him at various courses. He solidified my thinking about brain harmonics with his discussion of the cortical dynamics of the "Mozart-effect." Simply stated, one special composition of Mozart, *Piano Sonata in D Major* (K.448), appeared to be as effective as anti-seizure medications. When this music was examined in patients with seizures, 79% of seizures stopped—even when the patients were in comas.

This research brought me to the concept of the brain's unique symphony and a book written by Jim Robbins titled *A Symphony in the Brain: The Evolution of the New Brain Wave Biofeedback*. This is a beautifully written and easy-to-read introduction to the complex field of neurophysics—a topic the writer refers to as *the symphony*. It seemed to me back in 2001 (when this part of my journey with autism began) as well as now on the eve of 2014 as I write this chapter, that the brain of autism was no symphony. It was instead as though the orchestra members had appeared on stage with neither sheet music nor a conductor to guide them.

Pascual-Marqui, Lubar, Hughes, and the Thompsons greatly influenced my thinking about brain physics and its potential application for sorting out the mysteries of autism. Without their influence, I wouldn't have been prepared for what was to come – TMS.

By 2004, I had performed over 400 EEG-QEEG-LORETA studies on children with autism. If you have been with a child getting an EEG, then you know just how complicated the process is. Needless to say, children with autism are not interested is sitting quietly and cooperating with the acquisition of the EEG raw data. We developed some in-house strategies with the help of some applied behavior analysis (ABA) therapists to ease the kids through the ordeal, but it was a whole lot of effort and stress for the child, family, and my staff. But that wasn't the end of the efforts. The raw EEG data was full of eye movement and muscle artifact. All of those bad EEG segments had to be carefully edited out of the actual quantitative EEG and LORETA input so we didn't get a wrong impression of the brain's activity.

Eventually, both my staff and I became frustrated with the process, but before that happened, I had learned a lot about the autism brain and its electrical harmonics. To explain this better, we first need a short primer on brain frequencies. Practically speaking, the typical EEG is capable of recording brain frequencies ranging from about 0.5 cycle per sec or 0.5 Hertz (Hz) up to 50 Hz, although some newer technology is extending that range. The typical energy driving the EEG is very small when measured via the skin on the scalp: about 10 microV to 100 microV in amplitude when measured with an external electrode. As such, contraction of the muscles of the face, jaw, and neck can generate huge interference with the ability to see the very small brain generated electrical impulses. In a similar way, the eye acts like a dipole magnet, and its motion can create large disruptions of the baseline – particularly for the more frontal electrode sensors.

By the time I sat beside Professor Manuel Casanova at an autism think tank in 2007, I had largely abandoned QEEG and LORETA for autism due to the complexity of getting clean, artifact-free signals. That was disappointing to me because I knew the "symphony" had to be a major key to the autism puzzle. However, Professor Casanova re-energized my interests in neurophysics. He made a bold statement that was particularly unpopular to the other members of the think tank. He was adamant that the autism brain displayed no evidence of inflammation – at least not in the traditional way we think of inflammation in the brain. Rather, he believed it was derangements of the brain's electrical microcircuits – called minicolumns – that resulted in the abnormal neurophysics. His data were very compelling, and over the years I have stayed in touch with Casanova and his research. He and his team went on to publish the first study of magnetic stimulation for treatment of autism (Sokhadze et al., 2009).

Through a series of persons contacting me regarding the Brain Treatment Center in Newport Beach, California, I ultimately connected with Professor Yi Jin. Following Grisaru and his colleagues from Israel (Geller et al., 1997), who first explored repetitive magnetic stimulation for schizophrenia and depression (1994), Professor Jin went on to enhance the process and focused on a particular frequency that had not been previously used for magnetic stimulation. Jin is a tireless researcher who has gone on to extend his particular protocol, now referred to as MRT™ (more to follow on this), to autism. Several of my patients had been treated with Jin, and, in many cases, the results were and remain dramatic. Ultimately, I went to California to see for myself. I am now the principal investigator for the MRT autism study currently in progress in Atlanta, so I think that speaks for itself. Further, all three of my children have been treated for various issues with MRT.

Let's get back to the core science of magnetic therapy. With special computer software, it is now getting easier to extract the actual brain signal and filter away the interference, but this is still a complex task. On a clean sample, we can see certain patterns of EEG activity, and we divide these into bundles of frequencies. You will need at least a superficial understanding of this to understand what comes next. First the common names we use for frequencies: delta (up to 4 Hz), theta (4 Hz up to 7 or 8 Hz, depending on form), alpha (7 or 8 Hz, depending on form, up to 14 Hz [usually maxes out at about 12 Hz in most individuals and is most noticeable in an eyes-closed yet awake state; Figure 1]), beta (generally these start at about 12.5 Hz, but may be higher at around 14 Hz and extend up to 30 Hz), mu or the sensory-motor rhythm (10-13 Hz), and gamma (above 30 Hz and have been recently measured above 100 Hz). There are variations on these, but for practical applications, these are sufficient to our discussions.

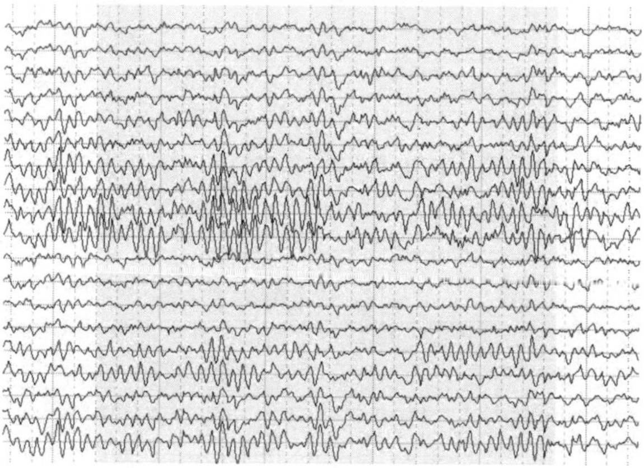

Figure 1 A normal pattern of eyes-closed alpha dominated EEG activity. You can see the large waves which cycle at approximately 11 Hz (11 wave peaks per second).

Delta [for autism] (Sokhadze, including Casanova, et al., 2009), delta [for autism] (Enticott et al., 2010), alpha-mu [8-13 Hz for autism] (Puzzo et al., 2013), and alpha [for schizophrenia] (Jin et al., 2006 and 2012) repetitive transcranial magnetic stimulation (rTMS) programs have been published. No study compares these various protocols to each other. Our unpublished observations regarding rTMS using an alpha protocol have been favorable enough for us to proceed to a controlled and registered study, and at the Brain Treatment Center in Atlanta, we will be well underway – or perhaps even finished (by the time this chapter is published) – with the first sham-controlled study of rTMS using a frontal alpha protocol for autism. With regard to the various other protocols, each operates on a different hypothesis of brain physics in autism or schizophrenia. Yet each protocol has yielded positive results in a significant subset of its subjects. More on the details of each in a bit.

Before discussing the unique features and results of each program, it is important to provide some sense of safety for rTMS or MRT™. Both rTMS and MRT™ consist of a cycle of magnetic pulses (train) followed by a delay until pulsing again (inter-train). The FDA defines times of safety for train timing as well as for the energy applied (motor-threshold). Following the establishment of safety guidelines since the mid-1990s, there have been extremely rare rTMS/MRT associated seizures. To the contrary, many of my autism patients with seizures have observed a decrease in seizure frequency following MRT™.

Motor threshold refers to the magnetic energy (power) applied to the motor cortex (the part of brain that works your muscles) that is sufficient to cause muscle contraction. Motor thresholds are established individually in each patient, and then the output of the machine is reduced well below the motor threshold for these types of interventions. In all the published studies and in my own experience with close to 100 children with autism, no serious adverse effects have been observed. Having said that, transient effects can be troublesome in the early course of treatment. Headaches both during the application of magnetic impulses and typically up to 30 minutes afterwards are relatively common. For anterior application of the magnet, eye pain can be experienced during the few seconds of the magnet pulsing each minute. During the first week while using the alpha protocol, it is common to see increased hyperactivity and/or agitation. This generally fades by the second week, and I have not observed it lasting beyond that more than once. Adjusting our protocol controlled the effect in that child.

The magnetic field generated by the technology I am most familiar with is maximally capable of generating at 4 Tesla (4T) pulse for about 3–9 inches, depending on settings and the magnet shape being used. The output strength of the TMS is actually much less as a result of the special treatment protocols employed. The typical magnets used in hospital MRI scanners range from 1 to 3T. Those magnets, however, generate a much larger magnetic field, which requires special shielding for the building around the scanner. If you have ever had an MRI, then you are aware of a loud banging inside the device while you are being scanned. The sound comes from the energy in the electromagnetic wires deforming rapidly as the current pulses on and off. With rTMS and MRT™, you will hear a noticeable – but not loud – clicking sound that corresponds to the frequency of pulses being applied to the head of magnet. Reproducing this sound for sham-controlled mock research actually created an engineering challenge, which, fortunately, has been overcome for our study. The magnets are safe for the operator holding the magnet as well as the subject as long as proper guidelines are followed. The rTMS and MRT™ magnets may be handheld or braced by the machine without any special shielding. With children, we have found handheld is best.

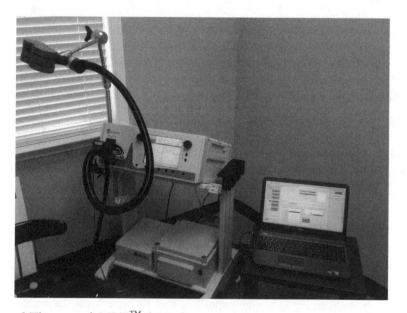

Figure 2 The research MRT™ device being used at the BTC –Atlanta Center.

The specific methodology utilized at the BTC centers in Atlanta, GA, and Newport Beach, CA, utilizes EEG- and ECG- (electrocardiogram) guided analysis of optimal harmonics for the brain. That process is complex, but Figure 3 gives you an overview of how it happens.

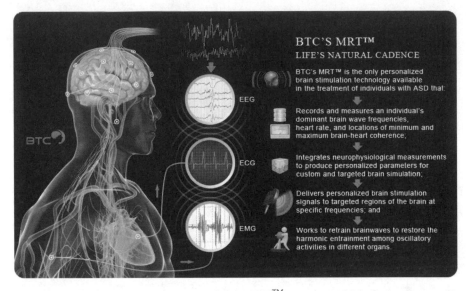

Figure 3 A diagrammatic overview of the MRT™ process, which finds a harmonic pattern in EEG, ECG and EMG (muscle tone).

The alpha protocol is linked to Jin's research evaluating the optimization of brain communication with that frequency, while Casanova's group is pursuing a different theory. His group theorizes that slow (delta) pulses will activate a special type of interneuron responsible for inhibitory regulation in the brain circuitry. This theory analyzes the absence of proper inhibition of noisy signals in the autism brain. This protocol resulted in approximately a 40% reduction in self-stimulatory behaviors and a 58% reduction in irritability. The study from 2009 was small, but certainly encouraging (Sokhadze, including Casanova, et al., 2009).

In a 2013 study, which is a bit similar to the MRT™ protocol, Puzzo et al. (2013) used stimulation in the same general range as Jin's protocol, although the magnet placement focuses on a different area of the brain (inferior parietal lobule). Uniquely, the Puzzo study applied the frequencies to neurotypical college students, with an objective of seeing if they experienced changes in sensorimotor function – with a further aim of using this methodology in the future to modulate the autism brain. They did observe changes in sensorimotor modulation, thereby indicating the treatment had a potential application for autism. Jin's protocol varies, but generally places the magnet at the frontal cortex.

In summary, rTMS and/or MRT™ show promise for the treatment of various symptoms of autism, and currently ongoing and future studies will help to define its best application to the individuals affected with autistic symptoms.

COMMUNICATION

31

AUTISMATE : PERSONALIZED FOR LIFE

By Jonathan Izak

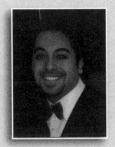

Jonathan Izak

Jonathan Izak is CEO of SpecialNeedsWare, a company inspired by his younger brother Oriel who is on the autism spectrum. He has a degree in computer science and engineering from the University of Pennsylvania and has guest lectured on AAC and technology at over a dozen of universities, regional conferences, and national conferences around the country.

Every student has unique learning needs. Some struggle with communication, others with daily living skills. Some need support in accessing school curriculum, while others are at a stage where they are learning vocational skills. We all have varying strengths and weaknesses that both shape and are shaped by our life experiences as individuals. Recognizing these differences and understanding that they have the power to either bind or unlock our potentials as human beings, is at the core of AutisMate; the personalized learning app for individuals with Autism.

The story of AutisMate began when Jonathon Izak, Founder and CEO of AutisMate, took an active interest and eventual critical role in his brother Oriel's learning and therapy programs. Diagnosed at the age of three with autism, Oriel was initially non-verbal and severely limited in his ability to complete daily living tasks independently. He spent the majority of his time with a team of therapists implementing the most advanced and effective behavioral and speech therapy techniques to teach Oriel daily functioning tasks, life skills, and eventually how to speak. Jon witnessed first hand how successful a personalized therapy program was for his own brother, as well as the difficulties and limitations faced in creating such a program. He thus set about creating a personalized application to facilitate learning, communication, and general wellbeing for individuals with autism.

Despite the large diversity of the learning styles and abilities, most autism professionals and family members of those on the autism spectrum will point out that those with autism tend to be visual learners. Years of research and clinical trials have demonstrated the effectiveness of using visual supports and visual strategies to help those with developmental disabilities communicate and learn. In recognition of these visual strengths, professionals around the world developed symbol-based supports as a central part of interventions for promoting communication, organization, appropriate behavior and learning. While symbols can be an effective way of representing concepts, it is difficult for many learners to understand these various symbols and even more difficult for them to learn how to string these symbols together to communicate successfully. Fortunately though, the mobile technology revolution of recent years has opened the door for a personalized adaptation to the use of visual learning. Today, we can have a computer, camera, GPS system, access to the Internet, multimedia player and more, sitting in our pockets in the form of an iPhone, iPad or Android device. Understanding the opportunity that the increased access to such cutting edge technology provides lead to the creation of AutisMate, a comprehensive app for visual supports, built in collaboration with Boston Children's Hospital, that can be easily personalized to each learner's needs and abilities in order to support their specific learning styles.

As previously noted, there are many well-researched strategies for supporting our learners with visual supports. Some of the primary visual supports for daily living skills, vocational skills, social emotional learning, cognitive skills, and behavioral skills include video modeling, visual schedules, and social stories. The primary visual supports for communication collectively referred to as Augmentative and Alternative Communication (AAC), include visual scene displays, grid displays, and keyboards with word prediction. All of these various supports are included within AutisMate, which utilizes the ability to take photos, take videos and record voice to personalize these supports with real images and sounds from the learner's own environment. The app even incorporates GPS to present the learner with the visual supports they need based on their current location so there is a reduced need to navigate through various locations. The combinations of these powerful supports allow learners to progress towards independence in everything from simple communication to vocational skills, and the use of GPS helps reduce the barrier of navigating to the right visual supports for those who are not yet at that level.

Picture a non-verbal learner who is just starting to communicate and struggles to understand the meaning of symbols, as many learners do. Now picture an interactive scene of the inside of your learner's own pantry or fridge filling a touch screen device. The learner sees the actual food items that he or she eats on a regular basis. Tapping on an item such as the milk will cause the phrase "milk" or "I want milk" to be played. Now consider a learner who is verbal and is working on vocational skills in an office setting. The learner sees an interactive scene of the office and taps on an icon on the mailboxes. A visual schedule pops up in which all the steps for sorting the mail are depicted using real photos of the activity of sorting the mail. As the learner progresses through each step, a video that models how to carry out that particular step plays on the screen so the learner can see exactly what needs to be done to complete it. After completing the step, the learner taps on the image for that step, a big check mark appears and the next step plays. These are just a few of the many real examples of how individuals are currently using AutisMate to become more independent in their daily lives. Videos of such success stories can be found on our website (www.AutisMate.com).

AutisMate provides a progressive and dynamic system of visual supports that help promote language and can be easily adjusted to grow with the learner and facilitate learning. The visual scene displays are a central part of the app for two reasons: First, the research behind visual scenes demonstrates that young children are better able to communicate using visual scene displays than grid displays due to their contextual nature. In addition to using scenes for this purpose, scenes are also used to provide visually intuitive access to the user's other visual supports. For example, I can place a symbol hotspot in a scene, such as a face-washing symbol, in a scene of my bathroom that brings up a series of videos depicting how to wash your face step by step. This both helps the learner understand the meaning of the face-washing symbol and provides the visual instruction needed to learn and independently carry out the activity of face washing. The importance of learning these symbols is to help the user progress from scene-based communication to symbol based communication, which provides greater access to spontaneous and generative communication, or the ability to say, "whatever they want, whenever they want." There are even a variety of visual tools provided to move beyond image based communication that focus on literacy learning and text based communication, foremost among these being the built in keyboard with word prediction that ties the predicted words to symbols that represent those words.

In creating AutisMate, SpecialNeedsWare collaborated with Dr. Howard Shane and his team at Boston Children's Hospital along with an advisory board consisting of leading behavior therapists, speech pathologists, special education experts, and assistive technology experts. In addition, we've also worked with hundreds of additional professionals and parents during the creation and have actively sought the feedback of thousands more once the product was released. This feedback led to the realization that, in addition to having the ability to personalize the visual supports provided to the needs and abilities of each learner, it is critical to provide practical access to these supports by every member of the learner's team in every environment whether it be home, school, or in the community. In responding to this need, we are currently building AutisMate 365, a cloud based version of AutisMate that allows every member of a learner's team to have access to that individual's visual supports from their own mobile devices and allows all of these devices to synchronize with each other. Thus, one subscription would allow full access to AutisMate and that learner's content on his parent's devices, school devices, behavior therapist's device, speech pathologist's device and personal device. This will allow the individual to be immersed in any environment in these visual supports for communication and learning, which is so important for our learners.

It is well recognized among augmentative communication specialists that learners need to be able to communicate expressively using these devices as if it is their own voice, which is promoted by having the supports on multiple devices. There is also a need for having these communication devices on hand at all times to provide a way for communication partners to communicate to the learner using visual supports. The way typically developing children learn to communicate is a great example of the need for communicating to learners through visuals if you expect that learner to use visuals in communicating with others. A mother holding up an apple and saying "apple" is an example of how children typically develop language. They learn through receptive communication, in this example the verbal communication of the label "apple." They are being communicated to using speech and are expected to model that communication in return. With individuals who are learning to communicate through visuals, the easiest way to do so is through receptive communication as well. Therefore, AutisMate allows you to display videos, photos, or symbols depicting "go to your room" or "Apple" to help provide this visual receptive communication. Allowing these visual supports to be shared among the learner's entire team ensures an immersive visual learning environment that enables this learning.

Autism intervention is a complex process whose successful implementation is dependent on professionals from various fields of expertise, and a deep understanding of the challenges faced by individuals with Autism and their supportive loved ones. Through continuous efforts to learn about the lives of those with Autism and improve upon the existing methodology on Autism intervention and education, SpecialNeeds Ware has successfully created a platform to help those with autism connect with others and live more independently. We at SpecialNeedsWare are proud of AutisMate, the app that can suit the needs of each unique individual on the autism spectrum and take a comprehensive approach that encapsulates the entire life experience of the learner.

32

RAPID PROMPTING METHOD

By Soma Mukhopadhyay

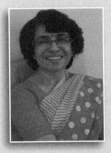

Soma Mukhopadhyay

BS Chemistry with Honors, MS Chemistry, BEd

Executive Director of Education
H.A.L.O. (Helping Autism through Learning & Outreach)
P.O. Box 303399
Austin, TX 78703
512-465-9595
www.halo-soma.org

A native of India, Soma Mukhopadhyay is a teacher and mother. Soma developed her trademark Rapid Prompting Method (RPM) to instruct her son, Tito, who is now a published writer and poet although he has severe autism. Soma and Tito have been featured on *60 Minutes II*, PBS, *Good Morning America, Scientific American,* the *New York Times, National Geographic, CNN,* the HBO documentary *A Mothers Courage* and more. Soma is the author of three books.

Soma has instructed thousands of students (youth to adult) with autism and similar disorders at the 501(c)(3) HALO Clinic located in Austin, Texas. Cornell University conducted a peer-reviewed study of Soma® Rapid Prompting Method titled "Harnessing repetitive behaviors to engage attention and learning in a novel therapy for autism: an exploratory analysis," which was published in 2011 in the journal *Frontiers in Psychology* (*see* www.halo-soma.org/files/news28_fpsyg_03_00012.pdf).

Rapid Prompting Method (RPM) was a method I developed when, as the mother of an autistic child in India, I was trying to educate my son, Tito Rajarshi Mukhopadhyay. Little did I know that I would cross continents and use the same techniques to teach my students here in the United States. While teaching my students, I am always learning something new and trying to improve my techniques as I work with them.

Rapid Prompting Method is **not an autism treatment.** It is a simple **educational approach** leading to communication. It empowers the student by providing a way to express his learning, reasoning, understanding and thoughts by utilizing his OPEN LEARNING CHANNELS during that instance of learning.

Like all typical people, autistic people have open learning channels.

- The **primary learning channels** are vision and auditory.
- The **secondary learning channels** are tactile and kinesthetic.

An RPM educator will assess the student based on these learning channels. Here are some student profile examples.

Vision:

- **Generalized vision**—when the student can look at a page or tabletop work and also focus his vision on a distant object *without becoming stressed*. This is the type of vision typical people have.
- **Selective vision**—when the student can look at his own preferred *selected object*— a DVD player or book or a few selected faces but cannot focus on other non-preferred objects and is unable or resistant to watch a new movie or look at a new book.
- **Global vision**—when students cannot focus on any specific environmental object, and their eyes keep continuously gazing at some unchosen aspect.

Auditory:

- **Generalized auditory**—when the student can follow any sound, conversation or noise or listen to any music. This is similar to typical individuals' hearing.
- **Selective hearing**—when the student selects a few sound aspects in the environment—e.g., selective music or own humming sound—verbally stimulating on the same selective words or phrases by requesting the same thing over and over again.
- **Global auditory**—when the student has difficulty in isolating any sound and does not react or show interest in any particular sound.

Examples:

A student who has selective hearing but generalized vision may look at the tabletop work but may become stressed if the teacher is trying to teach a concept. He will have better imitation skills and social language but after a while may stop accepting new concepts and recycle the same words and phrases he learned from years back when he was a child.

A student with generalized hearing and selective vision may not be stressed by a new concept that the teacher is trying to explain but may not be able to imitate or visually look at a picture the teacher has presented on the table. This student may not have imitation skills and may look for some chosen visual object to find visual respite in an overwhelming situation.

A student with a selective tactile learning channel may not find it difficult holding an object of comfort like a blanket, cloth or string but may find it difficult holding a pencil or touching the letters on the letter-board.

A selective kinesthetic student may feel comfortable moving his body by rocking, pacing or fidgeting his hands but may find it difficult with other generalized movements like how to move his hands appropriately to write.

A generalized kinesthetic and tactile student with selective auditory may have better posture control and physically adapt to any new environment and have better handwriting or drawing skills but may become "stuck" writing the same list of words.

Rapid Prompting Method ADAPTS to all kinds of students.

The best way the teacher **identifies the open learning channels** is through the stims (self-stimulatory movements) of the student.

RPM does *not see a stim as behavior* but as a **self-defensive mechanism** the student performs if the sensory challenges become overwhelming.

There are **external components** of the environment like the sound, sight, smell and temperature (tactile aspect) of the environment. Then there are the **internal components** like memory, obsession, pain and anxiety.

All factors—external and internal—**compete** with equal intensity. An autistic person may not be able to **shield** himself or herself from stimulations from external or internal environment.

Hence, as a defensive mechanism, he or she begins to engage in a self-stimulatory activity (or "stim") to minimize the overwhelming feeling.

The teacher who uses RPM must know the difference between the **excitatory stim and the calming stim.**

- **Excitatory** stim can be recognized when the student shows a facial expression—smiles, giggles or exhibits extreme anxiety (e.g., requesting the same request and expecting the same answer from someone). The teacher competes with excitatory stims through her voice, speed and choice of topic accordingly because excitatory stim can inhibit learning and slow the student's performance.
- A **calming** stim, on the other hand, is a passive involvement and does not involve emotional display. A student may passively hold a comfort toy or string and yet continue to participate in the lesson presented by the teacher. The teacher allows a calming stim because it does not interfere with learning.

In an RPM session, the teacher does not categorize a stimulatory activity with behavior.

Unlike a stim, **behavior** (escape or aggression) is a carefully planned activity arising from a flight/fight situation. The teacher works through the behavior by choosing the right lesson to extinguish it (e.g., teaching about force and impact or muscles and movements or an Aesop's fable with some moral if the student hits or kicks the teacher). The teacher prearranges the room for students who try to elope by limiting their exit paths (e.g., positioning the student's work area facing away from the door or entry way).

Every RPM session follows four goals:

Cognitive goal:

Because RPM is an educational method, the teacher makes sure that there is a new topic (poetry, story, science, history, philosophy or mathematics base) in each session, depending on the student's age, exposure and interest.

The teacher is required to take some time and prepare a lesson plan to meet the cognitive goals for the student. If not, then the student will only recycle his previously learned topics and as an RPM session, the session will remain incomplete.

The world is a jargon of concepts, and language defines every aspect of the world. It is the teacher's responsibility that the student finds the world with its concepts to be a friendly place. RPM is a language- and concept-based approach, and we teachers do not shelter our students from concepts. We are ambitious for the students' cognitive growth.

Spelling goals are embedded under cognitive objectives, whereby the student learns how to spell using phonics rather than memorizing sight words.

The teacher follows a "state and ask" method to alternate between the teacher's participation (stating from the planned lesson) and the student's response (the teacher asks a question based on the lesson statement she just stated to make sure the student attended to the topic).

The student responds either by choosing one from two written choices offered by the teacher or by spelling the answer on the letter-board or stencil-board (if his or her motor skills are good).

Skill goal:

Every student has different motor skill ability. The teacher adapts the student's response based on the eye gaze, mobility and posture of the student. Unlike other methods, it is *not important* for the student to sit in front of the table and work. If the student is tactile defensive to sitting at the table, then the teacher can adapt to the student's posture and continue the RPM session. It is okay if the student opts to find learning easier while sitting on a bean bag or even a sofa.

Some students may begin the student response by choosing between two written choices offered by the teacher, while others who have better motor skills may move on to learning how to spell on a set of three stencils, with large letters divided into letters A through I; J through R; and S through Z; however, there may be others who would not hesitate to spell on a full A through Z lettered stencil-board or letter-board.

The pictures of these stencil-boards are found on the website www.halo-soma.org. The teacher aims to improve the skills of the student graduating from two choices into spelling on the full lettered stencil-board or laminated letter-board.

The teacher determines how to present the choices—a visually defensive student whose eyes are not adapted towards looking at the paper choices may need to know their positions to make a selection. So the teacher may tap them if they are on the table (stimulating the student's auditory learning channel) to let the student know their positions or hold them up in air and shake each choice (stimulating the student's visual attention through the movement of shaking) while saying them aloud to make it easier for the student to locate their position.

Tolerance goal:

Every new situation is unique for most students with autism. There is the new voice of the teacher, a new way of learning, new demands from the teacher to get a response, new learning concepts, aiming at the right letters and spelling a word—everything needs growth in the tolerance level. Through practice and consistency, the student grows his tolerance skills in each of those areas.

Communication goal:

Communication develops through cognition. RPM expects a student not only to express his needs but also to reason why he wants something. It helps the student participate in a conversation, develop creative writing skills and, if necessary, explain to a doctor or specialist which part of the body needs to be examined. RPM aims towards language communication versus picture communication to avoid the longer neural pathway that is associated towards translating pictures into language versus directly using language through learning how to spell.

As the developer of RPM, I must admit that I am still learning and perfecting my skills. Is RPM the best **educational approach**? Many say it probably is.

AUGMENTATIVE AND ALTERNATIVE COMMUNICATION

By Patti Murphy

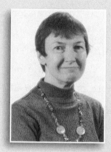

Patti Murphy

Patti Murphy writes for DynaVox Mayer-Johnson in Pittsburgh, Pennsylvania. She has written on disability issues for nearly 20 years, specializing in augmentative and alternative communication (AAC) for the past decade. Her work has also appeared in *ADVANCE for Speech-Language Pathologists, Closing the Gap, Exceptional Parent Magazine,* the *Pittsburgh Post-Gazette* and the former *Pittsburgh Press.* She thanks the clinical and product development staff members at DynaVox for the expertise, insight, and direction they offered to make this chapter possible: Jill Detwiler, MS., CCC-SLP, Clinical and Product Applications Specialist; Marleah Herman-Umpleby, MS, CCC-SLP; Bethany Diener, MS, CCC-SLP and Jeffrey Dobos of the Clinical AAC Content Team; Robert Cantine, Symbol Assets Manager; and Lisa Kehoe, Director of Educational Content. Thanks also to Carol Heilman, the parent of a child with autism and a former special education teacher, for taking time to read the draft.

To the many young people who use AAC, their parents, siblings, teachers, and therapists who over time have graciously shared their unique experiences—thank you. Collectively, you speak with one voice.

DynaVox (www.dynavoxtech.com) is the leading provider of speech-generating devices and symbol-adapted special education software used to assist individuals in overcoming speech, language, and learning challenges.

The technologies involved in augmentative and alternative communication (AAC) use have grown and changed in unprecedented ways since I contributed an overview of what AAC means for people on the autism spectrum to the 2012 edition of this book. While the chapter that follows addresses such developments, it will focus on human elements of AAC use that remain the same—and must, for it to work well—as the technology evolves.

Two interwoven topics will be highlighted: Social communication skills development through AAC use and the role of AAC in everyday or major life transitions including transitions that may occur during a communication exchange. After a discussion of challenges pertinent to those areas and technology's role in possible solutions, real examples of improvement enjoyed by young people with autism, their families and others in their support systems will be presented.

Challenges

Communication is possibly the most familiar challenge of autism. Roughly 25 percent of those with the condition are non-verbal, compared to nearly 50 percent a generation ago, a decline attributed in part to an increase in early intervention and rising awareness of milder forms of autism. (SFARI, 2013) It is believed also that AAC use may encourage, not deter, speech development (Silverman, 1980; Berry, 1987; Daniels, 1994), though it has long been said that up to one half of individuals with autism may never be able to use speech as a primary means of functional communication (Millar, 2009; Peeters & Gillberg, 1999; Light, Roberts, DiMarco & Greiner, 1998; and Mesibov, Adams & Klinger, 1997). Lines between non-verbal, minimally verbal, and non-verbal individuals with autism, however, remain blurry. The research lacks consensus on what constitutes those three levels of expressive communication.

Individuals with autism who can speak also experience difficulties with expressive and receptive language regardless of their intellectual abilities. Communication is very complex and filled with behavioral expectations. The mere expectation of interaction with another individual can unduly overwhelm some individuals with autism, shutting down their auditory processing and word retrieval abilities while triggering anxiety, aggression, or withdrawal. Sometimes behavior considered socially unacceptable becomes the equivalent of communication for the person. It may also be the surest way to get attention, which is reinforcing even when it is negative attention. Or it ensures permission to have a desired item, perform a desired activity or to be left alone. It is through AAC device use that many children learn how to make polite requests. Basic lessons may also include introducing oneself, addressing others by name, or remembering when to say "Excuse me, "Thank you" and "You're welcome."

Once children reach the milestone of learning to communicate for fulfillment of wants and needs, then what? Progress beyond that, with or without the aid of a speech-generating device, is uniquely challenging. Conversation for its own sake may not be as motivating as having a request honored. More than that, those with autism often struggle with unfamiliar people and nuances of social interaction—interruptions, turn-taking and changes in someone's tone of voice, for instance.

There is a consensus (Borg, 2010; Pease, A. & Pease, B. 2004) that a higher percentage of our interaction is nonverbal than spoken—that we say more through body language, facial expressions, eye contact, and our physical proximity to conversation partners, for example, than with our words. Understanding such cues is often problematic when autism is part of the equation.

It is common for those on the spectrum to be quite literal about language, a tendency that varies in frequency and intensity from person to person. The person, for instance, may not recognize anger, humor, or sarcasm in something a communication partner said, and a case of taking spoken words literally can become a barrier to interaction.

There is a strong tendency for individuals with autism tend to have very specific, and often very narrow, interests. Their focus on an interest, whether a particular type of music, trains, or running the vacuum cleaner, may be so intense that it precludes communication involving other topics. A body of research (Aspy, R. & Grossman, B. G., 2011; Leekam, S. R., Prior, M. R., & Uljarevic, M., 2011) supports that problems with social communication may have more do with this interest factor than with misunderstanding the etiquette of conversation.

Problems may arise when random changes occur in the communication environment. New people join or leave the conversation, for example, or the subject changes. Surroundings grow noisier or quieter, busier, brighter or darker. Even momentary changes can be unsettling for some individuals, blocking their ability to communicate.

It is important for communication partners to remember that while autism can prevent a person from engaging in social interaction for a variety of reasons, it does not mean they lack the desire to.

Solutions

Every individual with autism, even those with significant challenges, is capable of improving their social communication skills through a good mix of human and technological supports, some of which you already may be utilizing.

It has become common in the past two decades for individuals on the spectrum to experience success with electronic voice-generating devices featuring visual displays they control themselves. This makes sense given the affinity for objects and order that many with autism show. The technology—notably, the language framework of its communication software—offers predictability and structure in ways that spontaneous daily conversation may not. Tangible representation of language (through drawings or photos) supplemented by speech is one of its potentially lasting benefits for a child with autism. Language organized by topics of personal interest, or as the person needs it for communication throughout the day, is another.

Cafiero (2004) said that an AAC device can be "a buffer and a bridge" between communication partners. For some individuals with autism, using the technology may be more motivating than communication itself. And yet, a device can be a catalyst for interacting in new situations, planting seeds for relationships, improving behavior, and strengthening self-confidence. Such outcomes are not new. A few successes shared with me long ago:

A young man about to graduate from high school put his vigilance into words using his AAC device, the first portable DynaVox model. Concerned about safety when his infant brother grabbed a ball and stick, the young man called "Come get the baby!" to their mother through the technology.

Through her use of a similar device, a girl whose parents had pursued early AAC intervention had a solid comfort level while playing with typical peers by the time she reached the primary grades, said the senior therapist on the girl's in-home autism team. Others saw the girl's personality and imagination when she said "Let's be lions! Roar! Roar!" or communicated other vivid messages.

Small steps equated to leaps for a boy who had a pattern of using visible frustration to communicate. That changed after he got an AAC device. His requests were not just polite but more spontaneous and complete, as when he uttered, "Sara, come here please" to a school aide.

While a device may be a communication staple, printouts of device content to use when the device is not available, a binder filled with pictures, gestures, writing and symbols including the alphabet, are among an untold number of tools and techniques that come under the AAC umbrella. All can complement device use and vice versa. The best, or the best combinations of methods, are those that work for the time, place, situation, and especially for the person. Honoring all methods of self-expression, including attempts to verbalize, is fundamental to the process. So is fostering an encouraging communication environment where communication partners give the person using an AAC device ample time to respond and are willing to wait. Speech-language pathologists I know like to say that people make AAC successful, not the other way around. Success may be fostered using partner communication techniques including partner-augmented input, a strategy in which the communication partner uses both the device and his/her natural speech to show the child how to use the device as opportunities for communication occur on a given day, without pressure to perform. Links to videos demonstrating partner-augmented input, and the chain of cues (a prompting resource) and positive communication environment techniques are provided in the reference section for this chapter.

As we move forward in our 30-plus year journey of developing communication solutions, DynaVox keeps the personal side of AAC front and center. Much of the content found within our AAC devices and support material reflects tools and techniques known to make communication—and life—easier and more fulfilling for those with autism, their families, friends and helpers.

This content includes positive behavioral supports, designed to help children manage daily routines and potentially stressful situations including transitioning between activities, as well as to better understand the consequences of their choices and actions. Relevant positive behavioral supports may be created for every personal communication topic in a grid or visual scene format in the DynaVox Compass communication software available on our DynaVox T-10 device or as a subscription app.

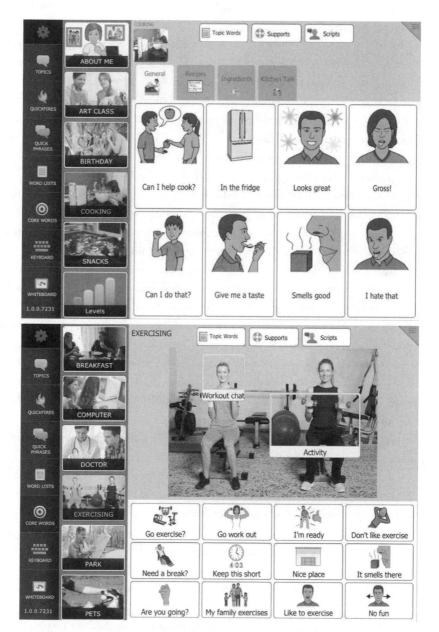

Figure 1 and 2 Topic-driven language content in the DynaVox Compass communication software is presented in both a grid format, as with this food-related vocabulary, and visual scenes, like the exercise scene. The Toolbar at the far left lets you move seamlessly between communication tools including topics and word lists. You can move between topics using the scrollable navigation bar (NavBar) between the Toolbar and the main page area.

Examples of positive behavioral supports:

- Contingency maps and "First (If), then . . ." pages. These related supports aid children in conveying more preferred/less preferred activities or items, and understanding the concept of good-better-best as it relates to their world. Contingencies can be simple if-then statements—"If I eat my dinner, then I can have ice cream," for example. The contingencies may be presented as a hierarchy, as in, "If I finish half my dinner, then I can have pretzels" or "If I clean my plate, then I can have a cookie," a perhaps more desirable treat. A positively reinforcing message ("If I set the table, then I can do puzzles") is often deemed more effective than one with negative overtones ("If I don't do my chores, then I can't play outside," for instance.) Social narratives benefit emergent communicators with a variety of developmental conditions who are ready to expand their language abilities and their communication partners. The narratives can help children with autism with self-regulation, understanding expectations and communication in new, difficult, or confusing situations such as transferring to a different school, visiting the dentist, or experiencing a power outage for the first time. Narratives are also helpful with transitions, which can be challenging when a child does not have a concrete frame of reference. The transition could be from home to school, a sunny morning to a rainy afternoon, or from a quiet car ride with mom to a crowded shopping mall. Generally short and easily tailored to individual learners, narratives integrate vocabulary with visual cues and help children respond appropriately in unfamiliar situations.
- Scripts similarly guide individuals through the beginning, middle, and end of a specific social exchange—introducing oneself or accepting a compliment, for instance. Like narratives, a script can help with self-management, clarifying expectations and following directions. Scripts may be dialogues or monologues, and may have visual cues or a text-only format.

The DynaVox Compass software includes templates for both social narratives and scripts.

- Visual schedules. Resembling a calendar or an illustrated recipe, these provide a concrete, often sequential, representation of activities the person will engage in, places they're going, or steps to tasks to be performed in the near future. Visual schedules are proven to reduce anxiety and increase independence. (Murdock, L.C. & Hobbs, J.G., 2011)

A link to a video on positive behavioral supports is provided in this chapter's reference section.

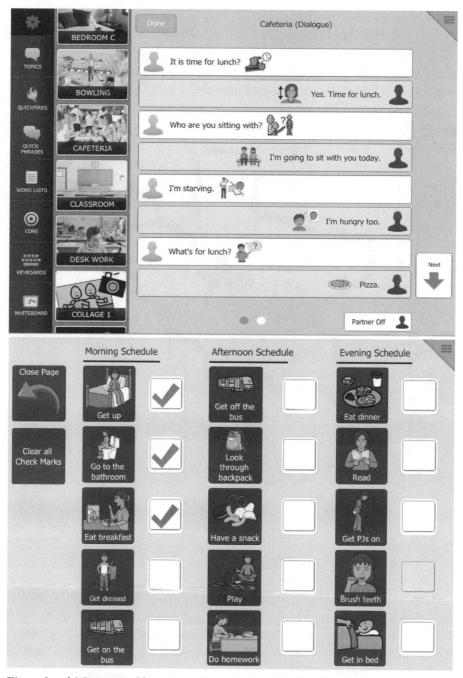

Figure 3 and 4 Customizable scripts and visual schedules like these help to ease everyday communication for individuals with autism and are included in the DynaVox Compass communication software.

The DynaVox Compass whiteboard is another tool for taking ownership of language. Like a blank piece of paper that you write or draw on with your finger, it can be used for drawing pictures, or to compose short messages and letters. Communication partners can use it together. Content created on the whiteboard can be saved in the device's cloud- based backup system for future use.

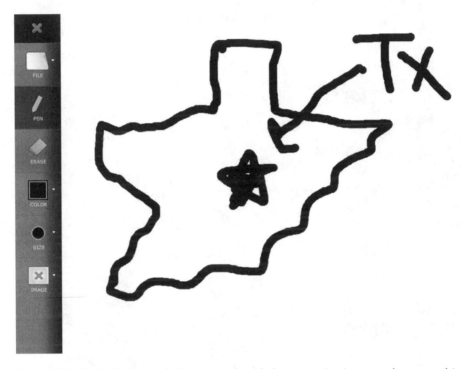

Figure 5 Individuals facing challenges with verbal communication can take ownership of language with aid from augmentative and alternative communication (AAC) tools such as this whiteboard on the DynaVox Compass software. Communication partners can use the whiteboard together, writing and/or drawing novel messages that may be saved for future use.

Sometimes those with good typing and literacy skills prefer to use the device keyboard to compose novel messages for in-person communication or emails, and its Internet capabilities to send and receive email, also viable ways of practicing social communication skills. It is often visual supports, however, that set communication in motion. Images—symbols, drawings, and photographs—lend visual representation that lets many folks with autism make sense of spoken language. Photos of familiar people, places and things, downloaded to or taken with a built-in camera on a device, provide meaningful context while symbols and drawings facilitate generalization. One boy shared his summer vacation plans through photos of the beach house where his family stays. His device also contains drawings of people shopping, which reminds him that shopping is an activity for everyone, not just people he knows.

With each generation of AAC technology come new motor planning solutions. The navigation pattern in our newest software moves forward instead of back and forth, eliminating the need to repeatedly open and close pages and pop-ups while conserving time and energy.

Support materials for school teams including storybooks and lesson plans are available. The online Boardmaker Achieve Community is a cloud-based venue for sharing original learning activities designed to facilitate meeting Common Core standards and individualized education program (IEP) goals including those related to social communication skills. Activities can be edited and saved in DynaVox Compass software. The Common Core State standards for each state also were part of the research to develop the software's core vocabulary.

Like many autism experts, our clinical and product development specialists believe modeling and role-playing, done in manageable steps, are optimal for teaching and learning social communication skills. In this best practice, technology is meant to be a catalyst, not a reason, for interaction. Onscreen interactive instruction or video self-modeling for expressive communication for children with or without AAC devices, for instance, can be a comfortable segue into modeling or role-playing one-on-one or in a small group setting.

Many of the tools and strategies described above are also effective for those with complex communication needs unrelated to autism. Their challenges may be associated with a congenital condition such as Down syndrome or cerebral palsy, or an acquired one, such as aphasia caused by a stroke.

Improvement

Alongside the ever-changing backdrop of AAC tools and technologies, personal desire for self-expression and nurturing communication partners are unchanging forces for lifelong communication skills improvement, as in the three examples shared below. The names of the individuals involved have been changed to honor privacy.

David used an AAC device throughout elementary school, drawing on his sharp visual and sequential memory to navigate its content. He usually responded readily when spoken to and developed a good vocabulary, but rarely initiated communication (even requests) and often seemed isolated in groups. Others gently and firmly encouraged his device use at home, school, and in community settings, to express his likes and dislikes, and to ask others theirs. Together they practiced the steps of a communication exchange before one actually took place. His school aide created pages on his device pages for sharing daily news with his family while his parents and siblings helped prepare "Last Night" and "Weekend" pages he used to tell classmates or teachers about life at home. He composed and sent messages using the email capabilities of his device to keep everyone in the loop.

Typical classmates formed a new bond with David over a Mystery State game during a fourth grade geography class. At his turn, David gave spoken clues as well as visual ones projected onto the interactive classroom whiteboard (not to be confused with the previously mentioned DynaVox Compass whiteboard) from the screen of his DynaVox Maestro AAC device. Peers saw him as one of their own and an academic lesson became a welcome social bridge.

As a child, Will often led his mother around by the hand, muttering in frustration until she understood what he wanted. She clipped pictures of his favorite foods and beverages from the packages so he could simply point to desired items. The DynaVox devices he used made functional communication easier yet. As he grew up, the adults in his life recognized opportunities for him to practice social skills. When company came, Will's mother asked him to share information with them through the device. He used the technology in high school work experiences. His job coaches made sure he had the vocabulary and free moments to ask coworkers how they were doing. On his days off, Will visited coworkers at a pizza shop during their lunch break just to chat.

At 18, Will reached an adult communication milestone on a visit to the Social Security office. Unhappy with the long wait to be served, he turned to a positive behavioral support on his device to tell the understanding clerk that waiting made him feel stressed. He told her that counting calmed him and proceeded to count, using the device, until his turn came. At one point, the clerk joined him in counting. Will expressed that he was hungry while meeting with the clerk, so she gave him and his mom directions to a nearby restaurant.

Will similarly kept a short conversation going through his device use when he met a favorite celebrity a few years later. He complimented her on her music videos and her looks as she autographed a T-shirt for him.

Robert, 28, likes hanging out with the other men at his group residence. He is equally comfortable saying, with the aid of his DynaVox Maestro, that he needs time alone. Robert then goes to his room where he may listen to oldies on the device's MP3 player.

The longtime house manager says the technology benefits staff, too. New employees who do not yet understand the body language Robert also uses to convey thoughts and feelings appreciate the access to concrete language the device offers. Robert likes routine and its visual tools help staff to help him stay on schedule. Just as she continually added pictures to his large childhood communication binder, Robert's mother regularly updates the device content, keeping his language skills fresh. It is Robert who best teaches others how to communicate with him, reminding them that he needs the device when he leaves home and showing them how it works.

David, Will, and Robert are fortunate that foundations for their communication success were set while they were young. Early intervention is ideal, but AAC planning is possible—and important—when it comes time for children move from school to the workplace, or to leave the place where they grew up for a new living arrangement. As parents and speech-language pathologists regularly remind me, a communication system with a device as its hub can mean the difference between days filled with inter-action and a life of silence.

34

FEEDING AND LANGUAGE STRATEGIES FOR MEALTIME

By Debbie Shiwbalak and Alpin Rezvani

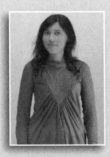

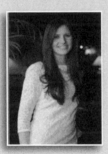

Debbie Shiwbalak, MA, CCC-SLP
Alpin Rezvani, MA, CCC-SLP
Gift of Gab Resources 1-855-SPEAK-HELP
www.giftofgabresources.com
debbie@giftofgabresources.com
alpin@giftofgabresources.com

Debbie Shiwbalak, MA, CCC-SLP, has a Baccalaureate of Arts in Speech Pathology and is a graduate of Long Island University-CW Post Campus, where she received a Master of Arts in Speech Pathology in 2001. She holds a Certificate of Clinical Competence (CCC) from the American Speech Language Hearing Association (ASHA) and is licensed by the state of New York to practice speech-language pathology. Debbie has 13 years experience as a speech pathologist in the New York City area.

Alpin Rezvani, MA, CCC-SLP, graduated from New York University with a Master's degree in Speech-Language Pathology. She holds a Certificate of Clinical Competence from the American Speech, Language, and Hearing Association (ASHA) and has New York licensure in Speech-Language Pathology. She has 7 years of experience as a speech pathologist in the New York City area and was an adjunct instructor at New York University.

Debbie and Alpin are co-founders of Gift of Gab Resources, which is a private practice that provides home-based speech therapy and evaluations. They provide workshops about speech and language development for parents and fellow speech pathologists throughout New York City at venues such as: NY Kids Club, Frolic Play Space, Preschool of America, and the Annual Young Child Expo & Conference. They also contribute monthly speech-related articles on various topics for parent groups called Mommy Bites and Big City Moms.

Mealtime for any family is extremely important—not only is it a time where you get vital nutrition for the day, but it provides you with a great opportunity to interact with each other. However, we know feeding your child may not always be easy. We know how tiring and frustrating it could be. Some parents refer to their children as "picky eaters" and this chapter is going to outline specific issues that can come up during mealtime. We will also provide strategies and techniques to help you generate feeding goals and learn how to assess your child's specific feeding issue. Feeding can be a stressful time for both parents and children; we hope this chapter will help to alleviate some of the anxiety related to feeding and mealtime.

When we eat, we do so with all of our 5 senses. You are SMELLING the food from the kitchen, then you SEE the food on the plate when it is presented to you. Some sights such as color, length, and shape might be more or less appetizing to certain children. Then, before you start eating you may TOUCH the food first. To some children, it may be too hard or too soft. Finally, you put it into your mouth and you are TASTING it. This of course can lead to sensory overload for many children. And then you take a bite and you're HEARING it. Due to all of the 5 senses interacting with each other, sometimes mealtime can last more than 30-45 minutes for a child.

Types of eaters

Difficulties with feeding may stem from a variety of issues, but can be categorized as sensory, behavioral, and/or physical or medical in nature. Sensory feeding can be determined when assessing patterns in a child's feeding behavior. Instead of using the term "picky eaters" we would like to go over 2 types of eaters that may have difficulty with mealtime. Some children can be "hypersensitive eaters" and some can be "hyposensitive eaters."

Hypersensitive eaters have a heightened oral sensitivity and may have high tone facial muscles. They are extremely sensitive eaters who prefer pureed or soft foods as well as bland or mild food with minimal texture. They avoid crunchy and chewy foods, and usually do not like their teeth brushed, etc.

Hyposensitive eaters can be defined as having less than normal sensitivity to food. Hyposensitive eaters often require feedback for his/her mouth and may pocket or hold food in the mouth due to decreased sensation. They prefer crunchy and flavorful foods (e.g., spicy, salty) and may also exhibit low tone of the facial muscles.

Once you've determined what type of eater your child is, you can begin to create a plan to slowly incorporate other tastes and textures into their diet. Following the 4Ts method below, you can begin to plan out goals for your child or client. Organizing goals into taste, temperature, tint (color), and texture can help parents and therapists target necessary problem areas.

The 4Ts method

Taste

There are four taste regions on the tongue as well as taste bud receptors, which respond to the type of foods we eat. We can assess what regions are tolerated based on a child's food preferences. Take note as to whether your child prefers salty, sour, bitter, or sweet foods. As speech pathologists, we have worked with children who prefer only one type of taste and the goal is to slowly add other flavors or tastes into the diet without overwhelming them. We proceed with caution and begin to experiment with adding more or less flavor to increase food variety.

Temperature

Some children are temperature sensitive. They may prefer to only eat cold or hot foods, drink water that is room temperature rather than right out of the refrigerator, etc. It is important to look at temperature when expanding your child's diet. Hyposensitive children often prefer very cold or very hot foods, while our hypersensitive children will restrict their diet to lukewarm meals and drinks. It is very important not to rush into a single temperature, but rather to work your way to expanding your child's diet. For example, adding one ice cube to a room temperature drink is a subtle way to tackle temperature, and then slowly build upon the temperature over time. If rushed, children may have adverse reactions to feeding and the building of trust between parent and child during mealtimes will have to begin again.

Tint (color)

Some children will refuse to eat based on tint or color. We worked with a child who would eat all of the rainbow colored goldfish crackers, except the green ones for fear it was a vegetable in disguise. When assessing your child's likes and dislikes about their meals, examine whether they are avoiding foods simply because of its color. If this is the case, there are lots of vegetables and coloring, which can change the color of a stew. We all try to avoid artificial coloring in our foods, especially when it comes to children, but there are healthier non-artificial options which can be added to meals to mask and change color.

Texture

The majority of our sensory feeding problems revolve around texture or how food feels. A child may have an aversion to food based on its visual presentation, as they are anticipating what the texture may feel like in their mouth. Textures can be broken down into liquids (water/juice), purees (pudding/yogurt), mechanical soft (banana/mashed potatoes), advanced solids (dissolvable crackers/cookies), and solids (chicken nuggets/apple). Our hyposensitive eaters will prefer foods that have a crunchy feel and they will avoid foods that provide little oral feedback such as purees. Hyposensitive eaters who also suffer from low tone often pocket their food, or hold food in their mouths between the cheek and gums, also known as the sulcus. Hypersensitive eaters will avoid most solids and gravitate towards softer, less orally offensive foods, as they have an aversion to too much sensory feedback. Increasing food variety based on textures can be a long process, and parents and therapists must be very patient, so as not to rush our sensory based eaters. Creating a feeding environment of trust and safety is very important. Now that you can identify the variety of textures, you can assess your child's problem areas. Begin to look at your child's feeding habits and patterns to determine what textures they prefer and which ones they avoid. Once you have created a list of target textures, you can slowly change texture. For example, if your child loves soft textures such as untoasted bread, slowly begin to toast it to change consistency over time and facilitate building your child's tolerance to harder textures. On the reverse side, if your child prefers crunchy toast and avoids purees or semi-solids, begin to add jam or butter to change the bread to a more pliable texture.

Medically based feeding disorders

Feeding issues may be medical in nature and this needs to be determined by a speech pathologist, an ear, nose, and throat doctor (ENT), or a gastroenterologist (GI). Medical issues can vary since so many factors can affect feeding and swallowing. Some of the more common issues include gastro-esophageal reflux disorders (GERD), metabolic disorders, low tone, high tone, or facial muscle generalized weakness, which may be secondary to a variety of syndromes and disorders. Our clients who are diagnosed with autism spectrum disorders often exhibit feeding difficulties, which may be medical in nature. For children with reflux, treatments can include medications prescribed by your doctor and/or eliminating foods that may cause flare-ups. Some families prefer to consult a nutritionist to determine appropriate diets for metabolic disorders, which are often associated with autism spectrum disorders. Behavioral issues can also surface as a result of allergies, reflux, metabolic disorders, etc. Children may develop an aversion to food based on their past experiences of discomfort when eating. Children who suffer from reflux often recall the discomfort and sensation of a flare-up. They begin to make the connection that they felt uncomfortable during or shortly after mealtime and will create a behavior to avoid food in general. It is important to consult an expert to determine the nature of a feeding and swallowing problem.

Steps you can take to make mealtime easier

Once you have consulted an expert to determine whether your child presents with a medical, behavioral, sensory, or a combination of feeding issues, you can move onto strategies to improve feeding.

First, conduct your own experiment. Try to determine a pattern to your child's feeding behaviors. For example, as speech pathologists, when we assess feeding behaviors, we try a variety of tastes and textures and document which foods your child will and will not eat until we have determined a pattern. We once conducted a feeding evaluation where the child refused to eat hard, crunchy foods. We told the parent, "You're child is a hypersensitive eater." The parent was relieved to have a label and a starting point for treatment.

Her following question was, "What do I do?" We explained that we do not expect our feeding clients to jump from purees to crunchy foods and vice versa overnight. It is a gradual process. Once you figure out what type of eater your child is, it's time to begin experimenting with foods that your child will not normally tolerate. Our advice is to always have fun with food, so do not be afraid to allow your child to explore and get messy with their food. Getting messy with food allows your child to eliminate their feelings of fear or food neophobia (fear of trying new foods).

Limit meal options to three, which should include two staple foods (foods your child will eat) and one new food item to explore. Keep in mind that most children with autism prefer to eat starches and often lack protein, so try to introduce foods that have significant protein content.

Once your child is ready to explore new foods, link the food with a subtle addition. For example, if your child loves crunchy toast, slowly add butter to the toast, then maybe some cheese, followed by vegetable or egg to ultimately lead to a sandwich. This can take weeks, and perhaps even months to achieve. It is important to think in terms of a hierarchy and it takes time to achieve the top echelon of this hierarchy, so be patient and this will help reduce stress for you and your child.

Children with autism often like routines. They prefer to follow a schedule for feeding and some children may not independently indicate hunger to their caregiver. Using visuals can allow your child to have a sense of order and provide much needed structure, which in turn reduces feeding anxiety. For example, present an after school picture schedule of homework, television, mealtime, and bathtime, so that your child knows what to expect in advance.

We strongly advise parents to never force-feed new foods. Forced feeding can create a negative association to mealtimes and possibly stress and fussing upon seeing a spoon, when placing a bib around their neck, or even when viewing their highchair. We include this as a feeding strategy because forced feeding can create new and more complex feeding problems, so it is best to approach feeding goals with caution and create a stress free environment for your child.

Language skills and mealtime

And last but not least, we want you to see mealtime not just as eating, but as a time to learn. There are many speech and language skills that you can target during breakfast, lunch, and dinner. To keep it simple we will continue to take a five senses approach.

HEAR: While making meals, there are many noises in the kitchen, so it becomes a great opportunity to comment on what they are hearing. Do not hesitate to make statements or ask questions to encourage commenting. For example, you can ask "What's going on in the kitchen?" while covering your ears to encourage your child to say "It's loud in there!" You may even talk about what you hear while you bite into the food (e.g., "I hear a crunchy chip"). Here is a sentence starter below along with possible adjectives.

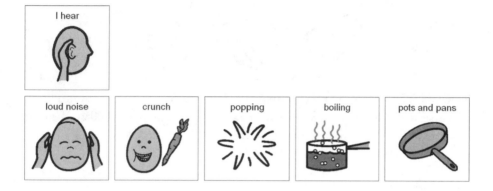

SMELL: When you are in the process of making something or when it is complete, say an open-ended statement to your child such as "Tell me about what you smell," or ask an open-ended question such as "What does it smell like?" If they have difficulty answering provide a model, "It smells sweet." Visuals for your child are below to encourage spontaneous productions.

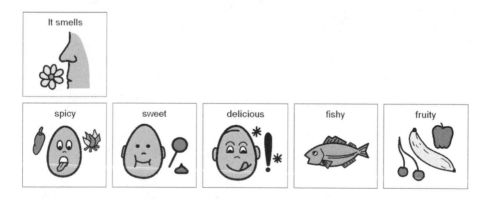

TASTE: A major part of eating is tasting our food, so it is a perfect time to spontaneously comment. Ask your child to "describe how it tastes." The visual of a sentence starter and various tastes are below.

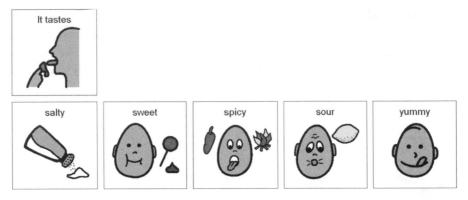

TOUCH: The moment a food is in front of a child, touching is hard to resist. This is, of course, perfectly fine since we encourage exploration. Offer your child open-ended prompts such as "Tell me about how the food feels . . ." Visuals below of a carrier phrase and various attributes can be helpful.

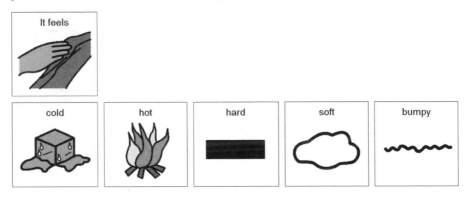

SEE: The whole act of eating is extremely visual, so feel free to talk about what their eyes are seeing. You can use a conversation starter such as "Can you tell me what your food looks like?" You may target commenting that involves color, length, shape, etc. You may use the visuals below as needed.

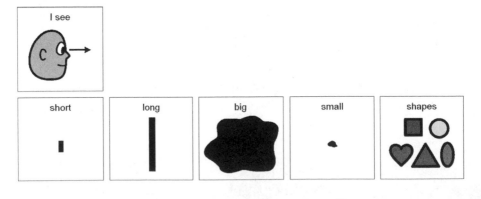

Additional language skills that can be worked on during mealtime include: initiating topics of conversation, maintaining conversation, recalling past events of the day (e.g., what they did at daycare), sequencing (e.g., the recipe, steps to setting the table), action words (e.g., stir, bake, eat, drink, etc.), requesting (e.g., "Help me open,"; "I want . . ."; "Can you pass the pepper, please?"), commenting using five senses, pointing to desired items, answering wh-questions and yes/no questions, etc.

Summary

Using our five senses approach, we hope that you have learned what type of eater your child is after reading this chapter. We hope that the 4Ts method—temperature, taste, tint, texture—will be helpful in expanding your child's palate. The key is to be patient and have fun—gradually you will see them grow into amazing eaters! We also encourage you to have your children be a part of all aspects of mealtime such as cooking and setting the table. If your child makes any attempt to taste, lick, or even touch a new food you should follow it with as much praise as possible so that he/she associates it with positivity. We wish you many happy and smooth mealtimes as a family!

35

AVANT GARDE APPROACHES TO LANGUAGE RESTORATION

By Dr. Harry Schneider

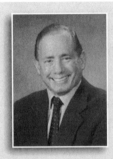

Harry D. Schneider, MD

146A Manetto Hill Road, Suite 207
Plainview, NY 11803
516-470-1930

491 North Indiana Avenue
Sellersburg, IN 47172
516-477-7682
hds7@columbia.edu or debra@harrydschneidermd.com
www.harrydschneidermd.com

- Advanced degrees in language and linguistics. Upcoming doctorate in Speech-Language Pathology
- World Health Organization, Pan American Studies and Research
- A neuroscientist at Columbia University Medical Center, where he has specialized in understanding the language circuits of the brain, having sent his research on these topics for publication to eminent peer-reviewed journals (www.fmri.org)
- A research fellowship in Neuroimaging at the Program for Imaging and Cognitive Sciences, Columbia University Medical Center, New York, New York
- Specialized training in diagnosing and managing autism at the Neurologic and Psychiatric Institute in New York, New York
- Investigational studies and clinical trials using novel forms of language therapy combined with investigational use of music, cerebellar-based physical activities, and neuromodulation (transcranial electromagnetic stimulation) to restore language function in minimally verbal ASD children

I have written three articles about cutting-edge technology we use to diagnose and treat language pathologies. To tell you that I am once again on the cutting edge sounds a bit like technological hubris—which I don't have—and which could conjure up pitfalls for all of us. I prefer to think of what we have been doing since the last "cutting edge" article as innovative and pioneering; new ways to study the brain for language functioning. Understanding how functional language is fully represented in the brain is no easy task. I need to understand the neural substrates of *all the features* of language: grammar (phonetics, morphology, syntax, semantics); the ability to use language to represent real-world situations; the ability to articulate something new;

the intention to communicate; arbitrariness of speech; linguistic interchangeability and socio-linguistic cultural transmission.

For children with developmental disabilities to learn all this must seem like an impossible task. There are no current therapies I am aware of that attempt to teach more than the rudiments of language. To accomplish what I need to do, therefore, I must delve even deeper into the workings of the brain. I aim to use a combination of imaging modalities, and then combine these images with our existing neuromodulation technology, transcranial direct current stimulation (TDCS). Such a profound understanding of language, as well as existing neuro-pathological representations (aphasia, autism), is the only way to truly provide efficacious, worthwhile, and useful treatment protocols to those in need of language repair—language therapies that are *sustainable* for children with developmental disabilities.

The cutting-edge imaging we have begun to explore is a form of "optical imaging," frequently called functional Near-Infrared Spectroscopy, FNIRS; it is one of the most promising imaging modalities to emerge in recent years. It is a truly noninvasive imaging technology, completely safe and benign enough so that it is now used to image infant brains. (Fig 1) FNIRS is helping to advance a wide range of research and clinical applications never thought possible. Applications derived from the science of linguistics include investigations of language and cognitive development over time in *infants*; those from the science of medical oncology include functional imaging of breast cancer at very early stages, even before the cancer is visible by x-ray. This optical imaging technology is now portable. It does not use ionizing radiation; the light from the NIRS unit emitted is LED

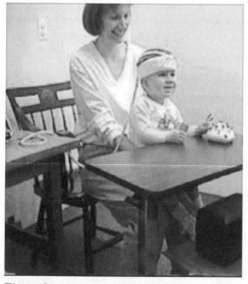

Figure 1

(light emitting diode) display light. This low-intensity red light has been used since the early 1960s in practical electronic components, such as displaying the digital time on watches. Devices containing LEDs are safe under all conditions of normal use and thus offer a host of advantages over other modalities. FNIRS has understandably recently attracted the interest of specialized professionals: cognitive medical neuroscientists like me, inquisitive surgeons, neurologists, and psychologists, among others. We all seem to have one common goal: early intervention.

We shall soon have the ability to map our brains from infancy to old age. This is the equivalent of a genome project for the brain. What if we also want to know what makes us become unnecessarily angry at our loved ones or unexpectedly not do well on a test at school? The best we can do now is measure behaviors externally—or go to the shrink. It is time to move beyond purely external measures and attempt to objectively test the behaviors we observe. With FNIRS , we could go about our daily business while brain mapping is being done using a lightweight band around the forehead. (Fig 2). We might be going about while daydreaming about becoming a billionaire or lamenting the loss of a loved one (Fig 3). We could then return home one-half hour later and review the images of our brain during this time to see what areas were activated or not activated but should have been. We have done bilingual testing along these lines—asking participants questions in their known languages— and noted the results. The brain activations in known language areas of the brain did not always correlate with the person's ability to speak that language. Regardless of the language output, we also noticed activity in other areas known to be associated with frustration. Brain areas for language ability and emotionality, or the frustration that sometimes accompanies speaking, were demonstrated to activate together. This led us to think about the importance of appropriate motivations and underlying feelings about speaking more than one language; it led us to think about different, sustainable approaches to bilingual education. We might stimulate multiple areas we believe will improve the weaker language and then acquire new FNIRS images to see if the stimulation affected both the language output and the emotion generated from its use. In essence, we can now image, treat, re-image, and re-treat ad infinitum any particular aspect of cognitive function using FNIRS and transcranial direct current stimulation (TDCS) together. I understand that solving the mysteries of genetics, black holes and using robotics to "operate" on inoperative brain areas are arguably cutting edge, but hypothesizing about what and where makes our brain function and then getting a real-time answer—is the particular edge I want. Having left Columbia University and now continuing on as a brain research scientist at Yale, I have temporarily put functional MRI to the side and am continuing to explore functional Near Infrared Spectroscopy. So, how does it work?

Researchers found 25-30 years ago that with the use of FNIRS, using light applied to and then detected from the scalp, useful information could be obtained from thick tissue samples, including the brain. This finding spurred the development of diffuse optics as a technique for human brain monitoring. All of the optical techniques are based on essentially the same concept: shine light onto the scalp through "emitting optodes" and then detect the light (with light detectors) as it exits the brain (Fig 3). We then measure the absorption spectra of light from specific light-absorbing molecules in the brain (called "chromophores") to interpret the amount of detected light as it

AND IT IS VERY PORTABLE!

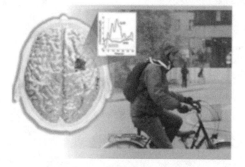

Figure 2

Here is what's under the headband:

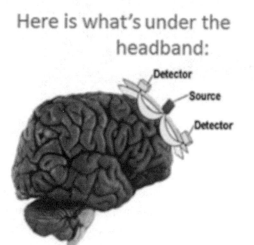

Figure 3

passes through them back to the scalp. In this case, just as with functional MRI, FNIRS detects the levels of hemoglobin (the main chromophores in the brain) *with* and *without* oxygen. The differential in oxygen consumption is the same BOLD signal (see article in cutting edge 1 and 2) as fMRI and tells us what parts of the brain are functioning for the task at hand.

Researchers had known, or rather believed, approximately 100-200 years ago that the basic idea of TDCS to stimulate an area of interest in the brain might be an appropriate, effective treatment for *everything* brain related, from depression to becoming really smart. Unfortunately, their investigations did not receive much attention at the time. When electroshock therapy (ECT) was developed for treatment-resistant depression in the 1930s and was found to be a relatively effective treatment to "re-boot"

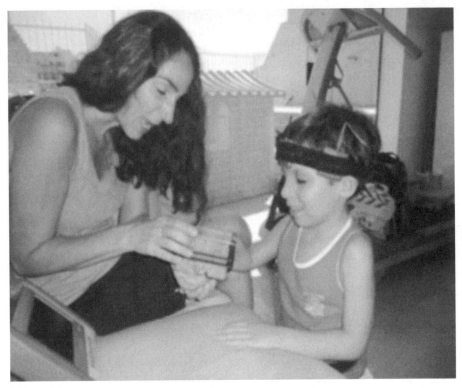

Figure 4

the brain, TDCS was completely abandoned. There are anecdotal reports that many patients viewed TDCS as a rather "Frankensteinian" approach, understandably so since the movie Frankenstein was released in 1931. Even today, parents ask me if I am going to "fry their childrens' brains" or make their brother look like "Frankenstein." Some thirty years later, there was another brief rise of interest in TDCS in the 1960s, for conditions such as depression, but at that time antidepressant medications were becoming available. A tuberculosis drug was found to make patients unusually cheerful. It was determined that the drug blocked one of the neurotransmitter systems—the monoamine oxidase system—resulting in increased levels of adrenalin-like chemicals and dopamine. This led to the development of MAO inhibitors, which today can be purchased OTC as an alternative medication in the form of St. John's Wort. Soon thereafter, there followed the tricyclic antidepressants, such as Elavil and Tofranil, and later the SSRIs like Prozac, which are still used today for depression. With the advent of new brain imaging techniques such as MRI and fMRI, which lead to a better understanding of basic brain functioning, TDCS is now finally at the center of attention. Medications were fraught with too many side effects for some and people were looking for non-pharmaceutical alternatives.

For those of you who have been following my "cutting-edge" reports, you already know that during a treatment session, the TDCS unit uses a very small electric current (unlike electroshock therapy): one thousandth of 1 ampere. "Electrodes," in the form of sponges soaked in salt water, are placed over certain parts of the head to conduct the electricity to where it is needed. The electrodes are held in place using a nylon or cloth headband. The direct current flows through the electrodes, from positive to negative, penetrating the scalp, creating a flow of electrical current in the brain. The only side effects are a slight itching or tingling sensation felt on the scalp under the sponge. These weak currents enhance brain activity under the site of the electrodes. The way in which they do this is complex, involving changes in neurotransmitter activity and synaptic plasticity, and is beyond the scope of this article. Since the last article I wrote for *Cutting Edge*, TDCS is now used all over the world in major universities in research programs: stimulation of the prefrontal cortex to improve learning and increase working memory; to the motor cortex to raise threshold for pain and make one more adept with the non-dominant hand; to parts of the left Perisylvian language area (in right-handed people) to facilitate language acquisition; to the parietal cortex to improve numerical reasoning; and on improving memory, math, language recovery in stroke, depression and most recently, even to reverse the cognitive decline in ageing.

I still concentrate mostly on language recovery/restoration in anyone who has lost it. Anyone who has lost it and then recovered it might tell you that was perhaps the most devastating time in their life; I never take not having language for granted. But remember that language is not just speaking. It's much more. Even the structure of the way we speak consists of subsystems: *phonology:* the smallest significant unit of sound in a language; *morphology:* the smallest unit of a language that has a meaning; *syntax:* the part of grammar that has to do with the arrangement of words to form phrases and sentences; and *semantics:* our lexicon (mental dictionary), which is the total stock of words in our language. For us to restore language fully, syntax is a must-have, a template onto which we must apply *sociolinguistics,* that is, how speech varies depending on a person's position in a social structure or relationship. And we must delve into some linguistic tongue twisters: haptics, the study and analysis of touch and how it affects speech; chronemics is the study of the different ways that cultures understand time and use it to communicate; proxemics is the study of the ways in which different cultures use space; and kinesics is the study of body movement, facial expressions, and gaze.

And last, but not least, we must explore the intricacies of pragmatics (social speech). We must know how to use three different kinds of pragmatics to socially interact gracefully. We must *use language* for different purposes, such as informing (e.g., I'm going to get a cookie) or requesting (e.g., I would like a cookie, please). We have to *change* language according to the needs of a listener or situation, such as talking differently to a baby than to an adult and speaking differently in a classroom than on a playground; and finally speakers need to *follow rules* for conversations and storytelling, such as taking turns in conversation, staying on topic, and how close to stand to someone when speaking, how to use facial expressions, and eye contact. Learning language is much more than repeating scripted phrases or amount of vocabulary! As I mentioned before, I must know which parts of the brain are involved in each of these features of language, in order to stimulate brain areas in harmony. When you have time, re-read the stuff I just wrote about language, and you will see that language, social interaction, emotions, passion, paying attention, decision making, making contact with each other—and on and on ad infinitum—all interact with each other!

After many investigations on using functional MRI to understand the autistic brain – and being a journal reviewer myself—I am now essentially approaching language restoration as a real-time combination imaging/treatment protocol. Infrared imaging does not give me a better image (it really is difficult to out-perform FMRI). FNIRS is more patient-friendly and can give me an image within thirty minutes. Our LFA (Low Functioning language in Autism) kids will not have to deal with the noise of fMRI, the radioactivity of PET or the x-radiation of CT machines. That being said, at Yale, we are preparing a research investigation that will compare the data and image quality from FMRI to that of FNIRS, because we have experience with both. We will show these two imaging modalities of the brain produce images that are comparable in quality. Detailed comparisons of the signals are done in both temporal (how fast we produce the image) and spatial (how fine is the detail) domains. It is thought that NIRS signals have a lower resolution (less detail in the images), but are nonetheless highly correlated with specificity of fMRI measurements. While fMRI has become the gold standard for in vivo imaging of the human brain in a laboratory or hospital setting, in clinical practice where kids are moving around and playing, FNIRS is noticeably more convenient and obviously a less expensive technology than fMRI. FNIRS can be an appropriate substitute for fMRI for studying brain activity related to cognitive tasks. I design studies for FNIRS that ensure that the spatial resolution—seeing enough detail within a brain area of interest—is adequate. The design protocols I use are the paradigms in which the order of instructions and tasks that the FNIR unit must follow. These paradigms can be done each time a child is evaluated or only when needed to follow a particularly new treatment modality. The application of FNIRS to image and then TDCS to treat (language) problems in the brain is sustainable way to restore language. We can see what happens in the brain during a language session, and see how those brain changes relate to what the participant did. What areas increased in intensity (showed signs of plasticity), what areas were underused, and did any unexpected areas become activated during the language-learning session? We have the obvious options of continuing or modifying our therapy approach each session, depending on what FNIRS imaging demonstrates. We can evaluate the cortical plasticity induced by the TDCS in real time and determine if we want this particular pathway to continue to develop long term.

The novel combination of TDCS, fNIRS and implicit-language offer insights into how cortical plasticity influences language task performance during and after interventions. Of utmost importance is continually making social contact with a child during each session and encouraging the child to want to enter into a world that is not yet theirs. We are attempting to document whether a child is acquiring a "theory of mind" by assessing the social areas of the brain's response to eye contact: the beginnings of social functioning. We are using brain areas known to stimulate emotional integration, which demonstrate the neural underpinnings of joint attention, during language therapy. TDCS stimulation of known language areas and concomitantly stimulating parts of the pre-frontal cortex enhances a child's "innate need" to make eye contact. This integrates initiating social contact and functional conversation. TDCS has been shown to modulate behaviors that may be more cautious or more risky. Neuromodulation of this type can influence cognitive processes involved in decision-making, which are at the core of human social and emotional function and dysfunction. These behaviors include not only risk taking, but reward seeking, impulsivity, and fairness consideration within correct and appropriate social interaction. When decision making is incorporated into language tasks, we generate the beginnings of *social* decision making—deciding to interact socially. This is the first time that such bimodal image/stimulation investigations are being done and the results are promising.

If someone's being at the cutting edge means their being at some position of the greatest advancement or the leading position in a particular field of study, then one has to continue learning. Learning is the beginning of health and the beginning of spirituality. Searching and learning is where the miracle process all begins. Walt Disney once said if you can dream it, you can do it. When a child speaks to me and gives me a hug of thanks, it makes me want to never stop learning.

36

COMMUNITY-BASED SPEECH LANGUAGE PATHOLOGY

By Alpin Rezvani

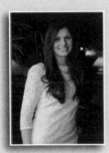

Alpin Rezvani, MA, CCC-SLP

Alpin Rezvani, MA, CCC-SLP, graduated from New York University with a Master's degree in Speech-Language Pathology. She holds a Certificate of Clinical Competence from the American Speech, Language, and Hearing Association (ASHA) and has New York licensure in Speech-Language Pathology. She has seven years of experience as a speech pathologist in the New York City area and was an adjunct instructor at New York University.

What is Community-Based Speech Language Pathology?

Our role as speech language pathologists, when working with any individual, is to mold them into effective communicators in society. In general, individuals on the autism spectrum have difficulty carrying over specific speech and language skills acquired during their sessions. As a result, it is often best to steer away from traditional one-to-one clinician directed therapy in a speech pathologist's office. Instead, it is best to venture out into the community while simultaneously encouraging clients take the lead. After all, the most effective way to learn is to practice by doing.

What are specific speech and language skills that can be generalized into the community?

- Labeling
- Producing Longer Utterances
- Topic Initiation
- Taking Turns
- Answering Questions
- Maintaining a Conversation
- Other Pragmatic/Social Skills
- Commenting
- Narratives

What are some settings or events that could help promote generalization of speech and language skills? What are some examples?

- Occupational Therapy—requesting a specific crayon color while practicing writing skills
- Physical Therapy—commenting on actions (e.g., "Look, I'm biking!"); counting the number of balls they throw
- Counseling—commenting on feelings
- School/Daycare—initiating "Good Morning"; singing along to songs; participating in academic lessons; taking turns in board games (e.g., "my turn"); asking to go to the bathroom; asking the nurse for their medication; commenting on feelings/states (e.g., "I'm thirsty!")
- Ice Cream Store—requesting a specific flavor with toppings
- Pharmacies—saying "Hi" to a cashier; ordering a prescription
- Libraries/Book Stores—asking where to find a book (e.g., "Where can I find the pop up books?")
- Zoo/Farm—labeling animals; asking permission (e.g., "Can I pet the rabbit?")
- Cooking—asking for help; sequencing steps to a recipe
- Museums—asking questions about the map (e.g., "Where can I find the dinosaur section?")
- Sports Activities—producing common phrases while interacting with peers (e.g., "It's your turn to bowl!"; "Ready set go!")
- Playground—initiating a game of tag; producing common phrases while interacting with peers (e.g., "Tag, you're it!")
- Bath Time—requesting a towel, Epsom salt, shampoo/conditioner; commenting on the temperature of the water (e.g., "Ouch! Too hot!")
- Story Time—directing the adult (e.g., "Turn the page"); initiating "wh" questions (e.g., "Why is he sad?")
- Art—requesting items necessary to paint
- Music—commenting on likes or dislikes (e.g., "I like that song! Play it again!")
- Computers/Video Games—engage in turn taking; commenting on status (e.g., "Yay! You're winning!"; "Go faster!")
- Watching TV—asking where the remote control is or to change the channel; holding a conversation about their favorite television show
- Walks—commenting on what they see, hear, etc. (e.g., "I hear a firetruck. It's so loud!")
- Restaurants—ordering food; using polite manners
- Post Office—buying stamps from the cashier; asking for a pen, tape, etc.
- Supermarket/Deli—asking about prices(e.g., "How much is this KitKat?")

- Movies—having a conversation about favorite scenes (e.g., "Did you like the scene where they were racing the cars?"); sequencing the main scenes; delineating the components of the film (e.g., main characters, problem, consequence, resolution, etc.)
- Taking Public Transportation—asking for directions
- Bank—asking for a lollipop
- Pools—commenting on the temperature of the water; asking for help while putting on their bathing suit; directing communication partner (e.g., "Go under and hold your breath for 2 seconds!"); playing social games (e.g., ring toss; "Marco Polo!")
- Trick-or-Treating—complimenting a friend's costume; telling a Halloween joke; initiating "trick or treat" and "thank you"
- Parades—commenting on what they see (e.g., "Wow, Mom, Snoopy is big!")
- Birthday Parties—singing "Happy Birthday"; giving a gift or saying "Thank you" for a gift
- Department Stores—commenting on clothing (e.g., "Pretty hat!")
- Fairs/Amusement Parks—initiating wants (e.g., "Let's go on ferris wheel!")

What can speech pathologists' role be in community events that they normally would or could not take part in with my child?

There are some instances in which speech-language pathologists may not be able to accompany children on their community adventures. This may include: doctor visits, haircuts, sleepovers, vacations, etc. In these cases, the speech-language pathologist can prepare them by making communication boards. For instance, if the child is going to an audiologist next month, you can make a board with core vocabulary such as "Hi," "Help Me," "Thank you," "Where's the bathroom?", "I'm finished," and activity-based words such as "Yes I hear it," "No I don't hear it," "Headphones please," "Too tight." By repeating target vocabulary and possibly acting out the future visit, your child will be equipped with the necessary language, consequently instilling him or her with more confidence.

What if my child is afraid to take part in certain community experiences?

Some of community experiences may be fear invoking, meaning children will be so anxious for the experience they may not be willing to participate. In these instances, we have found that social stories work best. These are personalized books that are tailored to each child to ease them into a social situation that initially made them feel uncomfortable. They can also be used to promote appropriate socials skills (e.g., private versus public behavior). The key is to maintain positive wording throughout the story and give them possible strategies to help them overcome their fear or issue. For example, if a child is anxious to go trick-or-treating on Halloween, while practicing you can use a camera to take pictures of the child to include in the book (e.g., putting on their costume, holding their treat bag, walking on the street, knocking on the door, internal reward of getting candy, looking through their candy, and ultimately eating their candy). Pages with strategies such as "If I hear a loud noise I can ask to put in ear plugs," "If I'm starting to feel uncomfortable I can do my breathing exercise," etc., can be incorporated into the book.

We must always remember that many of our children are visual learners. Therefore, creating a visual schedule of what to expect may also be a helpful technique in these instances. Some children have general schedules of what they will expect during the day (e.g., brushing teeth, getting dressed, breakfast, school, etc.), but in this case you can create an embedded schedule. Therefore, if for instance, trick-or-treating was on the child's general schedule, you can make a more detailed schedule of trick-or-treating only. The following pictures or symbols may be needed: costume, face paint, treat bag, walking, knocking on door, trick or treat, candy, thank you, searching candy, and eating candy.

Lastly, a technique called video modeling would also be a helpful form of perceptual support. This has been a great method to use when modeling and visual aids such as pictures and symbols were not successful strategies. Children are shown videos of targeted behavior (e.g., appropriate pretend play, playing tag, sharing bubbles, playing hide & seek, etc.) and the majority of the time they begin to imitate it. A mother of a boy with autism created DVDs called "Watch Me Learn," which shows children interacting in community based activities. If you are not able to get a hold of such videos you may try creating your own to personalize the video or simply look up similar YouTube videos.

How can AAC be incorporated into Community-Based Speech Language Pathology?

The ultimate goal of a speech-language pathologist is give our children the skills to become functional communicators—that includes verbal and nonverbal communication. Low tech (e.g., PECS) and high tech AAC (e.g., computerized devices) can undoubtedly be intertwined into the child's daily routines at home, school, and in the community. At times, this may take advanced planning (e.g., printing out necessary symbols or making a new activity page on a computerized system), but in the long run it pays off since the child will be prepared to take into any future setting. The key to helping a child generalize the use of their AAC system is to train individuals that work with the child. This includes the family members, classroom teacher, paraprofessionals, physical therapist, occupational therapist, counselor, other instructors (e.g., swim, piano, etc.), etc. The speech-language pathologist can play a huge role in turnkeying this information and there are also many free trainings offered by companies if your child has a high-end device. We must remember that AAC devices are our children's inner voices. Therefore, devices recommended for our children should be durable and easily portable to make sure they can be brought to all community activities.

How can an iPad, iPhone, or iPod Touch be a child's communication system?

Proloquo2go is an application that can currently be purchased for $189.99. It contains professionally made boards with audible messages. It also allows you to edit and custom make communication boards in order to personalize it to the life of the child. Others include TouchChat by Silver-Kite and SoundingBoard by AbleNet. Respectively, they are priced at $149.00 and $49.99. The latest version of SoundingBoard includes auditory scanning, which is utilized for children whose fine motor skills do not allow them to access buttons via touch. To increase durability of the iPad, it can be enclosed in an iAdapter case that has a handle, which was created by AMDi. The latest version is sold for $265.00 and includes amplified speakers.

What are other speech-language therapy related applications on the iPad, iPhone, or iPod Touch that are rich in language and that can promote communication?

- Focuses on **eye contact**: Fizz Brain; Look in my Eyes
- Concentrates on **pragmatics** and **social cues**; Provides practice in interpreting **feelings**: Touch & Say; Smile at Me; Super Duper What Are They Thinking; The Social Express; iTouch Learn Feelings
- Helps children retain **basic information** (e.g., school name, address, birthday, phone number, favorite items, etc.): All About Me
- Promotes taking **conversational turns**: Conversation Builder; Conversation Starters
- Helps build **vocabulary**: Learn to Talk; Speech with Milo; Pogg; House of Learning; Starfall
- Promotes **longer and more complex utterances**: iStory; 60 Story Starters; More Pizza!
- Targets **receptive language**: Preposition Remix; Splingo's Language Universe; My Playhome; Cupcake Corner
- Provides **communication boards** that can be adapted: Grace Picture Exchange for Non-Verbal People
- Targets appropriate **behavior** in various community settings: Model Me Going Places; School Skills

- Geared toward **language and drawing**: Doodle Buddy
- Helps children prepare for **dental visits**: My Healthy Smile
- Contains **visual schedules, routines** among other items: iCommunicate
- Provides picture-based prompts to guide in **transitioning** from one activity to the next and improves focus: iPrompts
- Targets **articulation** skills: Articulate it!; Articulation Station; Artic Pix; Smarty Speech

For more ideas, go online and search for Therapy App 411, Geek SLP, or SLP Sharing. There is also a list of Android applications available online for children with special needs created by special education teacher Jeremy Brown.

Will my child automatically generalize learned language skills into the community?

Generalizing speech and language skills will be a gradual process. A speech-language pathologist may initially use maximal verbal, visual, and physical prompting, but as the child becomes a more independent communicator, the once necessary prompts will be faded or completely eliminated depending on the child.

After years of experience working with children on the autism spectrum, we feel that best practice includes doing speech-language therapy in the home and eventually generalizing acquired skills into the community setting. Whether your child communicates via verbalizations or with an AAC device, it is crucial to make each teachable language moment salient so that it has a greater chance of remaining in the child's repertoire. Saliency is increased when we work with children in their natural environments. Our goal for this chapter is for readers to realize how children learn best and what we can do to provide the necessary support for them to communicate in the community. It was also to teach readers to "think out of the box." While traditional one-to-one therapy still has its place, we must recognize the benefits of carryover into the home and community. The only way this goal will be reached is to increase awareness in society and have our children get as much practice in the real world as possible. In the end, we hope to have helped your children make their needs known, participate in social exchanges, develop long lasting relationships, and hopefully even become productive members of society.

37

JOINT ACTION ROUTINES (JARS)

By Lerone Kamara, Jessica Goldberg, and Alpin Rezvani

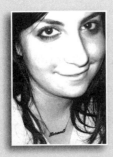

New York City Department of Education
District 75
http://schools.nyc.gov/Offices/District75/default.htm

Lerone Kamara, MA, CCC-SLP
lerone.kamara@gmail.com

Lerone Kamara, MA, CCC-SLP, received her Bachelor's Degree in Speech-Language Pathology from City University of New York's Queens College. She graduated from Long Island University C.W. Post., with a Master's degree in Speech-Language Pathology and additionally earned a certificate as a Teacher of Students with Speech and Language Disabilities (TSSLD). Lerone has New York State licensure in Speech Language Pathology, as well as her Certificate of Clinical Competence (CCC) from the American Speech, Language and Hearing Association (ASHA). She works in conducting evaluations, and developing treatment plans for children with mild to severe developmental disorders including intellectual disabilities, autism spectrum disorders, and emotional disturbance.

Lerone has been working as a Speech-Language Pathologist for the New York City Department of Education and District 75 since September 2008. For the past four years she has been working with elementary age school children classified with having intellectual disabilities, autism spectrum disorders, and emotional disturbance. Lerone has been trained in and utilizes a wide range of therapeutic techniques including Joint Action Routines (JARs), Picture Exchange Communication Systems, Sounds in Motion, and the multi-sensory SMiLE program. She works closely with classroom teachers to collaborate and implement these practices into her therapy program, while addressing the speech, language, and feeding needs of her students. Additionally, she implements instructional mealtimes and instructional yoga at her school.

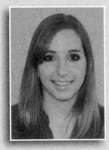

Jessica Goldberg, MA, CCC-SLP
jessicagoldbergspeech@gmail.com

Jessica Goldberg, MA, CCC-SLP, graduated from the University of Maryland at College Park with a Bachelor's degree in Hearing and Speech Sciences and a Concentration in Education, and from New York University with a Master's degree in Speech-Language Pathology. Jessica has New York licensure in Speech-Language Pathology, holds the Certificate of Clinical Competence from the American Speech, Language, and Hearing Association (ASHA), and earned her degree as a Teacher of the Speech and Hearing Handicapped. She specializes in the evaluation and treatment of children with moderate to severe developmental disorders including autism spectrum disorders, emotional disturbance, and intellectual disabilities.

Jessica is a Speech-Language Pathologist for the New York City Department of Education. She currently works in a District 75 school for children diagnosed with autism spectrum disorders. Jessica holds a position on her school-based Augmentative Alternative Communication (AAC) Evaluation Team. Jessica implements a variety of techniques as part of her therapy practices, including Picture Exchange Communication Systems, SMiLE, Sounds in Motion, Therapeutic Crisis Intervention, and Joint Action Routines.

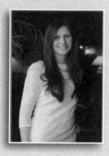

Alpin Rezvani, MA, CCC-SLP
ilovespeech@gmail.com

Alpin Rezvani, MA, CCC-SLP, graduated from New York University with a Master's degree in Speech-Language Pathology. She holds a Certificate of Clinical Competence from the American Speech, Language, and Hearing Association (ASHA) and has New York licensure in Speech-Language Pathology. She has 7 years of experience as a speech pathologist in the New York City area and was an adjunct instructor at New York University.

One of the challenges we face as speech pathologists is encouraging social interaction with peers and siblings. Rather than instinctively communicating with those who are close to their own age, we often find that children with special needs are drawn to interactions with adults. The reason for this is that adults are more likely to respond to their wants and needs. Many times, with an adult communication partner, the adult is able to infer what the child wants. The adult naturally responds so the child is able to cope using minimal joint attention skills. Joint attention refers to the ability to identify what another person is attending to or the ability to draw another person's attention toward something of interest to them. This can be accomplished either verbally (i.e., calling someone's name) or nonverbally (i.e., eye contact). Interacting with peers and siblings demands joint attention skills, and therefore, more independence from the child.

Joint attention is extremely important to social, cognitive, and language development. Development of these skills are closely related because language is usually performed in a social, interactive context; communication occurs naturally. Sometimes, however, our children do not acquire the skills necessary for social interaction without help. It is difficult to plan for these types of interactions to occur. The use of a routine is a valuable approach that can be implemented in the classroom, therapy room, home, or in the community. A Joint Action Routine (JAR) encourages joint attention, language, and a meaningful social interaction.

What are Joint Action Routines?

Joint Action Routines (JARs) are a powerful strategy for teaching communication and other skills through naturalistic, interactive activities and routines. It was created at the University of Kansas, Parsons Research Center, under the direction of Dr. Lee Snyder-McLean. It can be used with children of all ages with autism, cognitive delays, and developmental disabilities.

JARs are structured activities that weave in *planned opportunities* for students to work on *communication/social skills* within a meaningful, functional, and enjoyable context.

To understand the elements of Joint Action Routines, the following is a breakdown of each component:

- Joint—children interacting with others
- Action—children actively involved
- Routine—repeated many times

These three crucial components allow for a way to improve social interaction and communication by using routine activities. All of these interactions do not need to be done verbally. You can use pictures, symbols, and/or communication devices for these interactions.

Who can use JARs?

Speech therapists, parents, caregivers, other family members, classroom teachers, and paraprofessionals can all implement JARs.

What are the critical elements of a successful JARS?

- *Clear beginning and definite ending*—Define the structure by indicating the start and end of an activity (i.e., sing a song to initiate and cleanup to finish).
- *Obvious unifying theme and/or purpose*—Choose a theme that will be functional for your child. For example, if you want your child to learn to order food at a restaurant, you can make that the theme of your JARs.
- *Logical sequence and clearly defined interchangeable roles*—Create a series of steps which will be carried out in the same order each time you engage in the routine; this allows for predictability. Once routines become familiar, roles can be switched around.
- *Based on an individual needs*—Build upon the child's emerging skills, and consider what you want them to achieve.

- *Motivating activities, materials, and prompts*—Select activities according to their interests and strengths.

- *Planned variations*—As the child becomes more comfortable with the routine, you can deviate from the script and add spontaneous language. For example, if you are doing a JARs based on brushing teeth, hide the toothpaste and let your child figure it out.

- *Opportunities for repetition*—Have participants consistently repeat the same actions and use scripted language while following the routine.

- *Structured for turn taking*—Allow for planned opportunities between participants to initiate and maintain conversation and/or share items throughout the activity (i.e., Announce "My turn" or "Your turn").

- *Joint attention*—Provide opportunities for shared interest and ways to seek the attention of a communication partner.

- *Variety of settings*—Routines can be set up at home, school, and generalized into community activities.

Why are JARs useful?

Since JARs allows for repetition, it provides our children the opportunity to practice skills over and over, which is the most effective way for those skills to become spontaneous. Typically, most activities are used one time. Doing an activity one time (i.e., building a snowman one day and cutting out a snowflake the next) does not give our children enough time to learn the activity much less the targeted skills. Repeated use of routines become predictable, so children are provided the opportunity to feel successful in a social environment.

As children become successful in following these predictable routines, a scaffold can be provided for learning new skills. For example, at first a child may ask a question using a written prompt (i.e., Do you want a plate?), but within several opportunities, he or she may independently ask the question to his or her communication partner, without any form of prompting. Ultimately, the goal is for our children to generalize the language and social skills they acquire while participating in JARs activities. By providing scaffolding while they learn new skills, we also provide the opportunity for generalization to occur naturally.

Many activities are adult-directed, and are not designed to promote interaction. For example, when creating a snowflake, the adult hands out the materials and advises the child what to do as the child passively listens. Communication is not necessary. During JARs, however, the child must be an active participant and the social component is essential for success.

Since JARs are extremely flexible and are based around an individual's needs, they can provide an excellent framework for working on other skills within a meaningful and functional context such as literacy, math, science, and job site skills.

How do you plan a JAR?

Determine the activity according to child's communication, social, and academic skills.

- List the steps required for the activity
- Decide what roles participants will assume
- Plan opportunities for participants to interact with each other
- Create a list of materials and props that you will need
- If there are a lot of participants, it may be a good idea to create a "job board," displaying each person's job using pictures and/or words
- Plan a regular time of day or week to plan the JAR
- Don't be afraid of repetition!

What are some examples of JARs?

Example 1: *Playing With Bubbles*

- A child plays with a bottle of bubbles alone.
- An adult comes over and sits with the child with the bubble container between them.
- The adult creates a predictable sequence of taking the cap off of the bottle and dipping the stick and blowing bubbles.
- Possible target communication exchanges could include: "open bubbles," "want bubbles," "blow bubbles," "more bubbles," "pop bubbles," and "bubbles finished."
- The adult says target exchange during each step. This is repeated many times the exact same way.
- Over time, pauses are implemented and the child fills in the scripts.

The child also begins to understand the expectations, as well as the "give and take" of communicative exchanges. Eventually, the child learns to become more spontaneous with words and actions.

Example 2: *Making Hot Chocolate*

- Steven looks at the job board and it says, "Give out cups."
- Steven asks his classmate, "Excuse me, do you want a cup?"

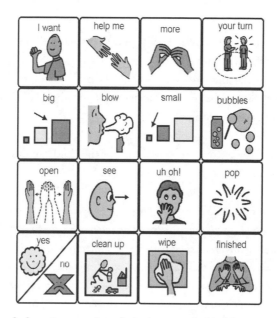

Figure 1: *The visual above is a speech-pathologist created aided-language board. The purpose is to provide the child with a visual support to aid in requesting and commenting during a particular activity. The board includes a variety of short phrases, nouns, verbs, exclamations, and concepts to make sure that the child is able to participate in the activity to the fullest extent. Aided language boards and visual always vary depending on a child's abilities. It is also important to note that often times an adult will need to model using the board in order for the child to become successful in understanding how to use the board appropriately.*

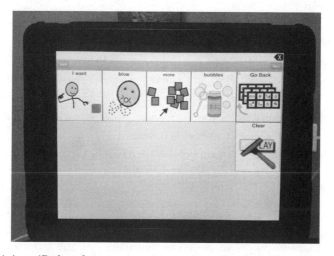

Figure 2: *This is an iPad used as a communication device for the bubbles joint action routine. Possible comments, questions, or answers the child may produce are preprogrammed in order for the child to be a proactive member of the activity.*

- His classmate answers "yes" or "no."
- If his classmate answers "yes," Steven puts a cup on his desk.
- Steven continues with this step until he has asked everyone who is present.
- Steven calls his classmate to look at the job board.
- The next jobs would be passing out napkins, hot chocolate, and marshmallows, until the sequence is completed.
- As the child becomes more comfortable with this, polite language such as "thank you" and "you're welcome" can be added or the child can deviate from the script (e.g., ask "Is that too hot?" or "do you like it?").

This delineates the sequence of the hot chocolate joint action routine for a classroom. It empowers each child by allowing them to be responsible for of a step. Their classmates give them a number, which they then match. They then look at the visual or written words to remind them of which step they perform. Natural communication acts are intermingled (e.g., if it is a child's turn to hand out marshmallows they may initiate questions like "Do you want marshmallows?" and wait for a "yes" or "no" answer from their peers; they may also ask "How many?"). The students take turns with their classmates until their end goal is reached.

Example 3: **Restaurant**

- Six friends each have a job including host, waiter, cook, second waiter, bus boy, and cashier.
- They take turns carrying out their jobs, utilizing routine language and social scripts.
- The host asks, "How many?" and takes friends to their table.
- The waiter asks, "What would you like today?" and writes down orders.
- The cook prepares the food, while verbally sequencing the steps of the recipe.
- The second waiter takes the appropriate order to each friend, and he creates receipts by adding up the cost of their order.
- The bus boy uses eye contact with his friends as he exchanges a picture of a plate for their empty plate. He then puts their plate in the trash.
- The cashier follows a social script to collect money.

Example 4: **Joint Action Routines for the Home**
   The visuals above are ideas for joint action routines you can perform at home that are related to activities of daily living and possible chores. You may use the given sequence or modify it to your needs.

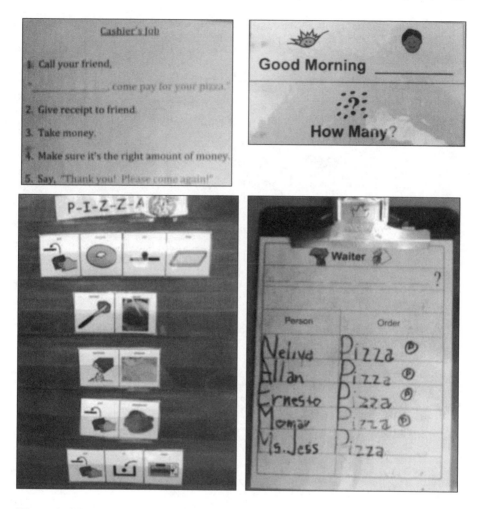

Figure 3: *The visuals included in this example were created to support the individual goals of one particular group of students. Some of the children in this class are able to read and write, as others use pictures to help them communicate. Support systems can be created in a various number of ways, as long as each child is able to actively participate in the cohesive routine.*

Additional examples of JARs to use:

JARs for younger kids:

- Nursery Rhymes
- Reading a familiar book
- Getting dressed

Examples of Joint Action Routines to Use at Home

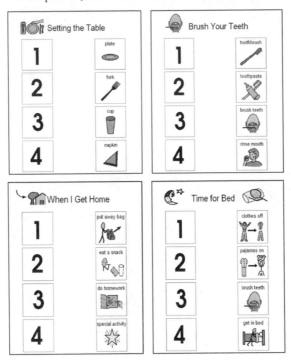

Figure 4: *These boards were created by speech pathologists using Mayer Johnson's Boardmaker.*

- Snack time
- Hand washing
- Ball games
- Tag/chase
- Building block tower

JARs for older kids

- Daily routines (e.g., brushing teeth, setting dinner table)
- Life skills (e.g., buying an item at the supermarket, taking public transportation)
- Greetings
- Board games or card games
- Gross motor games (e.g., playing catch, Simon Says)
- Cooking activities

Concluding Comments

In this chapter, we have provided a brief overview of the Joint Action Routine strategy. From personal experience, we have seen children at various levels make considerable gains. It provides an appropriate, functional, and motivating way to build upon language and pragmatic skills, in a naturalistic setting, during everyday activities. In many instances, children begin to rely less and less on adult prompting and grow into more independent, spontaneous communicators. We highly recommend implementation of this valuable program to any family or school team looking to expand on language, communication, and social skills.

DIETARY

SPECIFIC CARBOHYDRATE DIET (SCD)

By Judith Chinitz

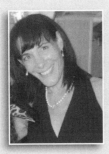

Judith Chinitz, MS, MS, CNC

New Star Nutritional Consulting
(914) 244-3646
www.newstarnutrition.com
judy@newstarnutrition.com

Following her son's diagnosis with autism in 1996, Judith Chinitz has spent the last eighteen years searching for answers. After saving her son's life through diet, and seeing firsthand the healing power of food, Judy earned a second master's degree in nutrition. She is also a certified special education teacher. Judy is the author of *We Band of Mothers: Autism, My Son, and the Specific Carbohydrate Diet,* which also contains commentary by Dr. Sidney Baker. She also assisted Dr. Baker in founding Medigenesis (available at www.autism360.org), an Internet-based, interactive medical database. Currently, Judy is volunteering to help set up a new company that will be providing a helminth for biome reconstitution.

For many years, the presence of gastrointestinal symptoms in children with autism was disputed by the medical community, until the publication of the paper, "Recommendations for evelation and treatment of common gastrointestinal problems in children with ASDs,"[1] was published By Dr. Tim Buie, et. al., in the journal *Pediatrics,* in 2010. Dr. Buie and his colleagues confirmed the presence of constipation, diarrhea, abdominal pain, and so on in many children on the spectrum. In 2013, Dr. Walker, et. al.[2] identified a specific variant of inflammatory bowel disease, similar to traditional IBD, but confined to those on the autism spectrum.

The cause or causes of these symptoms and pathology is not yet confirmed. However, in 2011, Dr. Buie, who is a gastroenterologist and researcher at Massachusetts General Hospital in Boston (Harvard's teaching hospital), was a member of a team which published another paper[3] that may have given us the best clue as to causation that we have. This study demonstrated that children with autism **have impaired carbohydrate digestion and transport, and bacterial dysbiosis.** The article states that children on the spectrum who have GI issues have a significantly lower level of the enzymes necessary to complete digestion of carbohydrates (80 percent of children in the study had deficiencies in two or more enzymes), and more than that, also have significantly lower levels of the transporters which permit carbohydrates to be moved by cells from the intestinal lumen into the body. "In total, 93.3 percent of AUT-GI [children with autism and GI symptoms] had mRNA deficiencies in at least one of the 5 genes involved in carbohydrate digestion or transport."

They go on to say in the discussion of their findings something that could have been taken directly out of Elaine Gottschall's book, *Breaking the Vicious Cycle*:

> Based on these findings, we propose a model whereby deficiencies in disaccharidases and hexose transporters alter the milieu of carbohydrates in the distal small intestine (ileum) and proximal large intestine (cecum*),* **resulting in the supply of additional growth substrates for bacteria. These changes manifest in significant and specific compositional changes in the microbiota of AUT-GI children. . . .** Metabolic interactions between intestinal microflora and their hosts are only beginning to be understood. Nonetheless, there is already **abundant evidence that microflora can have system-wide effects and influence immune responses, brain development and behavior.**" [emphasis added]

What does this mean exactly? **Some as yet unknown environmental trigger changes the children's ability to digest and absorb carbohydrates. This in turn causes undigested carbohydrates—which are just sugars—to remain in the intestines, providing plenty of food for bacteria, leading to measurable changes in the quality of the gut flora. These gut bacteria are crucial to good health, normal immune functioning and NORMAL DEVELOPMENT.**

Breaking the Vicious Cycle[4], by Elaine Gottschall, lays out the elements of what she called The Specific Carbohydrate Diet. After saving her own daughter from a lifetime of a colostomy bag after she was diagnosed with ulcerative colitis as a little girl by changing what her daughter was eating, Elaine spent most of her life researching and then promoting the idea that what we eat influences what grows in us, and that, in turn, affects our health to staggering degree.

At the Defeat Autism Now! Conference in April 2010, Dr. Jeremy Nicholson, an eminent researcher at Imperial College in London, presented a paper he had just published in the *Journal of Proteome Research*[5]. He and his colleagues examined the organic acids in the urine of 39 children with autism and compared the results with those from controls. They found multiple abnormal metabolites that could only be produced by abnormal gut bacteria. The concluding words of his talk were something along the lines of, "Almost every abnormality we find in children with autism—the digestive issues, the immune system irregularities, the developmental problems—can be explained by damage to the developing gut flora." (See article by Judith Chinitz on Biome Depletion in this book.)

The human body contains approximately 10 trillion cells and 100 trillion microbes. Our microscopic flora outnumber us 10 to 1. We are more other than we are ourselves. Our intestines contain billions and billions of bacteria that are absolutely crucial to health—and to life itself. At birth, we are meant to begin to acquire our "old friends" (as those in the field now refer to our symbiotic residents) who will help us digest our food, make vitamins for us, keep pathogens from populating our digestive systems, develop our immune systems by regulating the process whereby we learn to differentiate good from bad, and self from non-self, and more. Seventy percent or so of our immune system is our digestive systems. Most germs enter through the nose and mouth and our first line of defense, therefore, are the immunological armies centered there. Developing a healthy population of old friends means developing a healthy body.

There is copious research supporting the fact that our good flora is responsible for the normal development of our immune systems, which happens mainly in the first two years of life. For example, a paper published a few years ago in the *Proceedings of the Nutrition Society*[6] states, "Commensal bacteria are important in intestinal homeostasis and appear to play a role in early tolerance to foreign antigens. . . . Dysregulation of this balance can contribute to the pathogenesis of numerous inflammatory conditions such as inflammatory bowel diseases." That is, a disruption of the development of the gut flora leads to a dysregulated immune system and potentially to gut inflammation.

And now, as stated earlier, research is also beginning to provide proof that these same intestinal microbes are responsible for normal development as well.

On January 31, 2011, a paper was published in the *Proceedings of the National Academy of Science*[7] in which researchers compared the development of control mice, which were exposed to typical microbes from birth, to a group of mice who were raised in a germ free environment. The latter group showed clear developmental abnormalities as adults. Interestingly, if the germ-free mice were exposed to normal microbes early enough in development, they too developed into normal adults. However, if the microbes were introduced when the mice were already grown, no improvement was noted. The study rightly concludes that this is an animal experiment and may not apply to human beings. . . . But it's certainly safe to say the data are incredibly compelling.

Just a few years ago, another paper was also published in the *Proceedings of the National Academy of Science*[8] in which inflammation was induced in rats via injection of lipopolysaccharides, which are the toxins from pathogenic bacteria. The researchers write, "We hypothesized that peripheral inflammation leads to increased neuronal excitability arising from a CNS immune response." As predicted, the rats developed, " . . . a marked, reversible inflammatory response within the hippocampus, characterized by microglial activation and increases in TNF-alpha levels." Inducing inflammation via exposure to toxins from bacteria caused inflammation in the brains of the animals. The microglia are the immune cells of the brain. Coincidentally—or perhaps not so coincidentally—such microglial activation has also been found in those with autism. "We demonstrate an active neuroinflammatory process in the cerebral cortex, white matter and notably in the cerebellum of autistic patients," writes Dr. Vargas and colleagues[9] as just one example of research in this area.

We know then that the brains of those with autism appear to have abnormal activation of the microglia and for almost a decade, we've also known that individuals with autism appear to have abnormal gut flora. In 2005 research was published in the *Journal of Medical Microbiology*[10] which showed high levels of clostridial species in the guts of people with ASD: "The faecal flora of ASD patients contained a higher incidence of the Clostridum histolyticum group. . . ." The paper goes on to say, "Clostridia are recognized toxin-producers, including neuro-toxins. Theoretically, toxic products may be over-expressed in the autistic gut, which may lead to increased levels in the bloodstream and thus exert systemic effects."

By the way, science is also now demonstrating that the more dramatic the shift in gut bacteria, the more severe are the symptoms of autism. In 2010, Dr. Finegold and colleagues studied the bacteria found in the stool of children on the spectrum and found that the differences in bacterial content were a predictor of the severity of autism: "Bacteroidetes and Firmicutes showed the most difference between groups of varying severities of autism. Bacteroidetes was found at high levels in the severely autistic group, while Firmicutes were more predominant in the control group. . . . Desulfovibriospecies and Bacteroides vulgatus are present in significantly higher numbers in stools of severely autistic children than in controls.[11]"

To repeat, then, what we know: individuals in this current autism epidemic have abnormal gut flora. We suspect that this is because, at least in part, an environmental trigger has caused a change in the way these people digest and transport carbohydrates into the body. We know that toxins from these bacteria are causing systemic effects. We know that toxins from bad bacteria can certainly cause inflammation in the gut, and even inflammatory bowel diseases. We know that in rats, toxins from bacteria cause activation of the microglia, and thus inflammation in the brain. And finally, we know that in mice at least, early disturbances of normal gut flora can cause developmental abnormalities. So, while we cannot draw any definitive conclusions at this point, the evidence is mounting almost daily that bacterial dysbiosis plays an enormous part in causing a child to develop autism.

So, what can we do to improve the gut flora of these individuals on the spectrum?

Referring back to the article in the *Journal of Medical Microbiology* which found high levels of clostridia in the autistic gut: "Strategies to reduce clostridial population levels harbored by ASD patients or to **improve their gut microflora profile through dietary modulation** may help alleviate gut disorders common to such patients." [emphasis added]

There is considerable evidence that inflammatory bowel disease is associated with abnormal gut flora and also a large body of research published on the benefits of a diet low in complex carbohydrates/sugars when treating inflammatory bowel disease. One example: in 2000, a paper appeared in the *Israeli Medical Association Journal*[12] which concludes, "Combined sugar malabsorption patterns are common in functional bowel disorders and may contribute to symptomatology in most patients. Dietary restriction of the offending sugar(s) should be implemented before the institution of drug therapy." Even as far back as the 1990s, researchers found a positive association between high sucrose (white sugar) consumption and inflammatory bowel disease— and a negative correlation between fructose (the monosaccharide simple sugar found in fruit) and IBD.[13]

A 2010 article in the journal *Nutrition*[14] lays out the best treatments we have to date for curing a small intestine bacterial overgrowth. Therapies involve, among other things, certain kinds of antibiotics, probiotics, and a diet low in foods that ferment (i.e. feed bacteria). "Therapy is usually directed toward reducing the bacterial load with antibiotics, but altering the functional properties of the microbiota by reducing or **changing the supply of fermentative substrate** or by the use of probiotics are promising alternatives".

Changing the supply of fermentative substrate, reducing the amount of foods that can be fermented (digested) by bacteria, is exactly what the Specific Carbohydrate Diet does.

Decades of scientific research are presented in *Breaking the Vicious Cycle* and in the eight years since Elaine Gottschall passed away, more and more evidence has piled up providing substantiation for her premise that the removal of complex carbohydrates from the diet can markedly help diseased intestines, and in many cases bring about complete remission of inflammatory bowel diseases.

Before proceeding to explain how to implement SCD, it is vitally important to make clear that even individuals with no overt bowel symptoms can benefit from the diet. If your child is on the autism spectrum, the likelihood is that he or she has abnormal gut flora. Often parents are stunned by the improvements made by even high functioning children who seem absolutely healthy. The only way to know if SCD is going to help is to do it.

How does SCD work? The prevailing belief is that bad bacterial microbes produce toxins irritating to the lining of the digestive system, which cause the tissue to try to protect itself by secreting mucus. (All gut bacteria, good and bad, produce acids in the process of fermentation.) A lot of bacteria means a lot of acid. Now think about your runny nose when you have a cold—one of our bodies' defenses is to wash out germs with mucus. Once covered by a thick layer of mucus, the intestines are unable to break down complex carbohydrates. The necessary enzymes (secreted by the enterocytes, the cells lining the intestines) cannot reach the food, leaving the undigested carbohydrates (sugars which cannot be broken down into digestible form) to fester and feed the bad bacteria. Fifty percent of carbohydrate digestion occurs on the brush border of the small intestine. Our intestines can only absorb single molecule sugars, like glucose and fructose, which supply energy to every cell in our bodies. All that undigested sugar (from the incompletely digested di-saccharides (2 sugar molecules attached together) and poly-saccharides (long strings of sugar molecules such as found in starches) feeds the bacteria, leading to an increase in the overgrowth . . . which in turn produce more toxins . . . which leads to more mucus . . . which leads to worse digestion . . . which leads to more food for more bacteria . . . Elaine's vicious cycle.

To quote directly from *Breaking the Vicious Cycle*:

In various conditions, a poorly-functioning intestine can be easily overwhelmed by the ingestion of carbohydrates which require numerous digestive processes. The result is an environment that supports overgrowth of intestinal yeast and bacteria. . . . The purpose of the Specific Carbohydrate Diet is to deprive the microbial world of the intestine of the food it needs to overpopulate. By using a diet which contains predominantly 'predigested' carbohydrates, the individual with an intestinal problem can be maximally nourished without over-stimulation of the intestinal microbial population.

And don't forget that we now know, since 2010, through actual biopsy that children with autism and gut symptoms produce less of the enzymes necessary to break down carbohydrates into single molecule sugars! As those researchers stated, all these carbohydrates sitting in the intestinal lumen produce qualitative changes in the flora in the gut.

By keeping nearly all complex carbohydrates out of the digestive system, the aberrant bacteria are starved to death. Of course, at the same time you're replenishing the gut with good flora in the form of probiotics: SCD-legal homemade yogurt and/or store-bought probiotics (which are available from a host of retailers).

SCD stops the vicious cycle of malabsorption and microbial overgrowth by removing the microbes' food: sugars, specifically di- and poly-saccharides. Single molecule sugars, like those found in fruit, vegetables, and honey do not require digestive processes, but are immediately absorbed by the intestine. Therefore, even diseased intestines can absorb them so that they are not available to feed the bad flora. Inflammation decreases as the bad microbial population dies out, toxin levels go down and digestion improves. (Of course, it now looks like children on the spectrum may even have difficulties with transporting single molecules of sugar as well. Certainly though, at the very least reducing the carbohydrates that require digestion makes a dramatic difference.)

SCD absolutely does work and often it works miracles. Someday, in the not too distant future, it will hopefully be accepted as what it is: **a fundamental treatment for bowel disease.**

In July, 2011, researchers (led by the University of California at Davis) presented a small pilot study at the International Congress of Mucosal Immunology, in Paris. Their paper was entitled, "Impact of Diet in Fecal Microbial Diversity in Patients with Crohn's Disease."[15] In a randomized, single-blind crossover study, they compared the bacteria found in the feces of six patients with Crohn's disease who were following either SCD or a Low Residue Diet (low in fiber and other foods that increase bowel frequency). Their findings: "The overall abundance and diversity of bacterial families was lower in Crohn's as compared with controls. Clostridia richness was observed to be twice that of Bacteriodetes in Crohn's patients. LRD diet was associated with a decrease in microbiome diversity with 11 bacteria belonging to 3 families disappearing. SCD increased diversity to include 376 bacteria belonging to 32 different classes." That is, SCD went a long way toward normalizing gut bacteria.

The Specific Carbohydrate Diet involves the removal of any food that contains di- and poly-saccharides (that is, double and multiple chains of sugars). "Illegals" (as they're called by SCDers) include white and brown sugars. lactose (the sugar found in milk), maple syrup, all grain, and all starch. Permitted are proteins (eggs, meats, poultry, fish, certain dairy products that have been fermented long enough that no sugars are left), fruit, most vegetables (except the starches, like potatoes) and honey. Cookies, bread, and cakes can be made with a variety of other flours rather than wheat: nuts, coconut, bean, and fruit flours. There are legal substitutes for most well-loved foods, but parents must understand that the French fries and Skittles are out. Instead, you will be feeding your child only foods that are nutrient rich, wholesome, and actually good for them. (There is a fairly comprehensive list of legal/illegal foods on Elaine's website: www.breakingtheviciouscycle.info.)

If your child is already a good eater—a rare thing in the ASD population—then switching to SCD won't be a problem. The foods are delicious. If, however, your child is a chicken-nuggets-and-French-fries-only kid, it may be a better idea to begin the diet slowly to avoid negative situations for both of you. Those considering SCD should also consider working with a professional who is experienced at creating an individual plan based upon tolerance levels, parental choice, what the child is currently eating, and so forth.

For difficult children, it may be best to start by substituting one food at a time. For example, if your child loves cookies, make some SCD legal ones and replace the old favorites. Three or four days later, make your next substitution. Continue this pattern for the next month or two and before you know it, your child will not only be entirely SCD legal, but you will have gotten rid of all the junk food in your house.

If you live close to a good health food store, you will be able to buy nuts free of additives and can grind them into nut flours if you want to start SCD right away. To make things easier though, many high quality nut flours are available via the Internet. www.digestivewellness.com and www.lucyskitchenshop.com both are great resources for SCD flours and other products.

Don't start SCD until you are comfortable with the foods you have in the house or you'll just end up frustrated. Good preparation will make the transition much easier. The first step: it is absolutely crucial to read Elaine Gottschall's book if you're considering SCD. She provides an eloquent and easy-to-understand explanation of the history of the diet and the decades of science that support its efficacy, as well as providing some of the best SCD legal recipes. *Breaking the Vicious Cycle* is available via Amazon.com and BarnesandNoble.com, as well as through some of the SCD websites. It is THE formative work on the diet.

Elaine and I planned to write a book together about SCD, autism, and her journey with the diet. Tragically, she died just as we got started with her project. I carried on alone and in 2007 published, *We Band of Mothers: Autism, My Son and The Specific Carbohydrate Diet.*[16] (available via Amazon.com) The book is both a guide for managing SCD with children on the spectrum, but also a tribute to Elaine who was truly a towering human being. (In her crusade to help people suffering with bowel disease, she touched millions of lives. *Breaking the Vicious Cycle* is translated into at least 7 languages, and has sold well over a million copies worldwide.)

There are many wonderful cookbooks available and multiple websites devoted to SCD legal products, yogurt machines, yogurt starter, and so forth.

1. www.lucyskitchenshop.com (which sells superior quality almond flour, cookbooks, a yogurt machine and starter, and other great products).
2. www.digestivewellness.com (which sells kosher SCD products, nut flours, apple chips, etc.).

3. www.scdrecipe.com—This website is owned by Raman Prasad, who is also the author of two wonderful SCD cookbooks. Raman, a former colitis sufferer, was cured via SCD and, being a fabulous cook, has collected many great recipes. His site also provides news updates, links, and other great resources.
4. www.scdiet.org—A library of SCD information, including news, links, recipes, and so forth.

One very important thing to know before you start SCD is that there are a series of regular regressions that may occur. No one knows why and not every child undergoes these regressions—but most do. Please remember: **the regressions are temporary. Do NOT stop the diet. You are doing nothing wrong!** The children tend to come out of the regressions better than ever. (For more information on the regressions, please refer to *We Band of Mothers*.)

One crucially important note: SCD is NOT a low carbohydrate diet. Unlike the Atkins diet, which limits the amount of carbohydrates consumed each day, SCD limits only the TYPE of carbohydrates eaten. Be sure to give your child plenty of fruit and vegetables every day, legal fruit juices, and honey (assuming there is no significant yeast issue). Even the pickiest children do eventually begin to eat a wide variety of foods that prior to the diet, they would never have touched.

Even if your child has food allergies—even to nuts—SCD is still a possibility. Granted, it's not easy. But it is most certainly do-able. Instead of using nut flours we use pumpkin seed, coconut, mango, or bean flours all of which work well. Again, no matter what the dietary restriction, SCD is manageable.

The beauty of the SCD is that it is not only incredibly nourishing (there is no junk food) but more, it is truly a healing diet. After a few years, many individuals can successfully go back to eating a completely unrestricted diet. Elaine Gottschall recommended staying on SCD for a year after the last symptom had vanished. The time required for healing varies radically from person to person, and diet is a slow healing process. It takes several years even in the best cases. However, it is also entirely safe, healthy, and works the vast majority of the time. The Autism Research Institute's data of parent reports on treatment (2009) has 71 percent of children showing improvement from SCD, topping all other dietary interventions. In fact, it ranks third of all treatments on the survey.

SCD has the weight of what science we currently have supporting it. While the task may seem daunting, hundreds and hundreds of parents have succeeded in making radical improvements in their children's health and autistic symptoms through improving their gut microbes. You can too.

COMBINED APPROACHES TO FEEDING THERAPY

By Erica Goss

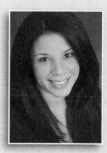

Erica Goss Goldstein, MA, CCC-SLP
Goss Speech, Language, & Feeding
74 East 79th Street, Suite 3C
New York, NY 10075
212-396-4133
info@gossslf.com
www.gossslf.com

Erica Goss Goldstein earned her Master's degree in Speech-Language Pathology from Temple University. Erica has worked in a variety of settings including hospitals, schools, early intervention and home care. Erica is PROMPT (Prompts for Restructuring Oral Muscular Phonetic Targets) certified and has specialized training in oral motor therapy and sensory motor based feeding therapy, behavioral feeding therapy, and sensory integration therapy. In addition, she has extensive experience working with children diagnosed with autism spectrum disorder. She is a certified Life Coach, holds a Certificate of Clinical Competence (CCC) from the American Speech-Language Hearing Association (ASHA), a New York state license, and is a member of the American Academy of Private Practice in Speech Pathology and Audiology.

What is Feeding Therapy:

There are many factors that influence a child's ability to eat/feed appropriately for his/her age. Feeding therapy is provided to help children who have difficulty feeding, or are picky problem eaters. It may involve sensory–motor therapy, behavior intervention, food chaining, or a combination of these approaches. Addressing feeding issues for children of all ages can prevent or eliminate nutritional concerns, growth concerns, unsafe swallowing and future poor eating habits and attitudes.

Feeding therapy is often recommended for children with the following disorders:

- Reduced or Limited Food Intake
- Food Refusal
- Oral Phase Dysphagia (Swallowing Difficulty)
- Food Selectivity by Type and/or Texture
- Oral Motor Deficits

- Delayed Feeding Development
- Food or Swallowing Phobias
- Mealtime Tantrums
- Gagging
- Food Stuffing
- Tube Feeders Ready to Transition to Oral Eaters as Medically Appropriate

There are several types of feeding therapy and feeding therapy programs. A thorough feeding evaluation will determine the best approach or combination of approaches for you child.

What to Expect During a Feeding Evaluation

A comprehensive feeding evaluation to identify your child's feeding needs will include the following:

- Case history
- Sensory evaluation
- Motor based evaluation
- Behavioral evaluation
- Trial therapy techniques
- Individualized feeding plan

Initially, you can expect to participate in a case history discussion with your evaluator. This discussion gives the evaluator background developmental information about your child and information about your child's ongoing feeding and mealtime behaviors. The following topics may be included in your case history discussion.

- Prenatal and birth history
- Medical history including allergies
- Family makeup and history
- Information regarding developmental milestones
- Types of previous or ongoing therapies
- Description of mealtimes and your child's food preferences

In addition, you may be asked for a 3-5 day food diary including what your child eats throughout the day, the times of each meal and/or snack, the amount your child consumes during each meal/snack, and any behavioral anecdotes that may be important to share. This 3-5 day food diary gives the evaluator a great deal of information regarding your child's sensory preferences, potential behavioral needs, and possible motor based implications.

Following a your case history discussion, a sensory evaluation will be conducted. A sensory evaluation identifies any sensory dysfunction your child may have that interferes with his/her ability to eat age appropriately. Sensory dysfunction occurs when the brain does not efficiently process information coming from the body or the environment. This may result in hypo-sensitivity, hyper-sensitivity or mixed sensitivity.

Children with hypo-sensitivity require increased intensity in taste, texture and/or temperature in order to process oral sensation. These children are often (but not always) described as having a "messy mouth," being "drooly," or as sensory "seekers." Children with hypo-sensitivity tend to prefer crunchy textures, and strong flavors. For children with hyper-sensitivity sometimes just a little input may be too much. These children are often referred to as tactile defensive. They are resistant to touch, tend to prefer bland flavors and textures and often have a hyper sensitive gag reflexes resulting in frequent vomiting. Children with mixed sensitivity often lack the appropriate motor skills to feed properly, yet require an increased sensory input to to process sensory information. Determining a child's sensory needs is crucial to creating an appropriate treatment plan for that child.

A motor based evaluation looks at the child's posture/trunk and oral muscle strength and oral motor planning skills. A motor based assessment may be done with the use of oral motor tools and/or clinical observation of ongoing feeding skills. Determining what motor limitations a child has is crucial to treatment planning. During the motor portion of the evaluation the evaluator access your childs ability to maintin an upright seated postion for feeding and the structure and function of your child's jaw, palate, lips, tongue, and cheeks. In addition the evaluator will access your child's motor planning skills and how they impact your child's ability to eat in an age appropriate manner.

Assessing a child's behavioral needs is often ongoing throughout the evaluation. Your evaluator will be able to assess what behavioral limitations your child has due to his/her "pickiness" or ridgity as new tasks, food items and activities are presented. A child who refuses to touch, taste or be in close proximity to a novel item may have these issues due to sensory dysfunction, poor motor planning and an unawareness of how or what to do with and item, or ridgity. At this time, the evaluator may try a few feeding techniques to see how your child reacts to different types of therapy. These techniques may include behavioral shaping and or motor planning training through appropriate tool or food placement.

An individualized feeding plan for your child will include pre-feeding techniques to get your child's gross sensory and oral sensory system ready for feeding. In addition, this plan will include any exercises necessary to teach your child the appropriate motor planing skills and develop adequate motor strength to develop age appropriate feeding skills. This plan can be done at home with a child's parent and or care taker and/ or in therapy sessions with your feeding therapist.

Treatment

The duration of feeding therapy will vary depending on your child's needs, the frequency your child receives therapy and the consistency that is provided throughout the course of treatment. Throughout ongoing treatment, your feeding therapist will continue to adjust your child's oral motor/feeding plan as new skills emerge. Your child's individual feeding plan/ongoing therapy treatment may include the following or a combination of the following techniques:

- **Sensory integration therapy** addresses your child's sensory dysfunction needs. In essence, helping your child organize his/her sensory system prior to and during feeding therapy sets the stage for clear communication, and the ability to move forward with therapeutic techniques.
- **Oral motor therapy** focuses on the use of specific tools for remediation of oral motor deficits.
- **Motor planning exercises** are exercises designed to target and teach specific motor planning skills necessary for speech and feeding. These exercises can be done with the use of oral motor tools, specific food items or a combination of tools and food items.
- **Food chaining** is a child-friendly treatment approach that builds on the child's successful eating experiences. Foods a child enjoys are described in terms of taste, texture and temperature. New foods similar to the ones the child eats well are used to create the food chains, formed between the foods a child accepts and the new, targeted foods to expand the child's food reptoire.
- **Behavioral shaping** refers to using successive, gradual steps paired with differential reinforcement to teach a child to interact with, experience and eventually eat or taste a novel food item.
- **Homework and carry over** are crucial to successful feeding therapy. Parent/caretaker participation during therapy sessions can facilitate the carry over of newly acquired skills into your child's natural environment.

Implications for Children with Autism Spectrum Disorder

Children diagnosed with ASD typically present with difficulty processing and integrating sensory information, or stimuli, such as sights, sounds smells, tastes and/or movement. Some children with ASD are hypersensitive to smells, touch and tastes.

Others are hyposenstitve and are observed to participate in "sensory seeking" to meet their sensory needs. Children with ASD often present with decreased muscle tone and or poor motor planning skills. In addition children with ASD are often described as rigid, having difficulty transitioning from what is familiar to new experiences including novel food items. Therefore it is common for children on the autism spectrum to be "picky" eaters. The combination of these limitations may interfere with your child's ability to receive adequate nutrition.

Since every child is unique, it is essential to establish an appropriate individualized feeding therapy plan to met your child's specific needs. In addition, feeding therapy for children with ASD should include appropriate strategies to facilitate clear communication. This may include visual support through the use of pictures, written words, and or lists. Ongoing feeding therapy for a child with ASD should be consistent allowing for your child to feel safe and clear as to what the demands are throughout the session.

The "Right" Feeding Therapist for Your Child

Feeding therapists often have a background in speech language pathology and/or occupational therapy with a specialty in feeding therapy. Given that every child is unique, it is important to find a therapist that is trained in a variety of approaches and is able to piece together the appropriate treatment plan for your child. In addition, it is critical to work with a therapist that builds an open, trusting relationship with your child and your family. Children ages 0-3 years may be eligible for feeding therapy through state funded programs such as early intervention. School age children may be evaluated through school based programs. In addition, if you feel your child would benefit from feeding therapy, you can ask your pediatrician for a referral to a seasoned feeding therapist.

THE HEALING POWER OF FERMENTED FOODS

By Dr. John H. Hicks and Betsy Hicks

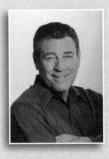

John H. Hicks, MD

Elementals Living
Medical Director
5411 State Road 50
Delavan, WI 53115
262-740-3000

www.elementalsliving.com

A renowned medical doctor and pediatrician for over thirty years, Dr. Hicks offers a unique integrative approach to health, incorporating medical, nutritional, emotional, and vibrational energy philosophies to create a customized treatment plan for each patient. This holistic approach draws clients of every age, in a variety of circumstances and from many different walks of life. As a result Dr. Hicks has gained broad and comprehensive experience in all kinds of health situations. In addition to diagnostic testing and analysis, expertise in natural supplements, and a strong focus on good nutrition, Dr. Hicks combines intuition with compassion for a highly successful program. Adding to his clinical practice as the Medical Director of Elementals Living, Dr. Hicks lectures nationally at workshops, classes, conferences and seminars throughout the country. His belief in the power of healing and good health inspires him to continue to seek out new and progressive methods of achieving good health.

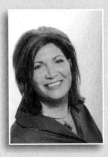

Betsy Hicks
betsy@elementalsliving.com

Elementals Living
Medical Director
5411 State Road 50
Delavan, WI 53115
262-740-3000

www.elementalsliving.com

Betsy Hicks is the CEO of Elementals Living, a holistic health and wellness center in Delavan, Wisconsin. Moreover she is an internationally known author, radio host, video anchor, and lecturer on a wide variety of health and wellness topics. Betsy has spoken at several international autism conferences including, the World Symposium in Dubai, Autism One in Chicago, and Spectrum Possibilities in Barbados. She is a regular host for Autism One Radio/Voice America. As the mother of an 18-year old with autism, Betsy's gift and passion for public speaking is both personal and practical. Her devotion to assisting parents find creative and useful solutions to overcome challenging eating habits, inspired her most recent book, *Picky Eating Solutions: Bringing the Joy of Real Food Back to the Table*. Betsy's unique understanding, her contagious enthusiasm and sincere empathy inspires all who hear her words, whether written or spoken, towards better health, wellness, and joy.

One glance at a person's face can speak volumes to the discerning eye. Over the past few years, I have travelled extensively, visiting six of seven continents. During my travels, I always look with great interest into the faces of the diverse nationalities I encounter, observing an array of shades, shapes, and colors. With attentiveness, I have noticed significant patterns pertaining to the general health of countries, cultures, and the foods that people eat. In the Middle East, eyes sparkle in complement to pure, sun-kissed fresh vegetables and unprocessed beans. In Thailand, dazzling teeth glisten from a diet that is naturally free of gluten, dairy, and preservatives. In Italy, complexions shine in appreciation of the benefits of heart-healthy fats. In the United States, in contrast, the standard American diet obscures the luster of vibrant good health in a growing population that is both overfed and undernourished. Certainly, there are exceptions to all generalizations of good health, yet here in the US, where the majority has an unhealthful diet, the exception may be the rule!

In this country, it is apparent that money and power have created a persuasive and unhealthful food industry that uses shrewd marketing tactics to yield incentives for profits. Both tradition and taste are eagerly sacrificed and cast off in favor of the convenient and cut-rate. Paradoxically, in our era of unlimited information, many North Americans are critically limited in their ability to understand and eat whole foods. It is not unusual for me to meet young adults (from many different places) who have never eaten a fresh vegetable or don't realize that fruit does not have to come from a can. Even when individuals are more informed, good-quality, wholesome foods can seem expensive and difficult to find alongside the budget-friendly but nutritionally empty processed foods that so abundantly line store shelves. Although processed and synthetically modified foods are marketed as being the best source of vitamins and minerals, they are often a page out of *The Emperor's New Clothes*—an eggshell disguised as an egg. For example, the once vital dairy industry now offers overly pasteurized, chemical-laden milk depleted of necessary digestive enzymes, which renders the milk indigestible and unusable to the body. Yet many people drink this adulterated milk erringly confident that they are choosing the best way to meet their calcium needs. Raw milk is a healthier alternative but can be extremely difficult to obtain if you don't own a cow!

In short, our country is at a crossroads. The children growing up today may be the first generation to have a shorter life expectancy than their parents. Because true health and vitality are built from the inside out, it is time to develop a deeper understanding of digestive health and look more closely at what we are eating and being fed.

The Role of Probiotics in Gut Health

When food enters the gastrointestinal (GI) tract, it begins a long journey through the body to become fuel and nutrition for all living cells. Everything we consume must be metabolically changed and broken down to a usable nutrient or identified as waste and eliminated. Food is digested and assimilated primarily in the small intestine. A protective barrier of epithelial tissue lines the lumen or inner wall of the gastrointestinal tract. These highly specialized epithelial cells (also called enterocytes) fit closely together and are connected by tight junctions that prevent unwanted substances and partially digested foods from leaking into the bloodstream. These absorptive enterocytes that coat the villi (finger-like protrusions) also allow needed nutrients to be picked up by circulating blood, carried to the liver for modification, and then distributed around the body to nourish cells and tissues. The food we eat must be digested, absorbed and then metabolized by our cells. Probiotics help prevent reflux.

Many factors affect the performance of digestion, including the type of food eaten, digestive enzyme activity, pH, and the condition of the internal gastrointestinal environment. When digestion and elimination are compromised, toxins and waste get stored in tissues and fat cells. A key element in the health of the gut (and, consequently, the immune system) is the presence of probiotics. These live microorganisms, which include hundreds of beneficial bacteria and yeasts, are found all over the body and are especially abundant in the GI and respiratory tracts. Overall, there may be as many as three pounds of microorganisms residing in the body. There are more probiotics in out bodies than we have cells.

Probiotics exist as many different species (for example, *Lactobacillus acidophilus*, *Lactobacillus casei*, and *Lactobacillus bulgaricus*), and within each species, there are a variety of strains. The word "probiotic" means "for life," which provides a significant clue regarding the crucial role that probiotics play in keeping the body in optimal health. Probiotics help regulate many metabolic functions within the body's various systems and work to maintain a healthy balance between good and bad organisms. Friendly flora do this by controlling pathogen levels and keeping pathogens from circulating in the body to build colonies and create disease.

Beneficial organisms also strive to control bodily pH to provide an environment that allows them to thrive, while limiting the growth of their pathogenic counterparts. Moreover, enzymes and proteins as well as vitamins and minerals are optimally absorbed at specific pH ranges. (Although there are different pH levels for different parts of the body, an overall range of 6.4 to 7.2 is considered healthy.) Outside of these narrow parameters, enzymes and proteins can be inactivated and minerals and vitamins left unabsorbed. When the body is too acidic, nutrients are not absorbed regardless of how healthy a person's diet may be. Probiotics support modulation of our hormones. They help reduce anxiety and depression; they support processing, focus and concentration and comprehension.

When Microorganisms Get Out of Balance

Epithelial cells and intestinal immune system dendritic cells use cell memory processing antigens to distinguish between beneficial and nonbeneficial organisms. Ideally, beneficial bacteria begin to colonize an infant's gut during the birthing process and soon after through breast milk. However, if pathogens outweigh friendly flora at this critical, initial stage of development, epithelial cells may fail to make the correct distinction between what is beneficial and what is not. If this occurs, an imbalanced environment is established where pathogenic organisms thrive without restraint.

Wherever there is an imbalance, infection and disease can occur. Food poisoning, epidemics, and pandemics become rampant in large groups of people when beneficial microflora are unable to protect against stronger and more virulent pathogens. As another example, pathogenic bacteria such as *Salmonella* or *Shigella*, when given the upper hand, will cause dysentery and severe diarrhea. These symptoms and consequences can be greatly lessened and even abated when there is enough probiotic protection in the gut. Probiotics offer protection by creating an additional barrier on top of the epithelial layer. Distinct strains of probiotic organisms make contact with the epithelial cells and trigger different responses to bring forth a variety of supportive reactions. For example, beneficial yeasts clean up partially digested foods to prevent them from entering the blood stream and, therefore, protect against food sensitivities and autoimmune disease. This includes *Saccharomyces boulardii* but is not limited to this form of yeast.

Overgrowth of pathogenic yeast can be prompted by a diet high in sugar and refined, processed foods. Moreover, antibiotics and antifungal medications kill healthy probiotics, causing further imbalance and loss of protection. If probiotic colonies are not repopulated, various strains can become extinct, thereby allowing pathogenic bacteria and yeasts to take over like weeds in an untended garden. When there is an overgrowth of yeast in the system, overgrowth of the *Candida* species can occur. This can lead to symptoms such as sugar cravings, weight gain, mood imbalances, and headaches, to name but a few.

Probiotics and the Immune System

In addition to the vital role probiotics play in digestion and assimilation of nutrients, they are considered the immune system's first line of defense. As well as residing in the intestinal tract, probiotics populate the lungs, nose, mouth, and sinuses, where they have primary exposure to foreign invaders. Along with surveillance B-lymphocyte cells, probiotics identify and interpret pathogens present in the body, communicate pertinent information to the immune system, and help to limit and control pathogenic populations. Probiotics determine the weakness of the pathogenic organisms and begin the attack and communicate this information to the rest of the immune system.

Signal transduction is a process of intracellular communication that elicits a direct response from the immune system for the purpose of clearing infected cells. Probiotics and lymphocytic cells use protein molecules called cytokines to inform the rest of the immune system about the weaknesses and strengths of specific pathogens so that eliminative efforts can be adequately coordinated and carried out. Cytokine signals bring forth either a cell-mediated response or an antibody response from the immune system.

A *cell-mediated response* involves NK (natural killer) and cytotoxic (cell killing) T cells. These cytotoxic cells activate whenever infected cells are present, identifying surface markers on cells in the body and labeling those cells for cleaning or destruction. This is accomplished by sending a molecular signal or vibrational message into a cell instructing it to either clear itself of the replicating pathogens and begin new processes or destroy itself entirely. An *antibody response* involves B-lymphocyte cells along with helper T cells, which are stimulated to produce specific antibodies in the presence of foreign invaders and pathogens. Antibodies are either secreted into blood and tissue fluids or are attached to the surface of the B cells. They function to survey for substances and organisms that do not belong in the body, identifying and neutralizing them. Using a lock-and-key method, they bind to the antigen (a unique part of the pathogen) and mark it for destruction. In this way, antibodies prevent pathogens from entering and damaging healthy cells. Antibodies eradicate foreign invaders either by destroying the invader themselves or marking it for elimination by other cells within the immune system such as macrophage cells.

An antibody response occurs when single-cell bacteria are independently free-floating in blood and bodily fluids, whereas a cell-mediated response is necessary when bacteria penetrate through membranes into the heart of cells. A cell-mediated response is the only way to clear organisms that enter cells; antibodies cannot penetrate and remove organisms. When probiotics are present in inadequate amounts, the immune system will elicit an antibody response erroneously. This can lead to continuous antibody overproduction. Similar to a teeter-totter, when the antibody production side of the immune system is overactive, suppression of the cell-mediated side of the immune system occurs. Over the long term, this imbalance may predispose the body towards autoimmune disease as the body begins to produce antibodies against substances and tissues normally present in the body. Chronic inflammatory diseases such as colitis, celiac disease, and rheumatoid arthritis are clear examples of an autoimmune response to an overproduction of antibodies.

A particular benefit of probiotics for females involves urinary tract health. Because our microflora are not limited to our GI tract and bacteria can travel and establish colonies, it is vital to ensure a strong probiotic presence throughout the body. For example, although *Escherichia coli* normally resides within the intestines, it can be discharged in the stool and can attach itself to the perineum. From there, it may travel to the urethra, settling in the urinary tract to create an infection. Helpfully, probiotics and fermented foods taken orally can migrate to all areas where they may be needed.

The Importance of Fermented Foods

When we take a close look around the world at indigenous peoples with an extensive history of longevity and good health, we encounter diets that are abundant in a wide variety of cultured foods. The first known case of fermentation dates back some 8,000 years. Although cultured or fermented foods initially developed as a means of preserving fresh foods beyond their growing season, they have since advanced to a place of medicinal nutrition, promoting health and wellness (see Table 1). Cultured foods and beverages intentionally use microorganisms to transform food and extend its usefulness and healthfulness. Culturing or fermenting allows healthy bacteria to convert sugars and carbohydrates into organic acids that act as preservatives. Foods containing lactic acid provide cofactors that support and improve cell energy.

Table 1. Benefits of cultured foods and beverages

Digestion	1.	Aid digestion and assimilation of nutrients from foods
	2.	Provide a wide variety of enzymes to assist with digestion and reduce stress on body processes
Internal ecosystem	1.	Restore the balance of beneficial bacteria in the body
	2.	Protect against and improve conditions linked to the lack of beneficial bacteria, including food sensitivities (such as lactose and gluten intolerance), constipation, yeast infections, allergies, and asthma reduce anxiety and depression; increase focus and concentration, processing and comprehension. They help eliminate biofilms.
	3.	Provide continual sources of probiotics that are inexpensive and easy to make
Food quality	1.	Increase vitamin content and flavor
	2.	Preserve food for longer life

Fermentation can also improve the nutritional profile of otherwise indigestible foods. For example, unfermented soy contains phytic acid, which binds to minerals (thereby preventing their absorption), and contains enzyme inhibitors that interfere with protein digestion. In addition, soy has several antinutrients that depress thyroid function and cause red blood cells to clump, interfering with proper oxygen absorption. Fermenting soy—in the form of tempeh (soybean cake) and miso (a paste often consumed in soup)—lends considerable benefits to soy by rendering it more digestible.

Fermented foods are numerous and vary with geography and culture (see Table 2). The Koreans are known for their kimchi (a cultured vegetable side dish); the Indian and Middle Eastern diets include mead (a fermented honey wine); the northern European diet features sauerkraut (fermented cabbage); and the Japanese diet boasts miso. Interestingly, Dr. Shinichiro Akizuki, director of Saint Francis Hospital in Nagasaki during World War II, theorized that miso helps protect against radiation. He and his staff worked with bomb victims just a few miles from where the atomic bomb was dropped without suffering any of the typical effects of radiation. Dr. Akizuki attributed this surprising outcome to drinking miso soup daily. This attribution subsequently was borne out by science. In 1972, a group of researchers discovered that miso contains dipilocolonic acid, an alkaloid that chelates and eliminates heavy metals. In the 1980s, a medical research group from Tohoku University in Japan found that miso also contains ethyl ester, a fatty acid that acts as an anti-mutagen, counteracting substances such as nicotine that change genetic material. Ethyl ester is formed only during fermentation.

Along the same lines, a study conducted by Seoul National University claimed that chickens infected with avian flu (H5N1 virus) recovered after eating kimchi. In May 2009, the Korea Food Research Institute, Korea's state food research organization, conducted a larger study on 200 chickens that supported the theory that kimchi can boost chickens' immunity to the H5N1 virus.

Table 2. Fermented foods around the globe*

Food/beverage	Description	Regions/countries
Dhokla	Fermented gram flour (from chickpeas), yogurt, and spices steamed together	India
Dosa	Fermented rice and lentils, similar to idli but smoother and usually prepared in flat pancakes	India
Idli	Steamed blend of rice and black lentils (urad dal) that is left out to ferment	Sri Lanka
Injera	Fermented flat bread made with teff flour	Africa
Kefir**	Fermented milk drink with a consistency similar to thin yogurt	Bulgaria, Russia, and many other parts of Europe
Kimchi (kimchee)	Combination of many vegetables, usually including Asian cabbage, onions, garlic, chili peppers, and ginger	Korea
Kombucha**	Beverage, often in the form of tea, made with a kombucha culture (or "mushroom") made up of yeast and bacteria	China, Middle East, Russia

Miso	Fermented soybean paste, developed by injecting cooked soybeans with a mold (koji) cultivated in either a barley, rice, or soybean base	Japan
Natto	Fermented soybean cake	Japan
Poi**	Paste made with taro	Africa, South Pacific
Pla ra	Fermented fish sauce	Thailand
Sai krok	Fermented sausage	Thailand
Sauerkraut**	Shredded cabbage fermented with salt and sometimes spices	Austria, Germany, Russia
Tempeh	Steamed, fermented, and mashed soybeans	Japan
Yogurt**	Made from cow, sheep, goat, yak, buffalo, and other forms of milk	Greece, Turkey, Middle East, and other parts of the world

*   Fermented foods have been used in every culture throughout the centuries. This table represents a small sampling of the fermented foods that still are being enjoyed around the globe by country or region of origin.

**   Found in more than one country or region

Introducing Fermented Foods

Oral probiotics provide a foot in the door and begin to dislodge pathogenic bacteria and yeast. Cultured foods implant, replicate and take up long term residence. These provide the long term benefit and repair that is required to eliminate leaky gut. For those who are new to the world of fermented foods, kefir drinks and raw cultured vegetables are a great introduction as they allow naturally occurring beneficial bacteria to grow and flourish. These powerfully immune-strengthening foods, full of many different strains of probiotic bacteria and yeasts, promote a strong and active response from the immune system to invading pathogens. Commercial fermented foods do not provide probiotic support because they are heat-treated, which kills bacteria and enzymes.

The probiotics found in naturally cultured vegetables and kefir drinks grow and colonize, inhibiting the growth of pathogenic organisms so as to regain control of the internal ecosystem over the long term. In contrast, isolated probiotic supplements typically dissipate in strength over time. Furthermore, many encapsulated probiotics are transient strains, meaning that they need to be taken on a continual basis as they do not self-populate or colonize. If supplementing, a probiotic that offers a wide variety of species and strains will offer better protection and activate a stronger immune response. (Note that each species and strain can have a distinctive action and response on the body, and these actions can be quite different from what is seen in laboratory testing. The specific action in the body will indicate whether or not an individual strain is helpful and, more importantly, under what conditions it is helpful.)

WATER KEFIR DRINKS

Water kefir grains digest added sugar and release a probiotic byproduct into the liquid. (Dairy kefir grains consume lactose and produce probiotic strains in milk. However, for individuals who have issues with casein, water kefir rather than dairy kefir will be the obvious choice.) For those who may be concerned that the sugar added to water kefir may increase yeast and stress the pancreas, it is helpful to consider that the sugar is broken down into fructose, which has a low glycemic index. Low glycemic foods, often recommended for those who have diabetes, break down more slowly and are less likely to create sugar highs and lows. Moreover, more sugar breaks down with longer fermentation. A standard 48-hour fermentation should consume close to 80 percent of available sugar. A second fermentation can be accomplished by removing the grains while leaving the liquid unrefrigerated for an additional 24 to 48 hours. Nonetheless, it is always prudent to start off drinking small amounts of water kefir to allow the body time to adjust.

To change the flavor of water kefir, fresh or dried fruit can be added for taste. Alternatively, instead of using pure filtered water, water kefir can be made with coconut water, which has antiviral, antibacterial, and anti-yeast properties. If coconut water is used, however, it is advisable to have backup grains on hand as anything antibacterial in nature will naturally weaken the probacterial properties of the grains. It is also possible to revitalize your grains with mineral-rich molasses.

CULTURED VEGETABLES

Infants can obtain the benefits of cultured vegetables from nursing or from drinking the juice of the vegetables. Multiple studies from all over the world show that babies who gain probiotics in this way develop fewer allergies and less asthma than children without any probiotic supplementation. Caesarian-section babies will get exposure in life through their interaction with things and people. Since they did not come through the birth canal, they are lacking the great implanting that usually occurs at birth; therefore, the composition of their flora will not be as beneficial until they are breastfeeding or receive probiotics in another form.

Fermented Foods and Autism

Many aspects of autism—such as food sensitivities, nutrient malabsorption, poor weight gain, lack of focus and concentration, and hyperactive immune responses—can be strongly and favorably addressed by building up the presence of probiotics in the body through fermented foods (see Table 3). For example, many children on the autism spectrum have difficulty digesting and assimilating sufficient nutrients to meet their needs, and they also tend to have difficulty converting B vitamins in supplements to their active, useable forms. Cultured vegetables contain small amounts of predigested B vitamins that are highly bioavailable and easily used by the body. Together with enzymes and probiotic bacteria, cultured vegetables and kefir drinks can assist in the digestion and assimilation of all other foods eaten. A few teaspoons at the beginning of a meal will greatly enhance digestion and assimilation. For focus and concentration concerns, cultured vegetables and kefir drinks also aid in the control and balance of pathogenic yeast and its resulting symptoms.

Table 3. Benefits of fermented foods for autism

1. **Increase probiotics** through live probiotic cultures that are implantable[1]
2. **Decrease inflammation** by decreasing proinflammatory cytokines[2]
3. **Decrease leaky gut** by decreasing the number of pathogenic bacteria and yeasts[3,4]
4. **Increase T-regulatory cells** (regulatory T-lymphocytes)[5] to decrease food allergies, food hypersensitivities, and environmental allergies[6]
5. **Decrease Th-2 shifts** to modulate immune system back to neutral[1,5,6]
6. **Prevent formation of autoimmune diseases**[5,6]
7. **Remove endotoxins** from intestines and liver and increase liver's ability to detoxify[1]
8. **Reduce constipation and/or diarrhea**[1,5,6]

Conclusion

In looking to the future, let us not forsake the helpful lessons of the past. Traditional, whole foods nourish the body and offer great support for healthy longevity. Probiotics play an important role in building and creating a strong, healthy foundation. They also protect against disease and sustain optimal metabolic functioning. Traditional foods such as kefir drinks and fermented vegetables provide the best sources of probiotic bacteria and have the added benefits of being inexpensive to make and delicious to taste.

EDUCATIONAL

41

HOW TO RECOGNIZE A TOP-QUALITY ABA PROGRAM

By Dr. Jonathan Tarbox, Dr. Doreen Granpeesheh, and Angela Persicke

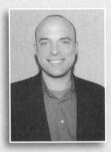

Jonathan Tarbox, PhD, BCBA-D

Center for Autism and Related Disorders
19019 Ventura Blvd, 3rd Floor
Tarzana, CA 91356
j.tarbox@centerforautism.com

Dr. Jonathan Tarbox is the Executive Director of Autism Research Group, as well as the Director of Research and Development at the Center for Autism and Related Disorders. Dr. Tarbox is a Board Certified Behavior Analyst-Doctoral, and he received his PhD in Behavior Analysis from the University of Nevada, Reno. His early career included positions at the New England Center for Children and the Kennedy Krieger Institute. Dr. Tarbox has conducted basic, applied, and interdisciplinary research and has over 50 publications in peer-reviewed journals, book chapters in scientific texts, and articles in popular media. Dr. Tarbox edited the *Handbook of Early Intervention for Autism Spectrum Disorders: Research, Practice, and Policy,* to be published by Springer Publishing in 2014, and co-authored *Evidence-Based Treatment for Children with Autism: The CARD Model,* to be published by Elsevier in 2014. Dr. Tarbox's areas of emphasis in research include behavioral approaches to complex language and cognition, the role of technology in treatment and training, and randomized controlled trials of autism treatment. Dr. Tarbox currently serves on the board of editors of The Analysis of Verbal Behavior, Behavior Analysis in Practice, and Research in Autism Spectrum Disorders and is affiliate faculty at the Chicago School for Professional Psychology.

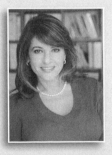

Doreen Granpeesheh, PhD, BCBA-D

Dr. Doreen Granpeesheh has dedicated over thirty years to helping individuals with autism lead healthy, productive lives. While completing her PhD in Psychology under Ivar Lovaas, she worked on the world-renowned 1987 study that showed a recovery rate of nearly 50 percent. Dr. Granpeesheh is a licensed psychologist in four states and is a Board Certified Behavior Analyst-Doctoral (BCBA-D). In 1990 Dr. Granpeesheh founded the Center for Autism & Related Disorders (CARD). CARD achieves success with every child through world-class treatment, staff training, curricula, and research. CARD provides services at 18 clinics in six US states, as well as sites in Australia, and New Zealand and partnerships in Dubai and Johannesburg. CARD employs over 800 staff and is a leading employer of BCBAs. Dr. Granpeesheh is on numerous Scientific and Advisory Boards for governmental and advocacy groups, and is the recipient of frequent honors, including the 2011 American Academy of Clinical Psychiatrists Winokur Award.

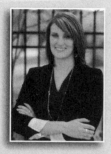

Angela Persicke

Angela Persicke received her master's degree in Psychology with an emphasis in Applied Behavior Analysis from California State University, Fresno, and is currently working on obtaining her PhD in Applied Behavior Analysis. She has been conducting applied research with children with autism for over 5 years and obtained her BCBA in 2011. Her research interests include behavior analysis of complex human behavior (e.g., language, cognition, social skills), dissemination of applied behavior analysis, early intervention and prevention of ASDs, performance management and staff training, and treatment and assessment for underserved populations. Her primary goal is to conduct and disseminate research that directly impacts the lives of all individuals affected by autism.

Treatment programs for children with autism based on Applied Behavior Analysis (ABA) have exploded over the last two decades, resulting in a dizzying array of terminology, acronyms, and brands. Many parents of children with ASD find it confusing and frustrating to navigate all of this information. This chapter expands on the chapter "What Makes a Great ABA Program" in the 2011 edition of *Cutting Edge Therapies,* and will provide a brief overview of the core defining features of ABA programs, as well as describing the major models, brands, and acronyms.

Core Defining Features of Top-Quality ABA Programs

Applied Behavior Analysis is a scientific discipline that applies scientifically validated principles of learning and motivation, and procedures derived from them, to solving problems of social significance. Autism is probably the best known problem to which ABA has been applied.

Principles

The basic learning principles that form the foundation of any good ABA program are: 1) reinforcement, 2) extinction, 3) establishing or motivating operations, 4) stimulus control, and 5) generalization. The principle of reinforcement refers to the fact that people continue to behave in ways that produce desirable outcomes—it's what motivates us all to do what we do. Extinction simply refers to the discontinuation of reinforcement—when reinforcement stops, behavior decreases. Establishing operations make reinforcement powerful, for example, being hungry makes food a strong reinforcer. Stimulus control is the process by which behavior becomes cued or signaled by the environment (e.g., the behavior of stopping at a red light). Generalization refers to how people apply what they learn in one setting to all relevant aspects of their lives.

Top-quality ABA programs are designed and supervised by clinicians with advanced training and knowledge of behavioral principles and how to apply these principles to teaching children with autism.

Procedures

There are many intervention procedures derived from behavioral learning principles, but the basic ones common to all good ABA programs for children with autism include: 1) prompting and prompt-fading, 2) preference assessment, 3) discrimination training, 4) shaping, 5) chaining, 6) explicit programming for maintenance and generalization, and 7) the provision of thousands of learning opportunities per day. All good ABA programs should have at least these seven features explicitly built into their daily operations.

Discrete Trial Training and Natural Environment Training

The vast majority of comprehensive ABA treatment programs for autism dedicate a large amount of time to discrete trial training (DTT), a teaching procedure that involves repeated practice of skills, gradually increasing in difficulty and gradually decreasing in structure and contrivance. DTT is still, by far, the most scientifically supported teaching procedure for children with autism. All good ABA programs today also incorporate a significant amount of naturalistic ABA teaching procedures, referred to as Natural Environment Training (NET). There are many different varieties of NET, including incidental teaching, milieu teaching, and Pivotal Response Training. Each has unique features, but all contain these basic elements: 1) all teaching is conducted in the natural environment (e.g., during play, while getting dressed, while making a sandwich, etc.), 2) teaching interactions are initiated by the child, 3) prompting is used when necessary, and 4) the natural consequence of the behavior is used as a reinforcer, whenever possible. Good quality comprehensive ABA programs do not choose between NET and DTT, they include both. For the vast majority of children with autism, both NET and DTT are necessary to ensure sufficient learning opportunities and effective generalization of skills. The specific proportion of DTT to NET implemented with any particular child should be customized to that child's individual strengths and needs.

A Functional Approach to Challenging Behavior

All good ABA programs are proficient at decreasing the challenging behaviors of children with autism and replacing them with other more adaptive behaviors. The best approach to decreasing challenging behavior is to first understand the function of the behavior, i.e., what the child wants when he/she engages in the behavior. Research has shown that in over 90 percent of cases, challenging behavior is motivated by: 1) getting attention from others, 2) getting out of doing something the child does not want to do (e.g., school work), 3) getting access to a preferred item or activity, and 4) automatic reinforcement (a.k.a., "self-stimulation"). That same source of reinforcement can then be used to teach appropriate alternative behaviors, such as asking for what one wants. Teaching a child to ask for what he wants instead of engaging in challenging behavior is called Functional Communication Training (FCT) and has been proven effective by a large amount of research. Positive Behavioral Supports (PBS) is a model of ABA treatment for challenging behavior that emphasizes arranging the individual's environment to avoid challenging behavior, as well as establishing other preventive measures, such as systems and family supports. PBS is not something different or separate from ABA, it is one area of emphasis within it.

Generalization and Maintenance

All good ABA programs place a heavy emphasis on generalization and maintenance of skills. This means that when a child learns new skills and/or his challenging behaviors decrease, these same improvements should also be seen in other settings, with other people (not just the therapists), and they should maintain across time. Good programs take explicit steps to encourage these outcomes, they do not merely hope for them.

Data and Accountability

All good ABA programs collect detailed data on child progress, in order to decide when to implement, change, or terminate particular treatment procedures. All good ABA programs assume that the teaching procedure is what causes learning, so if a child is not learning, it is unacceptable to blame the child or the diagnosis. The data must be used to evaluate procedures and the procedures must be changed until something effective is found.

Training and Supervision

All good ABA programs place a heavy emphasis on training and continued professional development for staff. A single brief seminar or "in-service" training for new therapists or teacher's aides is never sufficient to establish excellent staff performance. Frequent supervision must be done by a supervisor who is an expert in designing ABA programs for children with autism, ideally a Board Certified Behavior Analyst (BCBA) with several years' experience in top-quality ABA programs for children with autism.

Relationship-Building

All good ABA programs focus on building a positive relationship between the therapist and child by relying on positive reinforcement and rapport-building, and by providing the child sufficient help to ensure success. All good ABA programs begin with the assumption that every child with autism is capable of learning and that every child deserves a chance at learning the maximum number of skills possible, in a positive and fun environment. A common misconception is that ABA programs are aversive and uncomfortable for children, requiring nonstop drills, but this is far from accurate. Top-quality ABA programs incorporate positive reinforcement into every aspect of treatment and children in these programs are often observed to be happy and excited during therapy.

Intensity

ABA treatment requires hard work. The research has clearly shown that the best gains are achieved when children receive at least 30 hours per week of one-to-one therapy, for two or more years. Many children require three or four years to reach their maximum potential. No discoveries have yet been made that allow a shortcut around this level of intensity. ABA treatment implemented for 30 or more hours per week, starting before the age of 4, and addressing all areas of deficit, is often referred to as Early Intensive Behavioral Intervention (EIBI), sometimes as Intensive Behavioral Treatment (IBT) or Early Intensive Behavioral Treatment (EIBT).

Curriculum

Good ABA programs must use a comprehensive curriculum that addresses all areas of human functioning, since every child with autism is different, and some require learning in every area of development. It is crucial for top-quality ABA programs to individualize any curriculum to each child. It is rare that a "cookie cutter" type of program benefits children on the spectrum so a curriculum must include every possible skill that a child may need to learn.

Parent Involvement

All good ABA programs require parental involvement. At a minimum, parents should attend regular supervision meetings, at least every two weeks. Parents must be taught the basics of ABA and are reminded that their child has an opportunity to learn any time he is awake, seven days per week. However, parent training is *not* a substitute for professional-quality therapy and supervision. No research has yet shown that professional therapy and supervision can be replaced with parent training. No one would even suggest such a thing for surgery, and ABA therapy is no less complex or difficult to supervise.

Models and Brands of ABA for Children with Autism

Lovaas Therapy

In 1987, Ivar Lovaas published the first controlled outcome study showing that ABA can produce robust treatment effects for children with autism, including recovery in a subset of cases. Virtually all contemporary ABA programs contain some elements of the original Lovaas approach. However, most contemporary programs have made changes to the original Lovaas approach, most notably including a heavier emphasis on NET. It should be noted that therapy based on the Lovaas approach is still the most scientifically supported treatment for autism in the world.

Pivotal Response Training

Pivotal Response Training (PRT) is a form of NET. It is not something different from ABA; it is one set of procedures *within* ABA. It is distinguished from some other forms of NET by the fact that it explicitly involves reinforcing child *attempts* to respond, even if the response is incorrect. A large amount of research has shown that PRT is an effective teaching tool, but it is not a comprehensive intervention. It is one critical piece of comprehensive EIBI programs. No controlled outcome studies have yet been published on the effects of treatment programs that include only PRT and exclude other ABA teaching procedures, such as DTT.

Verbal Behavior

There is currently a lot of confusion about what verbal behavior is and how or whether it should be part of ABA treatment for children with autism. In the last decade or so, some groups (perhaps unintentionally) have spoken and acted as though verbal behavior is something different from ABA. This idea is highly uninformed. The term "verbal behavior" comes from B. F. Skinner's analysis of language in terms of behavioral principles, which yielded the concepts of the "verbal operants:" mand, tact, echoic, intraverbal, and so on. All good ABA programs should be thinking about and teaching language from the standpoint of behavioral principles and this is all that the term "verbal behavior" properly refers to. Skinner's verbal operants are useful tools for analyzing a child's language development and more basic verbal operants should be taught before more advanced ones (e.g., teach mands before intraverbals). The terms "Verbal Behavior Analysis" (VBA) and "Applied Verbal Behavior" (AVB) are not something different from ABA, they refer to ABA programs that place a heavy emphasis on incorporating Skinner's verbal operants into their programs.

Picture Communication and Sign Language

All good ABA programs should include some provision for establishing language in children who have particular difficulty in learning to speak vocally and/or learning to respond to vocal speech. In these cases, most programs will either teach basic sign language or some form of picture communication system. The most researched form of picture communication is the Picture Exchange Communication System (PECS).

PECS involves teaching children to exchange symbolic pictures in order to communicate. Research shows that both PECS and sign language are effective for children with autism, when implemented by clinicians who are experts in ABA.

CARD

The Center for Autism and Related Disorders (CARD) model of ABA intervention for children with ASD is a comprehensive approach to EIBI. The CARD model includes all major ABA principles and procedures described above, and customizes the proportion of each procedure for each child, based on his/her individual strengths, deficits, and preferences. The CARD curriculum is the most comprehensive curriculum available for children with autism and the CARD model is known for placing significant emphasis on higher-order skills, such as perspective-taking, executive functions, and derived relational responding. The entire CARD system is available online and is called Skills™. A significant amount of published research has demonstrated the utility of various aspects of the Skills system, including the validity and reliability of the Skills curriculum assessment, the effectiveness of the Behavior Intervention Plan Builder component, and the effectiveness of several of the advanced teaching lessons, including detecting sarcasm, metaphorical reasoning, detecting deception, rule-following, shifting attention, and working memory.

CABAS

Comprehensive Application of Behavior Analysis to Schooling (CABAS) is a comprehensive model of ABA instruction, based largely on Skinner's analysis of verbal behavior. The model focuses heavily on establishing concept formation ("generalized operants") and has a well-developed, but not publicly available, curriculum.

What's Coming Next

It is always difficult to predict the future but a few areas of development are worthy of special mention. First, it is likely that in the next several years, an additional certification will be created for ABA practitioners in autism. The BCBA certification assures foundational knowledge in ABA but not with respect to autism, in particular. Many parents of children on the spectrum have been demanding an additional guarantee of expertise in ABA treatment for autism and it is likely that such a certification will come about in the near future. Finally, the global demand for ABA services and the severe shortage of expert clinicians has created a need for faster training and dissemination of ABA expertise. It seems likely that information technology will play a part in meeting this demand, with university training systems moving increasingly to online education, as well as organizational communication systems moving toward web-based meetings and teleconferencing. The coming decade is likely to be a critical period for designing systems for training and dissemination that will increase efficiency without sacrificing quality, in order to meet the ever-increasing demand for ABA services around the world.

Technology and ABA

With advances in technology it is inevitable that technology will play an increasingly prominent role in various aspects of ABA programs. Data collection programs allow for easy and efficient means of making program data available in real time to others interested in viewing client progress such as clinical supervisors, parents, teachers and even funding sources. Web-based assessment and curriculum development tools allow clinicians to design comprehensive treatment programs that are linked to assessments and track client progress through the individualized program. Tablets equipped with various applications and games that assist in language and other skill development are becoming a common component of treatment programs. Not to mention the use of tablets or personal computers as a means to provide various reinforcing activities. It's likely that in the next few years educational games and programs presented on tablets or computers will be used as a supplemental treatment programs to provide more learning opportunities to individuals on the spectrum who do not receive the recommended number of treatment hours due to a lack of funding or availability of quality ABA programs with experienced clinicians. Moving forward, it is crucial that treatment programs ensure high quality despite the imminent changes that may occur with technological advances.

42

EMOTIONAL VOCAL EXPLORATION: A REVOLUTIONARY MODE OF COMMUNICATION

By Amanda Friedman and Alison Berkley

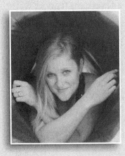

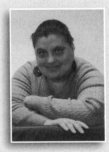

Alison Berkley, MsT
Alison@emergeandsee.net

Amanda Friedman, MsEd, SBL
Amanda@emergeandsee.net

Emerge & See Education Center
164 W 25th St Suite 7R
New York, NY 10001
212-256-0846
info@emergeandsee.net
Facebook: Emerge & See Education Center
and Social Groups
YouTube: EmergeandSee2012
Twitter: EmergeandSeeEdu

Alison Berkley, MsT, began working with children with special needs from the young age of 14. Since then Alison has worked with children of all ages and abilities. She earned her BS in psychology from New York University where she graduated on the Dean's List and was awarded a Dean's Scholarship to complete her MsT at Pace University. Alison has taught in both ABA and DIR/Floortime schools gleaning broad and intensive experience in varying educational methodologies. Throughout her career Alison has implemented data collection and analysis techniques and systems which informed and helped create Emerge & See's multi-disciplinary and comprehensive curriculum for children with ASD. This data-driven curriculum truly individualizes each comprehensive educational program for every student and will be a cornerstone of the future Atlas School. Alison co-founded the Emerge & See Education Center in 2009 with Amanda Friedman, and has been serving families and children with special needs in New York (and beyond) ever since!

Amanda Friedman, MSEd, is a special education teacher with over 10 years experience within the educational field. She has completed the Administrative Certification Program from the College of Saint Rose/CITE and is awaiting approval of her SDL and SBL license. She has worked with students ranging in age from 3–25 years old with an array of differences including autism, mental retardation, emotional disturbances (PTSD, schizophrenia, oppositional defiance disorder, etc.). She has acted as the vice president for the Hudson Valley Autism Society, sat on several Walk for Autism Committees, and is a parent advocate for families at CSE and school meetings. Amanda has been through certified trainings in ABA, TEACCH, BART, and multiple trainings in DIR/Floortime.

Emotional Vocal Exploration (EVE) Mission Statement:

To empower intellectual and emotional growth in students with complex verbal skill-sets through dynamic choice-making and independent thought. To validate internally motivated and self-initiated responses which expand interests and ideas through conversation and promote the power of voice.

Disclaimer: EVE breaks barriers and reforms previously held ideas of what "communication" means. We implore you to delve into this with an open mind and to explore a novel methodology and a new definition of what it means to "talk." Ready yourself for a revolution in *communication.* Read this chapter and fully imagine the real-life sensory experiences described. Walk with us now along the road our children walk every day. **Warning:** This chapter is laden with emotional content as are the lives of our students. Readers, accept our invitation to understanding and hearing their voices for the first time. **Thirst:** Imagine it's a regular day at school: you've been sitting in class for hours without a break from your deskwork, listening attentively to your teachers and completing tasks diligently. As your mind wanders away from the papers spread on the desk in front of you, you realize something. You are thirsty. Your mental energy has been so focused on the work, you simply didn't notice that nagging thirst until now. Your mouth is dry, your throat is scratchy and a nice, cold glass of water sounds like just the thing! You open your mouth to politely request, "May I have a glass of water?" Nothing. Not a sound comes out. You take a moment and try again. This time, your lips move and an unintelligible noise peeps out, but it is far from what you intended to say. You stop and give yourself a moment to think of the words you were trying to say in hopes that this time around your mouth will do what your brain so urgently wants it to. Yet, not a word passes your chapped lips. Your dry tongue sticks to the roof of your mouth as you try to move all the parts necessary to form the sounds and syllables. The next attempt brings another failure. And then another. This goes on and on . . . and on. Your internal, mental frustration becomes external, visible. Your brow furrows and your muscles tense. You feel your cheeks flush from both the embarrassment of not being able to say a simple sentence and the frustration of not already having the satisfaction of chugging that enticing glass of water. Your heart rate starts to pick up pace as you strain your body in an attempt to formulate those words. You try to simplify things a bit to see if that helps, maybe one word will be more manageable. "Water," you think, and then try to say. Nothing. You feel your palms get sweaty and salty beads of perspiration start to form on your forehead. Your facial expression turns to one of scrunched-up exasperation. The teacher in the room sees this and quickly offers you some of your most favorite things: lemonade, soda pop, a snack, a treasured toy; doing whatever they can trying to help you. Your friends and classmates join in to make this a group effort and now everyone around you is trying anything they can think of. Yet, it doesn't cross anyone's mind except yours that **you want water**. What do you do? How do you feel?

Empty Glasses: With even a miniscule amount of the simplest of molecules, that precious H_2O, life can form and grow and flourish. As social beings, communication in all its variety can be thought of as our life force, for without the ability to communicate, we become isolated and solitary. If you can imagine the above scenario that highlights one moment of one day existing in that uncomfortable and unnatural isolation from others, perhaps you can go a bit further and conceive of an entire lifetime in that kind of existence. Try and envision what it would be like living in a world void of both simple and complex communicative interactions: a world full of empty glasses. The plethora of ideas sprouting forth inside your mind could not be expressed, no matter how vigorous and creative your efforts to do so may be. Any and all attempts to convey your thoughts in myriad ways fall into an abyss that grows deeper and wider each time you try to speak; engorging the blackness of misunderstanding between you and other people. A social chasm is created; effective communication is broken down. Think of how your experiences would be limited. How your relationships with every single person in your life would be impacted. How your confidence and self-esteem would be deflated. How you might get frustrated and angry after all that hard work and all those failures. How you might just give up entirely, finding yourself alone and parched with no rain clouds overhead or even on the horizon.

Teachers come and go, years pass and still your mouth, tongue, and lips feel numb and act as though they are immune or impervious to the neural signals relentlessly sent by your brain. Those electrical signals fail to be interpreted or understood in a way that allows your mouth to form complex movements that, when combined, should form sounds and then words and then sentences. Your body, too works against you, refusing to send signals or communications that are understood by others: your facial expressions belie your true feelings and intentions. This is the life lived day in and day out by a vast majority of those deemed "non-verbal" or "less verbal" who are diagnosed with Autism Spectrum Disorders, Apraxia, and Speech and Language difficulties. These are our students, our children and our inspirations. They are the reason Emotional Vocal Exploration (EVE) was created. When we partner together in a new mode of thinking and approaching our children for whom communication seems an insurmountable obstacle, we can lovingly offer them a full glass and help quench their thirst.

Drink: Can you imagine what you would *do* and how you would *feel* in that classroom and living in a life-long drought? For us, the answer to that question has come bit by bit and, at times, painfully slowly. With over twenty years of combined experience in the field of special education we have traveled a long and arduous road exploring and experimenting with already established yet incomplete approaches, failed methodologies and inadequate ideas. Our previous trials-by-fire turned into some successes for our students that, while substantial and significant, left us educators wanting and needing more in order to help. We yearned for the "best of the best": a single idea or curricula or program that could help *all* of our students achieve without ceiling or limitations. EVE was born out of this desire, countless student sessions, research on any and all effective and current methods, piles of academic papers plowed through, specialists observed in action and experts consulted upon and debated with. EVE is the amalgamation of all those years of experiences, numerous failures and subsequently renewed and revised attempts. It is only through the support of our families and the trust and love of our students that we were able to reach this point. While EVE is still in the research phase at the time of this publication, its proof is in the pudding, so to speak: its ability to break barriers of communication motivated us to dedicate this chapter to sharing some of it with you now. We couldn't wait, and neither could our students.

The Science of Water: To align the science with the heart, we brought in Amanda Leeder to assist us in this process. She is currently a doctoral candidate in Fordham University's Applied Developmental Psychology program. Before attending Fordham, Amanda received her MA in General Psychology at New York University and has six years of experience implementing and researching therapeutic interventions for the ASD population in home and school settings.

Amanda has written the following synopsis to address her experience and understanding of the Emotional Vocal Exploration model: "EVE is a communication approach developed by the co-founders of the Emerge & See Education Center, and designed for individuals on the autistic spectrum with linguistic and social difficulties. The approach prides itself on the high level of respect therapists have for learners, which is inherent in the former's expectation for the latter to be active participants in discussion. These expectations are based on individualized sensory, physical and cognitive profiles of learners that are assessed at the baseline level before therapy begins.

EVE integrates the developmental basis of DIR/Floortime™ and the literacy focus of RPM™ (Rapid Prompt Method), but distinguishes itself according to its focus on teaching people with autism to communicate and advocate for their emotional, physical and intellectual needs and desires through the power of choice. EVE is designed to empower individuals with social and linguistic challenges by encouraging them to choose from a continuous array of topic choices that either switches the conversation topic or delves further into a topic that the learner has previously chosen. The therapist uses the choices of the learner to better direct the conversation, and the expectation is that the learner will utilize the tools afforded to them in order to converse within a topic that motivates them. Choosing topics that are honored by the therapist allows learners to value the utility of language in supporting self-advocacy and learning, thereby becoming active discussion participants."

EVE is a revolutionary use of the basic concept that *all* people are empowered by choice. As Dr. Stanley Greenspan, founder of DIR/Floortime™ stated time and again in his lectures and consultations, "There is no greater feeling than that of being understood!" With that statement ringing in our ears, it became evident that the community needed to understand this method and the doors it opens to building relationships, modifying curriculum and assessing students' true knowledge base as well as the expression of their personalities. It is imperative for this program to work for the individual communicating via EVE and that they be honored for what they are saying. EVE fundamentally encourages students to speak their mind: students are able to change the topic, to complain, or to say what they need to. We do not shy away from tough topics, emotions or personal interests. Similarly, we do not insert our own beliefs or agendas into the EVE sessions, thus creating a space for mutual trust, respect, and honesty.

The Data Dam: Handing a single glass to a single student was insufficient to meet our long-term vision of EVE. We believed that from the very beginning we needed to create a veritable reservoir that *all* students of EVE could access. Many highly effective programs could not gain traction due to lack of qualitative studies addressing efficacy and validity. We want to ensure people (parents, teachers, administrators, etc.) do not fall to cynicism in deciding whether or not our students are *authentically* sharing their true feelings and answers. We do not want doubt to circumvent celebration and engagement and, thus, from the birth of EVE's mission until now scientific reliability and valid assessment have been key factors in our process. As we actively work and collaborate with a speech therapist and research specialist we have been looking for those outside expert perspectives to inform our practices. Reliable data collection, analysis, and reflection are key components not only in the creation of the EVE methodology but also in aiding the progress of our students and the different arenas in which it will be implemented.

The initial research of EVE is currently under way. Its structural concept, execution, and ability to help students engage, build confidence, and communicate beyond the means of concrete requesting is being closely examined. The study will be used to inform staff development and instructions for caregivers eager to generalize EVE into the student's home and community lives as well. Amanda writes further, "The formative evaluation of EVE will assess the performance of five Emerge & See participants during six EVE sessions spanning over a three month period. Indicators for success are based on whether learner's performances reveal that they know how EVE works, as well as whether the discussion topics presented or chosen are shown to be interesting or useful to the learner. In addition to a quantitative analysis of these indicators for success (listed below), a qualitative analysis of therapists' suggestions/reflections/notes from post-session questionnaires will inform future improvements to EVE in preparation for a wider implementation of the approach."

Indicators for Success:

1. Increased number of consecutive back and forth interaction between therapist and learner (therapist offers choices→learner chooses one→therapist offers new choices based on previous selection by learner→learner chooses one)
2. Use (but not abuse) of the "something else" option
3. Choose paper without needing prompting (though repeated presentation of choices is allowed and encouraged)
4. Decrease in incidents wherein learner chooses a topic that conflicts with his/her expressed interest in a different topic (picking one piece of paper and saying the words from a different piece of paper, choosing one paper and then protesting against that topic, failing to choose correctly when simple/mastered factual questions are presented)
5. Decrease in tantrums, decrease in aggression, decrease in attempts to leave room during session
6. Increase in length of sessions
7. Increases in discoveries of newfound interests/abilities of the learner (therapists know the learners very well and for many years)
8. Increase in initiation of topics by verbal participants
9. Increase in therapists' ratings of learner performance during sessions, increase in therapists' ratings of implementation quality
10. More performances perceived by therapist as typical or better than average, compared with those perceived as worse than average

The Next Stage: It should be noted that there are particular prerequisites required in order to successfully enter into an EVE program. However, the adaptability and individualized nature of each unique EVE program (each one is slightly different based on each students profile and skillsets) enables us to overcome smaller obstacles in order to achieve greater results. For instance, a student must have symbolic thinking but they do not need to be a fluent reader (decoding words on a page). Three pieces of paper are laid out in front of you, I touch each one, and as I do I pair a different sound with each piece. You hold these symbols and sounds in your working memory and make your choice by giving me the piece of paper. As I touch the first piece of paper, and say, "A" you mark in your mind that that one is "A." Then, I touch the second one and say "B" and then "C" for the third. This is a simple example of EVE's sequencing and how choices are presented and then selected. Once the options are given, you now know that each piece of paper I touch corresponds to a particular letter or sound. You do not need to be able to read Shakespeare or even know your phonics yet. You simply need to know that each paper relates to a particular sound. Each sound, or in this case letter, can easily be swapped for a longer sound or a word. Once you show that you can give correct responses to concrete questions (i.e., "hand me 'B'"), you are ready to get into the student-directed phase. In this next stage, I present to you the same three pieces of paper and slowly touch each one and present the following three words in succession, "cat," "dog," and "cow," for example. You can then hold in your mind that the three pieces of paper now represent three different animals. Here is where conversation begins. Essentially, we are pairing concrete visuals (pieces of papers) with simple and/or complex sounds (letters and/or words). We are teachers after all, and our job is to teach and instruct, so in EVE, we write the word on the paper so that if you are a reader you can also pair the word with the paper visual and the auditory sound, and if you are not a reader yet, you can begin to learn some sight words in that when she touched the first one, that C-A-T combo sounded like that, and slowly the brain starts to put it all together. Conversation typically revolves around personal interests and motivating topics. Instead of demanding that you hand me "cat," for instance, I *ask* you, "which is your favorite animal?" Your chosen response is the one *you* want, which then creates an opportunity for us to have a conversation about animals, why you love that animal, and maybe I will tell you a story of my experiences with that animal. We talk, we listen, and we communicate! Focus and attention, physical readiness and auditory processing abilities are required in order to sit with us and actually hear the instructions, word pairings, etc. This is why the building and assessing of individual student profiles is so vital and crucial to the success of EVE. You cannot put the cart before the communicative horse. We always create an educational program that strengthens the student's brain-body connections first and *then* implement an EVE program that appropriately fits their individual needs and style.

It is imperative that all parties involved feel encouraged by, trust, and respect the validity of this communicative system. If the individual implementing the process is skeptical the warmth and significant amount of work the person trying to communicate is exercising becomes negated and the opportunity for a sincere back and forth dialogue is tainted by uncertainty. This process is not one of "right or wrong" answers but a forum for concept exploration, emotional outpouring, and idea development. We are building skyscrapers not knocking down a house of cards!

So now you know there's water to quench the thirst for communication and respectful conversation. Let's go over the prescription plan for EVE and if you have questions consult your intuition. Be sure to trust in your child/student/self. Should you need us, we are also here anytime at info@emergeandsee.net to answer as best we can!

Who should take this?

Individuals with pragmatic language challenges, apraxia, autism, executive functioning difficulties, selective mutism, etc. People eager to communicate with semi-verbal and non-verbal individuals in a respectful and sincere manner that enhances confidence, expansion of ideas, and personal relationships.

What are the side effects?

Some students may have an emotional response to their own success in communicating and being truly heard outside of basic requests and gestures. Often times there is a cathartic response to the liberation brought about by being aware of their own thinking and ability to be held accountable and to hold others accountable as well. Students will explore their own creative and multi-modal thinking and begin responding to both personal and learning based/academic questions on a regular basis, thus aiding them in creating stronger relationships with their peers, educators, therapists, and families.

Interactions

EVE can be implemented in conjunction with any and all modalities of effective educational and behavioral therapies. Albeit, during the sessions it is imperative that the interactions be student driven and it is evident the reinforcement for engagement is the EVE process and not token boards, edibles, etc. The relationship is key to the interaction and it is vital that the instructor's affect match the content of the session and is directly connected to the demeanor of the student.

Generic alternatives

EVE has no generic alternative. Emotional Vocal Exploration is a process unique to the individuals brought together either as family, student and teacher, or friends. It is the only process by which choice making, symbolic thinking, and a theory of "no ceiling" are integrated. EVE uniquely allows for trust in intelligence and eventual expansion into writing or actual vocalization of thoughts in a natural structure between equally responsive parties.

When to discontinue?

Never.

CARD eLEARNING™ AND SKILLS®: WEB-BASED TRAINING, ASSESSMENT, CURRICULUM, AND PROGRESS TRACKING FOR CHILDREN WITH AUTISM

By Dr. Doreen Granpeesheh and Dr. Adel C. Najdowski

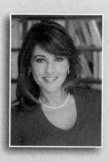

Doreen Granpeesheh, PhD, BCBA-D
Center for Autism and Related Disorders
19019 Ventura Blvd, 3rd Floor
Tarzana, CA 91356

Dr. Doreen Granpeesheh has dedicated over thirty years to helping individuals with autism lead healthy, productive lives. While completing her PhD in Psychology under Ivar Lovaas, she worked on the world-renowned 1987 study that showed a recovery rate of nearly 50 percent. Dr. Granpeesheh is a licensed psychologist in four states and is a Board Certified Behavior Analyst-Doctoral (BCBA-D). In 1990 Dr. Granpeesheh founded the Center for Autism & Related Disorders (CARD). CARD achieves success with every child through world-class treatment, staff training, curricula, and research. CARD provides services at 18 clinics in six US states, as well as sites in Australia, and New Zealand and partnerships in Dubai and Johannesburg. CARD employs over 800 staff and is a leading employer of BCBAs. Dr. Granpeesheh is on numerous Scientific and Advisory Boards for governmental and advocacy groups, and is the recipient of frequent honors, including the 2011 American Academy of Clinical Psychiatrists Winokur Award.

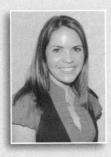

Adel C. Najdowski, PhD, BCBA-D

Dr. Adel Najdowski graduated from the University of Nevada, Reno, in 2004 with her doctorate in psychology. She is the co-creator of Skills,™ a comprehensive assessment and curriculum for children with autism, and currently serves as the Director of the Skills department at the Center for Autism and Related Disorders. She has served children with autism for 16 years. Dr. Najdowski has taught multiple undergraduate and graduate level courses in psychology. She served on the editorial board for the Journal of Applied Behavior Analysis in 2009 and has been a National Board Certified Behavior Analyst (BCBA) since 2003. She has six first-authored publications, 18 co-authored publications, and has been an author on 63 presentations given at conferences. Her current research interests include teaching higher level skills to children with autism, assessment and curriculum design for children with autism, and feeding disorders.

CARD eLearning™ is a web-based program for training individuals to deliver ABA-based intervention to children with autism spectrum disorders (ASD). Skills® is a web-based program for the assessment, curriculum design, and management of ABA-based intervention programs for children with ASD. CARD eLearning and Skills were developed by the Center for Autism and Related Disorders, Inc. (CARD).

Center for Autism and Related Disorders

CARD was founded by Dr. Doreen Granpeesheh in 1990 and provides behavioral intervention to approximately 1,200 individuals with ASD using an approach called applied behavior analysis (ABA). CARD currently has 19 offices across seven states within the United States, two offices internationally (New Zealand and Australia), and one affiliate site (South Africa). In addition to servicing children at these physical sites, CARD provides intervention to children on all continents using a consultative workshop model.

In the course of treating children for 20 years, CARD believes that children can recover from ASD and has published research on the recovery of children. While recovery is possible for a group of children with particular characteristics, it is not the only goal of intervention. The goal is to help each child achieve the most they can and live life to the fullest potential.

Over the years, CARD has become well-known for their robust therapist training program and for having the most comprehensive curriculum for teaching skills to children with ASD in the world. Given the rising incidence of ASD, CARD has experienced a tremendous increase in the demand for treatment services. This increase is what led to the development of both CARD eLearning and Skills. The two programs were created with the goal of helping as many children and their families affected by ASD as possible in order to fulfill the mission of providing global access to the highest quality of ABA-based intervention in the world. Both CARD eLearning and Skills can be accessed on the world-wide web at www.skills-forautism.com.

CARD eLearning

CARD eLearning is based on the didactic classroom portion of the therapist-level training provided at CARD. The development of CARD eLearning was initiated in 2002 and was completed in 2010. Also, in 2010 and 2012, research was published demonstrating that CARD eLearning is an effective tool for increasing academic knowledge of individuals on the principles and application of behavior analysis to the treatment of ASD.

CARD eLearning is an online training program designed to facilitate the provision of effective intervention for children with ASD by equipping users with foundational knowledge in autism, ABA and research-proven intervention techniques. CARD eLearning currently consists of 9 modules, equivalent to 40 hours of training. Each learning module focuses on a topic such as: "What is Autism?", "Applied Behavior Analysis (ABA)," "Skill Repertoire Building," and "Behavior Management." Each section of the CARD eLearning program is organized with teaching objectives, explanation of terms, examples of methodology, video demonstrations, printable study guides, online note-taking, quizzes, and other learning tools.

Upon completion of CARD eLearning, users are provided with a certificate of completion. Furthermore, organizations using CARD eLearning to train their staff can obtain reports about the performance of their staff. They can view the quiz and test scores of each user, determine which portions of the training were most difficult for the user to acquire by viewing how many times the user had to take a quiz to pass it, and compare the performance of staff with one another.

Skills

Skills is the online delivery of CARD's comprehensive assessment and curriculum and is also a globally accessible repository for data storage and analysis. While the CARD curriculum has been in continuous development and usage at CARD for 20 years (with new phases released annually), the development of Skills was initiated in 2003 and the product was completed in 2010. Since its launch, a network of behavior analysts and many school districts have started using Skills as a comprehensive assessment and curriculum helping to provide consistency in programs delivered to children with ASD across the world. Skills involves four basic steps: (1) assess the child, (2) choose activities to teach, (3) start treatment, and (4) track progress.

FOUR STEPS

In the first step, the user interacts with the Skills assessment, which is not only the most comprehensive assessment of child development ever created but has also been demonstrated to have high test-retest and inter-rater reliability for its Language subscale. Using this tool, the user assesses the child's skill level across all areas of human functioning and across every possible skill that develops between the ages of 0 and 8 years.

The Skills assessment provides basic "yes"/"no" questions that are relevant to the child's chronological age. The questions are organized by eight developmental areas: social, motor, language, adaptive, play, executive functions, cognition, and academic skills. Within each of these developmental areas, questions are further organized by concepts (e.g., within the developmental area of "social skills" there are concepts such as "apologizing" and "initiating a conversation"). Questions are provided in the order of typical child development and are presented in an "intelligent" fashion in order to maximize efficiency.

Following completion of the assessment for any given developmental or concept area, users can view bar graphs depicting the percentage of skills in the child's repertoire in comparison to how he or she should be performing at his or her age. In addition, Skills provides users with a pool of available lesson activities directly linked to the areas identified (by the assessment) as needed to be focused on during teaching. This now enters into the second step of the Skills program wherein users choose activities to teach.

For the process of choosing activities, there are five tools available to help users make good choices. First, each lesson is assigned to a teaching level between 1 and 12, with level 1 being the most basic and 12 being the most advanced. Teaching should generally begin at lower levels before moving to higher levels. Second, activities are organized by the age in which they are observed in typical child development. Users should start by teaching younger skills before moving to older skills. Third, activities are presented and numbered (starting with 1 and moving forward) in the order in which one would usually teach them. Users should generally start by teaching activity 1 and progress forward in order. Fourth, each activity specifies the other activities that are considered prerequisites. Prerequisite skills should generally be mastered first. Finally, each activity is given one of three possible designations: (1) building block, (2) fundamental skill, or (3) expansion skill. Fundamental skills are the milestones and building blocks are considered steps toward learning fundamental skills. Building blocks are not required for every learner. Children who learn quickly might be able to skip past the building blocks, whereas other children may rely on the building blocks for learning fundamental skills. Expansion skills are also not necessary for every child because they are not required for day-to-day functioning but can enrich a child's level of functioning within a particular skill area.

Once the user chooses lesson activities to place into the treatment plan, the user enters into the third step of the Skills program which is to start treatment. The user is now presented with an array of teaching materials to use during treatment. Each activity comes with a printable activity guide that provides step-by-step instructions, examples, teaching tips, and ideas for ensuring that what is learned is maintained and generalized in the child's daily life. The user is also provided with a series of printable handouts such as target checklists (e.g., targets for the activity of learning the recognition of emotions include "happy," "sad," "angry," etc.), teaching guides, worksheets, visual aids, and data-tracking forms. In addition to all of these materials, users can view a short video clip of each activity being conducted by a therapist and child.

It is in the "start treatment" phase that the user has everything he or she needs to begin teaching, using the resources provided by Skills as well as the knowledge acquired from CARD eLearning. As the child learns and masters targets and activities, the user checks them off as being mastered within the Skills treatment plan which automatically feeds data into the Skills database, generates printable bar graphs, and plots data onto a multidisciplinary timeline.

The bar graphs show both progress within developmental and concept areas and depict a comparison between what skills the child had in his or her repertoire during the assessment and how far he or she has come during treatment. The multidisciplinary timeline is a line graph that shows the child's acquisition of targets and activities over time. The key feature of the multidisciplinary timeline is its ability to allow users to enter in other life events. With this ability, the child's entire treatment team (e.g., special educators, speech language pathologists, occupational therapists, medical doctors, etc.) can evaluate the effects of their interventions on child progress. For example, if the child starts a new biomedical intervention, it can be entered onto the timeline and its effects on the child's mastery of skills can be evaluated. Other behaviors and events can also be added including challenging behavior (e.g., stereotypy, tantrums, aggression, etc.) and events such as when the child's treatment hours change or the child is ill.

ANALYTICS

In addition to receiving graphs depicting the child's progress while using Skills, data in the Skills database can be used for the purposes of prediction of probable outcomes, team evaluation, and cost analysis. Given certain child parameters, Skills will be able to predict each child's expected best outcome from receiving ABA-based intervention in terms of his or her expected level of functioning as a result of treatment. Likewise, Skills will be able to predict how much of the Skills curriculum the child will learn given a hypothetical number of hours of treatment provided per week and in turn will be able to predict the length of time the child will need treatment at said number of hours in order to achieve the child's predicted best outcome.

In addition to predictive models at the child level, the analytics piece allows interested parties to contrast the performance of children within the same treatment supervisor as well as to contrast the performance of different treatment supervisors or treatment agencies with one another.

Given the child predictive model and the ability to conduct evaluations of the treatment team, treatment supervisors and agencies will be able to be given a ranking in terms of their effectiveness. Now, interested parties will be able to conduct a cost analysis on each case by correlating predicted best outcome for a child with supervisor/agency rankings.

SUPPORT

In addition to all of the features above that Skills offers, the website also comes with many tools for support. This includes a video library of tips for success, navigational tutorials, live chatting, a support community (where users can ask questions, share ideas, and/or give praise), and access to an exciting new interactive web show called Skills Live (also viewable on the world-wide web by visiting www.skillsliveonline.com) which airs segments on topics such as autism news, interviews with experts, and tips for autism assessment and while also allowing viewers to ask questions during the show.

Conclusion

In conclusion, CARD is among the largest autism treatment organizations in the world. CARD's state-of-the-art services, global reach, and comprehensive scope are matched by none. Two features that set CARD apart from others is our world-class training and insistence on a comprehensive application of ABA-based intervention to every imaginable skill a person with ASD may need to learn.

CARD is now in the position to share its 20 years of knowledge and expertise in providing treatment to children with ASD (and in many cases, recovering children with ASD) with the world. Neither quality nor quantity can be compromised in our mission to extend top-quality behavioral treatment to the maximum number of individuals with ASD possible. CARD eLearning and Skills have been released to achieve this mission and both self-improvement and fine-tuning will continue until this mission is accomplished.

DRAMA THERAPY

By Sally Bailey, MFA, MSW, RDT/BCT

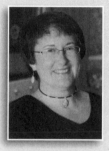

Sally Bailey, MFA, MSW, RDT/BCT

109 McCain
School of Music, Theatre and Dance
Kansas State University
Manhattan, KS 66506-4702
(785) 532-6780
sdbailey@ksu.edu
www.dramatherapycentral.com

Sally Bailey is a professor of Theatre at Kansas State University where she directs the drama therapy program. She is author of *Barrier-Free Theatre: Including Everyone in Theatre Arts Regardless of (Dis)Ability, Wings to Fly,* and *Dreams to Sign.* She has used drama therapy with clients on the autism spectrum for the past twenty-five years. A past president of the North American Drama Therapy Association, she is a recipient of NADTA's Gertrude Schattner Award for distinguished contributions in the field of drama therapy and Accessible Arts' Distinguished Service Award in Arts and Disabilities.

Drama therapy applies techniques from theatre to psychotherapy. Instead of entertainment, the focus is on helping individuals grow and heal by taking on and practicing new roles, creating new stories through action, and rehearsing new behaviors which can later be implemented in real life. Drama therapy involves participants in informal drama processes (games, improvisation, storytelling, role play) and/or formal products (puppets, masks, plays/performances) to help clients understand their thoughts and emotions better, improve behavior, and learn social interaction skills.

Drama therapy is effective because it involves action methods which can be rehearsed or repeated until a skill is learned. An embodied, concrete experience makes skills easier for clients on the autism spectrum to grasp, remember, and implement (Bailey, 2007, 2009b). While literature on autism suggests that people with ASD are not creative and have little interest in connecting with others, drama therapists find that ASD clients they work with are imaginative, highly motivated to participate in dramatic activities, and crave social connection, but are not sure how to make those connections on their own. Drama therapy helps in this connection process because drama is all about human relating and relationships.

Neuroscientists looking at the arts, learning, and the brain have discovered that the arts are motivating for children because they create conditions in which attention can be sustained over longer periods of time (Posner, Rothbart, Sheese, & Kieras in Ashbury & Rich, 2008). An additional benefit of the arts, particularly drama, is that participants receive immediate feedback in the process of enacting a scene from the other actors and from the audience, as well as soon afterwards when the group discusses the scene and/or when they replay the scene with corrections (Bailey, 2009a; Jensen & Dabney, 2000; Posner et al, 2008).

Temple Grandin (2002), a professor of animal science who has autism, says when she was growing up, she viewed many cultural customs and behaviors of neurotypical people as ISPs – Interesting Sociological Phenomenons. Role play can be the perfect way for people with ASD to come to a better understanding of the neurotypical world's ISPs. Practice putting themselves in another person's or character's shoes can become the first steps toward understanding how the rest of the world feels, thinks, and relates.

Drama strongly engages the mirror neuron system in actors and audiences alike (Blair, 2008; McConachie, 2008). Some neuroscientists believe that our empathic abilities and our abilities to learn cognitively and emotionally through observation relate directly to our mirror neurons (Iacoboni & Daprette, 2006; Iacoboni, et al, 2005; Oberman & Ramachandran, 2007), and there are others who suspect that autism may relate to deficiencies in the mirror neuron system (Ramachandran & Oberman, 2006). If this is true, then drama therapy could be extremely effective in promoting repair of weaknesses and disconnections in the mirror neuron system.

Drama therapy has been developed by a wide variety of practitioners. Most trained originally in theatre, then after recognizing the healing powers of drama, they trained in psychology and psychotherapy. Early twentieth century Jacob L. Moreno in Austria and US Peter Slade in UK Vladimir Iljine and Nicholai Evreinov in Russia. Late twentieth century Gertrude Schattner, Eleanor Irwin, David Read Johnson, Renee Emunah, and Robert Landy in US Sue Jennings and Marian Lindkvist in UK (Bailey, 2006).

In the early twentieth century, drama was used by occupational therapists in hospitals and by social workers in community programs to teach clients social and emotional skills through performing in plays. The field began to integrate improvisation and process drama methods, emerging as a separate profession in the 1970s. In relation to treatment of clients on the autism spectrum, drama was one of the very first techniques used. Hans Asperger, the German doctor who first described Asperger's syndrome in 1944, created an educational program for the boys he was treating which involved speech therapy, drama, and physical education (Attwood, 1998). Sister Viktorine, director of the program, was killed when the ward on which she was working was destroyed in an allied bombing attack in World War II, so no record of exactly how she incorporated drama survives (Attwood, 1998). This early use of drama indicates an appreciation for the strengths it offers as an intervention. Currently, many drama therapists across the US and internationally are involved in the use of drama therapy with children, teens, and adults on the autism spectrum.

Success Rate

Lee Chasen, PhD, RDT created an effective drama therapy program for children on the autism spectrum, detailed in his book *Social Skills Emotional Growth and Drama Therapy: Inspiring Connection on the Autism Spectrum* (2011). He incorporates video-taping to provide visual and auditory feedback for students. Bullying issues that the children are experiencing are addressed as well as developing of social connections and building friendships with each other.

Grady Bolding (2007), a drama major at Kansas State University who is on the autism spectrum, says about his experience in theatre, "The world of theater helped bring me out of my shell, since I got free crash courses in interpersonal communications with every script. Today, I speak like anybody else" (Bolding, 2007, p. 3). He reports that his theatre training helped him learn how to make eye contact, show emotional expression during conversations, and read the emotional messages in others' voices and bodies. The characters that he played on stage and the script analysis he did taught him how to carry on a conversation off stage. He has been able to take that understanding and apply it to the real people he encounters in everyday life. He says, "I can interpret the way someone else is feeling somewhat—just a little bit now. Back then [before drama training], people were just objects" (Personal communication, 2009).

Many theatres are beginning to offer drama classes geared toward students with ASD; however, when the drama activities are led by a trained drama therapist who knows how to target specific therapeutic goals, even more success can be achieved. The mother of an adolescent with ASD who I worked with told me:

> I have seen the child we knew was inside, but which we rarely saw at home, come out on stage. . . . On stage she is at her most confident, most assertive, her most centered self. Being in the plays gives her something *entirely* her own. . . . Most adults tell our children to be quiet—they don't want to hear what they have to say. But [in drama therapy] what they have to say matters. . . . It's very hard for kids with special needs to have a large group of friends. They tend to be very isolated. I see her involvement [in drama therapy] as a great social experience. . . . At the end of the year she has created and maintained many social relationships and she has a sweet taste in her mouth, looking forward to *next* year. (Personal communication, 1993)

Depending on the age, functioning level, and abilities of the client, drama therapists use puppets, sandtrays, role play, masks, videotaping, and many other dramatic activities to help clients safely and meaningfully practice new communication, social, and expressive skills. Kansas State University students trained in Applied Behavior Analysis have discovered that drama therapy fits perfectly with ABA therapy, serving as an educational tool and a reinforcer.

Risk and/or side-effects

Drama is not for everyone, just as playing basketball is not for everyone. Not all people on the autism spectrum will want to participate in drama therapy, but more may than might at first be expected. See the documentary *Autism: The Musical,* if you have any doubts. If a child is open and willing to participate in drama therapy, there are no risks or negative side-effects.

THE FLOORTIME CENTER

By Jake Greenspan and Tim Bleecker

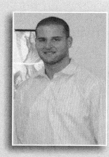

Jake Greenspan
jake@dirss.com

Tim Bleecker
tim@dirss.com

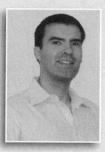

The Floortime Center™
4827 Rugby Avenue,
Bethesda, MD 20814
301-657-1130
info@dirss.com

Jake Greenspan and Tim Bleecker are the co-directors of The Floortime Center™ in Bethesda, Maryland. The Floortime Center is a child development center specializing in the use of the DIR®/Floortime™ model. With the help of Dr. Stanley Greenspan, they developed evaluation and intervention programs based on all aspects of the DIR model. Since the start of The Floortime Center in 2004, they have worked with over 900 families, and have presented 1 to 4 day workshops for various health and educational organizations.

Workshops include:
-Training the entire Special Ed. District of Maui, HI in DIR/Floortime
-Working on an ongoing basis with 5 Special Ed. Schools throughout the U.S..
-Training numerous special needs organizations in DIR/Floortime

Floortime is a developmental approach that focuses on strengthening the whole child through improving the ability to regulate their nervous system, to attend to their environment, to relate with a broad range of emotion, to communicate physically and verbally, and to think logically—the developmental ladder. Mastering these functional capacities in the developmental ladder enables children, and all of us, to learn, to socialize, and to think. This happens first at basic levels and eventually at higher levels of abstract reasoning. By using the principles of the Floortime approach, parents and other caregivers can help a child progress to higher and higher levels of social and emotional cognition.

It is the social interactions that start at birth that help wire the brain so that we learn from new experiences and move up the developmental ladder. Children with Autism have difficulty learning through social interactions and from their environment. Floortime harnesses children's motivation so that their thinking ability can build on the richness of human interaction and new experiences.

Floortime is based on three main principles:

- To follow the child's lead identify emotional interests;
- To challenge the child to move up the developmental ladder; and
- To expand on those challenges in a dynamic fashion so that the child is always creating and experiencing something new.

Following the child's lead allows us to join their world and establish a mutual trust. Once we have established that trust, we can gradually draw the child out of his world and into ours. By joining him and discovering what interests and motivates his, we can learn which of his interests will hold his attention sufficiently for his play partner to eventually challenge—to create a game around activity or toy that involves him in a relationship and provides new experiences. If the child invites you into his world and is happy to have you join in, it may not be necessary to become more challenging right away. However, if a child is more avoidant or self involved often joining the activity is insufficient for connecting with them. We need to challenge children to climb the developmental ladder voluntarily. This means that we create challenges, based on using their developmental capacities, which they are motivated to overcome.

Through following a child's lead we can also identify sensory activities that his body and nervous system need to function at a higher level. Whether he is on a swing, trampoline, or ball, we can gain an understanding of the types of stimulation that help regulate his nervous system. Without having a regulated nervous system, a child will have difficulty interacting and be willing to have new experiences. If we have rhythmic patterns in our activities where we start and stop and start and stop, always paying attention to the child's response to us, we will see that children will begin to attend and engage and even begin to interact—exactly what the child needs to reach higher levels. Because of the importance of a regulated nervous system in the early stages, Floortime will emphasize movement and physical activities during those interactions, and consequently, Floortime may seem different when helping a child work on the earlier developmental milestones than when working on the later ones.

Example 1—Johnny

Two-year old Johnny came into the office for the first time, upset and clinging to his mom. According to his parents, he had a problem with transitions: he didn't have the problem at home, only at new places. They also said that he had problems playing with toys appropriately and didn't look at or communicate with them.

Once we settled into a play room, Johnny began moving from object to object, looking at each one for a second before moving to the next. In this very fragmented and disorganized manner, he moved around the room, not engaging with any person. Once he had made many circuits around the room, he began a particular self-stimulatory behavior—finding small objects, looking at them very closely, and waving them in front of his eyes. In further talking with Mom and Dad, I learned that he liked to play games that involve tickling and moving through space, such as being tossed up the air. However, if left on his own, he tended to find small objects that move, and wave them in front of his face or spin them.

In order to follow his lead it was important to understand his sensory system to know which sensations he enjoyed and which to be cautions of. As I observed Johnny moving around the room and talked with his parents, I learned that he had under-reactive tactile, proprioceptive and vestibular systems. That is, he needed and would sometimes seek out certain touch, pressure and movement. He also exhibited a sensitive visual-spatial system: he had difficulty understanding the organization of new spaces and could get overloaded and distracted by lots of visual detail or changes to familiar details.

While we were talking, Johnny, true to form, had picked up a piece of ribbon and was waving it in front of his face. To join the play, Dad got down on the floor near Johnny (but not right in front of him) and picked up one of the ribbons that Johnny had discarded. Dad waved it in the air and said with excitement, "Wow, I'm waving this ribbon. Look at it move. This is great!" Dad's enthusiastic ribbon waving elicited a quick glance from Johnny, but nothing more. He immediately turned back to his own ribbon. Unfortunately following Johnny's lead with high affect was insufficient to establish shared attention. Johnny was too self-involved.

I instructed Dad to become a little more playfully obstructive with Johnny and gently involve himself in the ribbon that Johnny was waving. First, Dad used the same high affect and enthusiasm to describe his intended actions, saying, "Oh boy, look at your ribbon, I want to see that one! I want to get it." Again, his enthusiasm gained little response. Since it was important for Johnny to understand what Dad was going to do, I coached Dad to reach in very slowly and to have his fingers crawl up Johnny's leg like a spider. As Dad moved up Johnny's body toward the arm with the ribbon, Johnny glanced at Dad and moved the ribbon away. Dad, giving a positive affective response to Johnny's reaction, said, "Oh, you don't want me to get that ribbon!", and let his hand fly backward.

Dad continued this same pattern of explaining his actions, providing tactile sensation (tickling) with his fingers crawling toward the ribbon and always accepting and responding to Johnny's response. As Dad persisted, saying, "I want to see that ribbon. Here I come...", Johnny began to look at him, sometimes with a little smirk flitting across his face as Dad reached for the ribbon and Johnny moved it away. Dad had enticed Johnny to play a game. Dad continued to challenge Johnny by reaching for the ribbon, but he also expanded on the challenge by moving further away from Johnny. In this way, as he said, "I'm coming to get that ribbon!" Dad could start at one end of the room and move slowly to the other side, all while Johnny was watching and anticipating when to move the ribbon away as Dad came nearer.

Over the next month Johnny's parents did hours of these games each day in 20 minute increments at home. The toy that Johnny would be interested in would change and so did the challenges mom and Dad provided. They reported that Johnny actually let them start to play a tug of war with different toys and eventually let them take the toy as he chased them to get it back. The more they played these games and challenged a little more each time, the more Johnny enjoyed these games, especially because he always won. His attention, connection to his environment and engagement with his parents improved significantly, which allowed us to start challenging him to use more complex communication.

Example 2—David

David was four-years old when he and his parents came to see me. His parents were concerned about his aggressive behavior and limited language. They reported that it was difficult for David to interact with them for any period of time. He was always bouncing around the room and became easily upset if they tried to start an activity with him.

This pattern quickly repeated itself at the clinic. David wouldn't sit still and, when approached, ran away. Mom and Dad resorted to leading him by the arm to an activity. When Mom playfully pulled him to the toy castle and began playing, he became agitated and hit her. He just wanted to continue running around the room, which he did with a big smile on his face.

I asked David's parents to change the way they were trying to engage with David. Instead of introducing an activity that he wasn't interested in, they could join his activity, that is, his running around the room. At first, they simply chased him around the room, which David seemed to enjoy. After about five minutes, I coached them to playfully challenge him by becoming a human fence with their arms stretched out so when he was in the corner, he had to figure out how to 'escape.' He began his escape by scooting under their arms. Mom and Dad quickly regrouped and put their arms lower so that he had to climb over their arms. When Mom asked David, "What should I do with my arm now?" David excitingly responded with, "Move arm!" Enjoying the escape game, David then ran to another part of the room so they could capture him again. During this game David's parents noticed him giving them more smiles and eye contact and using more language. He did not have another aggressive outburst, such as his hitting Mom earlier, for the rest of the 45-minute session.

David's parents learned that his body needed certain inputs such as movement and deep pressure (that is, vestibular and proprioceptive inputs). David became more regulated, emotionally connected and interactive with his parents when they followed his lead and gave him the sensory inputs, such as movement, that his body needed. Over the next few months David's parents were able to turn these simple chase games into more complex games. They incorporated stuffed animals that both chased and were chased in simple imaginative play. Slowly, David's back and forth interactions became longer and included more language. He also had a significant decrease in negative behaviors because his parents were constantly giving him the sensory support he needed by joining his active world.

The key to David's success was his parents' learning the Floortime principles that helped them 1) join him in his preferred activities (ones that helped him regulate his sensory system), 2) playfully entice him to stay connected for longer periods of time, and 3) eventually challenge him to expand his play and interactions. Gradually David increased his language and progressed to higher levels of thinking.

Example 3—Sally

Sally was diagnosed with autism at the age of three. By age seven she was still self-absorbed, unable to expand her usage of language and ideas, and lacked interest in creating relationships. Her favorite activity was scripting: repeating memorized segments, such as lines from a favorite movie, in her case, Disney movies. Her concerned parents reported that Sally preferred to be self-absorbed in her fantasies rather than interact with them or her older sister.

At home Sally would go to the corner of the room with the same toys and repeatedly reenact a scene from a movie or favorite TV show. She ignored Mom and Dad when they tried to join her play. Although she had some meaningful language, she used rote language in most of her interactions. Additionally, she craved certain movements and would often spin herself in a circle. She also easily became overloaded by her sensory environment such as loud noises and many types of tactile inputs.

Typically, Mom and Dad had tried to get Sally's attention by using a loud, excited voice. They had not realized that increasing the volume would overwhelm her sensitive auditory system and create less interaction. Her parents also had attempted to stop her scripted activities by trying to involve her in a different activity that they thought she would enjoy. This strategy rarely worked and Sally always went back to her scripts.

Mom and Dad started using Floortime therapy in order to find a way to reach Sally and help her develop stronger relationships with her family. Their goal was to learn how to join her play by following her lead while not overwhelming her sensitive sensory system.

A Floortime therapist coached Sally's parents on the fundamentals of joining her scripted activities—basically to pretend to be the characters in her Disney dramas. Mom and Dad were surprised by this suggestion because they thought that this would reinforce her scripting behaviors. The therapist suggested that Dad get on the floor with Sally, follow her lead and join her script by becoming the prince in her movie. Sally did not seem to mind Dad joining in because he did not try to introduce a different activity. He was also coached to use a quieter voice and move at a slower pace.

Over the next few sessions Sally began to enjoy having her parents become the different characters in her dramas. She initiated play sessions by telling Mom, Dad and her older sister which characters she wanted them to be. Within a few weeks Mom and Dad began gradually challenging Sally to expand her play. For example, they had their character do something slightly different from the usual scripted storyline. Sally did not become avoidant or self-absorbed because her parents helped her expand her play at her own individual pace.

Mom and Dad learned to tailor their interactions to Sally's unique profile so they could join her world and help her climb the developmental ladder. They also became aware of her unique auditory and tactile sensitivities so they could keep her regulated, join her play and eventually challenge her to expand on her ideas and language. After a year of intensive Floortime therapy Sally looks forward to having other people join her play. She often develops new and creative ideas and rarely depends on her scripts. She is also starting to show some interest in playing with her peers at school. Sally still has areas that need work, but most importantly she now enjoys connecting with her parents and sister with warm smiles and is not self-absorbed in her own world.

More professionals are agreeing that a parent centered approach is ideal for children with autism. Floortime strengthens the most important relationships in a child's life, it gives the parent control over their child's development, and it integrates into everyday life. As a result Flootime helps children progress all the time, not just when in a therapy session. Floortime has the ability to improve the core deficits of autism of relating and communicating and can be applied to children of all ages and developmental abilities. Floortime never assumes that there is a limit to what children with autism can achieve, and instead continues to challenge each child to rise to their true developmental potential.

INTEGRATED PLAY GROUPS®
(IPG) MODEL

By Dr. Pamela Wolfberg

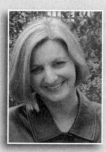

Pamela Wolfberg, PhD

Professor
Autism Spectrum Graduate Certificate and Related Studies-
Department of Special Education
San Francisco State University
1600 Holloway Avenue
San Francisco, CA 94132

Wolfberg@sfsu.edu
Office: 415-338-7651

Pamela Wolfberg, PhD, is Associate Professor and Director of the Autism Spectrum program at San Francisco State University and co-founder of the Autism Institute on Peer Relations and Play. She received her doctorate from the University of California, Berkeley. As originator of the Integrated Play Groups (IPG) model, she leads research, training and development efforts to establish inclusive peer socialization programs worldwide. She is widely published and the author of *Play and Imagination in Children with Autism* and *Peer Play and the Autism Spectrum: The Art of Guiding Children's Socialization and Imagination*. She is the recipient of several distinguished awards for her scholarship, research, and service to the community.

Integrated Play Groups® (IPG) is an empirically validated model for addressing core challenges in socialization, communication and imagination in children and adolescents on the autism spectrum while building relationships with typical peers and siblings in natural settings (Wolfberg, 2009, 2003; Wolfberg, Bottema-Beutel, & DeWitt, 2012).

IPG aims to maximize the developmental potential and intrinsic motivation of individuals on the autism spectrum to engage with typical peers in mutually engaging play, recreation and cultural experiences (i.e., sensory, constructive and imaginary play, drama, visual arts, filmmaking, physical movement and other culturally valued activities that are of high interest for diverse ages).

The IPG model is grounded in current theory, research and practice pertinent to addressing core challenges in autism that impact on social and representational facets of play development. Embedded in this model are methods for observing, interpreting, and building on children's play interests and social communicative abilities, and for designing environments conducive to social and imaginative play.

Conceptually, the IPG model is described as multi-dimensional, encompassing developmental and ecological features that are framed in sociocultural theory (Vygotsky, 1966; 1978). In practical terms, an IPG brings together children or teens with autism (novice players) in mutually engaging play, recreation, and cultural experiences with more capable peer play partners (expert players) while guided by a qualified adult facilitator (play guide). Each IPG is individualized as a part of a comprehensive educational and therapy program. IPG programs take place in natural settings, including in the home, school, and community. Group members range from 3 to 5 players with a higher ratio of expert to novice players. Each group meets twice weekly for 30–60 minutes sessions over a 12-week period or longer. Play sessions are tailored to the unique interests, developmental capacities and sociocultural experiences of participants.

Drawing on finely tuned assessments, the IPG intervention (guided participation) provides a system of support for maximizing each individual's developmental potential and intrinsic motivation to play and imagine, socialize and form meaningful relationships with other children. Equal emphasis is placed on guiding the typical peers to be more accepting, responsive and inclusive of people who may present differing ways of playing, imagining, communicating, and relating to others. Moreover, novice and expert players are encouraged to mediate their own interactive experiences with as little adult guidance as possible.

Primary Developers

Pamela Wolfberg, PhD, (Professor of Autism Spectrum Graduate Certificate and Related Studies at San Francisco State University and founding director of the Autism Institute on Peer Socialization and Play) is the originator of the IPG model. In its early conception, Dr. Wolfberg worked in close collaboration with the late Adriana Schuler, PhD, (Professor Emeritus, SFSU) and Therese O'Connor, MA. Over the years, the model has continued to evolve and expand owing to the collective efforts of many other remarkable professionals, family members and the children themselves participating in local, national and international training, research and development initiatives.

History of Development

The IPG model was first initiated as a pilot research project in an urban elementary school with a small grant from the San Francisco Education Fund (Wolfberg, 1988). Based on the preliminary success of this project, the IPG model was expanded through a model demonstration and research project that was supported, in part, through a grant from the United States Department of Education (Wolfberg & Schuler, 1992). In

2000, the *Autism Institute on Peer Socialization and Play* was established with the mission to "advance the rights of individuals on the autism spectrum to derive the joy and benefits of social inclusion in play, recreation, and cultural experiences" through training, research and global outreach efforts.

Introductory and advanced level training in the IPG model is provided via the *Autism Institute on Peer Socialization and Play*. Introductory Seminars are open to practitioners and family members to obtain a foundation in the IPG model's principles and practices. The IPG Apprenticeship offers advanced training and supervision to professionals to become qualified IPG Providers whereby they are endorsed to deliver the IPG model as a program or service. Advanced training comprises a competency-based curriculum that draws on the foundational book: *Play and Imagination in Children with Autism* (Wolfberg, 2009) and the IPG Field Manual *Peer Play and the Autism Spectrum: The Art of Guiding Socialization and Imagination (Wolfberg, 2003)*.

A growing number of schools, clinics, community, government and non-government organizations have adopted the IPG model at the local, national and international level. The expansion of programs around the globe coincides with the IPG model having gained widespread recognition as among established evidence-based practices for children on the autism spectrum (American Speech-Language-Hearing Association 2006; Disalvo and Oswald 2002; Iovannone 2003; National Autism Center 2009). This is consistent with the recommendations of the National Research Council (2001), which has ranked the teaching of play skills with peers among the six types of interventions that should have priority in the design and delivery of effective educational programs for children on the autism spectrum.

Success Rate

The IPG model has an established and growing research base documenting ample evidence of a high success rate. A series of small and large-scale studies have been and are currently being conducted to evaluate and replicate the IPG model (Bottema-Beutel, 2010; Bottema-Beutel, in review, Bottema-Beutel & Smith, in review; Fuge & Berry, 2004; Gonsier-Gerdin, 1993; Lantz, Nelson & Loftin, 2004; Mikaelan, 2003; Julius, Wolfberg, Jahnke & Neufeld, 2012; O'Connor, 1999; Richard & Goupil, 2005; Wolfberg, 1988; 1994; 2009; Wolfberg & Schuler, 1992; 1993; Wolfberg, Turiel, DeWitt, Bottema-Beutel, Young & Nguyen, 2012; Yang, Wolfberg, Wu & Hwu , 2003; Zercher, Hunt, Schuler & Webster, 2001). Most investigations have been focusing on the effect of the intervention on the social, communication and play development of children with autism representing diverse abilities (ASD Level 1, 2 and 3), ages (3 to 11 years), settings (community, home, school), geographic locations (Asia, Europe, North America) and languages (English, French, German, Chinese). Social validation measures assessing parent perceptions of the impact of the intervention on their children with autism have also been included.

Overall, outcomes for the children with autism consistently show relative gains in social, communication, and play development. Specifically, decreases in isolate and stereotypic play have been noted along with collateral gains in increasingly socially coordinated play and representational play (functional and pretend). Language gains also have been noted in several cases. Further, the evidence suggests that skills may be maintained after adult support is withdrawn. The data also supports evidence of generalization beyond the specific IPG across peers/siblings, settings, and social activity contexts.

The attitudes, perceptions and experiences of the expert players have been explored through observation and interviews with play guides and the children themselves. Findings to date suggest that the peers developed greater sensitivity, tolerance and acceptance of the novice players' individual differences. They also articulated a sense of responsibility as well as an understanding of how to include the less skilled players by adapting to their different interests and styles of communication. Novice and expert players also reported having fun while forming mutual friendships extending beyond the IPG.

Risk and/or side-effects

There are no known risks or side-effects associated with the IPG model when implemented with fidelity.

INTEGRATIVE EDUCATIONAL CARE

By Dr. Mary Joann Lang

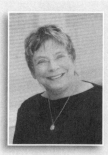

Mary Joann Lang, PhD

Beacon Day School
24 Centerpointe Drive
La Palma, CA 90623
714-288-4200
Fax: 714-288-4204
www.beacondayschool.com

Dr. Mary Joann Lang founded Beacon Day School in June 2004 for students with autism spectrum disorder (ASD) and related disabilities. Dr. Lang also founded Beacon Autistic Spectrum Independence Center, an in-home therapy-based program for children with ASD. Throughout her career, Dr. Lang has worked with children diagnosed with ASD and has lectured widely on the topic. She has been involved with the care of children for more than 25 years, first as a nurse practitioner and educator, then as an educational psychologist. Dr. Lang has many professional publications.

In 1988, Dr. Lang graduated from the University of Southern California with her PhD in educational psychology. A Diplomate of the American Board of Neuropsychology, Dr. Lang has been a practicing, licensed neuropsychologist since 1991. A member of several professional organizations, including the National Academy of Neuropsychology, Dr. Lang is also an associate professor at Azusa Pacific University.

Using an innovative model that will enhance learning is critical to academic, social-emotional, and motor development. An integrated approach to learning will provide students with more learning opportunities and thus be able to generalize their knowledge, social skills, and motor ability. Understanding this approach is critical to educational planning. The goal of education in a student's life needs to focus on the whole child versus simply the results of standardized testing, which may skew the teacher's perspective of the student's ability.

In order to understand the whole child, the following areas need to be considered in planning for a child's education: cognition, educational achievement, adaptive behavior, social roles, health, and context. Since schools primarily look at cognitive functioning and academic achievement in terms of placement, teaching strategy, and therapies, these cognitive functions need to be understood in greater depth.

Definition and Need

Traditional models of education are not effective for children with an autism diagnosis as they have challenges in communication, adaptive behavior, social skills, and self-regulation. Behavior issues arise because of these deficits. Integrated educational care has been gaining new ground in recent years. An integrated educational model is necessary for children with autism in order for them to reach their highest potential. A model like this looks at both strengths the child possesses and challenges they face. Understanding these will help to identify areas in need of support, informing the educator as to how to enhance the child's learning environment.

An integrated educational model focuses on many different subjects and goes beyond the traditional classroom that uses textbooks to teach children concepts and ways of doing things. For example, Beacon Day School uses this approach in teaching students with autism and related disabilities. At Beacon Day School, integration is used on two different levels: 1) integrating necessary therapies such as speech and language, physical, and occupational therapy into the student's day; and 2) integrating academic skills in order to enhance generalization.

This integrated educational model incorporates flexible schedules and student groups in order to cater to individual learning and what the individual child needs most. Rather than looking at just the student, an integrated curriculum focuses on all the facets that connect and influence the world of the student. In an integrated educational model, the focus is on cognition (attention, memory, language, visual/spatial functioning, reasoning, and coping strategies), educational achievement, adaptive behavior, social skills, and health, with all of these examined within the context of the child's home, school, and community. With all of this in mind, the focus can be on the whole child and the surrounding spheres of influence.

The concept of integrated curriculum has been around for quite some time, but has only recently been applied within the educational setting. According to Humphreys, Post, and Ellis (1981), integrated educational care is "one in which children broadly explore knowledge in various subjects related to certain aspects of their environment" (p.11). In this sense, learning and teaching are seen in a holistic view that is interactive. Within an integrated educational care framework, there are many levels of integration. It can include implementing objectives that overlap with goals listed on the child's Individualized Education Program (IEP), implementing model lesson plans that involve activities across assessments, enriching or enhancing students' abilities through specific activities that focus on communication skills and ways of relating to others through community based instruction, and implementing assessment activities that examine a wide range of functional capacities (Palmer, 1991). An integrated model with this basis will provide students with unified knowledge, while still encouraging them to learn new things. With an integrated educational model centered on these principles, the student will be prepared for lifelong learning.

Educational Planning

As was mentioned previously, in order to understand the whole child, the following areas need to be considered in planning for a child's education: cognition, educational achievement, adaptive behavior, social roles, health, and context. It is important to understand how these areas function, what behaviors and symptoms arise due to challenges in these areas, and what interventions and accommodations can be utilized to help the child grow in these areas.

Cognition

Cognition involves many different areas of functioning that include: attention and information processing, sensory-motor function, language, executive function, memory and learning, social skills, and emotional function. Parents and teachers need to be aware of the individual child's limitations in these areas and emphasize their strengths that will help them overcome these limitations.

ATTENTION AND INFORMATION PROCESSING

In order to function in everyday life and complete schoolwork successfully, a child needs to have good attention and information processing abilities. Attention involves selective attention (choosing what to listen to), shifting attention (moving from one stimuli to another), divided attention (splitting attention between two things), and sustained attention (staying focused on one thing for a long period of time). If a child has poor attention and information processing, they may have difficulty initiating focus, sustaining focus, and maintaining a train of thought. Difficulties in processing information may involve the need for repetition of instructions and an extended time to complete assignments and tasks.

Therapies and accommodations that are focused on these two areas of functioning should start with structuring the learning environment and eliminating distractions. This involves a set routine/schedule so that the child knows what is expected each day. Different sheets can be developed, such as note sheets and flow charts, in order to help the child visualize and take in information as well as keep information manageable and in limited quantities to avoid information overload.

SENSORY-MOTOR FUNCTION

This area of functioning includes a child's gross- and fine-motor skills. Gross-motor skills involve large muscles working to accomplish a task and include balance, body posture, and coordination. Fine-motor skills involve more specific ways of functioning, such as holding a pencil and writing letters. While some children with autism may be particularly strong in this area, many have great difficulty with these aspects of functioning due to underdeveloped muscles. Examples of difficulties in this area include sensitivity or lack of sensitivity to touch and textures, poor pencil grip, poor hand-eye coordination, impaired speech, and poor balance.

Physical activities should be encouraged for children with autism in a structured setting. Occupational and physical therapists can aid in helping children with autism to develop gross-and fine-motor skills. Additionally, sensory integration therapy can help by implementing a sensory diet, focusing on sensory-based activities, and applying pressure to joint areas in order to provide a calming and soothing environment.

LANGUAGE

Language involves many different ways of communicating, including speech, listening, reading, writing, and interpreting information. Different ways of processing language include auditory processing (understanding speech sounds), oral expression (linguistic competencies and oral vocabulary), and receptive language (listening to and interpreting information). Challenges in any one of these areas associated with language can result in not listening, difficulty with word problems, limited vocabulary, and difficulty with interpreting information.

Visual cues can be incorporated in order for lessons and instructions to be well received by the child. Careful attention should be paid to words and meanings in order to increase vocabulary. Study sheets, outlines, and note pads can be incorporated to aid in attention and learning of new words and meanings. Time extensions may be necessary for tests and assignments in order to make sure the child is optimally learning the material. Necessary information should be reinforced and repeated to stress importance.

EXECUTIVE FUNCTION

Executive function is considered to be the "conductor" of many different cognitive processes. It involves planning, organizing, flexibility, abstract thinking, rule acquisition, and self-regulation. Children with autism have a difficult time organizing, multitasking, and prioritizing information. They have difficulty planning for due dates of homework assignments and dates of upcoming tests.

Teachers, parents, and mental health professionals should provide children with autism structure in their daily activities. They can be taught responsibility for personal items through reminders and modeling done by the adult. Organizational tools can be provided that will help the child gain more order and control in their assignments and general life.

MEMORY AND LEARNING

Memory is comprised of four different groups: short-term memory (recall up to a minute without rehearsing material), long-term memory (information remembered for a long time), working memory (separation of different information such as visual and verbal), and comprehensive knowledge (information that is rehearsed and able to be recalled). These aspects of memory make it possible for the individual to receive, recall, store, and hold information. Challenges in this area take the form of inattention, inability to recall information, frustration, and difficulty following long, detailed directions.

Interventions may involve repetition of information to increase storage of information. The teacher should break up information into small parts and provide cues to assist in recall of information. Lists and charts can help students to remember information. The learning environment should be relaxed in order to alleviate pressure.

SOCIAL SKILLS

Positive ways of relating to others aid in developing friendships and avoiding being mistreated by others. Social skills involve communication, tone of voice, sense-of-humor, and the ability to take on another person's perspective. Nonverbal social skills are also important and involve active listening, relaxed manner, and confidence. Individuals with autism tend to lack social skills, including difficulty recognizing social cues and being unaware of boundaries.

Different recreational activities like clubs and sports teams can help facilitate communication and development of friendships. The environment should be enjoyable and non-threatening to boost communication skills.

EMOTIONAL FUNCTION

Being able to regulate one's emotional state helps to prevent an over–or under-reaction in a situation. Instances that may bring about an emotional reaction are requests to complete assignments, reacting to separations, and relational conflicts. Challenges in this area may include: blaming others for problems, tantrums, pulling away from others, clinging to others, frustration, and restlessness.

Discussing thoughts, feelings, and behaviors could help in regulating emotion. Role-playing different situations can help prepare an individual for an emotionally-charged situation. Teaching children to discuss their feelings helps them feel understood. The student should be able to retreat to a calm area that avoids overstimulation.

Educational Achievement

Individuals achieve at different rates. Individual education plans can help identify areas in which a child needs to grow as well as areas of strength. Outlining specific areas of need will help the team to collaborate on what interventions to use for the student. Teaching strategies and interventions are tailored to the individual child's strengths that can help them overcome areas of weakness.

Adaptive Behavior

Adaptive skills are necessary for helping a child thrive within their home, school, and community. Having the skills to adjust one's behavior in a particular environment or situation will help to prevent disruptive behavior. This can be achieved through community-based activities, vocational activities, and implementation of coping skills.

Participation, Interactions, and Social Roles

Understanding one's role in society and ways of acting appropriately are synonymous with social skill development. Specialized guidance can help children learn how to interact appropriately with others. Team building activities can help children understand ways of relating to others and recognize the perspectives of others.

Health

Individuals with autism have a variety of health issues that include allergies and seizure disorders. These issues can hinder educational progress. Teachers should be aware of medical conditions the child is suffering from and stay current on their medical treatment plans through collaboration with the family and primary care physician. Dietary interventions and implementation of medicines may be used to help with health issues.

Context

Intervention should be implemented in the home, school, and community environments. Continuity of care is important in enhancing overall development. This can be a time of learning and collaboration among parents, school staff, and health professionals.

Even with the best intentions and interventions, disruptive behaviors may occur in the classroom. The best intervention strategy for managing behaviors is applied behavior analysis (ABA). Behaviors may occur that might inhibit the use of an integrated model in the classroom. Therefore, some effective classroom environmental strategies need to be considered. There are several examples that include:

- Establishing rules and expectations for appropriate classroom behavior.
- Developing rules and procedures that are practiced by students with the help of teachers.
- Making students aware of the rewards for following the rules as well as the consequences if they do not.
- Create a warm and inviting learning environment.
- Implement a daily educational schedule that provides structure to the classroom.
- Design and model positive alternatives to challenging behaviors.
- Monitor behavior and, if problems arise, alter interventions to meet the needs of the student.

Beacon Model for Integration

Consideration of challenges in functioning aids in the establishment of a supportive environment that enhances self-esteem, recognizes individual strengths, and identifies areas in need of support. Parents, teachers, children, and professionals should work as a team in order to try to achieve established goals. Growth and learning occur at all times of the day and positive reinforcements should remain consistent throughout the day, both at school and at home. Conferences, IEP meetings, home visits, and informal meetings should all be utilized to enhance communication and collaboration between team members.

Regular reports about behavior and performance in school should be provided to parents. It would also be helpful for parents to share information about the child's behavior outside of school. Progression in all areas of development is dependent upon structure and consistency in the home, school, and community.

The child is understood in context. This means that each area of development: communication, social skills, motor skills, academic accomplishment, and others will be related to the cognitive functions discussed above (memory, emotions, attention, language, visual-spatial skills, executive function, and health) to ensure that all is functioning in a way that promotes development. A main focus is on identifying areas in need of growth and support that affect the overall performance of the child. Attention to detail is important, especially when looking at specific areas of cognition.

Autism influences cognitive, emotional, physiological, and social development. Each area needs to be addressed when looking at the whole child. Therapies and interventions are selected for the individual child so that they can function at their best within the home, school, and community. An integrative model that focuses on the whole child in context goes beyond what the IEP addresses and looks at all of the contributors to the diagnosis of autism. Identifying these will help the team to develop positive ways of influencing the child's overall condition. As one area of functioning improves, other areas will follow in the path towards positive developmental growth.

Why Integrate?

An integrative educational model provides an opportunity for collaboration among students, teachers, and parents. It engages students in the learning process and is an exciting change to the traditional educational model. Approaching the whole child promotes continuity in functioning across a wide range of contexts. The integrative educational model is designed to be enjoyable and motivating, not only for the student but for their surrounding support system as well. Gaining support from the community and utilizing resources within the community encourages development of a partnership and erases stigmas. The goal is to promote optimal functioning of the individual student in many developmental areas in order for the student to thrive within the home, school, and community.

INTEGRATING ABA WITH DEVELOPMENTAL MODELS: MERIT

By Jennifer Clark

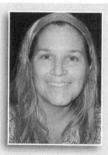

Jenifer Clark, MA, PhD (c)

New York, NY
212-222-9818
clarkjenif@aol.com
JeniferClark.com

Jenifer Clark has been working with children and families for over fifteen years. She received her master's in psychology from NYU and is completing her PhD in clinical psychology at CUNY. She has worked as an ABA therapist and consultant since 1992. She specializes in working with children with autism and has taught atypical development at Hunter College. Currently, she is the director of Boost!, an afterschool program for children with autism. This program focuses on teaching socialization and leisure skills to children on the spectrum, incorporating typical children as peers and social models. Ms. Clark is the co-founder and therapist for Sibfun, a support group for siblings of children with special-needs. She consults at special needs and typical schools and continues to consult with children and families.

There is a tremendous need for a treatment model which attends to autism in its entirety: one which successfully integrates the incredibly effective remediation, repetition, and hierarchical teaching common to ABA with a developmental model that focuses on the equally important emotional development of the child. As ABA satisfies the need to remediate the core deficits of autism, mentalization emphasizes the need for a mutual acknowledgement of inner states. Mentalization describes the process in which we attend to the thoughts and feelings of another (Fonagy et al, 2002). Mentalization based therapies provide a way of conceptualizing our interactions with children with autism in a manner that consistently takes into account, and reflects back to them, their inner world.

Despite the wide base of empirical data that supports ABA in the treatment of autism, there are critics who express concerns over the impact that this treatment has on the emotional life of the child. Many argue that it is antithetical to design an intervention that would give a child with autism repeated experiences of having their distress ignored. Some are concerned about the impact these experiences have on a developing sense of self and the child's capacity to attach and increase relatedness. Parents can be put off by the data driven nature of the ABA methodology. Many families have shared with me their stories of seeking to embrace a more developmental model but feeling as if they are failing to offer their child much needed remediation during a critical period.

It is clearly the case that children with autism struggle with the concept that it is worthwhile to communicate their needs to another person. This being the case there are significant detrimental effects that can evolve from repeatedly ignoring distress. If a child with autism is deprived of the experience of having their feeling states acknowledged — which is a precursor to acknowledging feeling states in others — how will they develop this capacity?

In response to these growing concerns, pediatric neurologists and developmental specialists are increasingly encouraging parents to use a blended intervention to treat their child's autism. They are recommending that parents set up a program for their child that incorporates ABA and other more developmentally based approaches. Many parents are at a loss for how to accomplish this integration however. Therapists tend to be deeply committed to either one philosophy or the other and there is considerable resistance to working cooperatively. Additionally, the dominant methodologies developed from two very different philosophies. They frequently contradict one another in terms of how the intervention should proceed and how to interpret the behavior of the child.

MERIT — Mentalization Enhanced Remediation — an Integrated Treatment is a hybrid treatment approach. The MERIT model accomplishes emphasizes the structured and hierarchical teaching that is a crucial component of remediation while incorporating a mentalizing approach in all interactions with the child.

The three most important aspects of this model are providing mentalizing experiences to forge a relationship with the child and establishing the initial phase of therapy, allowing mentalization to inform the treatment on a regular basis, and remediating the cognitive as well as the social-emotional areas that prevent the child from progressing in this area of development.

Initial Phase of Treatment

In the initial phases of treatment the therapist engages in mentalization in order to understand and forge a relationship with the child. As the therapist comes to understand how this child thinks, learns, and even how they cope with anxiety, all of this information will be influence how the therapist interacts with the child. This intimate relationship, which involves learning a child's likes and dislikes, as well as challenges and strengths, is, in fact, critical in using mentalization to treat autism.

It can be challenging to make sense of the inner life of a child with autism and therefore mentalization plays a pivotal role in the treatment. We cannot relate first-hand to a child who experiences sounds as painful and sensory issues as completely preoccupying. And yet, this process of being understood is an undeniably crucial aspect of development. A therapist must pose the question: How is this particular brain processing information? A therapist's job is to put him or herself in a child's place and to try to understand what it is the child is experiencing. A therapist must be able to determine the most constructive experiences to help a child with autism learn and be able to relate. This understanding will be a powerful guide to the therapy as well as a tremendous source of reinforcement and motivation for the child.

In this phase of treatment, reinforcement will be based on preferred activities, foods or toys. Initially the schedule of reinforcement will be more frequent so the child with autism comes to understand the expectation and the system. Most children with autism can quickly move to a token system. This is a system in which the child earns tokens for emitting correct responses. Once the child has earned a predetermined number tokens, they receive the agreed upon reward. These reinforcement systems are motivating to children with autism for two reasons. They continue to be reinforced with preferred items when a predetermined number of tokens have been received and they can see how many responses are expected. When working on a difficult task, such as verbal imitation for the autistic child with apraxia, the token board provides a clear visual for when they will have completed the task. It is hard work for these children. You can see it in their faces. They are summoning all that they can remember about how to properly pronounce a word and they are looking carefully at my mouth in order to imitate my movements. Occasionally their eyes dart to the token board or a check off sheet I sometimes use. "How many more?" they would ask if they could verbalize this question. The visual of the tokens provides an answer. It is not too dissimilar from a person in occupational therapy struggling to regain motor skills. Each step might take all they have in terms of effort and the physical therapist would be very clear about her expectation. Children with autism also need clear information about the expectation and in actuality these very behavioral techniques are providing the child with autism with an invaluable communication that reflects an understanding about the child. This system acknowledges how difficult it would be to work without an end in sight and most importantly it is a communication they can comprehend. As the child with autism progresses, modification can be made in terms of tokens and the types of reinforcement used. I will always move away from food and videos as quickly as possible as other preferred activities are more social and valuable in terms of expanding leisure skills.

The Remediation

Children with autism are often unable to profit from traditional educational approaches and may not learn readily. They require interventions specifically designed to take into account their unique capacity to learn. Although this observation pertains most notably to the acquisition of language and cognitive skills, it should also be a critical component of any therapy designed to improve an impaired child's ability to socialize, relate and connect to others. The heterogeneous nature of autism means that although all children with autism can be helped by remediation, it is dire that individual differences be taken into consideration. Failure to do so can result in disengagement both from the work and more importantly, from the therapist.

Traditional ABA programs that target areas such as verbal imitation, visual imitation, fine motor tasks and expressive and receptive language skills are incorporated into the treatment. The way in which concepts are introduced and the interactions before, during and after each discrete trial are profoundly influenced by the therapist-child relationship. This relationship is distinct from the relationship in some developmental programs in that the MERIT therapist will be directive. The MERIT therapist has an agenda and that is to remediate the areas of core deficit exhibited by that particular child. The heterogeneous nature of autism means that although all children with autism can be helped by remediation, it is dire that individual differences be taken into consideration. Failure to do so can result in disengagement both from the work and more importantly, from the therapist.

While engaged in their work, it is important that the child, despite their potentially limited capacity to understand language and gestures, feels understood. The therapist can increase communication through the use of language, gestures and visuals. Additionally, the work itself should evolve in such a way that it reflects an understanding of the child. Even if the child has a limited ability, initially, to process the world around them, presumably they can take in the experience of being less frustrated than they had been in their previous interactions with others. They can begin to trust that they can be successful. The nature of the relationship can be one of trust that nothing will be asked of this child that they cannot do (with some help). Ideally these interventions begin to remediate some of the areas of deficit which make it difficult to benefit from interactions with another or to process communication. The work builds upon itself. With each passing week the child develops more skills which allow him to better engage in social exchanges but in the meantime the relationship, which is critical to the work, is continually growing.

At a certain point, when the child has developed some of the core skills necessary to learn, they can begin to work on the specific skills that are so closely linked to the capacity to mentalize. There is not a clear temporal distinction between learning basic skills such as language, visual attention, imitation, attending and emotional processing and improving some of the capacities that have been linked to theory of mind and mentalization. In fact there is considerable overlap between these teachings.

My model is increasing the capacity for symbolic representation and integration, and thereby allowing the child with autism to become more organized. It is not, in my view, a case of either ABA or developmental interventions but rather ABA moving towards and allowing for the success of more developmentally based approaches. Cognitive remediation for the difficulties with abstraction, generalization, and symbolization in autism allows for the development of cognitive structures in the context of a highly dynamic exchange. This is the basis for the development of symbolization and language.

The repetition seen in discrete trial learning is not merely the repetition of cognitive exercises, but is additionally the repetition and re-internalization of experiences with a responsive other. Along a developmental trajectory, a child with autism must build a basic capacity to achieve early concept formation such as same and different, categories and relationships. These are precursors to the development of language and the development of these skills is very organizing to the child with ASD. In the case of autism it is not that these achievements cannot occur; they just fail to happen without appropriate intervention.

Treatment Evolves

By teaching and encouraging skills that enhance joint attention, I can reinforce the child while simultaneously strengthening our connection and their relational skills. It is through strategic implementation of a hierarchy of reinforcement that the work evolves beyond the classic ABA stance of evaluating reinforcers, and using token boards. I can instead engage in preferred activities or play with the child in between and then say "it's time to do some work." It is at this phase of the treatment that the teaching begins to mirror more typical teaching of a young child. Parents might engage with their child and occasionally pause to teach them something. One of the primary differences however, is that most children with autism need to be taught in a very specific way. Depending on the child's needs I create a list of goals. Each of these goals is translated into a program and each program has multiple steps. I incorporate traditional ABA programs that target areas such as verbal imitation, visual imitation, fine motor tasks and receptive language skills. I design programs using structure, hierarchical teaching, visual support, and contrived reinforcement in the initial phases of therapy. Each of these behavioral concepts is valuable both for the remediation that it enables a therapist to provide as well as the message that this methodology can communicate to the child if done from a mentalizing stance.

The Value of Structure

The structure of applied behavioral analysis serves to organize many children on the autistic spectrum. They are taught language and leisure skills and through this learning they are able to relinquish some of their maladaptive behaviors. Many children with autism engage in what have historically been referred to as "self-stimulating behaviors." These behaviors may have been misnamed as it appears that children with autism actually use these behaviors to reduce anxiety and to calm an overstimulated nervous system (Rapin, 2001). Remediation allows children with autism an opportunity to engage in an activity (structured learning) that is incompatible with many of their "self-stimulating behaviors." The child that has learned to draw pictures cannot flap as they draw. The child that has learned to have a conversation is less likely to moan and shriek as they do so. The value of teaching children with autism goes beyond replacing problematic behaviors, or even beyond the value of the skill learned (as precious as that might be). These children's brains are becoming more organized. Their self esteem is increasing as they begin to realize that they are capable, that they can learn and maybe most importantly that there is someone teaching them that believes that and is helping them to achieve these goals. The following vignette illustrates the impact these integrated interventions can have.

Josh: The Relationship

Josh was fifteen when I met him and had a forty-hour ABA program through his preschool years. I was called in to consult because of Josh's increasing "non-compliance." Josh was refusing to follow his schedule at school and refusing to follow the rules at home. If changes couldn't be made, his school had threatened to expel him.

Josh was skeptical to begin working with a new therapist. Being an adolescent, he was struggling with issues of autonomy and resented the high level of directedness that he assumed the therapy would have. I met Josh at school and observed him with the other teenagers. He was attending a program in which he was integrated with other high school students who did not all have autism. Some of the teens had learning disabilities or physical handicaps. While there were many advantages to being in an integrated setting, one aspect that Josh found quite difficult was observing some of his peers enjoy more freedom and independence than he was allowed. His less disabled counterparts were given appropriate freedoms at school and Josh resented this distinction. Additionally, Josh had an older sibling who had also been allowed more age-appropriate independence in adolescence.

Josh and I connected very quickly and he soon came up with a nickname for me. Initially he called me "Mickey" and he wanted me to call him "Pluto." He wanted to talk to me in a Mickey voice during this phase. When I shared this with his mother, she was very touched and said that he used to call his first baby-sitter "Mickey." She had cared for him for the first ten years of his life and he was very close with her. She was surprised that he had remembered that pet name and felt that it was indicative of his attachment to me.

As our relationship evolved, I came to see it was important for Josh to engage in activities that he enjoyed and that allowed him to experience more age-appropriate independence. We began riding bikes in Central Park. We would plan ahead and Josh would bring some of his own money. He would go to a stand and buy water or a snack for himself while I waited close by. During these activities the most critical factor was how I spoke to and interacted with Josh. There are very behavioral ways of increasing independence (with visual schedules and specific reinforcement). In Josh's case I could see that this level of facilitation was unnecessary and that Josh would be put off and even insulted by a more classic ABA approach. It was the normalizing of these activities that Josh needed and appreciated the most. By meeting him at home, I was able to model these interactions for his parents and speak with them about his need for increased autonomy.

Josh was asked to guess what might happen next in the novel he was reading with his English class. He refused to answer the question and was distraught when he was sent home with the assignment. I was able to talk with him about the question and what made it so difficult. "I don't know what is going to happen!" he responded furiously and incredulous that he was being asked such a ridiculous question. Acknowledging that this was a symptom of his disorder and not merely "non-compliance," I was able to implement an approach that simplified the task. I came up with three ideas of what might happen next and asked him to decide which one he thought was most likely to happen next. He was able to do this and proceed with the rest of his assignment.

Afterwards I was able to talk with Josh about how it made him feel to not know; to have to make a guess when there is no rule or to have to accommodate when an old rule doesn't seem to be working. Josh was able to convey that he feels nervous and sometimes angry. We then talked about ways that might help. We talked about what it means to guess. We think of a few answers that could be right and pick the one that seems best. He could tolerate this process and appreciated the step-by-step description. I think this example reflects the part that remediation can play in preparing an individual with autism to engage in and benefit from psychodynamic interventions. By offering another system or rule which appeals to the autistic mind I can help diffuse anxiety and disregulation and in some ways I am teaching a coping mechanisms or a more appropriate defense.

Josh continued to benefit from our relationship and the unique design of the intervention. I was able to engage in mentalization with Josh with regard to his life experience and his autism. His autism limited his ability to communicate and when this was exacerbated by heightened affect, it was crippling. I began to put some of Josh's life experiences into words. He would listen intently and look relieved to be "understood." Using a more structured approach, we talked about how much Josh liked rules and had a hard time accepting exceptions. We discussed the idea that exceptions could be their own rules.

Josh soon stopped talking to me in a Mickey voice. He abruptly stopped calling me Mickey and began calling me "Partner." This change represented a shift in Josh's conceptualization of our relationship. I had gone from caretaker, to a partner in helping him make sense of his experiences.

Additionally, I initiated changes at home and at school to increase Josh's independence without jeopardizing his safety. I was able to help Josh review and interpret which of his social behaviors were appropriate and which needed to be reflected on. He did not shut me out as he did to others because of how I presented the constructive criticism. I might begin by identifying with Josh's experience. "That guy was acting so crabby, huh?" Josh would relate immediately to that piece because he had perceived that as well. I could then speculate about why someone might have responded to him a certain way and then explore other options or different approaches he might try next time. These explorations seemed to help to reduce Josh's rigidity. I can't emphasize enough the importance of the delivery and the relationship in facilitating these interactions. Josh came to trust that I was attached to him as well and that I had his increased independence as a goal too. I truly was his "partner" in accomplishing his goals.

Josh looked forward to the time we spent together. One summer day, Josh called me up and said, "Partner—where are you? My bike is waiting for your bike!" It was safer and more comfortable for Josh to displace our relationship onto our bikes. He could talk more freely about his bike missing me and wishing to spend time with me. Although, there was still the goal of helping Josh to be able to express his own feelings without displacing them onto inanimate objects, he had come such a long way. I could suggest to Josh, "It sounds like you are looking forward to our ride together," and Josh (although awkwardly at first) was able to accept these interpretations and become more emotionally expressive over time.

This vignette emphasizes the need for an integrated approach. Mentalization and relational interventions were used in collaboration with remediation and structure. The result was an impressive improvement in behavior, relational capacities and cognitive growth. The integrated approach that MERIT offers was ideal in helping this boy. His adolescent struggles were complicated by his developmental disability. MERIT allowed him to increase his independence, improve his flexibility, and make significant strides in his ability to relate and connect with others.

RELATIONSHIP DEVELOPMENT INTERVENTION

By Laura Hynes

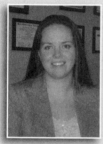

Laura Hynes, LMSW, RDI Program Certified Consultant

Extraordinary Minds, Inc.
4 University Place
Staten Island, New York 10301
(347)564-8451
LauraHynes@extraordinaryminds.org
www.extraordinaryminds.org
www.RDIconnect.com

Laura Hynes graduated from Stony Brook University with a bachelor of arts in psychology and a minor in child and family studies in 2001. She obtained a masters in social work in 2005 from New York University and is a licensed social worker in the state of New York. In 2008, Laura became certified in Relationship Development Intervention. She is the president and founder of Extraordinary Minds, Inc., where she currently provides RDI services to families.

Relationship Development Intervention is a unique approach to treating autism spectrum disorders. Developed by Dr. Steven Gutstein, RDI is based on the most recent research in autism spectrum disorders (ASD), neurology, and developmental psychology. The RDI theory is based on the premise that autism spectrum disorders prevent a child from providing their parent with adequate social-emotional feedback, thereby disrupting the typical parent-child relationship. The loss of this relationship results in the child's limited acquisition of dynamic intelligence.

The RDI Program has two major elements; restoration of the guided participation relationship and improvement of dynamic intelligence.

RDI provides a second chance for parents and their child to reestablish that parent-child relationship. It is a parent-based approach, whereby a trained RDI consultant teaches parents how to change the way they are communicating and interacting with their child to reestablish the disrupted guided participation relationship thereby improving the child's dynamic intelligence. The program is broken down into systematic and workable objectives. Because it is a parent based intervention, parents work on their own objectives prior to the assignment of any objectives for the child. As parents move through their own objectives and as they change their behavior, many child objectives are inadvertently addressed. Thus early on, from the very beginning, observable improvements in the child's dynamic abilities are often noticed.

Because an RDI program is based on typical development, it is an appropriate intervention for individuals with autism of all ages and levels of severity. All individuals with autism regardless of severity, co-occurring conditions or age will benefit from addressing deficits in dynamic intelligence and revisiting missed developmental milestones.

To best understand dynamic intelligence, one must understand static intelligence. Most individuals with ASD are quite proficient in static areas. Static intelligence is anything that has a right or wrong answer, that is unchanging and always produces the same outcome. Labeling, requesting, social scripts, academics, following directions, and memorization are all examples of static skills, and likely what a child with ASD is adept at.

Dynamic intelligence is the ability to manage situations that present themselves with elements of uncertainty. Examples of dynamic skills include the ability to problem solve, share experiences with others, curiosity, empathy, and taking another's perspective. All of these things are uncertain, in that there is no wrong or right answer, and no way to predict what specific outcome will occur. This type of intelligence is what is most often lacking in individuals with ASD.

Traditional behavioral interventions for ASD focus primarily on strengthening static skills; increasing language, teaching scripts to navigate social situations or following a schedule. These types of skills are merely compensating for deficits in dynamic thinking.

- Is increasing one's vocabulary improving the ability to share experiences and communicate with other people?
- Is teaching a child a social script for the playground preparing them for what to do when they don't get the response they were taught to expect?
- Is creating a picture schedule teaching a person to be flexible and manage the real world, where unexpected things happen all the time?

Years ago, the scientific community believed that the brain was unable to change. The only way we knew how to teach individuals with ASD was to give them the skills to compensate for their brain's difficulty managing uncertainty. We know now that the brain is an experience dependant organ; it changes and grows based on the types of learning experiences it is exposed to on a day to day basis. It is not only possible to but critical to begin addressing and remediating the deficits of ASD instead of merely working around them.

Neurotypical individuals begin thinking dynamically very early in life. The guided participation relationship is critical for the development of active thinkers and communicators. Guided participation is found cross-culturally, in every society, since the beginning of time. Children act as cognitive apprentices to more skilled and competent adults who provide them with ongoing challenges and the support necessary for them to be successful with life's challenges. Guides balance teaching various skills with a more important goal, providing the foundations for active thinking, learning, and cognitive growth.

Consider a young child raking leaves with his/her father. The father is not teaching his child to rake the leaves in a way that he would expect the child to go out and independently do this the following weekend. The father is teaching his child the goals beneath the goal; the foundations for learning. The child is learning how to collaborate with his father, how to flexibly manage problems and come up with solutions, and how to anticipate and communicate to one another about what they are doing.

Unfortunately, when ASD is added to the guided participation relationship, the child provides the parent with poor social and emotional feedback, leaving the parent with inadequate information to provide the child with opportunities to learn in a dynamic way. This is where RDI becomes so valuable.

Dr. Gutstein, developer of the RDI program, looked closely at the guided participation relationship between typically developing children and their parents and how parents provide their children with opportunities for dynamic growth. He was able to identify where the breakdown in this relationship occurs with children with ASD. The RDI program is designed to reestablish the guided participation relationship, thereby improving the child's ability to function in a dynamic, ever-changing world.

Through his extensive research on autism and the guided participation relationship in autism, Dr. Gutstein identified several core areas of dynamic intelligence that are lacking in individuals with ASD. These elements of dynamic thinking are incorporated into guided participation objectives that make up the dynamic intelligence curriculum.

One of the major deficits that affects individual with autism is social coordination, the basic to and fro of social interaction is often severely impaired. In typical development, social coordination occurs in infancy. Infants and very young children are able to take on active, participatory roles in social games such as peek-a-boo, pat-a-cake and other reciprocal games that require both partners to take responsibility for the activity.

Often times, individuals with ASD are either passive and prompt dependant or controlling and rigid. To establish social coordination with a passive partner, the parent must help the child to understand that he or she can bring something to the interaction without being told what to do. To establish social coordination with a controlling child, the parent must provide the child with an authentic role that allows the child to provide suggestions for enhancement without the usual controlling features. This often takes time for an individual with autism to master however, developmentally, it is the foundation for all social interaction. Without it, individuals with autism will continuously fail in social situations. As the individual with ASD understands and participates in basic social reciprocity, many new opportunities for interacting and communicating occur.

Many people think of communication and language as interchangeable. Communication is so much more than language. Much of our communication as humans is non verbal. In typical development, infants and very young children are proficient communicators prior to having any language. There are two types of communication, instrumental and experience sharing communication. Instrumental communication is used to obtain something and a specific response is expected. Examples of this would be requesting a toy, asking a question or providing a direction. Once the desired objective is received, the question answered, or the direction taken there is no longer a need to communicate with the other person.

Experience sharing communication, by nature, does not require a specific response. When you express what you like or dislike, what you are feeling or describing about your day, you will expect a relevant but not right or wrong response. Think about all the things that have to be considered in order to successfully have a conversation. We must interpret the other person's language, his or her non-verbal communication; gestures, facial expressions, intonation change, pauses and innuendo; and we decipher all of that simultaneously.

The value of language in the human experience is to communicate and share experiences with others. In an RDI program, parents look at what type of communication they are using with their child. Is it mostly instrumental; asking questions or providing directions or is it mostly experience sharing; commenting, sharing preferences and ideas? Parents are taught to strive for a balance of instrumental and experience sharing language that is found in conversational language among most people. To do this, parents increase their experience sharing language and decrease their instrumental language with their child with ASD. By providing the child with ASD language that does not require a specific response, parents are teaching a child the true value of language, to share with others. Parents find that by changing their own communication to become more experience sharing in nature, their child with ASD soon follows suit and begins commenting and sharing experiences spontaneously and independently.

The RDI program also teaches parents to create an environment conducive to the development of non-verbal communication. Using and reading non verbal communication is inherently difficult for individuals with ASD. Often times, parents and professionals compensate for this deficit by using language as the primary and often only form of communication. Individuals with ASD do not naturally monitor their communication environment, resulting in parents and professionals prompting them to attend and/or make eye contact. Instead of trying to change their behavior, parents are taught to consider their own. If we are always providing individuals with ASD auditory information, they never have the need to look or monitor their environment. By reducing language, prompts for eye contact and incorporating more non verbal communication into everyday experiences, parents create a need for the child to look, monitor, become a more active communicator and improve their ability to read social cues.

By utilizing non verbal and broadband communication, parents are also increasing the child's opportunities to reference. Social referencing, the ability to seek out information from a parent or guide when wary or unsure, is in place by twelve months of age in typically developing children. A twelve month old, exploring child who is feeling uncertain will reference his mother to see her emotional reaction. If mom appears encouraging and calm, the child will continue in his exploration. If the mother appears distressed, the child will cease exploration and may seek comfort. Individuals with ASD have great difficulty using social referencing to manage uncertainty. When faced with a situation that is uncertain, they will often respond with fight or flight, meltdown or withdrawal. Referencing, often a deficit, is a better option. The goal is to allow the child to discover that there is value in looking to their more competent guides for information, to borrow their perspective when they are unsure as how to process information.

The RDI program teaches parents how to create moments of productive uncertainty that create just enough curiosity without being so uncertain that the child feels anxious. The productive part of productive uncertainty will vary for every individual. For example, parents can create productive uncertainty by merely stopping while walking together. Some individuals will however require a more deliberate or extreme approach to productive uncertainty such as pulling a hammer out of a washing machine while doing laundry together.

By teaching the value in looking to more competent guides for help processing information, we are actually teaching them how to become more effective problem solvers. True independence begins with a healthy dependence on a parent or guide. No child is born into the world with the knowledge as to how to navigate it. Many individuals with ASD never develop a healthy dependence on their parent which results in great difficulty managing uncertainty, inability to appraise social situations and inadequate problem solving skills.

The RDI program teaches parents the value in helping their child to become more active thinkers and problem solvers. There are many ways to do this on a day to day basis, but the first is to look at areas where they may be overcompensating, perhaps doing things for their child that he or she is likely capable of doing. To create a feeling of competence in a child, the child needs opportunities to be successful at thinking, considering and problem solving. Take a simple everyday example of a child who wants a drink. Mom holds the juice and places the cup in front of the child, upside down. By just waiting and not providing the solution to "turn over your cup," mom has created an uncertain moment where she is asking the child to monitor his/her environment, think about and consider the situation, and take some kind of action to fix it. If the child is unable to figure out what it is that the mother is asking of him/her, mom can use a statement such as, "I don't think I can pour the juice yet," or "Your cup is upside down!" This type of statement is stating the problem instead of the solution, allowing the child the opportunity to think and problem solve on his/her own. The RDI program teaches parents how to identify opportunities and create dozens of moments such as these throughout the day.

Most of us are lucky enough to not have to think about memory and its substantial impact on our day to day functioning in the world. Individuals with autism are often thought of as having good memories as they can often remember facts and details a person without autism would never be able to retain.

Episodic memory is a type of memory that is a representation of specific experiences, events or situations that one has been involved in. This type of memory also allows you to reflect on past experiences, consider how to appraise and problem solve a current situation and consider a future experience and how you would manage it. Individuals with autism have an extremely difficult time creating episodic memories. They often do not see the big picture and get caught up in the details of an experience, leading them to miss opportunities to learn from their environment. A person with autism may remember the events of an experience, the people that were there, the things they saw, what time they arrived and left. Episodic memory puts in the forefront of your mind, what made you laugh, how upset you were when you had to leave, and how it was so great to see an old friend.

RDI teaches parents how to create situations that will create this type of memory for their child with autism. Positive episodic memories equal motivation. If a person with autism can begin having positive experiences with relationships through reciprocal interactions, experience sharing communication, productive uncertainty and being afforded the opportunity to think, consider and figure things out on their own, they will be more competent and motivated to participate in the world around them.

The RDI program is a unique and invaluable resource to families. It values parents as the most important influence in their child's life. Parents are provided the skills and direction to become successfully reconnected with their child. Knowing that their child's growth is due to their own guidance empowers parents to persevere through difficult times and look to the future with a great deal of hope.

Research

A study on RDI in the journal *Autism* in 2007 looked at 16 children prior to and at the end of 30 months of RDI therapy. At baseline, all children met the ADOS/ADI-R criteria for autism. At outcome, none of the 16 children met the autism criteria on the ADOS/ADI-R. Six of the children moved one diagnostic category to autism spectrum and the remaining ten did not meet any criteria for autism or autism spectrum.

The parents of the children were given a flexibility interview at baseline and at outcome. After 30 months of RDI, twelve children moved from the least flexible two categories to the most flexible two categories in at least one area. Prior to treatment, over half of the children were placed in special education classrooms. At outcome, 10 of 16 children were functioning in mainstreamed classrooms without an aide.

A new study being conducted at the Tavistock Clinic in London is showing extremely promising preliminary results. The study looks at 18 children that participated in RDI for about 18 months. The parent-child dyad was looked at prior to the intervention and at 18 months using the Dyadic Coding Scale (DCS: Humber & Moss, 2005). The participants were also assessed using the Autism Diagnostic Observation Scale (ADOS) at baseline and again at 18 months.

The study is looking at several things.
- Do differences in quality of parent-child interaction correspond with the children's social-communication impairment as measured by the ADOS
- Does the quality of parent-child interaction change over the course of an RDI Program
- Are observed changes in parent-child interaction accompanied by changes in the children's social-communication

The baseline measurement of the sample of children with autism showed their scores on the DCS to be much lower than a sample of typically developing children and similar to the scores of another sample of children with autism. After 18 months of participating in RDI, all parent child dyads showed significant improvement on the DCS and their scores were more similar to the typically developing group.

The ADOS administered at both baseline and 18 months are currently still being coded.

ASYNCHRONOUS TELEHEALTH TECHNOLOGY FOR AUTISM SPECTRUM DISORDER

By Dr. Mary Joann Lang and Ronald Oberleitner

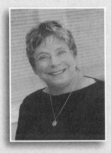

Mary Joann Lang, PhD, ABPN, BCBA-D

Beacon Day School
24 Centerpointe Drive
La Palma, CA 90623
714-288-4200
Fax: 714-288-4204
www.beacondayschool.com

Dr. Mary Joann Lang founded Beacon Day School for students with autism spectrum disorder (ASD) and related disabilities. Dr. Lang also founded Beacon Autistic Spectrum Independence Center, providing social skills and in-home therapy-based programs, and Beacon Life Project, created to serve the needs of adults. Dr. Lang has been involved with the care of children for over 25 years, first as a nurse practitioner and educator, then as an educational psychologist. Dr. Lang has many professional publications. She graduated from the University of Southern California with her PhD in educational psychology. A Diplomate of the American Board of Neuropsychology, Dr. Lang has been a practicing, licensed neuropsychologist since 1991. www.BeaconDaySchool.com

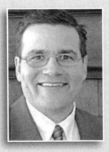

Ronald Oberleitner, MBA

Ronald Oberleitner is the CEO and founder of Behavior Imaging Solutions, which develops solutions to facilitate the observational, analytical, and collaborative needs of behavior healthcare and special education professionals. Behavior Imaging Solutions' award-winning technology enables remote assessment and consultation between patients/students and professionals through enhanced video capture and a secure health record or special education assessment record application that allows users to store, share, and annotate video and other files. Prior to Behavior Imaging Solutions, Mr. Oberleitner served as the president of e-Merge Medical Technologies, creating TalkAutism, a leading web portal and provider of autism resources. In 2005, he founded AutismCares, a coalition of organizations supporting families through natural disasters. www.BehaviorImaging.com

Introduction

Telehealth technology is a tool that allows behavior professionals and others to make valuable observations, gather data, and propose more targeted, appropriate remediation for areas in which an individual with an autism spectrum disorder needs to progress. This tool can be used across natural settings of home, school, and community, and it has practical applications including use in classroom observation and Individualized Education Program (IEP) meetings. The capability of telehealth technology to serve children and families remotely means that parents of children in rural settings can receive more frequent and consistent services from a greater variety of professionals.

This chapter will look at

- Defining telehealth
- Asynchronous telehealth for autism (Behavior Imaging® technology)
- How Behavior Imaging® can help professionals observe problem behaviors in the classroom for the purpose of remediation within an applied behavior analysis (ABA) framework
- How the results of this observation can aid at the Individualized Education Program (IEP) of a student with an autism spectrum disorder (ASD)
- How telehealth technology further helps IEP team members
- Case study
- Beacon Day School project

What are telemedicine and telehealth?

According to the American Telemedicine Association (2012),

> *Formally defined, telemedicine is the use of medical information exchanged from one site to another via electronic communications to improve a patient's clinical health status. Telemedicine includes a growing variety of applications and services using two-way video, email, smart phones, wireless tools and other forms of telecommunications technology. . . . ATA [American Telemedicine Association] has historically considered telemedicine and telehealth to be interchangeable terms, encompassing a wide definition of remote healthcare.*[i]

California's Bill AB 809 (2013) concerning telehealth defined it this way:

> *"Telehealth" means the mode of delivering health care services and public health via information and communication technologies to facilitate the diagnosis, consultation, treatment, education, care management, and self-management of a patient's health care while the patient is at the originating site and the health care provider is at a distant site. Telehealth facilitates patient self-management and caregiver support for patients and includes synchronous interactions and asynchronous store and forward transfers.*[ii]

The American Psychological Association (APA) "Guidelines for the Practice of Telepsychology" (2013) define telepsychology as follows:

> *... the provision of psychological services using telecommunication technologies. Telecommunications is the preparation, transmission, communication, or related processing of information by electrical, electromagnetic, electromechanical, electro-optical, or electronic means (Committee on National Security Systems, 2010). Telecommunication technologies include but are not limited to telephone, mobile devices, interactive videoconferencing, email, chat, text, and Internet (e.g., self-help websites, blogs, and social media). The information that is transmitted may be in writing, or include images, sounds or other data. These communications may be synchronous with multiple parties communicating in real time (e.g. interactive videoconferencing, telephone) or asynchronous (e.g. email, online bulletin boards, storing and forwarding information). Technologies may augment traditional in-person services (e.g., psychoeducational materials online after an in-person therapy session), or be used as stand-alone services (e.g., therapy or leadership development provided over videoconferencing). Different technologies may be used in various combinations and for different purposes during the provision of telepsychology services. For example, videoconferencing and telephone may also be utilized for direct service while email and text is used for non-direct services (e.g. scheduling)....*"[iii]

Telehealth for autism

There is a pressing need for diagnostic and intervention services to support the rapidly growing population of children with ASDs. Direct observation of the child remains the gold standard practice in diagnosis, assessment, and treatment planning for children with autism and related developmental disabilities. Moreover, the literature is now clear in supporting early screening to ensure that children are referred for diagnostic assessments sooner and that timely evaluations of eligibility for services result in immediate implementation of appropriate early intervention. In many poor and rural communities, care of children with ASD is marked by lack of access to autism-specific expertise among professionals in mental health, primary care, and education. Even in urban communities where services are more widely available, timely access to diagnostic and intervention services is often hampered by long waiting lists at centers and clinics.

A partnership between parents, providers, and teachers is necessary to address the challenges of early diagnosis, treatment, and care of children with autism. A technology platform is available that can provide the critical components for evaluating, diagnosing, and treating autism in children efficiently, conveniently, and securely – via asynchronous telemedicine. A video capture and personal electronic health record platform allows autism families to document their child's abnormal behavior and share this information confidentially with remotely located healthcare providers who can then provide each family with guidance regarding their child's behaviors and health condition. The technology is simple to use and provides parents with support during times of crisis. The platform meets the security, privacy, and control requirements associated with the multifaceted legal landscape of the USA. Preliminary surveys indicate that application of this type of platform in classroom settings as well as in the home environment are being received favorably by parents, educators, and healthcare providers alike.[iv]

With this technology platform, travel can be greatly reduced, remote specialists and professionals are able to see more clients and patients in a shorter time, while continuing to provide quality service. The video-based system is superior to non-video methods of data collection since the professional is able to actually see what is going on, instead of relying on non-natural-environment (in-office) observation or frequently inaccurate oral accounts. Furthermore, the data is more useful since it is easier to collect the needed behavioral information, and it can be collected in the "natural" environment of the child such as the home or school. Additionally, data storage, organization, and archiving are simple and intuitive.[v]

Behavior Imaging® technology

Ron Oberleitner and team developed an asynchronous, store-and-forward telehealth system referred to as Behavior Imaging® (BI). This system consists of software/hardware technology to capture video evidence of behavior in natural environments (Behavior Capture™) and a secure, HIPAA-compliant online telehealth consultation environment (Behavior Connect™) where the video data of behavior images can be easily uploaded for a clinician or other professional to review confidentially either onsite or remotely.

Asynchronous (store-and-forward) telehealth technology, such as Behavior Imaging® technology, is demonstrating how contextual video capture and a complementary online consultation platform effectively address the need for observation of the child by a professional who can make more timely clinical decisions regarding diagnosis and treatment. Beyond the potential for such technology to improve access to care for remotely located children (rural areas, military bases, etc.), it can also enable clinical centers around the country to shorten their wait-lists by facilitating more timely communication with families about the nature and range of the child's symptoms and needs. There is great potential in enabling these centers to quickly gather initial clinical impressions of the child by reviewing videos collected by caregivers in the home, and then to more effectively triage cases into those that are clear cut and those that require more extensive in-person assessment.

How telehealth technology can help observe problem behaviors in the classroom for the purpose of remediation within an applied behavior analysis (ABA) framework

Telehealth and ABA

ABA draws heavily on the use of Antecedent-Behavior-Consequence (ABC)

- **"A"** = **antecedent** = event or activity immediately preceding problem behavior
- **"B"** = observed **behavior**
- **"C"** = **consequence** = event that immediately follows a response

The use of telehealth technology in the classroom allows us to see the possible antecedent event(s) that precipitate a problem behavior. This allows us to takes steps to prevent a problem behavior in the future. The technology also allows us to see and assess consequent variables.

This also allows quicker implementation of strategies for more positive behaviors to build upon for the student's future.

The advantage of telehealth technology in a classroom setting vs. a clinic setting

Classroom	Clinic
Behaviors captured as they occur in natural settings	*Specialized room at a clinic may produce reactivity effects*
A key component of treatment planning involves understanding the function of the behavior	*The stimuli that evoke the behavior as well as consequences that maintain it in the natural environment may not be observed in an artificial setting like a clinic*
Clinical value of using Behavior Capture™ at home and in school to record the child's behavior along with its naturally occurring antecedents and consequences, to support educational and clinical assessments	

Better functional behavior assessments (FBAs)

Functional behavior assessments (FBAs) are processes to identify the functions of a behavior. FBAs are often required from teachers to document the problem behavior of a specific child to facilitate the process of expert analysis and corrective steps. FBAs can be very effective if they are accurate, complete and consistent. However, even the most conscientious and observant teacher will encounter these three drawbacks to traditional "pen and paper" FBAs:

- They rely on the teacher's direct observation of spontaneous, and sometimes fleeting, behavior events.
- They rely on the accurate recall of the event and the communication skills of the teacher writing the report.
- There is no way to determine exactly what caused the behavior event.

The specific detail leading up to a behavior event is even more essential for corrective measures than the event itself or the consequences of the event. The ability to capture the cause—and not just the effect—of disruptive problem behavior is resonating with teachers and behaviorists across the nation. Autism educators are especially interested in the ability to capture, store, and view the trigger of behavior events. Behavior Capture™ provides the an automated way to capture on video clips the cause that many times cannot be adequately observed as it's happening, and thus facilitates more accurate, more beneficial FBAs.

In one study, funded by the National Institutes of Health (NIH #2R44HD052340-02),[vi] the use of Behavior Capture™ resulted in 43% fewer data collection errors when collecting behavioral assessment data.[vii, viii] In this study, users across eleven clinical sites captured behavior data on video with Behavior Capture™, annotated it, and shared it online. The technology was found to increase awareness of children's classroom activities and allow experts to assess more students in the same amount of time.

How the results of telehealth technology observation can aid at the student's IEP and further help team members

With proper consent, Behavior Capture™ video images can be shared with IEP team members via Behavior Connect™ for an invaluable first-hand look at behaviors when they happen.

Behavior Imaging® telehealth technology can help overcome scheduling challenges of team members and caregivers. Professionals who were not able to be present before but who have important information about the student can now participate in the IEP meeting (e.g., psychiatrist who prescribes medication) and receive feedback from parents and teachers who monitor the student daily (e.g., as to behavioral or other effects). This fosters integration of services (e.g., connecting parents, teachers, school counselors, psychiatrist).

How this helps the IEP team

In general, the use of this asynchronous telehealth technology facilitates coordination of professional expertise throughout the overall program, thereby supplying other therapy team members with vital information for their treatment plans.

Communication and dynamic interaction among all team members can even be accomplished in a "real-time" format, with team members receiving the same contextual behavior information, thereby making the understanding of the student's program more contextual, with fewer misinterprations, and in a less fragmented fashion.

The visual documentation and delivery of information via the technology provides enhanced knowledge and understanding to parents, teachers, and mental health care members about the student's behavior and behavior management needs as well as about the urgency and time frame in which to address behaviors.

All of these factors result in more efficient, timely care to the student, thus producing more positive student outcomes in behavior and academic performance.

Case study: the advantage of telehealth technology in a home and community setting

Using Behavior Imaging® technology, the caseworker with Ron Oberleitner's son is able to capture examples in the community and school on video, which a behavior professional can then receive, study, and use as a guide toward better techniques going forward. For example, this data can capture perseverative behavior like repetitive hand washing. When Ron's son is supposed to be washing dishes, the data shows why the perseverative behavior is there (A—antecedent—there is an affinity to water); what the behavior is (B—behavior—washing his hands instead of the dishes); and this suggests a remedy for the behavior (C—consequence—a timer to time washing a dish).

This illustrates the use of technology to help professionals remotely supervise treatment that's working. Students'/clients' treatments are constantly able to be improved, showing the challenges and then the successful intervention strategies.

Beacon project

Beacon Day School conducted a pilot study assessing school district personnel and caregiver attitudes toward Behavior Capture™ and Behavior Connect™ technologies and their use during IEP meetings, also assessing the effectiveness of using this technology. There was a significantly positive response to the survey questions on the part of parents and school district personnel. Importantly, insight was added to the IEP process toward writing student IEP goals.

Conclusions

➤ Given that ABA is increasingly being implemented in classroom, home, and community settings – some of which are rural — and that there are a limited number of certified professionals to supervise such programs, applications of telehealth technologies provide promising potential alternatives or augmentations.

➤ Technology to capture behavior events in the classroom as they happen is an invaluable tool in understanding, and then remediating a student's problem behaviors.

➤ For current IEP teams in place, Behavior Imaging® technology allows greater participation of professionals, therapists, and family members to engage in a dynamic, more efficient process for the student's benefit.

51

THE RAMAPO APPROACH: FOSTERING RELATIONSHIPS THAT MOTIVATE BEHAVIORAL CHANGE

by Lisa Tazartes, Mike Kunin, and Jennifer Buri da Cunha

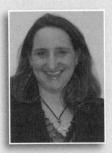

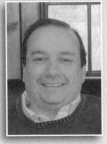

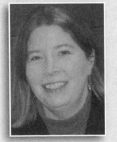

Lisa Tazartes, Director of Ramapo Training
ltazartes@ramapoforchildren.org

Mike Kunin, Director of Camp Ramapo
mkunin@ramapoforchildren.org

Jennifer Buri da Cunha, Director of Staff Assistant Experience
jburidacunha@ramapoforchildren.org

Ramapo for Children
Website: www.ramapoforchildren.org
Facebook: www.facebook.com/ramapoforchildren
Twitter: @Ramapo4Children

New York Office:
49 West 38th Street, 5th Floor
New York, NY 10018
212.754.7003

Rhinebeck Office:
PO Box 266
Rhinebeck, New York 12572
845.876.8403

Lisa Tazartes is a founding director of **Ramapo Training**, which provides professional development to educators and youth workers through training workshops and on-site, one-on-one coaching. Ramapo Training serves over 300 schools and agencies and more than 10,000 individuals annually. Trainers—who are veteran teachers, principals, and leading experts in youth development and education—work to bridge the gap between teachers' formal training in instruction and the daily challenges of managing a classroom. In addition to being a member of the Ramapo staff for more than 15 years, Lisa is a graduate of the Executive Level Program of the Institute for Non-Profit Management at Columbia University and holds an undergraduate degree in Psychology from

Swarthmore College. Her career has been devoted to building the skills and capacity of educators and youth-service professionals. She is the 2007 recipient of the prestigious Zella Bronfman Award, in recognition of her role as a change agent who is helping to transform the delivery of services to people with disabilities.

Mike Kunin started working at Ramapo in the summer of 1978 and, as the director of **Camp Ramapo**, oversees the organization's Rhinebeck campus and heads the summer camp program. Camp Ramapo is a residential camp that serves children ages 6 to 16 who are affected by social, emotional or learning challenges, including autism spectrum disorders. The program provides a traditional summer camp experience for children who have difficulty building and maintaining healthy relationships with peers and adults and would struggle in a less supportive setting. Camp Ramapo is structured to help children with special needs learn to live within a group, form healthy friendships, make good choices, develop self-confidence and experience success. Before taking on his executive role at Ramapo, Mike taught special education in public and private school programs, spending several years working in the New Haven, Connecticut public schools. He is a graduate of McGill University in Montreal and received his master's degree in Special Education from the University of Connecticut.

Jennifer Buri da Cunha heads Ramapo's **Staff Assistant Experience**, a residential transition-to-independence program for young adults with social, emotional or learning challenges who are ready to learn to navigate the challenges associated with disabilities such as Asperger's/other spectrum disorders, learning differences, and ADHD in order to transition to employment and/or college coursework. Based at Ramapo's Rhinebeck campus, the program is designed for young adults who have struggled in other, less supportive environments and helps participants to practice vocational and life skills in a community that includes typically developing peer role models, mentors, and coaches. Jen has worked in direct service and supervisory roles at Ramapo since 1991. Prior to overseeing the Staff Assistant Experience, Jen taught in public and private schools in New York City, and she holds a master's degree in Special Education from New York University. In addition to her current role, Jen also serves as an instructor for Ramapo's undergraduate level fieldwork course in special education.

Working with children, whether as a parent, teacher, or caregiver, is an inherently social process. This is no different when we are talking about children on the autism spectrum. In order to impact children with ASD, the adults in their lives need to employ a set of activities, strategies, and skills that form a strong adult-child bond as the basis of any intervention. This requires that we see autism not through the lens of social skills deficits, but rather with the understanding that children with autism actually seek comfort from and desire interaction with adults. In fact, the stress and anxiety that social situations trigger for the child with ASD actually heighten his or her need for meaningful relationships with caring adults.

Personal relationships are very often the catalyst for motivating behavioral change and are therefore a key component of good teaching. Once rapport is developed, a budding relationship between an adult and child becomes as reinforcing as any tangible reward used to manage behaviors and teach new skills. When this relationship is mutually enjoyable for the child and the adult, the child wants to exhibit behaviors that receive positive recognition from the adult and the adult is able to intervene effectively when maladaptive behaviors are exhibited.

All children with ASD want to learn social skills in a fun and relaxed way, but they need a facilitator to help navigate social situations. Unlike many typically developing children who learn to socialize though imitation or trial and error, children with ASD lack a road map for navigating social situations and need clear and deliberate models. Models are comforting and offer support, helping to dissipate stress and anxiety associated with such interactions and allowing the process of true social learning to begin. Regular caregivers can be very effective instructors for modeling behavior because they are uniquely positioned to promote social learning and generalizing skills in a natural environment.

Relationships, of course, affect both parties. Children with ASD have much to offer the caregiver in the form of support and comfort as well, though it may look different than other relationships. When the adults in a child's life stop acting as passive or reluctant receptors of autistic behaviors, and instead feel comfortable intervening and shaping interactions, the adult-child bond becomes richer and mutually beneficial. There is greater opportunity for both members of the relationship to appreciate—and even celebrate—the perspectives, preferences, and ideas that are unique to each other.

The value of building relationships with children on the autism spectrum goes beyond instruction. It also forms the basis for better communication and significantly impacts how effectively adults manage difficult behaviors.

Interestingly, many parents and professionals dealing with children on the autism spectrum frequently underestimate their child's ability to communicate their needs effectively. ASD children, regardless of their level of functioning, recognize acutely their need to communicate well and they often perform this function quite capably, even as others around them may not notice. ASD children express all of the major emotions—happy, sad, angry, and scared—with remarkable fluency. Body language is often used to indicate levels of comfort (both high and low) with a person or activity. Facial expressions, gestures, and body positioning are all key indicators of a child's willingness to participate in an activity or to be with someone. Even acting out behaviors are often simply an attempt to communicate, though they are rarely interpreted as such. Adults often see challenging behaviors as something separate and apart from the matter at hand—an expression of free-floating anxiety, a bad mood, or the perpetuation of a negative habit. In fact, difficult behaviors are the language children use to communicate when the demands of their environment are misaligned with their social, emotional, or adaptive capacities. Adults significantly increase their chance of managing such behaviors successfully when they take the time to correctly interpret the driving forces that are motivating them.

Amongst our program offerings, we run a residential summer camp for children with special needs. When a family is considering enrolling their child for the first time, and that child is nonverbal, parents are often concerned that he or she will not be able to tell them whether or not they liked it. Our response is that their child *will* tell them—loud and clear. In fact, nonverbal children provide us with the best feedback on how our staff are doing in their jobs, sometimes even better than our staff supervisors. They let us know very clearly who they have identified as helpful to them and who they have dismissed as relatively disinterested. They are the true experts at deducing who is sensitive, dedicated, competent, resourceful, and effective—because they need to be.

The more vulnerable a child is (or the more limited their verbal communication is), the more they seek out those individuals or venues that can best meet their needs. Adults who interpret a child's negative behavior as an attempt to seek assistance, adapt to a new situation, or communicate effectively can then help strengthen the child's ability to do all of these things by employing coaching and cues that foster more positive behaviors. This enhanced communication also helps the adults in their lives be more aware when children are adapting or coping well, enabling us to give credit for a job well done.

Relationship Building Strategies

No two children with an autism spectrum disorder are the same, and building an effective relationship requires taking the time to understand a child's uniqueness and special interests. A carefully designed plan that utilizes elements of this special interest to engage them in other, more productive activities is critical to nurturing a relationship and, ultimately, to building valuable skills. It sends a powerful message that we are willing to meet a child where he is, and value his contribution to a shared activity. By gradually decreasing the role and frequency of the child's special interest when engaging in other activities, adults can also reduce the exclusionary effect of this interest, and help him engage in more appropriate behavior.

To illustrate how such a plan can work, we draw from the experience of one of our campers, a 12-year-old girl named Camille who has a special interest in fairies. Whenever she was allowed to have her fairy dolls with her, she would isolate herself from people and activities to play with them. Camille resisted going over the daily schedule by screaming and putting her hands over her ears. Camille also had a lot of trouble taking a break from stressful or escalating situations, and engaged in a variety of other challenging behaviors that adults and peers found off-putting. The team of staff that worked with Camille designed an innovative way of addressing these issues: her daily schedule would be "delivered by fairy mail" by having a counselor put it in an envelope decorated with pictures of fairies and place it in the notch of a tree. She could start her day by getting her "mail" and reviewing the schedule with a counselor. To help her take a break when needed, they reframed such situations by inviting her to go on a "fairy hunt" one-on-one with a staff member, and away from the stressful activity. Then, in addition to giving her short, pre-arranged times to play with her fairy dolls by herself each day, she could earn up to 5 minutes of time playing with them at the end of each activity period by meeting behavioral expectations, as long as she included another person in her play. Before each activity, a staff member reviewed Camille's schedule with her and reminded her how she could earn time with the dolls, then let her know in the middle of the activity if she was on track to get the extra time.

Once Camille had developed some success with the plan, the staff began to gradually fade the fairy references and to increase the expectations for earning playtime with the dolls. By the end of the session, Camille had significantly decreased the amount of time she spent playing alone with her dolls, limiting play to socially appropriate times and regularly including others. She no longer resisted reviewing her schedule, was spending much more time participating in her group's activities, and had made a friend who motivated her to behave more appropriately.

Using a special interest to help effect behavioral change is just one part of the Ramapo strategy. It is also important for adults working with children on the autism spectrum to be skilled at projecting confidence, commitment, and caring, particularly when situations are stressful for a child. At Ramapo, the staff who build the most productive relationships with children on the spectrum demonstrate a genuine appreciation of the camper; they are active, assertive, highly prepared, and good at letting a child know that they want to participate in shared experiences often and in various ways. Since many children on the spectrum have difficulty interpreting or accepting behaviors such as smiling, making small talk, high fives, etc., adults can show that they care by being sensitive to a child's preferences in the tone or volume of a person's voice, physical proximity, and gradually engaging them with eye contact, verbalizations, and activities.

It helps for adults to think of themselves as "tour guides" for children on the spectrum, helping them navigate experiences that are often unfamiliar to them. And like any qualified "tour guide," these adults must demonstrate that they are confident about the course of action and capable of handling any issue that arises. Even children with very little language and great difficulty interacting with others adjust more quickly when they sense that there is a structure to follow and someone to lead the way. Certainly, working with children on the spectrum can be disorienting and unpredictable at times, and adults may not always feel confident in their ability to handle situations. However, it is vitally important that they make every effort to appear in control, because the absence of confidence in adults leads to great anxiety in children with ASD. Adults must be prepared to lead experiences for children on the spectrum without hesitation, display facial expressions and body language that indicate self-assurance, and initiate appropriate transitions to new experiences. Frequently, these children's restlessness and anxiety increase whenever there is a pause in the flow of the day, even a small one, so it is important to provide a steady stream of appropriately presented information to help smooth the transition from one activity to another. At Ramapo, there is a marked difference in the behavior of campers in the presence of staff who help them transition to new activities by talking to them (verbal prompt), placing a hand on their shoulder (physical prompt), and introducing props or materials (visual prompt) for the activity compared to those who hang back and hesitate to direct the transition.

Adults must also demonstrate a commitment to their plan and find appropriate ways to help children adjust to new routines and expectations. Difficulties usually occur when staff allow a child to direct all aspects of their time together, have not organized their resources and materials well, or abandon the planned activity at the slightest indication of reluctance. Although it can sometimes be beneficial for children on the autism spectrum to engage in self-directed behavior, having adults provide a predictable structure prepares children for what is coming next, reduces anxiety, and lets children focus on learning new skills. For example, if adults plan for every block of time to have a distinct beginning, middle, and end, the child will become more accustomed to the routine. Instead of worrying about what will come next, children can relax and be open to new ideas.

Youngsters on the autism spectrum may experience significantly higher levels of anxiety about seemingly routine tasks than their mainstream counterparts. That's why adults interacting with ASD children should always be mindful of the need to keep stressors to a minimum in most situations in order to encourage success. One of the best ways to do this is through the strategic use of humor: Joking around and taking a less intense, more easygoing tactic with kids is always a good idea. Kids can pick up your overall mood and affect and will use this information to help decide how to react to a particular set of circumstances. Lighten the mood, ease the tension, and smile. Use humor (not sarcasm) and be upbeat, especially when trying something new or introducing something that could produce anxiety. Be mindful about expressing exactly what you are feeling at the moment. Ironically, it is most important to appear relaxed and confident about a situation when you are not actually feeling that way yourself. Make sure the child is not sensing that you are stressed about his potential inability to succeed.

Remember, you are the educator in all scenarios. You are training your child to be at ease in certain situations, he is not training you on when to be tense. Assume competence—in both yourself and your child.

About Ramapo for Children

Ramapo for Children's philosophy is built around the simple and profound belief that all people want the same things in life: to learn, to feel valued and to experience success. When children (or adults) exhibit behaviors that are at odds with these goals, it reflects some combination of unmet needs and underdeveloped social or emotional skills. Ramapo works to help people align their behaviors with their aspirations.

At the heart of Ramapo's approach is our ability to equip educators, caregivers, and youth with the skills they need to build trusting relationships, serve as effective role models, handle challenging behaviors constructively, and improve continuously through reflective practice.

With over 90 years of experience in direct service youth programs and training for adults, Ramapo has developed a unique model for promoting skill acquisition, positive behavioral change, learning and personal growth among young people who must overcome significant challenges—including autism spectrum disorders—to achieve their goals.   Through a multifaceted and comprehensive approach that involves students, caregivers and educators, Ramapo works on behalf of children and young adults who face obstacles to learning, enabling them to succeed at home, in the classroom and in life.

The Ramapo Approach has been developed and implemented through four main programs:

- **Camp Ramapo:** a residential summer camp in Rhinebeck that serves over 550 children with a range of cognitive disabilities and behavioral challenges, including children affected by autism spectrum disorders.
- **The Staff Assistant Experience:** a transition-to-independence program for young adults aged 18 to 25 who seek independence, but have been unable to overcome the challenges associated with their disabilities, which include Asperger's Syndrome and autism spectrum disorders. The program helps participants to practice vocational and life skills in an inclusive residential community.
- **Ramapo Training:** providing educators, youth workers, and parents with practical tools for managing difficult behaviors and fostering environments that support success. In 2012, Ramapo served more than 300 schools and agencies and trained over 10,000 educators, youth workers, and parents.
- **Ramapo Retreats:** short-term, adventure-based experiences for young people, educators, and community-based organizations that give participants a greater appreciation of their own potential as well as strategies for successful communication, teamwork, and leadership. Ramapo works with over 150 schools and agencies each year, serving over 8,000 participants.

HOLISTIC

52

THE HOLISTIC APPROACH TO NEURODEVELOPMENT AND LEARNING EFFICIENCY (HANDLE®)

by Carolyn Nuyens and Marlene Suliteanu

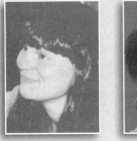 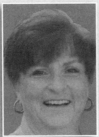

Carolyn Nuyens
Marlene Suliteanu, otr/l

The HANDLE Institute
7 Mt. Lassen Drive, Suite B110
San Rafael, CA 94903
415-479-1800
www.handle.org

Carolyn Nuyens, executive director of the HANDLE Institute, has extensive personal and professional experience in the autism community. She is a certified HANDLE practitioner and instructor. She traveled to India in 2005 with the creator of HANDLE, Judith Bluestone, to introduce HANDLE to the autism community there.

Marlene Suliteanu, OTR/L, also a certified HANDLE practitioner and instructor, with a therapy practice serving southern California, is Judith Bluestone's sister. Judith authored *The Fabric of Autism: Weaving the Threads into a Cogent Theory* as a semi-autobiographical, in-depth explanation of how HANDLE understands autism.

HANDLE is a unique **paradigm** for understanding human functionality, based on an observable sensory, motor, and processing hierarchy matched to neurodevelopment.

When anything within that hierarchy is irregular or underdeveloped, individuals experience mounting frustration, trying to "learn" to "do" tasks that come naturally when the body/brain/spirit has those prerequisite skills. Repeated experiences of frustrated effort, missing those functional sensory, motor, and processing systems, lead to a self image of defeat. It's those prerequisites, therefore, that a HANDLE program supports.

Stated differently: The end-points or products of that interactive hierarchical set of systems are the skills and behaviors the community at large expects and for which there's a "standard" of acceptability. HANDLE programs do not address those skills and behaviors, but rather support the irregular or underdeveloped systems lower on the hierarchy of sensory, motor, and processing systems, so function is spontaneous and matched to capability. That is, when the prerequisite systems serve the whole, coordinating with each other smoothly and efficiently, the skills and behaviors show up on their own. Less frustration and less stress are two of the most often named outcomes of any HANDLE program.

Nothing good can come from a recurring expectation of failure. HANDLE enlists the client's brain/body/spirit as an ally, to ready itself to take on life challenges. HANDLE practitioners have only one dogmatic "rule" for all activities: *Gentle Enhancement.*® When stimulation never exceeds the person's ability to use it—the activity stops at the first sign of distress—then irregular systems can develop, strengthen, and come into alignment with related systems; otherwise, they're always "defeated" at the same level. This key to the "A" of HANDLE, Approach, extends into every sphere, most importantly starting as a guide to relationships. *Nonjudgmental respect* conveys **trust in the client's behavior as communication**, always; trust without the kind of condemnation implicit in descriptions like "melt-down," "stimming," "oppositional defiance," or "noncompliance."

Contrary to a frequent misconception, HANDLE is not a set of effective therapeutic activities, though of course it includes those; nor is it a "method" taught to clients and families as if there were anything standardized about the program offered. There isn't. The paradigm, HANDLE, is the strategy for the tactics deployed as individualized recommendations.

So now let's look at some specifics about this paradigm and its resultant programs: how we understand the autism spectrum, and how we support function.

Characteristics, commonalities

Although each person on the spectrum is unique, neurodevelopmental characteristics shared by many individuals with autism are:

1. **Hypersensitivities**, especially auditory, tactile, and vestibular—which means bothered by sounds and irritated by imposed touch sensations (think: seams in socks, tags in shirts, hugs and kisses), and "gravitational insecurity" because the vestibular system tells us how gravity is acting on our bodies. All behavior and task response depends on how input from all these systems is processed; inaccurate or

unreliable *input* yields behaviors (*output*) incongruent with the community standard of acceptability.

2. **Low muscle tone** (throughout the body)—which limits the readiness for a motor response to task challenges, of which the first and uncontrollable one is gravity itself; impedes the ability to modulate movements (how fast, how hard, etc.); and sacrifices smooth rhythm and coordination.

Another experience shared by many on the spectrum: **digestive disorders**. HANDLE practitioners consider it likely that hypersensitive ears contribute to that, because the jaw is next to the ears. When chewing anything sounds very loud (which it does to hypersensitive ears), we avoid chewing, and thus don't start the digestive process soon enough for the stomach to know what enzymes to create. This is only one simple example of how irregularities in one system can cause irregularities in others. There are typically multiple contributing factors to digestive problems that individual's on the spectrum experience, including dietary influences such as gluten and casein.

A commonality considered vital is **language**, especially related to interpersonal relationships; it is also considered vital because it affects how some professionals gauge intelligence. Producing intelligible and appropriate language is probably the most complex task anyone achieves: It requires oral-motor precision and learned patterns of movement, synchronized with breathing. Each of those three contributors—oral-motor accuracy, kinesthetic memory, and breath control—depends on proprioceptive acuity and functional muscle tone. Remember that auditory issues and low muscle tone recur among many individuals on the spectrum; either or both can limit effective spoken communication. Adding in the need to partner right hemisphere (ideas) with left hemisphere (words and sentence structure) complicates the more "physical" elements significantly.

There is another crucial one (we referred to it at the start): **stress**. When life is difficult—proportional to how challenged anyone feels at any given time—there is an internal experience of distress. For essentially everyone on the autism spectrum, the body/brain/spirit baseline level of stress is very high. Anything added to systems already struggling to create and maintain stability can be overwhelming. "Anything" can mean perfumes, crowds (especially of children), household cleaning products, even medications, and always includes performance and behavioral expectations beyond the person's ability.

Because HANDLE practitioners know that, they understand that a "tantrum" or "meltdown" is actually a call for help, a plea to notice that the stress level has overflowed its container. A word of caution to family members: Try to identify what pushed your loved one beyond endurance—and don't expect it to always be the same thing. It could be noise in high-ceilinged supermarkets; or maybe it was the crowds, or smells, or any combination of these things. Always trust that there *is* a precipitating cause.

Who provides HANDLE services? Where?

The HANDLE Institute in San Rafael, California, confers the credential of Certified HANDLE Practitioner on individuals who have completed (1) a sequence of post-graduate intensive and explicit training programs; (2) a supervised internship, the duration of which is not time-based, but competence-based, and therefore varies in length from nine months to several years; and (3) an exam for which there are no "right" answers, but rather there is engagement of the intern in processing and reasoning from the HANDLE perspective, and to applying neuroscience creatively and always individually. There are also certified HANDLE screeners, but their more-limited training generally does not qualify them to address clients on the autism spectrum.

The practitioners represent diverse backgrounds: There are educators, counselors, occupational therapists, osteopaths, and even a chiropractic neurologist, among others from diverse fields of endeavor. There are practitioners on every continent. Two Canadian provinces have certified practitioners: Ontario and British Columbia. The environment in which HANDLE services occur varies as well but has in common the interpersonal relationship foundation of nonjudgmental respect, and a "physical" manifestation of *the core HANDLE premise: stressed systems do not get stronger*. So each site in which you encounter a HANDLE practitioner will strive to minimize the sensory load. Practitioners even wear only all-natural clothing without dramatic patterns or harsh colors, and no scents. The site limits visual and olfactory distractions. Work surfaces are wood. And you won't find reflective surfaces like mirrors, or dangling mobiles.

What is a HANDLE program?

Although there are slight variations specific to the practitioner and the site, basically, the program consists of a three-part start-up sequence, followed by six about-monthly program review visits.

The start-up sequence:

1. Evaluation

Each client family completes a detailed intake questionnaire prior to the initial appointment. The HANDLE practitioner then provides a comprehensive and sensitive evaluation (employing the copyrighted Learning Foundations Inventory if appropriate) involving interactive tasks; assessment of specific neurodevelopmental functions; and an extensive interview of the client, plus, in some cases, parents and other caregivers, to gather information about particular concerns such as health problems, nutrition, sleep, and pertinent details of the developmental history. The initial evaluation is typically scheduled for two hours, but varies depending on the complexity of the situation and the client's participation. The clock is not a factor!

The HANDLE practitioner observes the individual's response patterns during this unique series of tasks and rapport-building activities. The client's responses are never judged, and do not result in any scores or diagnostic labels. Instead, the responses provide information to help the practitioner see how the body/brain/spirit (whole) system is working. The practitioner analyzes how the client takes in, processes, and uses information. Seemingly perplexing behaviors come together like pieces of a puzzle, as the HANDLE practitioner analyzes both the individual systems and how the systems interact with each other.

Among the functions and systems considered are:

- Olfaction and gustation (smell and taste)
- Tactility and kinesthesia (touch and movement)
- Vestibular functions (balance, proprioception, muscle tone)
- Visual functions, including tracking, convergence, accommodation, and light sensitivity
- Oral motor functions (dental factors, speech articulation)
- Hearing and auditory processing (sequence, syntax, meaning)
- Reflex inhibition and differentiation of movement/response
- Rhythm and timing (includes coordination)
- Lateralization (right-versus-left leader: hand, eye, possibly foot)
- Midline crossing and interhemispheric integration
- Receptive and expressive language skills
- Visual discrimination and memory
- Visual-motor integration
- Visual-spatial processing
- Temporal-spatial organization
- Attentional priorities

2. Instruction: *neurodevelopmental profile and recommended program*

The practitioner assembles the findings of the evaluation into a chart of those interactive and interdependent sensory, motor, and processing systems: what's serving him/her well, and how it does; and what's getting in his/her way, interfering with efficient function. This image is the neurodevelopmental profile. Based on that profile, the practitioner recommends an initial program of seemingly simple activities, each of which is complex neurologically and addresses several aspects of what interferes with the client's ability to satisfy life's demands efficiently. Two examples: a Crazy Straw, used as instructed, supports focused vision, even bowel and bladder continence, as well as the more obvious oral motor skills; face tapping stimulates the trigeminal nerve to integrate all five senses, affecting speech and auditory sensitivity (especially important to folks on the spectrum). Nutritional recommendations may be made, as well as suggestions for environmental or lifestyle changes to improve functioning and reduce stress.

HANDLE routes each person toward his/her full potential with an individualized program of activities that require virtually no special equipment to gently enhance functioning. The client is guided through each activity to help his/her brain-body system process and organize information more efficiently. Each HANDLE program is customized for effective implementation in the client's home or other supportive setting. The program usually requires less than half an hour daily to complete and preferably is not done all at once, or even in a certain order. Some activities may require support from a helper.

The certified HANDLE practitioner gives the client materials as needed to do each activity, including written instructions. Both the assessment and the presentation are recorded, and the client receives a copy as a DVD.

As we said at the outset, among the key distinctions of a HANDLE program is the one principle guiding every kind of activity and other recommendation. It is called "gentle enhancement." The objective of each recommended activity is to provide organized stimulation without producing distress. Weak, disorganized, damaged, or immature systems need to be "gently enhanced." The parent or caregiver is taught to recognize the signs of a stress state change and deal with them swiftly, in a respectful manner; the client learns how to identify how the body conveys its needs, to respect them too. Gently enhanced systems get stronger; stressed systems shut down. It's a near-reflexive way that the brain fulfills its primal directive, namely to keep us safe. Honoring the body's signals of what input it can use and what exceeds its tolerance—at all times—earns from the body a comparable kind of respect: The client stabilizes, to enable him/her to function more efficiently.

3. Fine-tuning follow-up

A week to ten days later the client returns for the practitioner to assure reliable familiarity with everything that was taught: *why* as well as *how* to implement the program independently. During this one- to two-hour appointment, the practitioner watches the client perform all the activities in the program, making corrections or adjustments as needed. Just as importantly, the client is encouraged to give feedback about the program and what was experienced. Often it surprises clients and families that changes have occurred within that first week, and the practitioner asks about those changes. Video recordings made of all clinical sessions provide the client and caregiver a tool for easy reference at home. When in-person visits prove impractical, and Skype contact replaces it (a very distant second best), of course, there's no such DVD.

Program review visits

After approximately one month of the client-family's implementing of the recommendations, they return to the practitioner to determine what changes have occurred due to the neurological reorganization, the creation of neural connections, and/or the kinesthetic learning—and how those changes warrant different activities. Often the initial program establishes prerequisites to higher level challenges. This sequencing logic applies thereafter. That is, as the client implements HANDLE recommendations, changes occur; those changes represent gains in systems that previously interfered with function; now those systems can accept additional challenges, toward full functional interaction with the other systems of the body. Program reviews are usually scheduled every four to six weeks, depending upon client needs. In some circumstances, clients choose to receive off-site program reviews via Skype, and/or e-mail discussion and DVDs.

What changes can you expect from a HANDLE program?

The most frequent report of post-HANDLE behavior changes are "more calm" and "sleeps better." Other gains: toilet training, eye contact, hair washing, balance, manual dexterity, organization, focus, communication skills (both receptive and expressive language), and sociability, including more broad a range of interests and more flexibility in general. Given the vast diversity among clients, there is no way to predict changes precisely. What always happens is a gain in the interactive dynamism of all the sensory-motor and processing systems, and that in turn enables more efficient functioning, which means less stress. With the combination of strengthened sensory-motor interaction with the client's application of the principle of gentle enhancement, it's easy to understand how a reduced stress level generalizes. Less stress clearly looks like a "more calm" life, and can allow the client to sleep better and feel less frustrated; it also often means better digestion, and a stronger immune system, making the client less susceptible to illness. And when the client feels more safe in his/her own skin, a whole world of social opportunities presents itself.

A book about HANDLE

You can find a more extensive explanation of the HANDLE understanding of autism, in *The Fabric of Autism: Weaving the Threads into a Cogent Theory,* by Judith Bluestone.

HOUSTON HOMEOPATHY METHOD FOR AUTISM AND ASDS: SEQUENTIAL HOMEOPATHY AND BEYOND

By Julianne Adams, Lynn Rose Demartini, Cindy L. Griffin, and Lindyl Lanham

Homeopathy Center of Houston
7670 Woodway Dr., Suite 340
Houston, TX 77063
T: 713-366-8700
F: 713-366-8710
www.HomeopathyHouston.com

Homeopathy Center of Minnesota
1660 S. Highway 100, Suite 500
St. Louis Park, MN 55416
T: 1-800-962-2594
F: 1-800-962-5204
www.HomeopathyMinnesota.com.

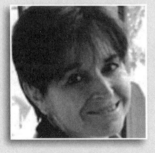

Julianne Adams, DSH-P, BCIH, BA (Psych), NST-CP

Julianne Adams has practiced homeopathy since 2001 and joined Homeopathy Center in 2005. She is also a certified practitioner of Neurostructural Integration Technique. She has successfully guided many children through the HHM to recovery from autism and continues to work with children with mild to severe autism as well as handling general clients outside of autism. Julianne completed numerous practitioner trainings through Defeat Autism Now!® and has studied with Thomas Rau at Paracelsus Biological Medicine Network trainings since 2006. She is board certified in integrative health through the AAIM.

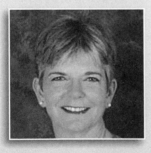

Lynn Rose Demartini, DSH-P, RN, HN-BC, LMT, BCIH, DCN

Lynn Rose Demartini has been a professional sequential homeopath since 2007, and joined Homeopathy Center in 2008. She is also a registered nurse, licensed massage therapist, holds several certifications and diplomas in holistic nursing, and has formally and informally studied nutrition, herbology, and reflexology. She attended practitioner trainings by Defeat Autism Now!® for several years. She is board certified in integrative health and a Diplomate of the College of Nursing through AAIM. Lynn has extensive experience in emergency medicine, having formerly been an EMT and ICU and ER nurse. Under Lynn's homeopathic care, several children have recovered from autism and many more have shown excellent ongoing improvements.

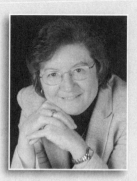

Cindy L. Griffin, DSH-P, DIHom, FBIH, BCIH, DCNT, FAAIM

Cindy Griffin has studied homeopathy since 1994, and has been a professional homeopath since 1998. She is co-owner of Homeopathy Center of Houston and Homeopathy Center of Minnesota and codeveloper of the Houston Homeopathy Method (HHM), a complex method developed and practiced exclusively by Homeopathy Center of Houston. Cindy attended the first practitioner training of Defeat Autism Now! ® in 2003, and attended annual sessions including the advanced practitioners trainings, until the group disbanded. The mother of three adult children, including one who has fully recovered from Asperger's Syndrome through the HHM, Cindy is a Fellow of the British Institute of Homeopathy, a Diplomate of the College of Natural Therapies, a Fellow of the American Association of Integrative Medicine and board certified in integrative health by the American Association of Integrative Medicine (AAIM).

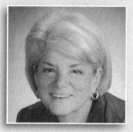

Lindyl Lanham, BS spec Ed, DSH-P, BCIH, DCNT

Lindyl Lanham has been a professional homeopath since 2001. She became co-owner of Homeopathy Center of Houston in 2003 and Homeopathy Center of Minnesota in 2014. She is the codeveloper of the Houston Homeopathy Method. Her work with autism began during college years in the 1970s, then professionally as a special education teacher of multiply and visually challenged children. Her background in special education and Tourette Snydrome spearheaded Homeopathy Center's move to develop a program for children on the autism spectrum. She also attended the first Defeat Autism Now!® beginning with the practitioner training in New Orleans in 2003, through the group's advanced practitioner trainings in San Diego. Lindyl is the mother of a son recovered through HHM from Tourette syndrome. Lindyl holds the Diploma of Sequential Homeopathy-Practitioner, is a Diplomate of the College of Natural Therapies, and is board certified in integrative health by AAIM.

Learning from biomedical research in autism to realize homeopathic solutions, the developers of the Houston Homeopathy Method (HHM) integrate the entire range of homeopathic methodologies to achieve improvements and even full recoveries in children on the autism spectrum. Sequential homeopathy provides the infrastructure to the approach, clearing to the cause of damage done by physical, chemical, medical and emotional traumas. Working through each client's personal history, these traumas are addressed in reverse chronological order with homeopathic remedies appropriate for repairing each impacting event. The Houston Homeopathy Method is a modern application of homeopathic remedies, based on sound homeopathic principles, but updated for the illnesses of toxicity of today's modern world.

History and Model of Homeopathy

For over two centuries homeopathic medicine has brought about recovery from acute and chronic health issues in a rapid, gentle, and permanent way for millions of people worldwide. Prior to the 1920s homeopathy accounted for approximately 25 percent of all medicine practiced in the United States. Today homeopathy is enjoying a resurgence of popularity in North America. It has long been known throughout the world as a therapeutic medical approach, and in many countries homeopathy is recognized as mainstream medicine.

Homeopathy is founded upon the Law of Similars, *Similia similibus curentur*, or "like cures like" Dr. Samuel Hahnemann observed from his experiments with cinchona bark, used as a treatment for malaria, that the effects he experienced from ingesting the bark were similar to the symptoms of malaria. Upon further experimentation, he realized that by inducing a similar "artificial disease" through the use of a tiny and diluted amount of cinchona (a homeopathic remedy) that recovery from malaria could be achieved. As another example, peeling an onion causes the eyes to burn, sting, itch, and water. These same symptoms are relieved by the use of homeopathic *Allium cepa* (red onion) during a cold or allergy attack.

Over time, Hahnemann discovered that even smaller amounts of the original substance as well as even greater dilution achieved greater therapeutic benefit, and that more highly diluted amounts of substances actually were the most therapeutic while doing no harm. Most homeopathic remedies today, made from minerals as well as botanical and biological sources, are considered "micro-doses" or "nano-doses" of the source substance. All of our homeopathic remedies are manufactured in homeopathic pharmaceutical laboratories under FDA scrutiny or international manufacturers which must meet comparable standards under international standards called current Good Manufacturing Practices (cGMP.)

Homeopaths believe:
* Health = wholeness
* True healing is self-healing—living creatures naturally seek balance and health
* Homeopathy's role is to support the re-balancing and healing process

Sequential Homeopathy

Our homeopaths consider current health complaints to be a result of impacts and burdens on the system. Each of these traumas can create a cell-level memory or retain chemicals or biological components that block the ability of the body to reestablish balance or homeostasis. Just as the rings of a tree record wet and dry years, infestations and disease, so the body retains a cell memory record of its impacts, as well as chemical or biological residue. Eventually these traumas weaken the resistance and bring about physiological changes in the body's regulation resulting in illness. The client's personal timeline provides clues to the current illness just as looking at the cross cut of a tree reveals the rings that record its history. By looking at both the current symptoms and the client's chronological history, a roadmap for healing can be developed.

Strongly influenced by the work of Constantine Hering M. D. (1800–1880), the "father of American homeopathy," and author of "Hering's Laws of Direction of Cure," sequential homeopaths focus on his three key principles of natural healing:

- The body heals from top to bottom
- The body heals from innermost to outermost
- The body heals in reverse chronological order

Sequential homeopathy draws its name from the latter principle. Working in reverse chronological order, the sequential homeopath focuses not only on the effects (symptoms) of each trauma in the client's history, but also on helping the body identify and naturally remove or undo the cell level memory of causational impacts in order to allow permanent repair of the damage and restoration of health. Sequential homeopathy uses multiple remedies to guide the body to "return to the scene of the crime," and to address the damage left behind by supporting the resources of the immune system to resist, eliminate, or destroy the offenders. Employing the natural balancing mechanisms of elimination, respiration, and inflammation (heat which will kill bacteria or viruses) the body will return to homeostasis (balance). Once balance is restored, the body can then re-establish wholeness (self-healing).

Sequential homeopathy is unique because it works with the natural laws of healing, supporting the body in the way it was designed to heal itself, like peeling the layers of an onion, one layer at a time. This process results in the deep but manageable release of pathogenic toxins, viruses and bacteria trapped in cells, and gradual reduction of the burdens and demands on the immune system. An individualized program of daily remedies becomes integral to support the elimination processes stirred by the sequential clearing process. In this way the HHM works in concert with the body itself to undo the damage left behind in a workable, natural, systematic manner.

Healing From Vaccine Impacts

Based further on the work of Jean Elmiger, who used homeopathic remedies to "clear" blockages to healing from vaccines, the Houston Homeopathy Method advanced beyond his "sequential therapy." The HHM broadened the use of isopathy (a homeopathic remedy made from an actual pathogen or toxic substance), applying it not only to the elimination of vaccine damage but also to the purging of heavy metals, environmental toxins, drugs, chemicals, and biological pathogens.

At the heart of the Houston Homeopathy Method lies the concept of vaccine injury and its reversal. Whether assessing blame to vaccines' role in autism is controversial or not, parents of children with autism very frequently observe and report that their child regressed significantly after the administration of one or more vaccines. The parents' reports are often confirmed when a specific vaccine or multiple vaccines are cleared homeopathically and old regressive behaviors return briefly. The behaviors normally last a few hours to 2–3 days, and are followed by a fairly immediate, and often dramatic improvement overall. For instance, often when an MMR is cleared, the child will break out with a mild rash on their cheeks for a day, have less appetite, followed within a few days by GI function improvements and broadening of food choices. The body releases not only the toxins and pathogens involved, but the cell memories of the emotions and behaviors from that insult layer. Then the body is able to heal the damage over time, sometimes gradually over weeks or months, other times fairly quickly and dramatically. This phenomenon has been observed repeatedly in hundreds of children who have worked with the Houston Center.

Physical Healing Requires Emotional Healing

For complete healing to occur, the body must heal emotionally as well as physically. When a child has limited or no speech, their trapped emotions can stall the healing process. A stellar point of the HHM is the inclusion of emotional support remedies to help promote emotional processing and release trapped emotions. If a child processes pent up feelings through dreams, artwork, behavior, or tears, the result will typically lead to further improvement. Physical and emotional healing frequently goes hand in hand. Emotional healing plays a key role in the child's current level of comfort as well as long-term recovery. The HHM is the only biomedical research-based autism therapeutic method to offer emotional support without the use of drugs which can bring on unwanted side effects or add to the difficulties and behaviors of autism by stunting or suppressing emotional processing.

Homeopathic Tools of the HHM

Most homeopathic practitioners do not study or accept the research from biomedical model of autism and employ only one single method, such as classical or constitutional homeopathy, CEASE therapy, homotoxicology or sequential homeopathy alone. The Houston homeopaths trained with Defeat Autism Now®, then developed the Houston Homeopathy Method based upon biomedical research learned there, as well as staying up to date with other research such as recent developments in GcMAF. The HHM encompasses and integrates the biomedical knowledge base, addressing the known problems with sequential homeopathy and additional homeopathic tools. These include oligotherapy, gemmotherapy, Cellular Re-Programming Therapy, Cytokine therapy and German Biological Medicine. As new research uncovers more functional problems, genetic snp anomalies, and biomedical disruptions in autism, new combinations of proprietary remedies are developed in ongoing efforts to enhance the efficacy of the HHM by supporting the correction or rebalancing of the problems. These combinations target problems such as dysbiosis, inflammation, pain, OCD, and low ATP production, and offer support for other areas such as Peyer's Patches for intestinal inflammation and the immune system along with various growth and macrophage factors.

What to Expect

Autism is not just one disease or syndrome that presents the same way in all children. There are as many combinations of physical and behavioral symptoms as there are individuals with autism. Individualization of the HHM program is achieved through the individual timeline as well as observations by caregivers that are noted and discussed with the homeopath each month at the consultation. Behaviors or symptoms that arise and their timing will offer important clues to the child's progress and guide the homeopath's next step in the HHM process. The caregiver is trained in what to expect, what to report, and how to handle old problems that can return briefly. While following the general plan of the timeline, occasionally the body may have a different priority that will manifest as unexpected or unusual symptoms. Each client's needs change from month to month, and no two clients will have the same exact experience. Because the consult is based largely on the observations of those who live with the client, consultations are interview style, and thus they can be done in person, via telephone, or by internet video anywhere in the world. Consultations are by appointment. The communication is a give-and-take style, so email consultations are not offered. If excessive problems arise during the interim period, there is a pager to provide after-hours help from one of our homeopaths.

Once the plan is determined for the next monthly interval, the homeopath will craft a package of remedies based on the client's needs. The office staff will individually label each item with the homeopath's instructions and recommendations; it will all be carefully packaged for shipment to the client's home or office, or made available for pick up in the Houston office for local clients.

Results from the HHM

Improvements have been achieved in many areas, including sleep, bedwetting, aggression, headache pain, lower abdominal pain, gastric pain, joint and muscle pain, constipation, diarrhea, speech, cognition, academics, social skills, OCD, stimming, tantrums, hyperactivity, spaciness, rashes, allergies, food sensitivities, and more.

We have seen documented improvements from lab tests* including porphyrin tests of mercury body burden, titers for Hepatitis strains, herpes strains, streptococcus strains, inflammation markers, dysbiosis markers, stool microbiology improvements, behavioral, social and cognitive tests and ATEC scores.

Most importantly, tangible behavioral and physical improvements are noted by parents, teachers, family members, therapists, psychologists, and school diagnosticians. Over 100 children are considered fully recovered by the Homeopathy Center's stringent standards.

Case Examples**

"George"

George had been developing normally until about 1 month after his MMR vaccination at age 12 months. He gradually started to become anxious, shied away from family with whom he previously been affectionate, covered his ears constantly in response to normal sounds, steadily lost his words and eye contact, while tantrums began and intensified. Sleep became fitful and unpredictable. He was diagnosed with PDD-NOS at age 14 months. He had lost all language and would simply stare when asked to do or say anything. He was not potty trained. He began working with HCH a few months later because the parents did not like the idea of pharmaceuticals, and he had previously shown negative reactions to antibiotics. Improvements began. About 3 months into the program improvements began showing, with fewer incidents of running from mom, crying, constipation, and skin rashes. He also improved his sleep patterns. Within 8 months of starting the program, he had regained a few words, stools were improved, he initiated play with friends, and eye contact was normal. Improvements are normally slow and steady rather than dramatic, and George continued to add a few words each month, finally graduating to 4–6 word sentences by 15 months with HCH. In two years, he was potty trained, and very verbal and expressive. His mother commented that he argued with her about everything "because he knows everything better than I do!" At 27 months into the HHM, the school diagnostician removed his diagnosis of PDD, and he entered Kindergarten fully mainstreamed, and without a diagnosis of any kind. Today he is an excellent student in middle school, in several advanced classes, plays on several sports teams, has many friends and enjoys good health. None of his friends or teachers knows he ever had autism. He is described as "chatty, happy and outgoing," making plans for his future in high school sports.

"Jimmy"

At 3 years old, Jimmy had only a few single words, and was not potty trained because he had 6 explosive bowel movements daily. He was a poor sleeper, extremely shy and fearful, and had multiple allergies. He was diagnosed with autism. After one year working with the HHM he was re-evaluated by the same psychologist who had tested him previously. The psychologist said he no longer fit the criteria for autism and pronounced Jimmy recovered. He began mainstream kindergarten in fall of 2013. Jimmy still has more clearing and healing to do in order to complete his timeline, eliminate the remaining allergic responses, and complete his gut healing so that he will no longer need special diets or remedies, but he has made amazing progress in just 1 year.

His mother wrote, "Thank you so much for giving my son back to me. I know Jimmy would not be where he is today without Houston Homeopathy. You are truly amazing."

Summary:

The Houston Homeopathy Method offers a complete alternative drug-free approach to autism's many problems. Its uniqueness is that it is a true stand-alone method integrating multiple homeopathic methodologies, and, unlike any other homeopathic method, it was created on the biomedical model and viewpoint of autism spectrum disorders. Geographical location does not limit clients' ability to avail themselves of the practice via telephone and internet. With four experienced homeopaths, the Homeopathy Center of Houston offers clients an effective, affordable, and non-toxic alternative whether recently diagnosed with autism or for older children who have undergone many other treatments with limited or no success. The HHM can also be an advantage for children sensitive to supplements, drugs or other conventional treatments for autism, because homeopathy is well-tolerated by all.

HOMOTOXICOLOGY AND BEYOND

by Mary Coyle

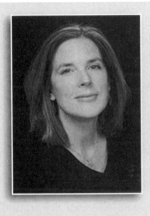

Mary Coyle, DIHom
Real Child Center
1133 Broadway, Rm. 1015
New York, NY 10010
212-255-4490
www.realchildcenter.com

Mary Coyle, DIHom, has been consulting with families of children with autism for over 12 years, and in 2009 she founded the Real Child Center in New York City. She works in collaboration with a number of DAN physicians, neurologists, naturopaths, nutritionists, classical homeopaths, and chiropractors in the surrounding New York area. She received a BSc from the University of Washington, and obtained her diploma in homeopathy in 2000. She has been personally trained by some of the experts in the field, including Jean Elmiger, MD, creator of Sequential Homeopathy and author of *Rediscovering Real Medicine* and German naturopath, Dr. Andreas Marx. Along with her colleague Sandra Stewart, Mary conducted an MPI teleconference entitled "Autism Solutions" and is co-creator of the Stewart-Coyle Holistic Practitioner Course. For two years she hosted an Autism One radio show covering bio-energetic healing, and has presented at LIA, Autism One, and the NAA in New York City.

As more research is devoted to the science of environmental health, toxicology, and epigenetics, vast new insights have been gained as to the effects of toxic exposures on human health, particularly as it relates to our children. Perhaps the question, "Is your child on the autistic spectrum?" might one day be replaced with, "How toxic is your child?"

Analyzing and addressing the impact of toxins on human health were the passions of Germany physician Dr. Hans-Heinrich Reckeweg, who developed the theory of homotoxicology over 60 years ago. Through integrating two well-established healing systems, the principles of homeopathy (like cures like) and medical science, Reckeweg created a systematic approach designed to stimulate the body's own defense mechanism of self-healing and self-regulation.

Derived from the Greek, "homo" meaning man, "toxico" meaning toxin, and "logy," meaning study, homotoxicology is the study of toxins on humans. Functioning as a holistic approach, homotoxicology does not merely focus on one particular pathogen or toxic metal. Instead, it systemically and holistically supports the body's own physiologically, enabling it to effectively manage its own pathology.

TOXINS AND HOW THEY RELATE TO THE CHILD WITH AUTISM

A national human adipose tissue study determined that all humans carry a toxic body burden of at least 250 chemicals. No matter how pristine a lifestyle *we think* we're living, there's simply no way of escaping them. Equally disturbing, this toxic load doesn't just sit quietly in our biological terrain. Scientific studies have proven that a portion of that toxic load is passed-down trans-generationally from mother to fetus, and is then further expressed through breast milk. As one out of every two American children is now diagnosed with a chronic illness, many questions as to the etiology of this escalating health crisis continue to remain unanswered.

TRAITS VS SYNDROMES

Scientists who research trends in our wildlife identify and observe *traits* such as IQ decrements, behavior aberrations, and physical malformations. However, when it comes to investigating human health, the model shifts to *syndromes,* which are then translated into diseases or disorders, such as multiple sclerosis, asthma, diabetes, and autism. Identifying syndromes simplifies and standardizes illnesses to assist the medical community in determining the most appropriate pharmaceutical or surgical intervention. But the rise in autism, and the comorbidity many share, such as gut dysbiosis, brain inflammation, food sensitivies, and immune dysfunction, are pushing the scientific community beyond this over-simplified syndrome/pharmaceutical model.

BEGINNING THE JOURNEY OF HOMOTOXICOLOGY

Homotoxicology approaches the various stages of health as it relate to the body's ability, or inability, to remove offending toxins, and views healing as a dynamic and active function. Reckeweg views disease as three main processes:

1. Excretion of the toxin: diarrhea, skin eruptions, mucus, fever, coughs
2. Deposition (deposits) of the toxins: warts, hemorrhoids, benign cysts, endometriosis

3.   Degeneration through the actions of the toxins: autism, diabetes, asthma, lupus, neoplasms

Reckeweg considered disease as the body's *meaningful* biological response to homotoxins and its attempt to actively remove them. He refers to toxins as homotoxins (toxins derived from the body itself, environmental pollution, or pharmaceutical interventions). The primary focus of his approach is determining of the cause (homotoxins) distressing the biological system, and not just reacting to the symptoms.

TABLE OF HOMOTOXICOSIS

Essential to the effectiveness of homotoxicology is the unblocking of the enzymatic system. Enzymes act as catalysts for the mobilization and excretion of the toxins. To avoid confusing a healing reaction for a disease state, Dr. Reckeweg developed the Six Phases table. This table functions as a guide to understanding the various psychological and physiological changes that may occur during the process of removing the toxins.

The humoral phases consist of excretion, inflammation, and deposition. These occur when the enzymes have remained intact, enabling the progression towards the natural removal of toxins (termed "regressive vicariation") through the various excretion pathways. The toxins have not yet reached a saturation point and remain in the extracellular tissues. The primary pathways of elimination include the skin, liver, kidney, intestines, mucus membranes, and lymphatic system. The secondary pathways include the nose, lungs, stomach, genitals, bladder, and pancreas.

The cellular phases consist of impregnation, degeneration, and neoplasm. These occur when damage has been done to the enzymatic system, and therefore, the toxins cannot be completely eliminated, leading to the development of deterioration (termed "progressive vicariation"). A saturation point of the toxin(s) has been reached, and the toxins have begun penetrating the cells.

THE CHILD WITH AUTISM AND THE TABLE OF HOMOTOXICOSIS

It's not uncommon to hear parents remark that their child with autism rarely mounts a fever, or that their skin is pale and translucent, even during the summer months; that their eyes are dull with dark circles underneath, and the pupils are often dilated (wired but tired); and that their bowel movements are embedded with undigested food, or are very hard. Therefore, according to Reckeweg's table, the child with autism might fall somewhere between the impregnation and degeneration phases. This is no surprise, as recent research has determined that a sub-population of ASD children suffer from an atypical form of mitochondrial function related to environmental toxins. A reduction in cellular metabolism could hinder the body from efficiently performing necessary metabolic functions, leading to a host of health problems. In short, it would appear that there's just not enough tiger in the ASD child's tank.

THE FLOW SYSTEM AND THE CHILD WITH AUTISM

At the turn of the century, biologist Ludwig Von Bertalanffy described every living system (man, bird, slug) as systems of flowing elements, designed to gain and maintain balance. According to the tenets of homotoxicology, substances that disrupt the flow system (homotoxins) will inevitably cause disease. Reckeweg stated that "Illness is the expression of the action of the greater defense system against homotoxins, or the organism's attempt to compensate for the damage caused by homotoxins." How the body effectively, or ineffectively, responds to these homotoxins relates back to disturbances in the flow system. Reckeweg developed his table to monitor these reactions.

If the "flow system" is severely blocked, sufficient energy production in the form of ATP is often negatively affected, resulting in metabolic acidosis. An acidic biological milieu acts as a perfect breeding ground for the proliferation of microorganisms—further damaging the terrain. Toxic waste products and microforms poison the body, increasing acidity. This compromised system enables microorganisms to become even more opportunistic, further reducing celluar energy and increasing inflammation. It is a vicious cycle.

HOMOTOXICOLOGICAL REMEDIES

Remedies utilized in homotoxicology are designed to activate what Reckeweg called the "greater defense system." This is a collective biological response to react, neutralize, and eliminate homotoxins. Drainage remedies are a staple in this model of healing and are designed to drain major organs, such as the liver, kidneys, lymph nodes, adrenal glands, and colon. Homeopathic cellular supports products are often employed to supply vitality and stimulate organ systems and immune function. Low-potency homeopathic homochords, specifically geared to assist the body's ability to remove toxins such as heavy metal, pesticides, chemicals, fungus, yeast, and parasites, are also common remedy tools applied in homotoxicology. In essence, the goal of homotoxicology is to assist the body's physiology to move the toxins out—without negatively impacting the active immune—as well as to facilitate more efficient blood flow, which instigates faster healing.

AND BEYOND....

Functioning as the template, and working in the systematic fashion, homotoxicology can incorporate other health strategies that support the biological terrain into its matrix to maximize therapeutic results. Since most ASD children, according to Reckweg's table, would fall under the degeneration phase, practitioners of homotoxicology consider it wise to start off slowly before instituting more aggressive detoxification measures. This is accomplished first through proper drainage of the eliminative pathways and concentrating on supplying the body with adequate cellular energy and support. Laser treatments can be an excellent method of increasing that much needed energy for cellular repair. Rebuilding with proper supplementation and nutritionals are also essential first steps.

TRACKING PROGRESS

What are some things to look for as your child begins to rebound in a positive direction through Reckeweg's table? Some parents reported better eye contact; improved receptive and expressive language; happier and greater interest in life and new things; greater comfort in the child's own skin; more integration and the feeling of grounding; longer and more deep sleep; improved bowel movements; tans and/or sunburns in the summer; catching the family cold or flu (garbage in, garbage out); more physical, emotional, and cognitive connections; the ability to gain weight and height; and better gross and fine motor skills. Some have even remarked that their child no longer seems to be functioning in "survival mode," is not as stressed-out out, and is therefore more available to learn. Lab tests are also excellent vehicles for tracking and verifying these improvements.

THE EVIDENCE

Homeopathy might best be understood as it relates to the concept of hormesis. This term corresponds to a biphasic dose response to an environmental stimulant. For example, a low-dose stimulation promotes a beneficial effect, but a high dose of the same stimulant produces an inhibitory or deleterious effect. Homeopathic remedies are designed to produce a beneficial effect through this low dose stimulation. The method of creating a homeopathic remedy is through diluting a substance in an iterative fashion, followed by vigorous shaking between each dilution. This process is referred to as "dynamization." The energized substance, in theory, acts as a signal, stimulating the body's own system to react.

One of the more notable articles includes "Critical Review and Meta-Analysis of Serial Agitated Dilutions in Experimental Toxicology," which states that "Four of five outcomes meeting quality and comparability criteria for meta-analysis showed positive effects from SAD preparations" (SAD being serially agitated dilutions). Authors include Dr. Wayne B. Jonas, former director of the Office of Alternative Medicine at the National Institutes of Health.

WHERE WOULD HOMOTOXICIOLOGY FIT INTO YOUR ASD CHILD'S PLAN?

I consider homotoxicology analogous to a degreasing agent. Addressing cellular toxicity is like taking the grease off cellular walls to enable subsequent therapies, such as speech, OT, and ABA, to stick that much better. One parent of a recovered child made the comment that homotoxicology kick-started her child's garbage disposal, and he began "detoxing autism—one bowel movement at a time."

LIVING ENERGY: USING THERAPEUTIC GRADE ESSENTIAL OILS IN THE TREATMENT OF AUTISM

By Dr. Shawn K. Centers

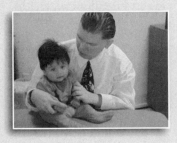

Shawn K. Centers, DO, FACOP

Shawn K. Centers, DO, FACOP, clinical director of the Osteopathic Center for Children & Families in San Diego, California, is a pediatrician and internationally known expert on osteopathic pediatrics, nutrition, and natural medicines as they apply to children. Dr. Centers has worked for the last 10 years as a staff pediatrician and osteopathic manipulation practitioner at the Osteopathic Center for Children & Families. Prior to this, Dr. Centers served as the pediatric chief resident for the Children's Hospital of New Jersey in Livingston, New Jersey, where he was very active in developing and integrating osteopathic principles into the educational program for residents and medical students. www.osteopathiccenter.org.

Background

Essential oils have been used therapeutically for thousands of years. In fact, many believe they were the world's first medicine. My own experience with the therapeutic uses of essential oils began a little over a decade ago. At that time, a patient I was treating had what was called by D. Gary Young, the dynamic and sometimes controversial founder of the essential oil movement in the United States, an "awakening." I will have more to say about that encounter shortly.

As a physician, integrative medicine practitioner, and herbalist, I was vaguely familiar with essential oils. Having studied with the late herbalist Dr. John Christopher, I learned that essential oils were volatile, aromatic compounds usually distilled or extracted from herbs or plants. I knew that essential oils had strong aromas, and they sometimes could be used to confuse the body's pain mechanism, relieving headaches and relaxing tight muscles. In medical school, I learned about the use of smell to stimulate the brain in cases of traumatic brain injury or coma. There were dozens of case reports describing how certain smells, such as cinnamon or lemon, had triggered comatose patients to awaken from their coma. Although doctors still did not really understand the effect of smell on comatose patients, the use of inhaled scents had become a standard therapeutic intervention in brain injury hospitals.

In my early years of practice, I toyed with essential oils, primarily utilizing the therapeutic benefits of their aroma. Drawing on what I had learned in medical school, I used the scents of mint, cinnamon, lavender, and other oils to stimulate the olfactory sense in children who had suffered from traumatic brain injury. However, I stopped the practice when one of my patients presented to the office with what appeared to be a second-degree burn with redness and blistering. The patient's mother had purchased an essential oil of lavender at the local health food store and had dowsed her child's neck and back with the oil, thinking to augment the office treatment. The fact that the child sustained a burn from what was labeled an "essential oil of lavender" is quite ironic since there are a number of case reports documenting the effectiveness of lavender essential oil in the treatment of severe burns. I will address this issue a little later. Concerned about further burns and possible allergic reactions, I followed the Hippocratic admonition to "first do no harm" and eliminated essential oils from my practice.

My next experience with essential oils came a year or so later when an adult patient came in for a routine osteopathic treatment and declared that she had discovered an amazing cure for a lifetime of depression and anxiety. She reported that after using a combination of essential oils obtained from a network marketing company, she had weaned herself from pharmaceutical drugs and was cured. Although the woman was enthusiastic and did not appear depressed, her claims seemed less than plausible to me. I instead attributed her extreme enthusiasm to the manic phase of a bipolar personality disorder. My leeriness grew when the woman wanted to sign me up to share the dream through the vehicle of network marketing. However, I had to admit that her brand of essential oils had a different feeling and scent than some of the others I had experienced. They also had intriguing names such as Valor and Joy. Nonetheless, I remained unconvinced at that time. (When I recently spoke with this patient, however, she reported that she continues to be free of depression and uses an essential oil regimen daily.)

Another year or so later, an older student whose experience I respected and valued began volunteering in our practice. She had recently finished all the prerequisites for medical school, intending to pursue a career in osteopathic medicine. At the time, she had already worked in the medical field as a holistic health practitioner for more than 10 years. I considered her a knowledgeable and accomplished healer and a dedicated student. One day during one of our discussions, she told me about her experiences with essential oils. Several of her patients with chronic illnesses such as fibromyalgia, depression, and mental disorders had made remarkable improvements after adding essential oils to their treatment regimens. I flashed back to the patient who had credited essential oils with healing her depression. The student also explained that many of the products labeled as essential oils in this country are actually adulterated, chemical look-alikes. This fact clarified why an oil purported to be successful for use with burns resulted in a burn to the patient mentioned earlier.

The student explained that contamination and adulteration were well-known problems with lavender oil especially. For example, the largest manufacturer of personal care products in the United States uses more lavender oil per year in its products than there are lavender plants on the planet. Obviously, there must be something more in the common ingredient "lavender oil" than just the essential oil derived from the lavender plant *(Lavandula angustifolia)*.

In fact, most of what is labeled as natural lavender oil in the US does not contain a single drop of pure lavender oil. Instead, most "lavender oil" is actually chemically altered lavandin *(Lavandula x intermedia)*, lavender oil's cheaper hybrid cousin. Lavandin is known to contain a high concentration of camphor, which is likely the cause of the burns frequently reported in connection with lavandin oil use. Lavandin is imported primarily from Russia, China, and Tasmania and typically is laden with petrochemical-based insecticides and pesticides. In addition, because lavandin on its own has a sour smell, synthetic linalyl acetate is added to make the oil smell sweeter. The mixture is then cut with colorless and odorless petrochemical solvents such as phthalates and propylene glycol. These synthetic lavender oils can be found in many products, including shampoos, deodorants, and even toothpastes.

Synthetic linalyl acetate, phthalates, and the petrochemicals found in pesticides all serve as endocrine disruptors. There have been several case reports of adulterated lavender-oil-containing hair gels and shampoos causing abnormal breast development in prepubertal boys. Some research suggests, moreover, that endocrine disruptors may play an inhibitory role in the elimination of heavy metals such as mercury (which is in and of itself an endocrine disruptor). Products containing synthetic lavender oil thus should be of particular concern to those involved with autism.

In the European Union, essential oil producers adhere to guidelines set out by the French Association for Standardization *(Association française de normalisation* or AFNOR) and the International Organization for Standardization (ISO). In the US, however, there is no regulation of essential oils. Therefore, use of therapeutic grade essential oils is crucial.

After the student volunteer and I spoke about essential oils, she began bringing one or two of the oils with her each time she volunteered and later brought her entire kit of about 150 different oils. We began diffusing oils in our treatment room, applied them topically, or simply had children smell them before or after their treatments. We noticed that certain oils seemed to enhance the osteopathic treatment, while others seemed to open up the child's energy pathways, and still others seemed to constrict or focus the body's energy on certain areas. We experimented with using recommendations from available texts to select oils related to each child's inherent need. We also experimented with having the child select the oil they wanted from my volunteer's full kit. Interestingly, the oil that the child randomly or intuitively selected often was either the exact oil indicated by our books for their particular complaints or the exact opposite of the oil indicated for their complaints.

Turning Point: An Awakening

It was by using this random selection method that I began to understand the true power inherent in essential oils. A 9-year-old boy came in one Saturday for a sick visit, presenting with a low-grade fever and a mild cough. Although I had never seen him before, he had been my partner's patient for several years. I examined him and did some osteopathic manipulation to help with his cold symptoms. The child remained quiet throughout the treatment. Toward the end of the treatment, I asked him to select one of the essential oils from the kit. The child quietly looked at several of the oils and selected a bottle labeled rose *(Rosa damascena),* which happened to be among the rarest, most expensive, and most difficult-to-obtain oils in the kit. The child opened the bottle and sprinkled a few drops of the oil on his hands, sniffed it, and took several deep, exaggerated breaths. He then said that the oil made him feel much better, adding that he liked it and wanted more. I sprinkled a few more drops on his hand. I then sent the boy on his way, giving his parents some instructions and telling them to contact the office if he did not get better.

Although I had noticed a subtle but distinguishable change in the boy's countenance after using the oil, the change appeared to go unnoticed by the parents. Whereas the child seemed to like the essential oil treatment, the parents seemed surprised by it and left saying very little. Because essential oils were not as popular then as they are today, I assumed that they found the essential oil component of the treatment unusual. My partner (this family's usual provider) was a homeopath, and her patients were, for the most part, unfamiliar with herbs and essential oils. I therefore expected to hear complaints about my use of essential oils from my partner after the family's follow-up visit.

First thing Monday morning, however, my office told me that the parents of the Saturday patient had called with questions about some kind of oil therapy. The office staff had no idea what the parents were talking about since essential oils were not yet a routine part of my treatment approach. When I reluctantly returned the call, expecting to hear complaints, the mother had a long string of questions. What was the oil treatment I used? What did the oil do? How did it work? Where could she get it? I was surprised and, furthermore, did not have answers for most of her questions. I had no idea where the oils were from or how to purchase them, and I had only an elementary understanding of how they worked or if they worked at all. When I asked the mother why she wanted this information, she took a deep breath and told me that her son had a type of autism. Before using the oils in my office, he had not spoken in over five years.

I, like the mother, was stunned. Having no immediate medical explanation for the response apparently exhibited by this child, I did an Internet search for medical research, case reports, or experiences with essential oils. I pretty much came up empty-handed, finding just one distributor's website that mentioned scientific studies on the brand of essential oils contained in my volunteer's kit. However, the website provided no information that would account for the dramatic response seen in our patient.

When I called the telephone number listed on the website, I was referred to the parent company that manufactured the oils. Several hours later, the company's president was on the phone explaining that essential oils were powerful healing tools. He said that using essential oils to heal was not so much about the aromas they produced or the plants they originated from but about the way that their energy signature interacts with the body. He explained that the energy signature of essential oils is produced by molecules found in the plant oil, including specific molecules such as terpenes and sesquiterpenes, which produce frequencies of energy that raise the vibration of the body. He described the body as a living energy field that, in some individuals, becomes damaged or "fractured." When the body is presented with the appropriate energy field—in the form of an essential oil—the fracture seals and the body's vibration increases. This executive reported that he had worked with technology (developed at Eastern Washington University in Cheney, Washington) that attempted to measure this energy field and demonstrate how application of essential oils changed the field within minutes.

In the case of the boy seen in my office, clearly something in the energy signature of the oil exactly matched his energy deficiency signature. In essence, the oil had sealed the fracture in his energy field. The company president did not find this surprising because he had imported the *Rosa damascena* oil from a region in Turkey where the energy frequency was the highest of any oil the company had ever tested. Interestingly, only the oil from this particular region had the high energy signature. He emphasized that it was the energy frequencies produced by the molecules distilled from plants that had such unique qualities.

I learned that while chemists have been able to duplicate plant aromas, it is impossible to duplicate the molecules found exclusively in the plants' essential oils. Moreover, if the oils are not distilled long enough (or for too long), if too much pressure is used, or if they are heated improperly, the special healing molecules in the oils are lost. According to this executive, most of the oils available commercially are mixed with synthetic chemicals or solvents; these adulterations greatly damage the molecules, making them useless for therapeutic purposes. Truly therapeutic grade essential oils must be carefully distilled under low heat and pressure from organically grown plants. By allowing the healing molecules to be preserved, the oils retain what this man called "living energy." The only way to know if the oils have these healing molecules, however, is to subject samples to gas chromatography and mass spectrometry analysis, which was standard practice for this company. This company followed and exceeded the standards set by AFNOR.

Rediscovering Essential Oils

As I learned more, I found that, in fact, thousands of studies have been conducted showing the efficacy of essential oils in treating everything from depression to the most virulent strains of methicillin-resistant *Staphylococcus aureus* (MRSA). I also learned about the work of D. Gary Young, a self-taught naturopath, botanist, archeologist, agricultural expert, inventor, farmer, and healer. Called a fraud and "snake oil salesman" by some, Young's work has been nevertheless endorsed by Dr. Terry Friedman, one of the founders of the American Holistic Medical Association, and by Dr. Ronald Lawrence, professor at the University of California, Los Angeles (UCLA). Both are well-known and respected experts in complementary and alternative medicine.

Young pioneered the medical use of essential oils in the United States and changed their use around the world after sustaining a crippling and near fatal logging accident in the Canadian wilderness in the early 1970s at the age of 24. Crediting the recovery of his ability to walk to the use of essential oils, Young set out on a course of self-directed study across six continents to learn about and understand the power inherent in the oils. In Egypt, he studied frankincense with Dr. Radwan Farag, biochemistry expert at Cairo University, and went on to learn about essential oil manufacture and distillation in Israel, Turkey, and Oman. In France in the early 1990s, Young rediscovered a little known and unique system of French medicine, *la médicine aromatique*, in which French medical doctors prescribed oral administration of essential oils to treat various medical conditions. While in France, Young also studied with Dr. Jean Lapraz and Dr. Daniel Penoel, recognized authorities of aromatic medicine.

Young subsequently brought many of these experts to the United States to conduct seminars and conferences, raising awareness of the value of essential oils as a healing modality. More importantly, he pioneered a unique form of holistic medical therapy that combines principles and techniques from French aromatic medicine, German and British aromatherapy, Tibetan and Chinese medicine, Native American lore, and Western herbology. This system uses essential oils to treat (1) *the mind and emotions* (by stimulating brain pathways that recall and release negative emotional patterns), (2) *the body* (by ingestion, massage, and inhalation of the oils), and (3) *disrupted energy patterns* in the body (by finding oils with energy patterns that match the deficiencies found in the patient).

Essential Oils as Carrier Oils

Essential oils have the unique ability to diffuse across cell membranes; therefore, they can act as carriers for other substances such as herbs or nutrients. In my own practice, I first explored essential oil supplementation around 2003. I noticed that when added to nutraceuticals (foods or food products that provide health or medical benefits), the oils greatly enhanced the effect of individual herbs or nutrients. One supplement I prescribed contained *Lycium barbarum*, reishi, zinc, melatonin, and orange essential oil, among other ingredients. The orange essential oil is composed of over 90% D-limonene (a component of the oil extracted from citrus rind). D-limonene, a powerful solvent of petrochemicals that is also known for its anti-tumor effects and uses in treating gastroesophageal reflux, makes an excellent carrier for nutrients.

Many children with autism, as well as those suffering from symptoms of attention-deficit/hyperactivity disorder (ADHD), have been found to have low melatonin levels, which corresponds with sleep disturbances and hyperexcitability. In the past, when I had tried using melatonin alone, many patients showed no effect from supplementation even after baseline testing identified low initial melatonin levels. However, when I began to use the melatonin supplement with the orange essential oil carrier, I noticed that children who had not previously responded to melatonin therapy began to respond. Parents of children with ADHD reported that not only did their children's sleep improve, but their ADHD symptoms also improved and in some cases disappeared. Moreover, when the supplement was given for a period of time (6-12 months), I frequently could wean the child off it quite easily; the child's sleep patterns and melatonin levels remained in the normal ranges, and the symptoms did not reappear.

Although these experiences helped me realize that supplements enhanced with essential oils greatly benefited my patients, I did not fully realize how significant the benefits were until 2005 when the enhanced melatonin supplement was temporarily unavailable. Our office received hundreds of calls daily for about six weeks until the supplement again became available. When I spoke to parents, many of whom had children with autism, each testified to the powerful and beneficial effect they had noticed since their child began using the supplement.

Essential Oils and Detoxification

Essential oil enhanced supplementation is powerful. However, direct ingestion of essential oils themselves can have an even more potent effect. When ingested, the molecules in essential oils can have various effects. Their lipophilic nature allows them to diffuse throughout the bloodstream, easily cross cell membranes, and cross the blood-brain barrier. The various molecules in the oils may stimulate antibody production, increase production of neurotransmitters, and interact with hormones and enzymes.

In 2003, D. Gary Young reported using an essential oil combination of *Helichrysm*, celery seed oil, and *Ledum* to detoxify and repair liver damage. Both *Helichrysm* oil and celery seed oil are on the generally recognized as safe (GRAS) list, and *Ledum* has been used safely for centuries in the form of Labrador tea. Subsequently, clinicians at Young's US and Ecuador clinics noticed that this combination could also be powerful and effective in chelating mercury from the body. Many essential oils have the ability to act as natural chelators, binding heavy metals and allowing them to be harmlessly excreted from the body. In addition, very few available substances other than essential oils are capable of neutralizing petrochemical-based toxins.

Case Study

To understand how essential oils are used in practice, it is worth describing one of my cases at some length.

AF was a three-year-old white male who presented with a significant medical history of developmental delay, loss of language, and elevated serum mercury levels. The child had received a formal diagnosis of moderate-to-severe autism at the age of 2 years and 9 months at the local children's hospital. He spoke at most 1-2 words (infrequently and inconsistently), was frequently lethargic, was sensitive to certain sound frequencies, and had difficulty in motor planning (such as catching or throwing a ball). He also had a history of birth trauma, with an unsuccessful occiput posterior (sunny side up) delivery that had resulted in an emergency Caesarean section and marked head molding and plagiocephaly.

The boy had experienced fevers over 104 and severe flu-like symptoms on three separate occasions after being vaccinated. His pediatrician dismissed these reactions as "unexplained viruses" that were unrelated to the vaccines. The pediatrician had run serum mercury levels to appease what he termed the mother's "irrational and hypervigilant concern" over possible mercury exposure secondary to immunization and its connection to the child's autism diagnosis. Because serum blood levels are the least likely tissue to display elevated levels of mercury, the pediatrician was at a loss when a series of blood tests showed elevated blood levels of mercury. The child was referred to a toxicologist who told the parents that there was no relationship between autism and mercury. Suggesting that the child's mercury levels were high because he likely consumed too much fish, he recommended that they halt fish consumption. However, the child did not eat fish in any form. Having heard that some physicians were reporting success with children with mercury toxicity via use of DMSA (a standard sulfur-based chelating drug approved by the FDA for treatment of lead toxicity), the parents consulted with a physician conversant in this protocol. During the first two attempts of DMSA use, however, the child became extremely ill with high fevers, flu-like symptoms, and worsening of behavior. After the second chelation attempt, the parents discontinued treatment and came to my office.*

At the time of consultation with my office, the child was eating a gluten-free/casein-free (GF/CF) diet, using topical glutathione, and taking a broad spectrum probiotic, enzymes, a nutrient support formula, buffered magnesium, and cod liver oil. All supplements had been obtained from a nutraceutical company preferred by many families touched by an autism diagnosis. Because the cod liver oil (which was also third-party tested for heavy metal contamination) had been started after the blood mercury levels were obtained, it was unlikely to be related to the elevated heavy metals.

I recommended osteopathic manipulation to the cranial sacral area to correct the cranial soft tissue injury caused by his birth. I also used topical applications of essential oils to stimulate the nerve pathways and address lower extremity hypotonia. In addition, because heavy metals seemed to be playing an important role, I decided to decrease the toxic heavy metal load by using the essential oil protocol suggested by D. Gary Young. To minimize possible side effects and better observe the effects of the essential oil treatment, I administered each round of essential oil chelation therapy for a 3-day period and then waited 11 days before beginning the next round of treatment. I started with a small test dose of 1 to 2 drops; once I determined that the dose was well tolerated, I increased the dose to 5-7 drops three times a day (during the 3-day chelation rounds) in a juice made from freshly squeezed lemons and agave nectar.

I obtained a standard metabolic profile, a complete blood count, and a liver function panel during every third 3-day chelation round. The laboratory values remained normal throughout the treatment. When I assessed urine toxicology for heavy metals, it revealed a marked increase in heavy metal excretion in the moderate toxic range (values similar to those that would be expected with DMSA chelation) (see Figures 1-3). However, unlike with the DMSA, the patient exhibited few side effects. The mother noticed that the child seemed slightly more irritable on the chelation days but also

---

* Editor's note: Many children, including some who have significantly improved or recovered, have benefited from this form of treatment. Please discuss your child's unique physiology and appropriate options with your child's treating physician.

Figure 1.

Initial urine toxicology showing elevated mercury level

POTENTIALLY TOXIC METALS					
METALS	RESULT µg/g CREAT	REFERENCE RANGE	WITHIN REFERENCE RANGE	ELEVATED	VERY ELEVATED
Aluminium	< dl	< 100			
Antimony	< dl	< 2			
Arsenic	24	< 200			
Beryllium	< dl	< 0.6			
Bismuth	< dl	< 20			
Cadmium	0.3	< 3			
Lead	< dl	< 5			
Mercury	11	< 5			
Nickel	0.4	< 20			
Platinum	< dl	< 1			
Thallium	0.2	< 1.1			
Thorium	< dl	< 1			
Tin	0.3	< 20			
Tungsten	0.2	< 2			
Uranium	< dl	< 0.3			

Figure 2.

Heavy metal screen six months after initiation of essential oil therapy

POTENTIALLY TOXIC ELEMENTS			PERCENTILE	
TOXIC ELEMENTS	RESULT µg/g	REFERENCE RANGE	68th	95th
Aluminium	7.1	< 8.0		
Antimony	0.041	< 0.066		
Arsenic	0.045	< 0.080		
Beryllium	<0.01	< 0.020		
Bismuth	0.089	< 0.13		
Cadmium	0.13	< 0.15		
Lead	0.45	< 1.0		
Mercury	0.06	< 0.40		
Platinum	< 0.003	< 0.005		
Thallium	< 0.001	< 0.010		
Thorium	< 0.001	< 0.005		
Uranium	0.063	< 0.060		
Nickel	0.33	< 0.40		
Silver	1.5	< 0.20		
Tin	0.13	< 0.30		
Titanium	0.68	< 1.0		
Total Toxic Representation				

Figure 3.

Heavy metal screen one year after initiation of essential oil therapy, showing an increase in excretion of neurotoxic aluminum

POTENTIALLY TOXIC ELEMENTS				
TOXIC ELEMENTS	RESULT μg/g	REFERENCE RANGE	PERCENTILE 68th	95th
Aluminium	26	< 8.0		
Antimony	0.042	< 0.066		
Arsenic	0.082	< 0.080		
Beryllium	< 0.01	< 0.020		
Bismuth	0.25	< 0.13		
Cadmium	0.082	< 0.15		
Lead	0.45	< 1.0		
Mercury	0.08	< 0.40		
Platinum	< 0.003	< 0.005		
Thallium	< 0.001	< 0.010		
Thorium	< 0.001	< 0.005		
Uranium	0.18	< 0.060		
Nickel	0.07	< 0.40		
Silver	0.15	< 0.20		
Tin	0.22	< 0.30		
Titanium	0.83	< 1.0		
Total Toxic Representation				

noted marked improvement in the boy's concentration, focus, and language. During the 3 days of the second round of essential oil treatment, the patient said his first 3-word sentence. Within six months, the child's vocabulary had increased to over 200 words.

At this juncture, it may be helpful to describe the most primitive part of the brain, the limbic or reptilian brain. The limbic system is made up of the hippocampus, amygdala, anterior thalamic nuclei, septum, limbic cortex, and fornix. These areas are involved in long-term memory storage and also process and interpret emotional input and the fight-or-flight response. At the time of birth, the amygdala is fully developed and functioning (the other structures that make up the limbic system, such as the hippocampus, do not develop until the age of 3). Thus, the fight-or-flight response is active even at birth, allowing extreme emotions to be processed and stored, including such emotions as horror, fear of death, and physical pain or trauma.

Research by perinatal psychologists suggests that birth trauma can result in later neurological and psychiatric conditions, including addictive personality disorder, schizophrenia, and autism and may even influence criminality. More recently, neuroscientists have examined size or volume changes in the limbic system. For example, increases in amygdala size have been found in children with an early history of trauma, including both birth trauma and neglect. To explain this, researchers have theorized that amygdala volume increases as a protective mechanism following trauma.

Increased amygdala size has also been observed in children with autism in numerous studies, including a study at the University of North Carolina that found that children with autism had a 13% increase in amygdala size compared with controls.

The olfactory sense is the only one of the five senses that has a direct neural pathway to the limbic system. Research done by New York University confirms that the sense of smell is one of the few avenues available to directly stimulate the amygdala and release deep emotional trauma. Stimulating the olfactory pathways with an essential oil application is believed to open up the neural pathways of emotion. By placing the body in the original position of injury using osteopathic techniques and presenting the amygdala with specific novel fragrances, the brain is able to process and release old trauma.

During osteopathic treatment with the three-year-old boy, I perceived a sense of deep-seated fear and loss as well as a sense that life was a struggle and that the boy was apprehensive about interacting with the outside world. I viewed this as a form of the "death urge" described in the work of Leonard Orr (rebirthing-breathwork practitioner) and French obstetrician Frederick Leboyer (author of *Birth Without Violence*). I speculated that deep-seated apprehension triggered by his birth difficulties and subsequent C-section was preventing the child from expressing his true nature and effectively interacting with his surroundings. To address this trauma, therefore, I applied essential oils topically to reflex pathways that are involved in emotional trauma. In addition, I placed therapeutic grade essential oils in a glass apparatus attached to a standard nebulizer (as used in asthma treatment) and diffused the oils during the osteopathic treatments. Thirdly, I instructed the parents to apply specific essential oils to the child at home to reinforce the office treatment. Applying essential oils in the home is a nonintrusive way of helping the family release their own accumulated trauma. In such cases, I generally assume that where a child has experienced trauma, the parents also have experienced trauma and will benefit from essential oil treatment (for example, the trauma of receiving an autism diagnosis). If there are siblings in the home, I additionally recommend that the parents apply oils to the siblings.

By the time my patient was 5 years old and had undergone 2 years of essential oil based therapy, he had made significant progress (see Figure 4). He had regained a vocabulary close to his peer group and was mainstreamed with an aide into a regular classroom. At age 6, he was re-evaluated, and no signs of autism were observed. At the age of 7, he entered a new school. The parents purposely withheld the records from the prior school, and the teachers had no knowledge of his history of autism. He performed at grade level and, by fifth grade, was on the honor roll. He excelled in both academics and sports and received a number of taekwondo awards. According to his teachers, he was one of the most well-liked children in his class and exhibited unusual and extraordinary empathy with his peers, especially socially slower peers and those with disabilities.

I recently spoke with the child as part of a yearly follow-up visit. He had no memory of his early medical diagnosis or the intensive aromatic therapy he had received. Although the parents have discontinued medical supplementation, the mother reported that they continue to use some essential oils because they are calming to the family and help maintain immunity in the winter.

Discussion

There are literally hundreds of essential oils. Although the exact mechanism of action of essential oils has not yet been fully explained, more and more research is being conducted into their powerful effects. In my practice, I have found pure, therapeutic grade essential oils to be profoundly beneficial in facilitating the healing process. Because of the amygdala and its response to olfactory stimulation, this is especially true in autism and brain-based disorders.

People often ask for a cookbook or protocol for various conditions. However, because essential oils are an energetic medicine, each individual reacts differently to any given oil. Selection of appropriate oils is both an art and a science and must also take into account an intimate and specific knowledge of the individual being treated.

Recognizing that the origins of essential oils are ancient, my method of application and use (based extensively on the work of D. Gary Young) is unique. This approach uses the energetic frequency of therapeutic grade essential oils to address underlying energetic disturbances in the body, brain, and emotions. This is accomplished through topical application, inhalation, and ingestion, supported by proper nutrition, removal of toxins, and attention to matching the appropriate oil with the appropriate individual. Although no one healing system has all the answers, essential oils can be a powerful and healing modality in helping children to reach their optimum potential.

Although I have chosen not to provide specific protocols in light of the need to match oils to individual situations and needs, I describe five oils that I have found enormously useful for my patients, particularly those with autism. Where such information is available, I outline the scientific and theoretical rationale for their use.

SANDALWOOD

Sandalwood has a long history of use and is often one of the first oils I use with an autistic child. It has a pleasant and exotic aroma that is unparalleled. Although products labeled as sandalwood can sometimes be found in perfume shops or health food stores, its rarity almost guarantees that these products are not pure plant oil. The pure essential oil has a starkly different and immediately recognizable aroma due to its high sesquiterpene levels.

Research at the University of Vienna has shown that inhalation of oils such as sandalwood that are high in sequiterpenes increases brain oxygenation by as much as 28 percent, resulting in a calm but alert state. Sandalwood has been found to especially interact with the amygdala and limbic system, which can be seen in SPECT (single photon emission computed tomography) scans. Other research has shown that, when the user is awake, sandalwood produces greater focus and alertness; when the user is sleeping, however, the oil promotes deeper rapid eye movement (REM) sleep, especially in individuals who are sleep-disturbed. In Ayurvedic medicine (the traditional medicine of India), sandalwood is thought to open the energy pathways at the base of the spine to release deep or cellular memory.

FRANKINCENSE

Like sandalwood, frankincense has a long history of use. The ancient Egyptians called it "holy anointing oil" and used frankincense to anoint the heads of newborn royalty. (It is likely that the oil's antibacterial effects prevented the royal infants from developing infections caused by head abrasions from difficult births.) Mentioned in the Judeo-Christian Bible, frankincense has been used by religious groups to stimulate focus and religious contemplation. In Eastern medicine, frankincense is known for its profound impact on the spirit.

Practitioners report that frankincense helps users to feel stable, grounded, and secure, both physically and emotionally, making it a good choice in autism. Like sandalwood, frankincense stimulates the amygdala and, because of its high sesquiterpene levels, increases brain oxygenation. Researchers have discovered a molecule in frankincense called incensole acetate (IA) that is liberated either by burning the resin or diffusing extremely pure essential oil. Researchers at Cairo University have found that the IA in frankincense stimulates a previously unknown neural pathway responsible for decreases in anxiety, which results in mood elevation and a feeling of well-being. Follow-up research on IA has found that it is also neuroprotective and stimulates dendrite growth. In animal models, mice subjected to traumatic brain injury who inhaled IA molecules displayed neurobehavioral and cognitive improvements.

VETIVER

Vetiver has a pungent, earthy aroma described by some children as the smell of an old tree. Traditionally, vetiver has been used to combat stress and feelings of sadness, and to release emotional trauma and shock. Vetiver is an oil to consider because of its grounding properties and high sesquiterpene levels.

In 2002, Dr. Terry Friedman completed a 2-year study comparing vetiver essential oil with lavender and cedarwood oils. Of these three oils, vetiver was associated with the greatest decrease in ADHD symptoms. The study evaluated participants with serial, real-time electroencephalographic (EEG) studies as well as the TOVA (Test of Variables of Attention), a standardized computer-based screening tool for ADHD. Dr. Friedman noted that whereas ADHD children typically exhibit marked slowing of brain waves in the prefrontal cortex (an area responsible for the brain's executive functions), this slowing halted, appearing closer to a normal profile, after administration of vetiver essential oil through inhalation, almost as if this part of the brain had been awakened. The post-treatment TOVA values also showed a marked improvement in the treatment group.

EUCALYPTUS BLUE

(Eucalyptol natriol azul spp. Eucalyptus bicostata)

Although previously thought to grow only in Australia, this plant species was newly discovered deep in the Andes Mountains near Guayaquil, Ecuador, by D. Gary Young. The Ecuadorian plant is used by natives to heal wounds and various other conditions. This oil has one of the strongest recognizable aromas of any essential oil. Even one small drop can be recognized from a great distance. This oil has a strong oxygenation capacity and frequently prompts those exposed to the oil to take deeper and more sustained breaths. It has an opening or expansive effect that is both calming and stimulating to the emotions.

PALO SANTO

Palo santo oil is in the same family as frankincense. Like frankincense, palo santo is known as a "spiritual" essential oil. South American shamans and native healers use it to cleanse negative energies from the surroundings and believe that applying the oil to the skin creates a protective covering. This oil, too, has a very distinctive aroma. Although there has been little research on palo santo, it likely has properties similar to vetiver and frankincense. I have seen palo santo be very powerful in facilitating the release of trapped emotions.

STRESS REDUCTION FOR PARENTS OF CHILDREN WITH AUTISM

By Karen Nourizadeh

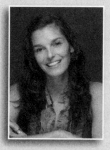

Karen Nourizadeh

Former New York City litigator, now a "recovering attorney," Karen Nourizadeh, has created a path of healing and health, after leaving the practice of law and Corporate America (pharmaceuticals, insurance, and executive recruiting), more than 15 years in. Karen has found a true calling teaching meditation and yoga to highly stressed New Yorkers at Pure Yoga, voted New York City's "Best Yoga" by *New York Magazine* (2009, 2010). Her sold-out workshops and workshop series at Pure Yoga East & West provide a comprehensive discussion of modern-day stress, its effects on the body-mind, and healthy management techniques, which combine Eastern and Western philosophies and methods. This holistic approach takes into account neuroscience, neuro-plasticity, energy medicine, quantum physics, epi-genetics, yoga philosophy and practice, meditation, energy psychology and spirituality in healing. Karen has developed a modern-day health perspective for both 'non-yogi' and 'yogi' looking for more daily balance and health. Karen holds an advanced 500-hour certification, through Pure Yoga and Sonic Yoga, with an emphasis on Tantric meditation practices and Yogic philosophies in addition to asana. For more information, please visit www.karennouri.com.

For families with children with autism spectrum disorders, each day can be emotionally overwhelming, stress-filled, depleting, and isolating. A child's behavior and the frustration of not being able to communicate or connect with their child can leave parents depressed, anxious, and/or feeling disconnected from themselves and the outer world. Many parents feel as if they struggle alone.

Most parents of children with autism have less time for themselves compared to the average parent, and the amount of stress in their day is significantly more than the average parent as well. Researchers have found that mothers of children with autism, in particular, have stress equivalent to the chronic stress of soldiers in combat (*Journal of Autism and Developmental Disorders,* by Marsha Mailick Seltzer, researcher at the University of Wisconsin-Madison, 2013). Parents of children with autism also struggle with frequent fatigue and work interruptions, which are associated with chronic health problems, affecting glucose regulation, immune functioning, and mental activity.

Another stressful aspect of parenting a child with autism is handling judgmental remarks, wondering why the child isn't under control. Unwelcomed comments are enough to engender feelings of blame, shame, guilt, embarrassment or anger.

Programs to help manage parents' stress are often lacking, beyond a family's financial resources, or not comprehensive enough. Unfortunately, the number of Autism Spectrum Disorder (ASD) cases is soaring. Statistics from the U.S. Centers for Disease Control and Prevention say that almost 1 percent of children have autism or another ASD, and therefore, more parents' state of health will be impacted.

Many parents have difficulty asking for or seeking out help because they fear that they might be admitting failure, or might be judged by others. Some cannot find ample or adequate child care, and are often depleted from having to do much of the work themselves.

In order to manage this often overwhelming stress, an understanding of stress is necessary.

Stress, according to Eastern philosopher and yogi, Swami Satyananda Swaraswati, can be defined as follows:

Stress=the number of stressful situations/ability to cope

Formulaically speaking, to reduce stress, one can either reduce the number of stressful situations, which requires some lifestyle changes or one can increase the ability to cope.

When a negative or limiting thought enters the mind, the brain matches a chemical to the emotion experienced. For example, if an individual believes that there is never enough time in the day, this thought produces an emotion, perhaps anxiety, and produces a threat to one's subjective well-being. The limbic system, the "feeling and emotional" portion of the brain, is responsible for coordinating behavior, autonomic and endocrine responses to environmental stimuli, especially those with emotional content, such as fear and anxiety. Once the brain identifies a situation to be a threat or a danger (whether objective or subjective), the endocrine system is signalled, which then triggers the production of stress hormones, such as adrenaline, norepenephrine or cortisol. Adrenaline, norepenephrine and cortisol are important stressor responses *when there is an actual danger* because it increases blood sugar and blood pressure, to help escape or fight the danger. However, even when there is no actual threat, but a "perceived" threat, the brain still triggers the production of stress hormones, which then creates a neural and nervous system response. If the stress is perceived repeatedly, the firing neurons wire together in the brain to create a neural pathway that trigger anytime a similar situation is perceived, whether it be based in reality or not. Once a neural pathway is wired, it fires in that manner, creating an involuntary autonomic stress response, which over time, wreaks physical and mental havoc.

The body's stress response transports blood away from the internal organs and out to the limbs to prepare the body to "fight" or "flee." Blood drains from the frontal portion of the brain, which damages clear thinking and reason. Sugar infiltrates the blood as well to sustain fight or flight. Over time, if this response is chronic, then the body's internal systems begin to malfunction and manifest as disease in the physical and mental bodies. Raised levels of stress hormones for prolonged periods weaken the immune system and the organs, cause cells to mutate or die, kick-start nervous, circulatory and inflammatory responses, and impair memory and cognitive ability. People with chronic stress also suffer from one or more of the following: insomnia, depression, anxiety, autoimmune and digestive disorders, migraine and tension headaches, asthma and ulcers.

How one reacts to one's environment is crucial to managing stress. The subconscious mind has been conditioned to react to stress based upon past experiences as well as our observing, then absorbing, how those around us reacted to stress. We then become wired in this way, without our consent or knowledge until around the age of seven. In past years, it was believed that these reactions were "hard-wired" by our genes, as were certain diseases thought to be "hard-wired." However, a relatively new science, "epigenetics" now demonstrates that we are not "hard-wired." Epigenetics tells us that a majority of a gene is affected by *how we react to our environment*. Therefore, if we change or manage the reactions, and our perception of events, we can change the genome, our cellular structure, our health and the future. Epigenetics helps us to understand that we can change our reactions, and thereby, our reality. Quantum physics tells us that infinite possibilities exist, but it depends on the observer's posturing that affects the perspective and the outcome.

Common limiting or negative beliefs such as "I am wrong or did something wrong," or "I need help," or "There is never enough time," or "Nobody understands," or "What will happen to my child after I'm gone?" constantly barrage subconscious and unconscious minds of many parents of children with autism. The conscious mind may be aware or wholly unaware of the subterfuge, but these types of thoughts set off a complex chemical, neurological and biological reaction, that become manifest in the physical body. In order to mutate the mental, and thereby the physical, we must eliminate or reduce negative and limiting beliefs, emotions, habits and behaviors that no longer serve us. In order to mutate the mind, we must relax the mind and body, then access portions of the subconscious and unconscious mind, in order to allow the negative and limiting impressions to surface. Once they surface, we can choose *to let them go* and create a new reality that works for our present day circumstances. Only then, can we wire new pathways that are healthy to our functioning, rather than sabotaging it.

Yoga Nidra Meditation, The Art of Conscious Relaxation, is a holistic system which is designed to relax both body and mind, and to access the subconscious and unconcious minds, where 90–95 percent of thoughts and beliefs are stored. Yoga Nidra is composed of various parts: 1) An intention/s; 2) Rotation of consciousness over the body; 3) Countdown of the breath; 4) Bilateral stimulation of the brain by pairing opposite mind states; 5) Visualization and; 6) Object imaging. With the application of Yoga Nidra, brain wave activity decreases from Beta (fully awake/alert) and vascillates between Alpha (meditation), Theta (dream) and Delta (deep sleep). When the brain wave activity has slowed, the mind is more receptive, and impressions from the past, stored in the subconscious or unconscious, can be released. Through repeated use, Nidra can actually help to re-structure the surface of the brain, and thereby, re-program the mind.

During Yoga Nidra, one is asked to create an intention for the day, phase of life and/or for life. Intentions align us with our purpose here on earth, and help maintain our focus in the midst of chaos. If we begin to value our own intentions for our lives, then we diminish the value of others around us who judge, confuse or frustrate us. Over time, beliefs, behaviors and decisions will be made that are in alignment with our resolve, and those that are not in alignment will eventually be removed from our attention and focus.

The daily intention is a statement of something that can be manifested in each day, such as, "I will eat a healthy lunch," or "I won't check my email prior to bed." The phase of life intention is a short positive phrase for the phase of life that one is in at the present moment, contemplating an aspect of life that the individual would like to improve upon, such as "I will sleep better at night, or "I will step into my own worth/voice/power." The phase of life intention remains until time that one is out of that phase. The life intention helps to identify one's life's purpose-who you are, why you are here. This may be challenging because many of us have never even considered our individual purpose in life. This intention should benefit the creator of it, but should be broad enough in scope, so that it benefits both creator and those around him or her. The life intention remains the same throughout life and does not alter. If we use the power of intention, it lifts us above that which is not of priority or in alignment, and will thus keep guiding us back to ourselves and our individual path of creating the life we intend to live.

After the intention, the praciitioner is guided through a rotation of consciousness over the body parts and a countdown of the breath. During this phase, the senses are withdrawn as the mind concentrates internally. The external world is filled with sensorial distractions that serve to dissipate our attention and fragment the mind. If the senses are withdrawn, and awareness is directed inward, then the individual is no longer pulled towards or repulsed by the object of the senses, allowing the mind to relax.

The rotation and countdown also serve to keep the mind focused, which help to heal the body. A concentrated mind also unlocks the ability to release past negative impressions and experiences, and anxieties about the future. One is then able to view his/her circumstances with clarity. When there is clarity, there is wisdom. When there is wisdom, one begins to align one's choices, decisions and behaviors with wisdom.

The system of rotating the consciousness over the body and counting backward with the breath also has demonstrated a physiological disconnect between the 'fear brain' and its endocrine, autonomic and emotional responses. It also slows down brain wave activity. Once the brain wave activity is slowed, the practitioner's subjective experiences can be brought to the surface and taken into context, without reacting to them.

Through pairing oppposite brain states (heavy/light, hot/cold, pain/pleasure), the mind begins to re-structure itself to balance, rather than pulled by extreme negative or limiting emotions and beliefs. Over time, the mind and brain will be less sensitive to stressful events, eradicatng or diminishing old neural pathways that create a "stress looping" response. New neural pathways will be created which help to balance the imbalances of both mind and brain.

In this deeply relaxed state, visualization and object imaging are introduced, and demonstrate the mind's subjective association to the visualization or object. In this way, the practioner is able to identify and understand more perceptively and objectively the associations that arise which adversely affect one's mental and physical health. With consciousness and repetition, these associations can be eliminated altogether, and new associations can be formulated. Visualization and object imaging also help to improve memory and cognition because parts of the brain that are normally dormant, the prefrontal cortex, are activated during Yoga Nidra.

Yoga Nidra can be practiced in full or in part, depending on the amount of time one has to devote to the practice. It can be practiced while in a supine or seated position, though lying down is preferential. A quiet dimly lit space is all that is required. Numerous scientific studies have demonstated the efficacy of Yoga Nidra, which has been successfully used to treat anxiety, depression, insomnia, circulatory issues, cancer, digestive disorders, and a number of other disorders of the body-systems. Many studies are referred to in the index of *Yoga Nidra*, by Swami Saraswati (Yoga Publications Trust, Mungher, India 1976).

Yoga Nidra helps to balance our focus towards abundance and creativity, rather than lack and limitation. If the focus turns to abundance and fulfillment, then transforming limiting and negative beliefs to expansive ones becomes not only possible, but realistic. Through repeated practice, Yoga Nidra helps to manage expectations and emotions. Each time an expectation is not met, it usually creates disappointment. Feelings of disappointment then turn to shame, blame, rage, guilt or embarrassment. Then the ego kicks in to make us feel either helpless or, at the other extreme, self-righteous. And the emotional cycle perpetuates. The practice of Yoga Nidra reduces the internal fear-cycle and negative backlash caused by expectations and emotions. ("If I don't get x, then I am not good enough, smart enough, loveable enough . . ."). We begin to grasp that we cannot control others, how they view us or how another acts or speaks, but we can do the work to control our own belief, decisions and thus behaviors, choosing love and fulfillment over fear and lack.

Once we begin to look inside ourselves, we can more readily accept the human condition. No one is perfect, and in seeking perfection, fragmentation of the mind occurs. You are human. You will stumble, you will make a mistake, but don't allow it to render you powerless, to fragment your energy. Ego will tell us, either "poor me, I am a victim" or "great strong BIG me, I am amazing." Go beyond ego, and find love for yourself. Find compassion for yourself. Once we are able to love ourselves, without condition, we can find compassion within for ourselves to be human, to not always be perfect. We can also make more rational choices, and keep unhealthy people and situations at a healthy distance.

Yoga Nidra is a complete practice to support a healthy mind and body, which creates a healthy environment for loved ones. Taking time to deeply relax body and mind is the greatest present one can give to oneself and those they love. From that healthy, grounded and centering perspective, parents can then feel more empowered to balance all that comes their way, while keeping the extreme autonomic, endocrine and emotional responses at bay.

For techniques on how to relax the mind-body systems through Yoga Nidra, upcoming workshops, or to book a workshop, visit The Recovering Attorney's website, www.karennouri.com.

OSTEOPATHY: A PHILOSOPHY AND METHODOLOGY FOR THE EFFECTIVE TREATMENT OF CHILDREN WITH AUTISM

By Dr. Shawn K. Centers

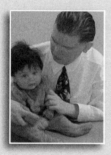

Shawn K. Centers, DO, FACOP

Shawn K. Centers, DO, FACOP, clinical director of the Osteopathic Center for Children & Families in San Diego, California, is a pediatrician and internationally known expert on osteopathic pediatrics, nutrition, and natural medicines as they apply to children. Dr. Centers has worked for the last 10 years as a staff pediatrician and osteopathic manipulation practitioner at the Osteopathic Center for Children & Families. Prior to this, Dr. Centers served as the pediatric chief resident for the Children's Hospital of New Jersey in Livingston, New Jersey, where he was very active in developing and integrating osteopathic principles into the educational program for residents and medical students. www.osteopathiccenter.org.

INTRODUCTION

Founded in the backwoods of the Missouri frontier at the close of the 19th century, osteopathy is perhaps the only uniquely American form of complete medicine in existence today. While other healing systems have fallen by the wayside, osteopathy as a profession has persisted. Moreover, after persistent national and international research, multicenter studies, and publication of clinical results in mainstream journals such as *Pediatrics*, there is now a renewed and heightened enthusiasm for the benefits of traditional osteopathic care for both adults and children.

Osteopathy was founded at a time when the scourges of cholera, smallpox, and dysentery were capable of wiping out entire families, and the primary treatments for such ills were mercury (in the form of calomel) and bloodletting. In the latter part of the 19th century, osteopathy offered a bold alternative, declaring that the body could heal itself and that every person, regardless of disease, had the potential to get better.

Early practitioners of osteopathy also stated openly that many of the day's medications did not work or, even worse, were potent toxins. This philosophy and approach to care set the osteopathic profession squarely at odds with its mainstream counterpart, represented by the American Medical Association (AMA).

Andrew Taylor Still, MD (1828-1917), is regarded by most medical historians as the founder of osteopathic medicine. Dr. Still was a frontier physician, considered by some a renegade and radical. Still reviled slavery, objected to the inhumane treatment of women and children, and admitted women to and graduated them from his medical school at a time when women's brains were thought to be "too small for intellectual pursuits but just right for love" (Sims, 1889). Although Still attended medical school in Kansas City and apprenticed with his physician father, he credited most of his medical learning to "the school of life" as well as careful and meticulous observation, tutelage from American Indians, and countless dissections and studies of human anatomy. Dr. Still also garnered considerable experience while working as a surgeon in the Civil War.

Although Dr. Still constantly sought to deepen his understanding of the world around him, it was only after the deaths of three of his children that he began to question the efficacy of the medical practices of his day. For weeks after their deaths, Dr. Still traveled hours on horseback to a university library to read medical texts and attempt to understand why conventional medicine had failed his children. One day, Still stumbled upon a text authored by Samuel Thomson (1769-1843), one of the forefathers of what is now called herbal medicine. Although more than three million Americans used Thomsonian medicine in the 1840s, "regular" physicians were not allowed to associate with Thomsonian physicians nor even mention Thomson's name or practices in their medical writing or correspondence. By 1860, Thomsonian medicine was specifically targeted for eradication by the AMA and, by the 1890s, it had been almost completely eliminated.

The Thomson text read by Still described the effects of calomel (mercury) poisoning. Dr. Still realized that disease had not killed his children—rather, the "medicine" given to cure the disease was responsible for their deaths. Stunned by the fact that available medical treatments were, in many cases, worse than the diseases they purported to cure, Dr. Still began to voraciously read everything he could about the medical profession. Returning to the original teachings of Hippocrates, Still realized that many practitioners had lost touch with Hippocrates' essential lessons regarding the need to "do no harm," the importance of harnessing the healing power in nature and the vital forces in the body, and the ability of the body to heal itself once balance is restored.

Drawing on Hippocrates' ideas and his own observations of nature, Dr. Still began to formulate a philosophy and methodology of practice to improve on the current system of medicine. Dr. Still called this new system osteopathy, from "osteo" (meaning "structure") and "pathos" (meaning "suffering or deepest need"). To guide this new approach to healing, Still formulated three fundamental osteopathic principles:

1. Structure and function are reciprocally interrelated.
2. The body is one integrated unit of function.
3. The body has an innate self-healing or vital force within.

FIRST OSTEOPATHIC PRINCIPLE: STRUCTURE & FUNCTION

The principle of the reciprocal interrelationship of structure and function is a basic teaching of the biological sciences. However, modern day medicine rarely applies this teaching with any real meaning or intent. In osteopathic science, in contrast, the structure-function principle is a foundational concept, teaching us that structure (whether through evolution or the infinite intelligence of the universe) has a purpose and that the purpose relates directly to function. Every structure within the body has a function, from the smallest microscopic or chemical level to the largest bone within the organism. If the structure is absent or impaired, proper function cannot occur.

As a simple illustration of the first principle on the chemical level, if the structure of the walls of a red blood cell is weakened because a glutamine molecule is present instead of a valine molecule, the red blood cell will fold over onto itself. As the blood cell tries to move through the capillaries, it will clog the capillaries and, if the capillaries are in the lungs, the red blood cell will interfere with the function of the lungs to such an extent that the patient may die. Although the red blood cell may function perfectly in every other way, in this instance its altered structure impairs its function. (In fact, we call this condition sickle cell anemia because the structure of the cell is like a sickle.)

A more complex illustration of the first osteopathic principle can be achieved by considering the skeletal tissue, which represents 70% of all body tissue. Every skeletal muscle has a vein that takes deoxygenated blood as well as toxins produced by the muscle back to the heart. If a muscle is injured and micro-tears occur in the muscle's fibers, the muscle will contract so that the micro-tears can heal (a situation described by physiologists as "hypertonicity"). If the hypertonicity is the result of acute trauma, it may remain for days, weeks, or—in some cases—years, resulting in compression and/or irritation to the venous structure underneath the muscle and, eventually, partial or complete occlusion of the vein. Just as a slight alteration in the circumference of a tube will dramatically decrease the amount of fluid that can flow through the tube, similarly, if less blood returns from a vein because of occlusion, the arteries will compensate by sending less blood back to the muscles. The inadequate supply of oxygen received by the muscle due to the decreased blood supply will then cause the muscles to use an alternative mechanism for acquiring oxygen (called anaerobic metabolism), which will cause further muscle contraction and an increase in toxins (primarily lactic acid) within the muscle.

To further elaborate on this example, one must consider that all skeletal muscles are covered by a white shiny tissue called fascia. (Dr. Still observed, "We begin with the fascia and we end with the fascia.") The fascia—the body's great organizer—covers all muscles, blood vessels, and organs and connects to every other structure in the body. If the consistency of the fascia is changed by a hypertonic muscle in one area of the body, it affects every other bodily structure. Fascia, made primarily of collagen, has the unique property of being a colloid, meaning that it can behave as either a liquid or solid. If a high velocity force impinges upon the tissue (meaning the fascia and anything that the fascia encases or is surrounded by) over a short period of time (as in the case of a traumatic muscle strain) or tissue is held in a constant position for a prolonged period of time (as when a baby's head is abnormally positioned in utero), then the fascia becomes more like a solid, resisting deformation or change in shape. If this continues for any length of time, the fascia (and the tissue beneath it) will retain the shape, position, and tone acquired at the time of the injury or trauma, a fact acknowledged by Dr. Still in his comments about tissue memory.

The tissue memory property of the fascia has to do with adhesions (called cross linkages) that form within the fascial layers as collagen fibers become intertwined and tangled. By observing the movement of the fascia and applying sustained pressure along the lines of the original injury, osteopaths have found that fascial adhesions can be untangled or unwound and resolved. If done over a period of 90 to 120 seconds, the unwinding of the fascial tissue will cause the muscle to return to its original physiological tone and will resolve the occlusion of the underlying venous structure. This, in turn, allows proper physiological blood flow to return to the affected areas and effectively eliminates the tissue dysfunction. Osteopathic physicians refer to this type of treatment as osteopathic manipulative therapy (OMT). OMT improves function by restoring proper physiological structural relations, which is the foundation of the structure-function principle.

SECOND PRINCIPLE: INTEGRATED UNIT OF FUNCTION

The second osteopathic principle perceives the body as an integrated unit of function, meaning that patients are greater than the sum of their parts. In today's economically motivated, protocol-driven, and "evidence-based" practice of medicine, this simple principle is too often ignored. Rather than equating patients with their disease label, Dr. Still encouraged osteopathic practitioners to view patients as marvelous human beings designed by a perfect architect and containing within them the blueprint for perfect functioning. Operating from a fundamentally different perspective than the conventional medical practitioners of his day, Dr. Still did not believe that isolated organs or systems were "stuck" or "broken" but instead examined the state of the whole body.

Supported by his understanding of anatomy, Dr. Still saw the body as a network bounded and made whole by the vast interconnectedness of the fascia. Viewed in this way, a disruption in one part of the body may have distant effects in an entirely different and unexpected area. Thus, for an osteopath, it would not be at all unusual to find that the source of shoulder pain or dysfunction might be in the big toe. In fact, pain referral patterns of this type are numerous throughout the body (as when heart attacks cause pain in the left arm, or gall bladder disease causes pain under the right shoulder blade).

In the 1930s, William G. Sutherland (1873-1954), a DO with a background in engineering (and another student of Dr. Still's), noticed that the cranial sutures (the spaces between the 32 bones that make up the skull) had alternating bevels. This suggested to Dr. Sutherland that the bones moved in a distinct physiological pattern, like gears in a watch. Sutherland experimented by creating a device that used gigantic wooden screws to apply sustained pressure to each of the separate skull bones. Sutherland noted that when pressure was applied to certain areas, the shape of the skull changed due to slight movements between the individual bones. Through careful study, he further discovered that it was possible to feel a slight and rhythmic expansion and contraction motion between the skull bones, occurring approximately 6-12 times per minute. This rhythmic motion was interconnected with the rest of the body, changing when trauma was present elsewhere. This meant that a trauma or muscle fascia imbalance in the pelvis would affect the motion felt in the head. Likewise, impairment of the minute motions of the skull could cause far-reaching effects throughout the rest of the body.

Dr. Still had reasoned that motion was the very characteristic of life. The inherent motion of the body, even when lying completely still, is caused by the beating of the heart, the rhythmic interchange of oxygen and carbon dioxide in the lungs, the slow rolling motions of the intestines, and the increase and decrease in pressure within the brain and spinal cord. Motion brings nutrients and allows for proper interchange of fluids to remove toxins. According to Dr. Still, if the motion of any vital organ stops, then the tissue begins to decay or die. Although most anatomists of the time still believed that the spaces between skull bones were remnants of fetal growth and did not move, Dr. Sutherland's findings confirmed the fact that the head, too, is in constant motion. To Sutherland, it was obvious from an engineering standpoint that the skull is designed for motion. In fact, every type of possible joint known to engineering occurs in the skull.

Dr. Sutherland went on to develop and teach techniques of precise palpation to detect the inherent motion within the head. However, although Sutherland described his initial findings regarding functional and dysfunctional cranial motion in 1936, it was not until 1956 that American anatomists published histological studies showing that slight movement occurred between the bones, even in adults. Later, others were able to demonstrate the inherent motion of the cranium through sophisticated physiological recording devices that continued to confirm Dr. Sutherland's 1936 findings noted through simple palpation. Newer technologies have continued to yield similar findings. Finally, in the late 1990s, Dr. Viola Frymann, a renowned osteopathic physician, and Professor Yuri Moskalenko, an internationally recognized pioneer in cerebral circulation, demonstrated that cranial OMT using Sutherland's techniques resulted in marked and quantifiable changes in cerebral blood flow. This proved that function (i.e., blood flow) could be influenced by manipulative techniques.

THIRD PRINCIPLE: INNATE VITAL FORCE

The third principle of osteopathy states that within the body, there is an innate vital force that pushes the body toward balance or healing. Dr. Still believed that physiological balance and proper nutritional resources allow the body to heal itself. Other measures to promote the body's natural healing include removing toxins, resolving structural inadequacies, and even changing toxic thoughts. By these means, the body can achieve physiological homeostasis and thereby heal itself.

As a simple illustration of the third principle, Dr. Still noted that physicians cannot heal a simple cut, but the body can (although physicians can bandage, clean, and place salve on it). Still also spoke of an inherent therapeutic potency that could produce its own medicines, defend against invading bacteria or disease, and alleviate pain and discomfort when necessary. Nearly 25 years before the discovery of the humoral immune system, 70 years before the understanding of endorphins, and 90 years before the concept of psychoneuroimmunology, Dr. Still taught that blood contained within it chemical "factories" that could produce antibiotics, analgesics, and self-regulating substances. In short, Still's osteopathic model of disease acknowledged that the body is constantly exposed to stresses but has innate healing forces that tend toward self-regulation and health.

If one recognizes that the body will always attempt to adapt to and compensate for stressors, then it becomes apparent that disease can only develop when stressors accumulate beyond the body's ability to compensate.

According to Dr. Still, three areas create stress and lead to disease: the mind (i.e., attitudes, beliefs, mental state); matter (physical exposures such as food, environment, or atmosphere); and motion (the fundamental characteristic of life as discussed earlier). Each of these aspects may affect an individual's health in a variety of ways. From the osteopathic perspective, we may add resources to the body through nutrients or freedom of motion and even a change in attitude, or we may take strain away from the body by removing toxins, resolving structural inadequacies, or changing toxic thoughts. Through these means, the body is allowed to achieve a more physiological homeostasis. With proper nutrition, removal of toxins, and a physiological state of balance, the body will, in turn, be able to heal itself.

In osteopathy, we do not believe that patients are inherently sick, stuck, or broken. Rather, we realize that patients may have symptoms of dis-ease as a result of strains placed on the internal homeostatic mechanisms. These strains (or "lesions" as osteopathy calls them) are not the disease but the precursors of disease. As such, these precursors are actually the best option for health that the body has at a given moment, representing the body's attempt to adapt and achieve homeostasis or balance. For example, if a muscle undergoes a strain, it contracts—thereby changing function—yet this is still better than if the muscle tears. In other words, a muscle strain is the body's mechanism for trying to compensate or heal itself.

From an osteopathic perspective, the roots of subsequent disease may be established at birth. Consider an individual who had a difficult, labored birth, causing compression of nerve tracks in the head and neck, resulting in early colic and increased work of the diaphragm. Perhaps this same person went on to have a poor diet as a child and, in addition, used a pacifier, causing the muscles in the posterior pharynx to become tight and rigid. This may have allowed sugar-filled foods to be sucked up the small tube in the back of the throat (which connects the posterior pharynx to the inner ear), leading to ear infections. Perhaps this individual then was given antibiotics. In addition to disrupting the flora in the intestine, the antibiotics may have placed the body under stress as it tried to eliminate the toxins in the medication. Imagine further that this person lives in an area with poor air quality and takes inadequate breaths, contributing to the development of asthma. Finally, imagine that this individual's parents divorce, causing mental stress. In this example, the body surely will attempt to compensate for each instance of stress. Eventually, however, the accumulation of physical, mental, and structural toxins overcomes the body's ability to adapt.

OSTEOPATHIC PERSPECTIVE ON AUTISM AND AUTISM SPECTRUM DISORDERS

All models of healthcare come with their own biases, opinions, and theories. The conventional model of healthcare focuses on the disease entity, teaching that the patient is

442   *Cutting-Edge Therapies for Autism*

sick, stuck, or broken. In this model, the provider's duty is to diagnose and "fix" the patient, attack the disease, prevent future occurrences, and decrease the burden to the overall population. As has been seen with autism, in the absence of a "magic bullet," conventional medicine has framed the "battle" as unwinnable, leaving practitioners with few apparent options other than to manage the condition.

How does osteopathy approach the child with an autism spectrum disorder (ASD)? First, rather than labeling and treating an "autistic child," osteopathic practitioners make the important distinction of treating a child who happens to have symptoms of autism. Osteopathy operates from the bias that healing comes from within and that the physician's job is to assist the patient in finding health. Osteopathy also views all children, regardless of diagnosis, as wonderful human beings who need to be helped to achieve their maximum structural, physiological, and emotional potential. Drawing on the three fundamental principles laid out by Dr. Still, osteopaths seek to determine the most effective treatment approach for each child by considering the child's medical, psychological, and spiritual needs as well as their age and developmental level. This requires careful attention to symptoms, past history, and psychological and social issues in relation to the child's family and caregivers.

The osteopathic approach also requires reaching agreement as to what defines autism. From the osteopathic perspective, autism is, first and foremost, a collection of symptoms—not a disease—found in susceptible children. Those working with children with autistic symptoms have noted four key symptom categories:

1. Disruptions in the ability to effectively communicate. This includes challenges with expressive language (i.e., the ability to communicate ideas, feelings, and needs) and difficulties with receptive communication (i.e., the ability to understand, relate, and process both verbal and nonverbal language).

2. Sensory dysregulation, which may manifest as increased or decreased sensitivity to sound, touch, pain, or light. When children with symptoms of autism flap their hands, cover their ears, or bang their heads, osteopaths believe that the behaviors are responses to pain or abnormal sensory stimuli rather than the result of dysfunctional mental aberrations.

3. Problems in auditory processing. Children with ASD symptoms generally have hearing that is within normal range but experience impairment in their ability to perceive sound and interpret language.

4. Gastrointestinal dysfunction. Children with symptoms of autism frequently have an early history of gastrointestinal dysfunction, including colic, diarrhea, and constipation. Such children may also have a history of sucking difficulties and may be hypersensitive to foods or environmental allergens.

Osteopaths also note that many children with autism have changes in muscle tone (hypotonia) and difficulty in motor planning (dyspraxia).

Many of these symptoms (for the most part ignored by the mainstream medical community) also occur in siblings of children diagnosed with classic autism, which was noted in the 1970s by the pioneering psychologist Dr. Bernard Rimland, himself a parent of a child with autism. In surveys and extensive interviews with families of children labeled autistic, Dr. Rimland discovered that many of the "non-autistic" siblings had similar hyper- or hyposensitivities. For example, where a child diagnosed with autism might display extreme sensitivity to loud noises, his non-autistic sibling might have the same hypersensitivity but without any other symptoms of autism. Dr. Rimland found that many of the "non-autistic" siblings also had other diagnoses or medical conditions (e.g., ADHD, obsessive-compulsive disorder, or a seizure disorder). Dr. Rimland concluded that the children all had the same disorder but manifested differing levels and degrees of severity. Moreover, what psychiatrists dismissed as stereotypical behaviors were actually signs and symptoms linking autistic children with an array of children suffering from other conditions. Conceptualizing autism as a spectrum of disorders, with severe autism on one end and perhaps seizure disorders on the opposite end, led practitioners to begin referring to those affected as children with autism spectrum features rather than autism.

OSTEOPATHIC TREATMENT GOALS AND TREATMENT APPROACH

The osteopathic approach to treating symptoms of autism begins with a detailed history from birth to the present. It is also essential that the osteopathic physician establish a true and meaningful rapport with the child. Observing the child at play and in a position of comfort can provide valuable information regarding the child's level of wellness, developmental stage, and attitude. Osteopathy is also a touching profession, involving the use of hands to palpate the inherent motion of the child's body. Because many children on the autism spectrum are resistant to touch and may refuse to lie down on a treatment table (particularly if they have had negative experiences with other healthcare providers or significant trauma within their body), osteopathic physicians may need to proceed cautiously. Osteopathic evaluation and treatment should begin with a total and complete focus on establishing a meaningful contact with the tissue under our hands, alongside a focus on the highest aspect of the child (i.e., "What is beautiful about this child?" or "What are this child's gifts?"). Initially, we may perform vibratory stimulation with a fast-moving device called a percussion hammer or palpate the body from distant areas such as the feet or hands. As we gradually establish a "dialogue" with the tissue through palpatory skill, children eventually will perceive the touch as safe and allow us to manipulate and unwind the tense and tight areas within their bodies. From this point on, we divide our approach into the three different areas of motion, matter, and mind. Each area is discussed in greater depth below.

IMPAIRED MOTION IN CHILDREN WITH SYMPTOMS OF AUTISM

Autistic children are 12 times more likely to have suffered birth trauma or complications than their non-autistic siblings. Medically induced deliveries are associated with birth trauma. In a British study describing children born in a London hospital (Stein et al., 2006), children had an autism rate 21 times higher than that of neighboring hospitals. Examination of the hospital's records revealed that the hospital had a policy of scheduling all mothers for elective C-sections one week prior to their due dates. Two other large studies in Sweden (Stein et al., 2006) and Australia (Glasson et al., 2004) failed to find a genetic basis for autism but found that birth trauma correlated highly with its subsequent development. In both studies, premature infants were excluded from the research.

Normal birth involves coordinated, efficient, involuntary contractions that lead to progressive cervical effacement, dilatation, descent, and delivery of the newborn baby. However, if the birth process is not coordinated, efficient, or natural, or if the labor is prolonged, complicated, and/or difficult, stress can become trauma. Normally, as a baby's head descends into the pelvis during birth, the pubic bone exerts pressure on the presenting part of the skull (usually the occipital area). If forces exceed the limit of the tissue, the soft tissues may become strained or bent. As the cranial bones override each other, this, in turn, can compress the venous structures within the skull, ultimately resulting in decreased blood to the brain. These changes in structure can affect the function of the brain and brain stem. Instrumentation such as forceps or vacuum extraction, although at times lifesaving, can further put babies at risk for cranial bone dysfunction. In addition, as a baby's head is delivered, the neck is frequently hyperextended. Obstetricians who are focused on getting the baby out quickly generally devote little thought to the possibility of injury. However, hyperextension of the neck can cause injury to the soft tissues at the base of the skull.

Cranial bone dysfunctions, including a misshapen head (plagiocephaly), are frequent findings in children with symptoms of autism. When providing a health history, parents often note that the child arched his neck repeatedly as an infant, was extremely sensitive at the base of his head, or refused to wear hats or constrictive clothing. Long-term studies of children with plagiocephaly suggest that they are at increased risk of subsequent neurological and developmental problems (for example, 40% of the children in a 2000 Washington University study) (Miller & Clarren, 2000) compared to their age-matched siblings.

In children with autism symptoms, injury to the back of the skull (where the first cervical vertebra attaches to the skull) results in the neck being jammed up against the skull base or occiput. This condition, in turn, results in injury to three groups of muscles that make up the suboccipital triangle. When these muscles and their fascia become contracted, they compress a space called the jugular foramen (literally, a hole in the skull). Several nerves as well as a large blood vein pass through this area. The jugular vein drains 95 percent of all blood coming from the brain. If the hole is compressed, the amount of blood that can flow through the vein will be decreased. (This is so because what goes in must equal what goes out to avoid brain swelling; when less blood exits the skull, the spinal cord "tells" the arteries to send less blood to the brain.)

The brain does not distribute blood equally to all areas; rather, blood distribution occurs in a specific order and sequence. The areas at the base of the skull (e.g., those used in movement, respiration, and hormone regulation) receive the greatest amounts of blood, while the peripheral areas (e.g., speech) receive less. (In other words, it is more important for the heart to beat and the body to take in oxygen and metabolize food than it is to speak.) As it happens, the areas that receive a decreased amount of blood flow are the same areas involved in autism.

The jugular foramen contains exit points for three cranial nerves (9, 10, and 11). Infants experiencing irritation to cranial nerve 9 will often display early difficulties in sucking. Irritation to cranial nerve 11 can cause tight neck muscles and, in some cases, a condition called torticollis where the baby holds his or her neck to one side. Cranial nerve 10 (the vagus nerve) is one of the largest nerves in the body and the body's primary parasympathetic nerve. Irritation and compression to this nerve can cause widespread problems, which may manifest in infancy as difficulty feeding, persistent and excessive spitting up, diarrhea and, later, constipation. Babies with this type of compression also typically have early histories of colic and abdominal pain.

Looking at autism spectrum disorders from a brain function point of view, some interesting correlations are apparent. In children with seizure disorder, for example, we find very fast abnormal brainwaves called gamma waves (from 30-100 cycles per second or cps) in the temporal lobes of the brain and the amygdala. In children with ADHD and hyperactivity, we typically find slowing of alpha waves (7-14 cps) in the frontal lobes and amygdala. In children with autism, very slow delta brainwaves (1-7 cps) are found in the frontal, temporal, and prefrontal areas and the amygdala. The commonality in each of these conditions is the presence of a unifying dysfunction within the amygdala. Moreover, nearly 90 percent of all nerve impulses occurring in the amygdala come from or go to the vagus nerve. In effect, vagal nerve dysfunction equals dysfunction in the amygdala. The amygdala, of course, is especially associated with emotions and aggression. (In fact, when removed in animals, the animals exhibit autistic-like symptoms.)

FIGURE

Ideally, the body should have a slight predominance of parasympathetic function (also called the relaxation response). When the body is under chronic stress, however, the sympathetic (fight or flight) function comes to predominate. From a structural point of view, then, the osteopathic physician's first objective is to restore motion in the area of the jugular foramen to decrease tension on the vagus nerve. Bringing the sympathetic and parasympathetic nervous systems (also called the autonomic nervous system) into balance has long been a core goal of osteopathic treatment, guided by studies done in the 1950s and 1960s confirming the benefits of osteopathic manipulation for autonomic nervous system functioning.

MATTER

The second component that osteopaths examine in a child with ASD is matter, that is, what the child physically puts into the body or toxins to which the child may be exposed. Osteopathic findings suggest that hyperstimulation to the vagus nerve through a problematic birth can result in hypersensitivity of the gastrointestinal (GI) tract, causing it to be more sensitive to various viral and toxic influences. If the tissue of the GI tract becomes dysfunctional, impulses will be sent from the intestinal tract back to the amygdala through the hypersensitive vagal nerve. These abnormal reactions may well be responsible for some types of seizures as well as autism symptoms. There is a well-known association between GI disorders and seizures, so severe in some children that it is referred to as abdominal epilepsy. Although Dr. Still did not address autism in his writings, he did address childhood epilepsy, which clearly is structurally and functionally closely related to autism.

Dr. Still also advised: "Be very particular to bring the third, fourth, and fifth lumbar far enough forward to give free passage of the nerve and blood supply to sacral and lower abdominal viscera. ...Fill the lower bowels with gruel, not starch, in order to take off any irritation that undigested food is producing because this irritation has much to do with infant convulsions." (Still, *Osteopathy Research & Practice*, 1910)

Still's advice foreshadows more recent reports (Murch et al., 1998) in which investigators found significant bowel pathology in 47 out of 50 autistic children. When subjected to colon cleansing, the children showed notable improvement in their autistic symptoms. (In fact, the gruel mentioned by Dr. Still, a poorly digestible oat preparation, was used in the 1800s for colon cleansing.) Since Dr. Still's time, there have unquestionably been enormous changes to children's diets. The impact on food quality from insecticides, pesticides, inorganic fertilizers, genetic manipulation, additives and preservatives, inappropriate farming techniques, chemical colorings, and food processing techniques have caused much of today's food supply to be of poor nutritional value. Studies published by the Food and Drug Administration and the Department of Agriculture actually show that since the 1920s, the vitamin and mineral content of fruits and vegetables has decreased. Although these nutrient declines are not well understood, scientists speculate that they are, at least in part, due to improper crop rotation and fertilizer use (Rutgers University, 1995).

When a hyperfunctioning intestinal tract damages the intestinal wall and makes it more susceptible to pathogenic viruses or bacteria, these, in turn, may damage the intestines' enzyme system and cause overgrowth of normally occurring yeast or bacteria. Although osteopathic treatment can restore proper neurological function through manipulation affecting the vagus nerve, improvements in function will not correct the underlying dysbiosis. Therefore, it is essential to also address the dysbiosis and digestive functioning more directly. Colon cleansing, enzyme therapy, and the use of probiotics and other nutritional factors may also be needed to help improve the dysbiosis.

MIND

In children with autism spectrum disorders, many of the stereotypical behaviors observed are related to autonomic dysregulation. With proper osteopathic treatment of structural issues, hypersensitivities to touch, sound, or light often will disappear. However, this is not always the case. In instances where the brain has adapted to dysfunctional sensory input over a number of years, it may not resolve even if the initial structural dysfunction causing the adaptation is resolved. This is especially true for visual problems. Many children with symptoms of autism will look from the side of the face instead of making direct eye contact. Yoked prism glasses that cause the child to focus in front of them, accompanied by treatment from an experienced developmental optometrist, can be exceedingly helpful for these children.

In cases where there are disruptions in the auditory system, a child may misperceive the sounds in his or her environment. One of the branches of the vagus nerve goes to the ear, supplying it with sensation. Abnormal firing of the nerve can result in abnormal reactions to certain sound frequencies. Many ASD children have poor or inadequate perception of high-frequency sound. The problem is not necessarily that the children cannot perceive high frequencies but, rather, they may be too sensitive to this spectrum of sound. In this situation, auditory reeducation, such as Somanas sound therapy or Tomatis therapy, may be helpful. These therapies involve filtering and reintroducing high-frequency sound patterns. In our office, we have a specially designed osteopathic treatment table that helps to address these needs while the child is being treated osteopathically.

CONCLUSION

Perhaps the most important aspect of working with ASD children is to never forget that we are treating a child, not a disorder or a label. Osteopathic physicians must endeavor to establish a meaningful contact with each child. If we treat such children like infants or speak about them in their presence, we do them a disservice. Children are very perceptive and will take on the expectations that others have for them. From the osteopathic perspective, *every* child is a gifted child. It should be our goal to unveil those gifts, regardless of diagnostic labels. Sadly, many of the ideas upheld by the prevailing model of healthcare are antithetical to the fundamental principles and approaches espoused by the osteopathic model. Given these two models of healthcare, both admittedly guided by their own biases, isn't a model that supports the integrity of the person better than one that conditionally assumes the worst? Dr. Still thought so. Osteopathy teaches us to point every child in the direction of health, irrespective of label or dysfunction, so that every child can achieve their optimum potential.

NAET EXPLAINED

By Geri Brewster

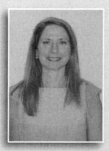

Geri Brewster, RD, MPH, CDN

Geri Brewster is a certified dietitian-nutritionist with a master's in public health from New York Medical College. Geri has advanced areas of study with the Institute of Functional Medicine. She also holds certificates of study in the areas of chronic fatigue, fibromyalgia, biomedical therapies, and weight management.

Geri has worked with children with developmental disabilities and autism for over 25 years, addressing complex nutritional needs. Her practice is maintained in New York City and Mt. Kisco, New York. She is the former director of nutrition at the Atkins Center for Complementary Medicine in New York City and currently assists families in the implementation of the modified Atkins diet for seizure control. A long-time advocate with the Better School Food movement and currently a volunteer with her local National Autism Association group, Geri speaks frequently on a local and national level on the subjects of children's health and nutritional needs. She is a contributor to a number of publications and has been quoted in numerous newspaper and magazine articles as well as featured on numerous radio and TV appearances discussing health topics. She hosts a monthly radio show on AutismOne Radio. Please visit www.geribrewster.com.

Introduction

NAET* is an acronym for Nambudripad's Allergy Elimination Techniques. Dr. Devi Nambudripad, a physician also licensed in chiropractic medicine and acupuncture, discovered her allergy elimination program almost 30 years ago in November of 1983, as she attempted to thwart an adverse allergic reaction to a vegetable she had just consumed. She found that stimulation of certain acupuncture points balanced her body with the substance, averting a full-blown reaction. In the aftermath of this discovery, Dr. Nambudripad began to explore energetic medicine.

NAET is based on the premise that we are electromagnetic beings and that everything has an electromagnetic field. Chinese medicine philosophy suggests that exposure to substances that are not compatible with one's energy results in energy blockages in

---

*   NAET is a registered trademark of Dr. Devi S. Nambudripad.

the body's meridians. Meridians are "any of the pathways along which the body's vital energy flows."[1] There are 12 meridians in the body. When energy blockages occur, they result in disease. Dr. Nambudripad broadly defines "allergy" as an outward manifestation of disease brought about by energy blockages.

Though NAET treatments are not well defined from the perspective of standard or conventional therapies, the premise of NAET is rooted in acupuncture and Chinese medicine principles. Informed by Dr. Nambudripad's multidisciplinary background, the NAET approach is geared toward reconciling the energetic pathways governed by the brain and nervous system to the body's organ systems in the presence of an allergen. Recognizing that the brain creates its electrical signals through a complex chemical process that cross-reacts with the immune system, Dr. Nambudripad theorizes that a person's sensitivity or allergy to a substance is rooted in neurochemical energy imbalances and that NAET's meridian balancing technique can result in desensitization and elimination of the reaction.[2] Similar to rebooting a computer, NAET operates on the premise that we can "reboot" our nervous system and overcome the adverse reactions of the brain and body that manifest as allergy.[2]

How NAET Works

Nambudripad's Allergy Elimination Techniques are noninvasive and use either kinesiological[3] or electrodermal screening techniques[4] to determine sensitivities or weaknesses to substances. If a weakness is determined through neurosensitivity testing,[5] it is balanced with the person's energy through stimulation of acupressure points.

NAET treatments are designed to balance the body with the substance being desensitized on the physical, chemical, and emotional levels. NAET desensitizes one allergen at a time. After balancing to the allergen, the person must avoid the item that was balanced for 25 hours; this provides the 24 hours needed for energy to travel through the body's meridian clock (see Figure 1), plus one additional hour for the energy to settle. The meridian clock is made up of 12 two-hour intervals, one for each of the body's meridians. Energy begins to circulate in the body at 3 am with the lung meridian and ends with the liver meridian 24 hours later. Within each major meridian, there are also micromeridians that generate energy to other meridian points. This energy can potentially interfere with full harmonization to the allergen if exposure occurs too soon. Thus, the 25-hour substance avoidance time is essential to ensure energetic compatibility with the allergen across all meridians.[6]

Persons who are not severely immune deficient generally need just one treatment to desensitize one allergen. Thus, a person with a mild to moderate number of allergies might require approximately 15-20 office visits to desensitize 15-20 food and environmental allergens. The initial visits focus on balancing about 15 basic essential nutrients;

Figure 1:

Meridian Clock

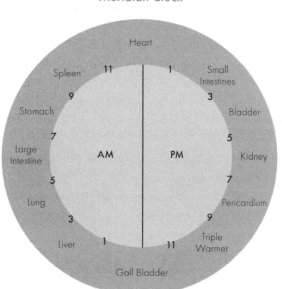

Source: Nambudripad D. *NAET Pain Relief*, 1st ed.
Buena Park, CA: Delta Publishing, 2008, p. 342.

when these are completed, treatment can then focus on chemicals, environmental allergens, immunizations and so forth.[7] On the other hand, individuals who have significant reactivity to a particular substance may require multiple desensitizations to both the substance and the chemical components comprising that substance or to combinations of one or more related substances (such as stomach acid, pancreatic enzymes, and cytokines).

Sensitive individuals react to even the basic components of the foods they ingest (that is, proteins, minerals and vitamins), meaning that anything they eat or supplement with can cause a reaction. Eventually, these individuals react even to foods that once were allowed or tolerated on elimination or rotation diets. NAET therefore seeks to build the body into compatibility not only with identified allergens but also with itself. Immune-deficient people and individuals with chronic illness, autoimmune disease and typical allergy-associated symptoms often appear as though they are allergic to themselves. In such cases, the body's energy is so disrupted that nothing these individuals try brings relief. An acupuncturist will find that the liver meridian is "on fire" or their chi (vital energy) is blocked, while a chiropractor may find that they are constantly out of alignment. In many instances, these individuals have suffered for their

452 Cutting-Edge Therapies for Autism

whole life and their "bucket" is so full that any additional drop into it causes a complete overflow of symptoms.

NAET balancing stops the downward spiral and (metaphorically) allows the water in the "bucket" to recede by energetically reconciling the body's energy to itself as well as the core components of foods. Accordingly, the order of the first 10-15 treatments is important. For example, the first few treatments address core nutrients from the majority of foods that we consume:

- Egg albumin (one of the highest bioavailable proteins for humans that closely resembles our own)
- Egg mix (egg yolk is rich in choline, cholesterol, B vitamins, vitamin A and minerals essential to our nervous system)
- Calcium (an essential mineral for bodily functions and musculoskeletal demands)
- Vitamin C (necessary for connective tissue, growth, and healing)
- B complex (necessary for nervous and endocrine systems)
- Sugar (primary source of energy)
- Iron (needed to carry oxygen throughout the body)

NAET and Homeopathy

As with all treatment options, individual responses to NAET vary. It can sometimes take multiple treatments to achieve desensitization to a single item. Recognizing that homeopathy has long been used to successfully reduce allergy symptoms and response, a NAET homeopathic protocol was designed to increase the efficacy of treatments and help reduce the possible need for multiple treatments for one allergen. The combination of the two modalities provides a synergistic remedy.[8]

Homeopathic allergy treatment functions by inducing the downregulation of the immune system in relation to an offending substance. Homeopathic remedies contain information about a substance that can re-teach the body not to react to the substance even though the allergen is not physically present in the remedy. This is similar to NAET, with the exception that homeopathic energy substances are generally taken internally, while NAET treatment is external. The use of homeopathy after a NAET treatment involves giving a person offending substances in homeopathic form in multiple quantities at different dilutions, thereby continuing to expose the body to the substance in an energetic form. This can improve the outcome of a single NAET treatment and reduce the possible need for multiple treatments to an offending or highly reactive substance.[8] The NAET homeopathics also contain seven paired meridian formulas specifically designed to optimize meridian flow and transfer of information throughout the body (see Figure 2 on the following page).

Figure 2

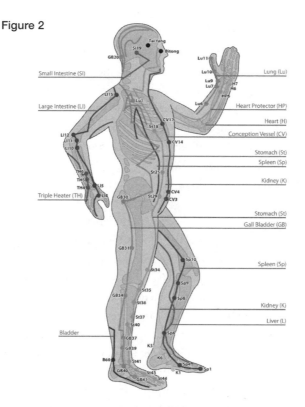

According to Dr. Bruce Shelton, the seven Paired Meridian Formulas are designed to prepare the meridians and their related organs to recieve signals and unblock and tone "stuck" meridians. The Basic NAET protocol has the practitioner locate the patient's most blocked meridian(s). If a meridian is blocked, the transfer of information through the Meridian System during the complete NAET treatment cycle may be compromised. These formulas are designed to maximize each meridian's ability to function properly.

The Paired Meridians are:
1. Bladder / Kidney
2. Gallbladder / Liver
3. Governing Vessel / Conception Vessel
4. Heart / Small Intestine
5. Lung / Large Intestine
6. Pericardium / Triple Warmer
7. Stomach / Spleen

Source: Shelton BH. Meridian formulas. Deseret Biologicals, Inc., 2006 - 2009 [cited 2011 June 22]. Available online from: http://www.desbio.com/NAET.html.

NAET and Autism Research

Dr. Nambudripad has conducted two studies examining the energetic balancing brought about by the effects of NAET desensitization treatments on autistic children.[9,10] She defines allergy-related autism spectrum disorders (ASDs) in reference to NAET's principle that allergy can manifest in any form of disease, and that reconciling the body to allergens will diminish or eliminate those symptoms.[11] According to NAET theory, autism is "a nutritional deficiency disorder causing biological, neurological and developmental problems in children."[10] Dr. Nambudripad suggests that children with autism may be suffering from allergies even if they do not manifest in a typical allergic response.[11]

The most recent study sought to determine whether NAET procedures are effective in restoring verbal and nonverbal communication in children 3-10 years of age with allergy-related ASDs.[9] The study hypothesized that children with diagnosed ASDs and related symptoms (such as no eye contact and/or inability to speak) would show a significant improvement over the control group in verbal and nonverbal communication after 50 NAET treatments focused on systematic desensitization to most food allergen groups, environmental allergen groups, childhood immunizations, and other relevant allergenic substances. In addition to supporting its hypothesis, the study's findings also demonstrated a reduction in autistic traits, including improved social interactions, improved play with other children, improved sleep, reduced restlessness, reduced irritability, and reduced abnormal body movements (such as flapping hands). The study's results also supported findings from a previous investigation conducted in 2005.[10] A third study, though not specific to autism, assessed milk allergy elimination with NAET.[12] All three studies are registered at ClinicalTrials.gov.

To support further research into NAET's effectiveness, Dr. Nambudripad recommends that individuals who are considering NAET receive conventional allergy testing prior to beginning NAET treatments. This allows for the possibility of collecting data to assess improvements in IgE-mediated laboratory results following NAET.

Conclusion

Guided by its underlying principles, NAET has been used successfully to reduce (often completely) the symptoms of illnesses other than typical allergic reactions. This is evidenced by support for NAET from well-known physicians working with autoimmune disease and chronic illness. For example, Dr. Jacob Teitelbaum, researcher in the field of chronic fatigue syndrome and fibromyalgia and author of *From Fatigued to Fantastic*, has described NAET as a beneficial adjunct to the therapies he recommends.

Similarly, Dr. David Brownstein discusses the benefits of using NAET with chronically ill patients in his book, *Overcoming Thyroid Disorders*.

As NAET receives more attention, it is important to note that Dr. Nambudripad cautions against modifications of her techniques. There are no shortcuts, and it takes time to positively influence a person's energy. In most cases, illnesses and sensitivities have built up over many years. In addition, any trial of exposure to a previously known allergic substance must be done under the supervision of a medical practitioner. Nonetheless, because NAET is a noninvasive energy-based modality that has resulted in or augmented the recovery of many individuals experiencing allergies and chronic conditions, it is a modality that deserves consideration.

PHYSICAL

CRANIOSACRAL THERAPY AND AUTISM

By Tami A. Goldstein

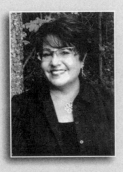

Tami A. Goldstein, WLMT, CST

A Therapeutic Touch by Tami LLC.
1513 Newport Rd.
Janesville, WI 53545
tel. 608 931-9488
Tami.CST1@Gmail.com
http://www.iahp.com/atherapeutictouch/

After learning her daughter was on the autism spectrum, Tami Goldstein began to intensively educate herself about supports and interventions. In 2004, Tami was state and nationally licensed in therapeutic massage and bodywork. She opened A Therapeutic Touch by Tami LLC. in 2004, where she facilitates CranioSacral Therapy. Approximately 40% of her clientele are individuals with autism. In January 2013, Tami completed her certification in CranioSacral Therapy. She is the author of *Coming Through the Fog,* an autism recovery story. *Coming Through the Fog* is the winner of a Reader's Favorite International Book Award. In 2005, Tami founded the Rock County Autism Support Group and became a community resource liaison for the SPD (Sensory Processing Disorders) Parent Connections Support Group. In 2013, she received an award for her advocacy efforts from the WOTA (Wisconsin Occupation Therapy Association). In 2014, Tami will begin teaching a continuing education course she developed titled *Applications of Upledger CranioSacral Therapy, Massage & Bodywork for Autism.*

CranioSacral Therapy (CST) is a gentle, non-invasive therapy that influences and makes corrections in the central nervous system. The craniosacral system is made up of the brain; the cerebral spinal fluid (CSF) that supports and protects the brain; all structures related to the production, absorption, and containment of the CSF fluid; the bones of the skull; the membrane system of the skull; the connective tissue structures intimately related to the membrane system of the skull; and the spine. This system gives off a rhythm that is like a heart rate or a pulse, but distinctly different. This rhythm can be evaluated anywhere on the body in order for the therapist to discern where the restrictions are located. The therapist uses light touch techniques to release restrictions and improve the rhythm, thereby freeing the central nervous system to perform at its best.

The existence of the craniosacral system was brought to mainstream awareness with the work of osteopathic physician and surgeon John E. Upledger, DO, FAAO, the "developer of CranioSacral Therapy." While CranioSacral Therapy had its roots in cranial osteopathy, and Dr. Upledger studied the work of William Sutherland, DO (1873-1954), CranioSacral Therapy is a unique modality.

Cranial osteopathy is a system of diagnosis and treatment that works with structure and function, and it is an osteopathic treatment that encourages the release of stress and tensions throughout the body, including the head. Dr. Sutherland was convinced that the cranial bones have a slight movement, and he hypothesized about how the brain functioned. Dr. Upledger performed clinical research between 1975 and 1983 at the University of Michigan, transforming Dr. Sutherland's original ideas. His research findings proved that the cranial sutures do indeed have movement through adulthood, the bones are slaves to ligament and muscle, and the craniosacral system functions via a fluid-based pressure stat type model. Dr. Upledger named his approach to correct the restrictions found in the craniosacral system CranioSacral Therapy.

CST differs from chiropractic care. Chiropractic care addresses the musculoskeletal system and neuromusculoskeletal system through spinal manipulation. With regard to CranioSacral Therapy, Dr. Upledger said, "The craniosacral system is intimately related to, influences, and is influenced by: 1) the nervous system, 2) the musculoskeletal system, 3) the vascular system, 4) the lymphatic system, 5) the endocrine system and 6) the respiratory system. Abnormalities in the structure or function of any of these systems may influence the craniosacral system. Abnormalities in the structure or function of the craniosacral system will necessarily have profound and frequently deleterious effects upon the development or function of the nervous system, especially the brain."[1]

Look at some of the characteristics of children with autism. Many have anxiety (nervous system), tics (nervous system), repetitive behaviors (nervous system) and motor planning issues (nervous system and musculoskeletal system). Many children with autism have circulation issues, internal inflammation, and gastrointestinal issues. Simply put, if the systems of the body are not working correctly, the brain is not working correctly. If the brain is not working correctly, it affects how the other systems work. But if you correct the restriction in the central nervous system (your brain), then you improve the functioning of the other systems in the body. In this way, the therapy allows the body to access its own healing processes.

Here's an illustration of how CST might improve the endocrine system. Let's say there is a restriction in the frontal bone (forehead). The restriction could impinge on the pituitary gland because of its relation to the frontal bone. The pituitary gland is part of the endocrine system and regulates the hormones that address blood pressure, sex organs, the thyroid gland, water regulation in the body, water balance as part of the reabsorption process for the kidneys, and temperature regulation of the body. It's like the motherboard controlling five major hormones in the body. The impingement can prevent the pituitary gland from functioning correctly and affect its ability to produce and/or regulate the appropriate hormones. As I facilitate CST, I may find a restriction in the frontal bone, the anterior membrane attachments, or other structures that touch the pituitary gland and that can cause an impingement. CST can release those restrictions, giving the pituitary gland the best environment to return to its greatest level of performance. This illustration can also apply to other systems in the body.

In 1985, the Upledger Institute began one-week intensive treatment programs for children with severe autism, and this intensive autism program is still in existence today. Some behaviors Dr. Upledger observed when working with autistic children are "attempts to change/correct physiological and/or anatomical dysfunctions that may be causing pain or discomfort." He referenced autistic children who are known to "bang their heads, chew on their wrists and/or base of their thumbs until deep tissue was visible." He also observed that when specific corrections were administered through CST, the behaviors "spontaneously" ceased. He testified that all of his examinations revealed that the intracranial membranes were very tight."[2]

I am one of the nearly 100,000 health care practitioners who have taken CST training with Upledger Institute International. For over ten years, I have been facilitating CST in my office. I specialize in autism and sensory processing disorders (SPD), with almost 40 percent of my clientele being children on the autism spectrum. I started training in CST after observing its benefits firsthand in my own child. My daughter, Heather, was a month shy of thirteen when she was finally diagnosed with autism, and she was deteriorating quickly. (Eight years of mental health supports had done nothing.) CST was recommended and facilitated by the occupational therapist (OT) who facilitated sensory integration therapy, and this OT was also certified in CST. This OT told me CST would help reduce the forty seizures a day my daughter presented with, help control her debilitating obsessive-compulsive disorder (OCD) symptoms, and reduce her high anxiety. And this therapist explained it would improve sensory, motor, and mental dysfunction.

I'll never forget that first CST session Heather had with her OT. Heather lay down on a massage table, and over her clothing, the therapist gently touched her head, back, neck, and shoulder and even pulled her ears. Heather said she felt nothing, but the change in her was profound. At the end of the session, Heather jumped off the table, hugged and kissed me, and thanked me for getting her help. It was then that I realized I had not touched or kissed Heather on the cheek since she was a baby. She was so sensitive to touch that I had learned early on to kiss her hairline, but never her face. She was now almost fourteen. After the session, Heather went into an 18-20 hour shutdown, but the girl who emerged was different. She could make eye contact; she was engaged; she was focused; she was open to conversation; the tic was greatly reduced; she could be touched; and the anxiety responses had greatly dissipated. We added CST as part of our approach to functioning recovery.

Neuroanatomy information has come a long way insofar as knowing what part of the brain a behavior emanates from. For example, many children with autism have sensory based motor planning issues, OCD, perseverative behaviors or thoughts, oppositional behaviors, cognitive inflexibility, and eating disorders. That tells me the part of the brain that is restricted is the cingulate gyrus, which is located behind the frontal bone (forehead).[3] I use the CST technique to release the anterior/superior membrane in the skull, and the behaviors reduce. Let's say a child has auditory or reading issues, word finding problems, anxiety, fears, periods of spaciness or confusion, or social skills struggles. These behaviors stem from either or both temporal lobes.[4] I use CST techniques to evaluate, verify appropriate movement of the temporal bones, and release the restrictions.

There are many reasons why you would seek out CranioSacral Therapy for your child. Conditions avoided or reduced by facilitation of CST may include attention-deficit disorder, attention-deficit/hyperactivity disorder, autism spectrum disorder, speech disorders, reflux and digestive issues, hearing problems, hydrocephalus, an impaired immune system, emotional problems, and many others. There are testimonials and case studies available from the International Association of Healthcare Practitioners, www.IAHP.com, explaining reduction in maladaptive behaviors associated with autism and increase in learned behaviors and brain function from facilitation of CST. Improvements have been seen in reading, writing, sleeping, overt behaviors, potty training, and math skills. Also reported have been reductions in pain and seizure activity. There has been improvement from and reduction of issues related to birth trauma. CST has a powerful effect on the nervous system, so it addresses issues like aggression, fight or flight, fevers, and proprioceptive issues (proprioception is the body's ability to sense movement). Correcting proprioception issues helps the body facilitate accurate motor planning or body awareness.

CST is individualized to the patient. Just like you can line up 10 children with autism and see 10 different presentations, a therapist can also see 10 different restriction patterns in the craniosacral system for children with the same diagnosis of autism.

Though they present with different restriction patterns, there are oft-seen differences associated with the brains of children with autism. Children are also continually growing, and puberty brings hormone changes; therefore, it's important to continue CST in order to accommodate changes in their craniosacral system and enhance function.

When looking for a craniosacral therapist, look for one who has multiple levels of CST training and who has completed a PEDS (pediatric) class. It is useful to inform the therapist about your child's triggers, such as sensitivities to light, sounds, or smells; this can help the therapist individualize the environment so it's best suited for your child. Since CST involves the nervous system, therapists are already trained to provide a quiet therapy environment while the child is on a massage table or even during play. Sessions can vary from between fifteen minutes to more than an hour. The parent would observe the therapist's simple, light touch, which exerts no more than 5 grams of pressure (the weight of a nickel). The Upledger Institute International provides the industry standards regarding CranioSacral Therapy training. You can find a qualified therapist by going to www.Upledger.com and clicking "find a therapist."

I've learned to be creative when working with children in the therapy environment. I have weighted toys, a visual timer so the child can see elapsed time until session ends, fiddle and vibration toys, and a portable DVD. The children I work with have exhibited some of the most gratifying results, attesting to the effectiveness of this therapy: toileting issues have been resolved and/or mastered; nonverbal children have spoken during a CST session; children have recited the days of the week or months of the year, with parents' excitedly telling me that they had been working on those skills for months or years.

One of my clients was a nineteen-year-old who had come very far with the therapies his parents had already provided and was high functioning, but who was floundering after high school. He was not working nor socializing, and he was regressing behaviorally. After facilitating six weeks of CST, the young man found a job, joined a social gaming group, started maintaining his own finances, and began working on independent living skills. No therapy other than CST was utilized during this time. Clearly, CST provides benefits as a standalone therapy.

My experience and research has taught me that functioning recovery for autism is a multidisciplinary approach, and CST should be included in that approach. I share my daughter's journey through autism and the crucial role CST had in achieving and maintaining that functioning recovery in *Coming Through the Fog*. Autism is about brain function and the nervous system. CST acts to improve brain and nervous system functioning.

DANCE/MOVEMENT THERAPY

By Mariah Meyer LeFeber

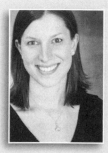

Mariah Meyer LeFeber, MA, LPC, BC-DMT, DTRL

Hancock Center for Dance/Movement Therapy
16 N. Hancock St.
Madison, WI 53703
608-251-0908
www.hancockcenter.net
mariah@hancockcenter.net
info@hancockcenter.net

Ms. LeFeber is a dance/movement therapist and licensed professional counselor living in Madison, Wisconsin. She embodies her love of movement in both individual and group treatment for children, adolescents, and adults affected by developmental delays and mental illness. Beyond her passion for the healing power inherent in dance/movement therapy, Ms. LeFeber further pursues her love of movement teaching yoga for children and modern dance in the University of Madison-Wisconsin's dance department.

Movement is a language. For children affected by autism, movement may be the only language they can rely on. Children with autism often have limited verbal abilities, making it extremely difficult for them to reach out to others (Hartshorn et al., 2001). When words fail, dance/movement therapy fosters a child's ability to relate, communicate, and connect on a nonverbal level.

Dance/movement therapy (DMT), which uses movement as a "universal means of communication," is a valuable form of communication for children with autism, especially those with underdeveloped speech skills (Erfer, 2005, p. 196). Dance/movement therapy provides the space for these children to explore and discover their bodies, while unlocking their potential for creativity. Children are encouraged to find themselves in a supportive environment where there is no "right" way to express or create (Canner, 1968).

As defined by the American Dance Therapy Association (ADTA), dance/movement therapy is "the psychotherapeutic use of movement as a process which furthers the emotional, social, cognitive, and physical integration of the individual" (American Dance Therapy Association, 2008). Dance/movement therapy is an effective form of treatment for people with developmental, medical, social, physical, and psychological impairments (Levy, 2005). This expressive therapy is a bridge, linking creative expression through movement with psychological theory (Kestenberg et al., 1999).

Dance/movement therapy emerged in the 1940s in the United States. Marian Chace, also known as "The Grand Dame" of dance/movement therapy, led the emerging field. Through her work teaching dance to people with varied abilities, Chace recognized the profound impact of the movement on various facets of her students' lives, and began to bridge her work in dance to the world of Western medicine. In 1942, Chace was asked to bring this work to St. Elizabeth's Hospital in Washington, DC. Here, psychiatrists also realized the benefits of this expressive and healing movement. In 1966, the American Dance Therapy Association formed, with Chace as the first president (Levy, 2005).

A second wave of dance/movement therapists emerged in the 1970s and 1980s. During this period, dance/movement therapy sparked the interest of many professionals, and therapists began experimenting with the use of the form with a variety of populations—including autism. In the midst of this, dance/movement therapy was also officially categorized as a form of psychotherapy.

In application, dance/movement therapy fosters socialization and communication in clients who otherwise might find it difficult to relate. The ability to engage fully through nonverbal activity sets dance/movement therapy apart from other forms of therapy. It creates an affirming environment for clients, where they are able to experience the value of belonging. Ultimately, dance/movement therapy provides both a bridge for contact and a medium for reciprocal communication for children with autism (ADTA, 2008).

A few basic principles form the guiding theory of dance/movement therapy. These overarching tenets of the field include the beliefs that behavior is communicative, personality is reflected through movement, changes in movement will eventually lead to changes in personality, and the larger an individual's movement repertoire, the more options individuals have when it comes time for them to cope with the environment (Kestenberg et al., 1999; Meekums, 2002). The actual practice of dance/movement therapy relies on the observation of movement behavior as it emerges in relationship, more specifically the therapeutic relationship between client and therapist. Dance/movement therapists are trained to understand, reflect, and eventually expand on the nonverbal expression of their clients (Adler, 2003). A consistent, supportive, and accepting atmosphere is used to begin the process of relationship formation, along with the following: mirroring (reflecting rhythms, patterns, and vocalizations expressed by the client), eye contact, touch, vocalizations, props, and rhythmic body action (ADTA, 2008; Erfer, 1995). In particular, props can be helpful with this population because they are very concrete and tangible, thus serving as a connecting medium between client and therapist.

In addition to the mirroring technique mentioned above, the approaches of both attunement and shape-flow adjustment (from the Kestenberg Movement Profile, one of many movement-analysis systems utilized by dance/movement therapists) help build the therapeutic relationship and augment the therapist's ability to make clinical choices. As described by Loman (1995), "attunement is based on sharing qualities of muscle tension, and Shape-Flow Adjustment is based on a similarity of breathing patterns and shape of the body between individuals" (p. 222). Within the therapeutic relationship, attunement builds a sense of empathy between therapist and client, while shape-flow adjustment builds trust in the relationship (Loman, 1995).

A constant priority, the initial and overarching goal for dance/movement therapists working with autism (or with any population) is to reach out and meet a client at his or her functioning level. Once this relationship has been established, it serves as a consistent guiding principle behind the work and emerges in the balance between the physical and relational. In the dance/movement therapy setting, relationships occur as a byproduct of the body in action, and physical movement flourishes because of the trust built within the therapeutic relationship. When the physical and relational aspects of the work are in balance, movement truly can serve as a language for universal communication.

When building treatment goals, each child with autism presents with specific needs and challenges, yet a handful of goals are generally applicable. The first of these goals is increasing sensory motor and perceptual motor development, directly targeting the motor deficits often faced by children with autism spectrum disorder (ADTA, 2008; Erfer, 1995). By working from both a functional and expressive standpoint, dance/movement therapists can use simple vocabulary and movement to stimulate perceptual, gross, and fine motor skills. An example of this is teaching children the perceptual concept of "in and out" by having them physically step inside of a space (i.e., a hula hoop) and then outside of that same space. Through the gross motor movement, the children experientially learn the concept, which can then be generalized to other areas.

The second goal for dance/movement therapists is to help clients improve their socialization and communication skills. As the therapeutic relationship builds, clients increase their ability to interact as part of a group and communicate (verbally or nonverbally) within that group. Steps toward these goals include: increasing eye contact, participating in shared rhythmic activities with engagement (and independently whenever possible), recognizing and responding to group members, increasing proximity to the group, decreasing a need for interpersonal distance, developing trust, and forming an understanding of "self" as opposed to the "others" outside of the self (ADTA, 2008).

Although these social and communication goals can be met through several modalities, dance/movement therapy is unique because the steps towards these goals can all be experienced on a kinesthetic level. For example, in group rhythmic activity, group members move together with similar rhythms, intensities, and physical tensions. This extension of movement throughout the body helps a client to integrate what may be a fragmented sense of self (Levy, 2005). Moving small movements into total body activity helps build cohesiveness and a sense of grounding, not only for the person as an individual, but also for his/her identity as a group member. The similar rhythmic and movement patterns allow each client to feel a sense of belonging on a nonverbal level.

Thirdly, building off of the growing understanding of self vs. others, dance/movement therapy works to foster body awareness and nurture a client's personal self-concept. By reflecting a child's movement nonverbally and then translating what is seen into simple language (i.e., mirroring the child in moving their head side to side, while verbalizing "I see you moving your head"), the dance/movement therapist positively verbalizes how the child appears, inherently improving his/her body awareness or body image. The simple verbalizations, or the "noticing" of what is going on, also help to structure the experience for the participant (Loman, 1995). As an added benefit, this verbalization of action naturally increases the movement repertoire of the client (applicable to goal one), as he/she is exposed to not only the conscious experience of his/her own movement, but also that of the others in the room.

"Body image is one of the most fundamental concepts in human growth and development and one that appears to be lacking in children who are autistic" (Erfer, 1995, p. 197). Standing behind this concept, body awareness and a positive body image are imperative, as the two combined form a foundation for a basic understanding of the self. Not only does the development of body awareness parallel sensorimotor development, but also the movement experience also helps children to orient to their space, their own bodies, and the others in the room. This orientation occurs on both an internal (self to self) and external (self to others) level. Because body image is formed from input from the vestibular, kinesthetic, proprioceptive, visual, and tactile systems, movement is an all-encompassing medium for the development of an individual's self-concept (Erfer, 1995).

A 1985 research study conducted by Enid Wolf-Schein, Gene Fisch, and Ira Cohen studied the use of nonverbal systems in children with autism and other developmental delays. The study came to the conclusion that "dance/movement therapy should be considered an intervention for persons with both autism and mental retardation since there are indications that deviations in nonverbal behaviors do contribute to the overall pathology of the individuals" (Wolf-Schein, Fisch, & Cohen, 1985, p. 78). This serves as an example of one of many studies indicating the potential for healing when combining dance/movement therapy and autism.

In more recent years, neuroscientists have been increasingly interested in the presence and impact of mirror neurons on mental health and relationships. Regarding this research, Cynthia Berrol notes, "a keystone of the therapeutic process of dance/movement therapy, the concept of mirroring is now the subject of neuroscience. The domains of mirror neurons currently under investigation span motoric, psychosocial and cognitive functions, including specific psychological issues . . . " (Berrol, 2006, p. 303). Dance/movement therapy inherently engages this mirror neuron system in the brain, for both those moving and those witnessing the movement of others. Since autism possibly relates to deficiencies in the mirror neuron system of the brain, dance/movement therapy has the potential to unlock and develop some of these deficient areas through the process of movement.

Risks and side effects related to dance/movement therapy are minimal. Movement may not be the preferred modality for expressing or relating for all individuals, although many who are open to trying the format find that it is a truly accessible approach to therapy. Like with any kind of movement, a person must be cautious and only do what is safely within their physical means in order to avoid any physical harm to self or others, within the process.

The American Dance Therapy Association (ADTA) is the professional organization for dance/movement therapists in the US and beyond. To learn more about the field or find a dance/movement therapist in your area, visit the website at www.adta.org or contact the national office by phone at 410-997-4040.

61

EXERCISE: THE GATEWAY TO BUILDING RELATIONSHIPS, SELF-ESTEEM, AND FITNESS

By David Geslak

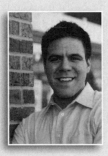

David S. Geslak, BS, CSCS, ACSM-HFS

David S. Geslak, "Coach Dave," has become widely recognized in the autism community for his affection to the community, dynamic presentations, and for the pioneering of structured visual exercise programs. He has trained professionals throughout the world on the Exercise Connection protocol, authored three books, hosts a TV show, "Coach Dave," on The Autism Channel, and provides jobs for individuals with autism, his Champions. The autism and special needs community has enthusiastically embraced Dave's message and is especially encouraged by his results.
www.ECautism.com

Many of you reading this may not recognize exercise as a type of therapy for individuals on the autism spectrum. That is good because exercise should not be labeled as such. One can assume the word *therapy* indicates that something is wrong, which in-turn means that something must be fixed.

There is no doubt that a children or adults on the autism spectrum face physical and cognitive challenges, but approaching them as *broken* is not how I have experienced breakthroughs with exercise. Establishing the relationship and building trust is vital to any successful partnership or program. However, this is often lost in a therapeutic setting with an emphasis put on clipboards and pluses (+) and minuses (-). When working in this community it is imperative to remember that they are children with autism, not autistic children.

Over the last ten years I have received many questions from parents about exercise. A common question from parents of adults with autism has been, "My child has been out of OT and PT for years and he is starting to gain weight. How do I get him moving?"

Occupational Therapy (OT) and Physical Therapy (PT) are absolutely vital for our children, but I have to stress that they are not the same as exercise. Each therapy session often varies in frequency and duration due to insurance coverage and/or your child's Individualized Education Plan (IEP). If you are a parent of a recently diagnosed child, these therapies may often end by middle school. If your child requires more support, such therapies may continue until high school and beyond.

Exercise, when taught appropriately, can be forever part of your child's lifestyle. And like OT, exercise can fulfill sensory needs. Dumbbell exercises (heavy work) can be a part of your child's routine and age-appropriately carry over until adulthood. Dumbbell exercises provide sensory feedback and can help to calm the body.

PT will aid to enhance movement patterns and improve muscular imbalances and so can exercise. Through the use of many bodyweight exercises such as yoga, bands, dynamic flexibility, and exercise machines, your child can improve his or her physical abilities.

Exercise, when done in groups or in a physical education class, provides your child the ability to work with their peers and build social skills while occurring in a realistic environment. Often in OT, PT, and speech therapies, the situations are structured around a protocol in an unnatural setting.

Having your child involved in exercise can help to improve any PT or OT goals, and many of those goals can be incorporated throughout an exercise session. This gives your child or student more opportunities for physical and cognitive development.

With over 30 percent of children with autism overweight or obese, I am not surprised that parents are looking for exercise programs. *We need to exercise more* has been the common pledge for our society. And as individuals, making exercise a part of our lifestyle is often only a New Year's Resolution. People are typically motivated, starting off strong and then are quickly overwhelmed, making the same resolution year after year.

Exercise is vital for every person, but the challenge, especially for those with autism, and the million-dollar question is, "How do I get my child motivated to exercise?" I wish I could give you one answer but there just isn't a cookie-cutter approach for exercise. The answers lie within you as a parent, teacher, and professional working with each individual child. The answers are often not independent of each. It takes a *team* approach to begin an exercise routine and carry it throughout your child's life.

When individuals begin to exercise and experience an increased heart rate, sweat, awkward yoga positions, dumbbells, and exercise bands, it can become overwhelming on the systems (nervous, endocrine, digestive, muscular & skeletal) of the body. We should not wonder why our children could become upset or may experience a maladaptive behavior with exercise. While it can be a challenge for your child to begin exercising, I urge you to focus on exercise's benefits and how it can provide your children and you a newfound hope and optimism.

After moderate aerobic activity, children with autism may experience increases in attention span, on-task behavior, and levels of correct responding (Rosenthal-Malek & Mitchell, 1997). Also, in children with autism, exercise can reduce stress and anxiety and improve sleep (Autism Research Institute, 2004).

While exercise has been proven to benefit children with autism, running an exercise class (physical education, park district, YMCA) can be challenging at best and organized chaos at worst. Think about this scenario: foreign objects (balls) being thrown and kicked in their direction, bright lights in a room, echoing sounds, and sometimes over 40 kids to a classroom with only 1-2 teachers . . . wow! Our children must have an exercise environment adapted to their needs.

One study states that a physical activity-based program is *easy* to implement and has been shown to be effective in controlling inappropriate behaviors associated with autism. (Alison, Basile, & McDonald, 1991; Elliot, Dobbin, Rose, & Soper 1994). While I have witnessed many children and adults become calmer, limit their stimulating (stimming) and maladaptive behaviors following an exercise routine, this study is a bit misleading because it is not, as it states, easy to implement a program. Unfortunately, you cannot just throw the kids a basketball and say, "Shoot some hoops," or tell them to run a lap or even line up. You need to have structure for them, and for you, and once established, then you can begin to make your job a bit "easier."

Implementing an exercise program takes proper visual and individual supports, planning, and motivation. If attempting this in a group session one must also have the ability to assess which children to pair together to not only reduce maladaptive behaviors but also to promote social interaction, ultimately, hoping to achieve an improvement in an individual's self-esteem and love for exercise. "Easy" is not the word I would have chosen, but in this chapter I will provide you tried-and-true guidelines to begin an exercise program.

Think of this chapter as your to-do list for teaching exercise, much like the daily schedule your children are dependent on. I want you to revert back here when you need a reminder of what you need to be focused on. Reread the stories that I share of my clients and always have hope because exercise is possible.

Children with autism are unique and deserve a higher quality physical education that meets their needs. They can and will exercise. But often it will take us, the parents and/or professionals, to set or change our expectations of when and how *it* will happen.

When working with Kevin, who was non-verbal, wore orthotics on his legs, and headphones covering his ears, I tried for months to get him to jump his feet together and then apart. I used nearly every visual support and strategy I could think of. After months of trying he was still unable. I would build different exercises into his routine he could successfully perform, and I tried not to focus on the one thing he couldn't do. Just as I was beginning to lose hope in my own abilities, six months later, he jumped his feet apart and together!

I do not know exactly why it "clicked" that day but it is a day I will never forget. As professionals we have to adapt our routines, lesson plans, expectations and sometimes our education in order to help our children. We need to think outside the box and most importantly, keep the passion we had on the very first day we worked with an individual with autism. In doing so, you must be flexible, and you will not only help to engage your children in exercise but forever transform their lives.

1. You Need To Establish Trust to Get Results

A study conducted by Dr. Mahoney, states that, "The facilitators (parent, other) having a visible affect of acceptance, enjoyment, expressiveness and warmth . . . are significantly related to increase in the child's language, social competence, joint attention and self-regulation." I find this to be one of the most important studies I have read in relation to autism.

Professionals in this field have chosen to be here because they want to help our children. However, as we go through the education system, we are told to follow protocols, take notes, record data, and measure results. This is absolutely important and should be done to assess whether a therapy or program is working. However, when you begin with exercise, I encourage you to put your clipboard down and put yourself in the child's shoes.

When I started with Roan he was 3.5 years old. He had the classic autism symptoms, no eye contact, "stimming," echolalia, and scripting. He wanted to play with his toys but that was only if he was not running from wall-to-wall. Talking to him did not help me to engage him. So, when he grabbed his trucks, I grabbed one too. For weeks this was the routine, although I always had a large exercise visual off to the side. When I got his attention I would point to the visual, next model the exercise, and then ask him to do it with me. And slowly he would begin to participate. After one year of sessions, one hour per week, he was not only choosing his exercises but maintaining better attention and focus.

His parents said when I would leave he would repeat, "right hand, left hand, right foot, left foot." The school OT and PT were not teaching him that or saying those small phrases. But he was able to learn more than exercise in our sessions, which will impact him for a lifetime.

Parents, it is important to recognize the relationship your child has with their instructors. Trust your gut. If you notice that your child is not responding to the therapy or intervention, it may not be the therapy you need to switch it may be the instructor.

2. A Picture is Worth a Thousand Words

If I were to tell you to perform a single leg hip extension, would you know what to do? How about if I asked you to do a scorpion? By simply placing an exercise visual (picture) next to your child while trying to do exercise, this can make all the difference. They don't necessarily have to hear you tell them because they can see it. The picture takes the auditory processing out of the request and pointing to a picture (with you modeling the exercise of course!), can be what helps to engage your child or student.

When Ben and I first began he was twenty-one years old and non-verbal. With Ben, I used large, 8.5" x 11" exercise visuals. He would attempt the exercise, for the given duration, and upon completion I always ended with the praise, "Great job, Ben." Because his parents had him involved in movement at a young age, he picked up some of my exercises quickly (after a 60 minute session). Challenging him for his capabilities, I would often try exercises that I did not have a visual for. This would cause him to get upset by "stimming" and biting his shirt. By the next session I would have the specific visual made and he would do it but with no more "stimming" and no more biting of the shirt.

Visuals supports can be implemented with individuals across the age range, beginning in preschool and extending through middle school. In elementary and middle school, visual supports such as schedules and picture cues have proven effective in reducing transition time, increasing on-task behavior, and in completing self-help in the home. (Bryan & Gast, 2000; Dettmer, Simpson, Myles, & Ganz, 2000; MacDuff, Krantz, & McClannahan, 1993). Also, effective visual supports in early childhood settings include visual schedules to increase task engagement, visual scripts to encourage social interaction, and picture cues to support play skill development (Krantz & McClannahan, 1998; Massey & Wheeler, 2000; Morrison, Sainato, BenChaaban, & Endo, 2002).

Parents may think that visuals are elementary and because your child or student is an adult, they do not need them. These thoughts are quite the contrary, especially with exercise. You may have to go back to grade school techniques in order to transition your child to an exercise routine.

While exercise visuals benefit the child you are working with, if you are a teacher with a limited exercise background and may be reliant on the dedicated work of paraprofessionals, visual supports can be just as important for you and the paraprofessionals as it is for your children.

3. You Need Structure to Transform their Lives

When establishing an exercise program, structure is crucial. Our children excel in a structured environment. Structure will provide your children with expectations. A beginning, middle and end are needed to complete a routine. And as your children or students progress in their program, structure will provide you an opportunity for change.

Structure will also help you as a parent or educator stay organized and not become overwhelmed. I suggest beginning with exercise stations. Start with two stations. Think of them as a first-then board, first beginning with something non-preferred activity such as hip extensions, and once this is completed, a preferred activity such as lying on a stability ball.

First-then image

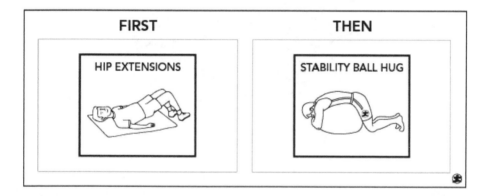

And please, do not make food the reward! Too many times, I have seen food be the common reward. Children should not be motivated by sugary, fatty foods especially in an exercise setting. It not only defeats the purpose following exercise, it begins to instill bad habits for our children. Establishing a familiar and consistent structure, positive feedback and educating them throughout, can keep your child engaged and limit your need to run to the pantry.

With many of my clients the beginning of each session has remained the same from the first day I began establishing structure. Ben, who I spoke of earlier, began by using the elliptical because he was used to doing that with dad. In doing so, I was establishing trust with him (not barking orders to do a new activity) and this became the structure. I started with him on the elliptical and then transitioned him to do exercises on the floor. To this day, we still begin with five minutes on the treadmill.

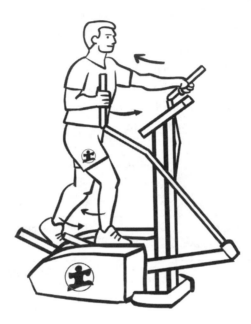

Brody, ten years old, limited verbal abilities, and a toe-walker, begins with an exercise story and/or a written schedule on a white board. He was used to this approach with private therapists and at school, so I was not going to change it. Changing the routine can be confusing for the child so try to make the transition to exercise as familiar and as easy as possible.

And with Rachel, who has Asperger's and was fourteen years old when we started, we began with exercises on the foam roller. When she started to exercise she had anxiety with her social communication with her peers as well as typical challenges with high school. I choose the foam roller exercise because it has the ability to reduce tension in the neck and shoulders, where most people hold their stress. The foam roller improves posture and provides sensory feedback, which many of our children need. Now, every session our days begin with the foam roller, but she is now further able to reduce her stress with a high intensity run!

Each child is different, but special needs or not, everyone needs structure and likes to know what is expected of him or her. You can create routines that are engaging, fun

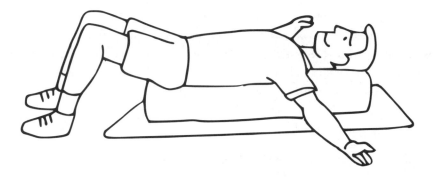

and are not dependent on food. Take your time and do not rush exercise. It's a lifestyle change. I promise you that your children will shock you at their abilities.

4. You Can't Afford to Push the Limits

Often many people believe the more they do, the better. This is incorrect, especially when beginning an exercise program. Some people push their bodies to the extreme while exercising, which can not only weaken the body but the mind as well. This mentality can often lead to physical injury and deter many people from exercise.

Remember, individuals with autism have heightened sensory systems and we may never experience the sensation exercise brings to their bodies. Using a "less is more" philosophy will reduce their risk of injury and prepare their bodies for exercise.

Three sets of 10 repetitions (3x10) of an exercise is a common protocol for what people think is getting an effective workout for an exercise. This would mean that you would perform an exercise 10 times, rest for 30–60 seconds, perform it again for 10 repetitions, rest and repeat for a third set of 10 repetitions.

Three x 10 is not the miracle equation to working out. If your child has never done, for example, a Hip Extension, 1 set of 5 repetitions can be beneficial! The key is setting realistic goals and expectations for your child and for yourself.

I was presenting at an autism conference and a mother came up to me after the presentation and said, "I took my son to a personal trainer at our local gym and now he won't go back because the trainer worked him too hard."

The trainer had no experience in autism and my assumption is that his education was average like many trainers are in the industry. Mom was absolutely doing the right thing and trusted in the "expert," but he was probably just a good salesman.

It may take weeks, even months, depending on your child's abilities to work up to 3 sets of 10 repetitions of an exercise. Start them slow, engage them in a few exercises a day, not a full hour, and build on that.

Many times when working with a child, I begin by doing one set of each exercise. I do not want them to get bored and, especially in the beginning of an exercise program, I want to keep their attention. With one set and one exercise at a time you can identify what exercises they like and excel at. Then the next time you workout together you can do more sets/reps or find new exercises similar to their strengths and interests that they can try. And when searching for the "expert" in exercise in your neighborhood, I would suggest you start by looking in the mirror.

5. Sports Are Not the Only Form of Exercise

Sports is what many believe to be the primary way to get exercise or participate in physical activity. I will agree that sports can provide a tremendous amount of physical benefits but also social and cognitive benefits. However, many children, special needs or not, do not want to be athletes or play sports.

Picture a child with autism who is non-verbal trying understand what to do with this black and white round object (soccer ball) and when she picks it up with her hands, she is told "NO."

In her mind she may have thought, *This ball goes in the orange round cylinder* or *I like the shapes and patterns on this ball.*

Sports for your child may be the exact way to get him moving and engaged in exercise, in which case, obviously, do not stop. But please remember that basketball, soccer, and some of the other team sports are predominately played with a group of children. At times, a large group of children can be difficult to find or your child may not yet have the social skills to be in this environment, which can ultimately lead them away from sport.

It is important to teach them lifetime exercises so they can incorporate them into their daily routine. By focusing on the Five Components of Physical Fitness for Individuals with Autism © (Body Image, Posture, Motor Coordination, Muscular Fitness and Cardiovascular Fitness) you can prepare your children's/students' bodies for sport, the classroom, and daily physical exertion. You also should educate your child who loves sports, that exercises focusing on the Five Components can allow them to throw the ball faster, hit the ball farther, have a stronger kick and even run faster during the game, ultimately encouraging them to do more activity, which all our children need.

When I was teaching at a school for children with autism one of the girls, Erica always had behavioral issues during soccer. Erica was more challenged, non-verbal and still in diapers at sixteen years old. She had poor proprioception but her smile and laugh was infectious. I knew exercise should be apart of her life because I had seen some many children experience positive benefits from it. When I taught my sport lesson plans, I assumed soccer would be good for her because girls play soccer, right? I was wrong. She would end up crying on the ground, hardly wanting to kick the ball, and when she had it in her hands she would throw it across the room.

Months later, as I bi-monthly rotated my lesson plans, I was on the football lesson plan. I watched Erica with her paraprofessional as she rotated through the stations and she had no maladaptive behaviors. I could not figure out why, but she was happy and so was I.

Her mother came to pick her up later that afternoon. I told her about Erica's challenges with soccer but that she was having great success in football. Her mom said to me, "That makes sense." I asked, "why?"

"Because her Dad and her watch football together every Sunday," she responded.

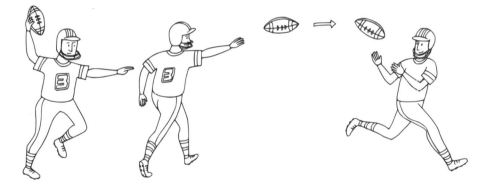

Sports may not always be a motivator for some children and for others it may not be the sport you would choose or assume. Keep your children moving in any way possible and be aware that as they age their likes and dislikes can change in exercise so you may have to as well.

Professionals, I have been in your shoes (bit, scratched, hit, hair pulled, changed diapers, etc.) and while it has been emotional I have never given up on my mission of incorporating exercise. I know that by using these tips and strategies exercise can help you to reach your mission with the children you serve.

Together we need to support each other by sharing experiences, strategies, successes and failures to help our children reach their full potential. Our children need us. The parents need us to support and encourage. In the end, our mission is the same, so let's work as a team and conquer.

Moms and Dads, I have witnessed many breakthroughs with exercise that go beyond the physical. Improvement in self-esteem, confidence and a smile is not easily measured but I can guarantee that when you begin exercising with your children you will learn something new about your child abilities.

62

EARLY INTERVENTION PHYSICAL THERAPY

By Dr. Allan Cuevas

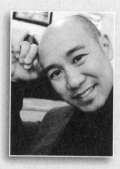

Allan Cuevas, PT, DPT, CSCS

allancuevaspt@hotmail.com

Dr. Allan Cuevas works as a pediatric physical therapist on the Upper East Side and East Harlem neighborhoods of Manhattan. He received his Masters of Science in Physical Therapy (MsPT) degree from Columbia University in 2001 and completed his Doctorate of Physical Therapy (DPT) degree at Temple University in 2007. He also completed training as a Certified Strength and Conditioning Specialist (CSCS) from the National Strength and Conditioning Association (NSCA) in 2001.

Dr. Cuevas treats infants and toddlers through the Early Intervention program of New York City. He makes his rounds around Manhattan using a speedy kick scooter, known as a Xooter, moving from place to place with a backpack filled with a variety of balls, toys, and games. He works in apartments, playgrounds, Early Head Start programs, and child care facilities. Dr. Cuevas has success treating his caseloads of infants and toddlers because he has the unique opportunity to directly teach and coach parents, nannies, and teachers; who can effectively carry-over activities into the child's daily routines. Dr. Cuevas also works effectively with his teams of Applied Behavior Analysis (ABA) Therapists, Speech Therapists, Occupational Therapists, Special Instructors, and Service Coordinators.

Dr. Cuevas has extensive experience in improving the gross motor problems related to Autism Spectrum Disorders, Tracheostomy, Torticollis, Toe-Walking, Down's Syndrome, Prematurity, Fragile X Syndrome, Cerebral Palsy, Hydrocephalus, and Developmental Delay. He utilizes his knowledge from evidence-based practice and skills developing exercise routines to specifically design fun and effective activities for his patients that tailor to the child's unique developmental delay diagnosis, functional limitations, personality, and immediate environment. His focus remains on initially gaining the trust of the child as a playmate, learning their specific fears that are negatively reinforcing the delays, and teaching the children gross motor skills through facilitation and support techniques utilizing multiple repetitions and feedback for optimal motor learning.

Early Intervention Physical Therapy (PT) is a unique way of touching the lives of individuals and families. The immediate months and years following a birth of a new baby are filled with happiness and excitement. However, there are situations where the caregivers of an infant or toddler may grow anxious because their child may not be developing at the same rate as their age group. Their child may not be independently crawling, sitting, standing, or walking when other children their age are able to do so without any difficulty. With the assistance of a pediatrician or childhood services, these delays in gross motor skills can be screened and the appropriate early intervention PT services can be initiated for initial evaluation and treatment.

The belief remains that if you are able to detect gross motor developmental delays in infants and toddlers early, then you can be more effective in improving the child's ability to learn and successfully perform age-appropriate gross-motor skills. Working with a child between 0-3 years, an early intervention PT would address skills such as negotiating their environment by crawling, walking or running, transitioning between different positions, stair climbing safely, negotiating playground equipment, and jumping in all directions. By improving the gross motor skills that are delayed, a PT can affectively improve the child's development to ensure that they can participate with their peers by the time they reach a classroom setting.

Major Milestones

During the gross motor development of an infant and toddler, there exists a certain step ladder of skills that should be accomplished in a pre-determined order. One skill at an earlier age usually serves as the building block for the next skill at a later age. For example, before a child learns the balance and strength needed to stand without assistance, the child must first learn the balance and strength needed to sit without assistance.

These gross motor milestones are not accomplished at a specific age. Instead, every child reaches certain milestones within a range of months. For example, the general age for walking without any kind of support is around 12 months of age. However, a child may be showing normal gross motor development even if it takes them until 16 months of age to take their first steps without any support. If the child continues to have difficulty walking independently into the 17th month and onward, the parent may seek professional guidance in determining if their child should be recommended for early intervention services.

Fear

The two basic concerns in contributing to the delay in gross motor activities in infants and toddlers have been traditionally a decrease in balance and a decrease in strength.

However, a third factor has expressed itself when approaching each gross motor milestone. This concern that usually goes undetected is fear. With each progressive milestone, new fears challenge the ability of a child to move forward with each advancing age-appropriate skill.

The most common fear remains the basic fear of falling. For example, after a child learns to sit independently, the next mobility skill to learn would be the transition from a sitting position to a crawling position on the floor. However, if the child does not overcome this initial fear of a controlled fall to the floor, the child will have a difficult time making this transition to grasp for toys out of reach.

Another example shows itself when a child begins to learn to walk without hand support. When a child shows interest to ambulate on their feet, they often begin by cruising furniture, pushing a walker/push toy, or walking while being held by a caregiver. At this point, the fear to walk becomes lessened because they are holding onto a support and do not have to rely on their own balance. If this child does not overcome this fear of walking without hand support, they will continue to creep along the floor and will only walk when given support. This fear of walking will prevent them from participating with activities with same-aged peers that can walk.

Support and Facilitation Techniques

Caregivers have the ability to participate in play activities with their infants and toddlers to help promote age-appropriate activities. To help infants and toddlers overcome fears, it becomes vital that caregivers and therapists learn to support and facilitate the movements of these infants and toddlers. By having successful supported movements, such as walking or stair climbing without fears, the child will eventually attempt to complete the assisted activity independently.

Every gross motor milestone requires a different set of skilled movement patterns. Acquiring these skills will involve multiple repetitions of the specific motor skills that will be guided by the caregiver or PT. The infant or toddler will need to practice repetitions to increase strength, to improve balance, and to learn from mistakes that will be made during the exercises.

Major Problems

Infants and toddlers tend to develop along an ordered line of gross motor milestones. However, when a child encounters a delay in gross motor development, they may encounter a major problem which may be difficult to solve without the guidance of a physical therapist. Without the appropriate assistance, the infant or toddler may be stuck in a particular stage of development and will perform movements with compensations that form very bad habits. These compensatory movements make moving around their environment easier and less scary, but prevent them from using the correct muscles needed to successfully achieve future milestones.

For example, a child who is fearful with transitioning to a crawling position from a sitting position can develop an alternative strategy for negotiating their environment. Instead of crawling, this fearful child may learn to scoot. Scooting involves moving along the ground in a seated position by using only their arms to propel themselves along the floor on their buttocks. Eventually, the child uses this strategy to scoot across a room and develops this motor pattern of scooting instead of learning how to crawl on the belly or creep on the hands and knees. This is problematic because although they may learn to walk, they will have trouble standing up from the middle of a room if they happen to fall down.

ASD Perspective

Autism Spectrum Disorder (ASD) does not directly affect the balance and the strength required to complete age-appropriate skills for gross motor development. However, the social impairments, communication difficulties, and repetitive behaviors can indirectly impact the acquisition of more advanced gross motor skills. A child with ASD can usually develop the basic balance and strength to be able to crawl, stand, and walk; but they usually have more difficulty acquiring more abstract gross motor skills, such as running, ball playing, and jumping.

A child without ASD can generally have normal gross motor development as a result of exploring their environment and engaging in play activities with other children and adults. As a result, a child with ASD may not participate in these complex activities and may not develop more advanced muscle strength and balance necessary for school aged activities. A knowledgeable early intervention PT will be able to teach the caregivers different activities and games to engage their child; while facilitating and supporting proper movements to strengthen muscles, to improve balance, and to learn motor patterns.

Gross Motor Development in the Infant and Toddler

I.   **Tummy Time**

   a.   **Major Milestone:** 4–5 months—An infant will lift up their head and bear weight on their forearms while lying on their belly.

   b.   **Fear:** Babies lying on their belly require more strength and effort in lifting their heads to explore their environment with their eyes. On the other hand, relaxing on their back requires little effort to see toys and caregivers.

Therefore, babies may cry when placed on their belly because this extra muscle strain to lift their head may frighten them.

c.   **Support & Facilitation:** During playtime, a caregiver can gently place them on their bellies on the floor to track and reach for toys. If the baby begins to cry, a parent can assist the baby with head lifting by laying the baby with their chest on the inside of a boppy pillow. While on the pillow, they will need constant supervision.

d.   **Major Problems:** Torticollis may occur when a child is left on their back for extended periods of time, especially in a bouncy chair or car seat. The infant will likely develop a flat spot on the back of their head and will sometimes develop a head tilt and rotation away from the midline position.

e.   **ASD Perspective:** The baby will not be diagnosed as having ASD at this time. It will be important for caregivers to continually attempt to engage the child in focusing activities requiring tracking toys while on their backs and bellies.

II.   Sitting & Transitions to the floor

a.   **Major Milestone:** 6–8 months—Sitting independently without help from parents.

b.   **Fear:** Often times, a baby will not grasp for a toy if it is out of arms reach for fear of falling to the ground.

c.   **Support & Facilitation:** To encourage exploration and using their own trunk muscles, the baby needs to be given support at their trunk when sitting upright. As the baby gets more stable, the support should be moved to only holding the legs in the sitting position. This forces the baby to use their trunk muscles to stabilize their upright position to prevent a fall.

d.   **Major Problems:** Babies will not move out of the seated position. They will grab for toys within reach; but will not attempt to grab toys that are immediately out of reach. They will have difficulty moving to the floor to crawl and creep forward to explore their environment. Eventually, these fearful babies will turn to scooting on their bottoms instead of making the fearful transition to the floor.

    e.   **ASD Perspective:** The baby will not be diagnosed as having ASD at this time. It will benefit the child for the parents to engage the child in supported and unsupported sitting. This involves playing with toys, tracking toys, or reaching for toys in a seated position with appropriate support on the trunk or legs.

III. Crawling & Creeping

    a.   **Major Milestone:** 8–10 months—Crawling forward while on their belly and creeping forward on their hands & knees.

    b.   **Fear:** Babies will have an initial fear of creeping on their hands and knees. By raising their body off of the ground, there is a greater chance for them to hit their face and head on the ground. In addition, the muscle strain from raising the body off the ground with the legs & arms can frighten them.

    c.   **Support & Facilitation:** To encourage crawling along the floor, the baby needs to be shown how to move forward by pulling with their arms/hands and pushing with their legs/feet. To encourage creeping along the floor on their hands and knees, the baby can be supported by holding the belly off of the ground while the baby attempts to move their hands and knees along the ground to obtain a toy.

    d.   **Major Problems:** Babies may prefer to crawl with their belly on the ground even at a later age. This movement is referred to as a 'commando crawl.' If a baby gets stuck with this movement pattern, they will not develop the extremity and trunk strength that usually results from creeping on their hands and knees.

    e.   **ASD Perspective:** The baby will not be diagnosed as having ASD at this time. It will be important for caregivers to continually attempt to engage the child in focusing activities requiring them to make crawling and creeping movements forward along the ground to reach for toys and explore their environments.

IV. Supported Walking

    a.   **Major Milestone:** 9–12 months—Pulling up to standing, cruising furniture to the left and right, and lowering to the ground.

b. **Fear:** After pulling up to standing by a table or chair, a toddler may develop a fear of lowering self to the ground from a standing position. The toddler will naturally straighten their legs while standing to achieve the most stability to prevent a fall. However, this leg stiffness to improve stability will also prevent mobility to move to the ground due to fear of falling once the knee is unlocked and bent.

c. **Support & Facilitation:** In order for a toddler to learn how to pull-up to standing, cruise furniture to the left and right, and to lower to the ground, they must be supported and facilitated at their hips and ankles. By supporting lower and away from their trunk, the toddlers will be more accountable for their movements and safety or else they will fall.

d. **Major Problems:** Toddlers will get stuck in a standing position while holding onto the furniture. They will often cry to be placed on the ground safely. In addition, the toddler may suffer from frequent falls when cruising furniture due to lack of recognizing dangers and lack of awareness of their bodies in space.

e. **ASD Perspective:** The toddler may be diagnosed as having ASD at this time. It will be important for caregivers to continually give assistance to the child to make standing transitions using furniture and lowering transitions back to the ground. The toddler will need practice with assistance to increase their strength, balance, and confidence with their abilities to make these supported walking movements.

V. Independent Walking

a. **Major Milestone:** 12–16 months—Walking, turning, & pivoting without support.

b. **Fear:** The biggest obstacle in teaching a toddler how to walk is their individual fear of falling when there is nothing to grab onto to stop a fall.

c. **Support & Facilitation:** The obvious support for a toddler would be to hold their hands. While this is the safest way to walk a toddler, this will also slow their learning to independently walk. The support and facilitation for walking is best accomplished around the toddler's hips and thighs. The most fearful part of walking is making the weight shift at the hips in order to pick up the leg. However, picking up a leg means having to lean to one side which usually causes the loss of balance and eventual fall.

d.   **Major Problems:** A toddler will continue to creep along the floor on their hands and knees and cruise around furniture to explore their environment. These non-walking toddlers will have difficulty participating in the walking games and activities of their same-aged peers. In some instances, they will not be allowed to enter a child care class of their same-aged peers because they cannot walk and keep up with the other children.

e.   **ASD Perspective:** The toddler may be diagnosed as having ASD at this time. It will be important for caregivers to continually give assistance to the child to make learn how to walk independently and be more aware of their body in space. There are new dangers when a child begins to walk and the consequences are much greater if the child falls or bumps into items when they do not pay attention.

VI.   Stair Climbing

a.   **Major Milestone:** 15–20 months—Supported stair climbs moving upward & downward using the wall or rail

b.   **Fear:** The biggest fear climbing upward on the stairs is not having the necessary combination of adequate lower extremity strength and upper extremity support to stair climb upward. If the toddler feels that this combination is not present, the toddler will put their hands on the stairs to ensure that they will not hit their face or head onto the next step. The biggest fear going downward on the stairs is falling down the stairs head-first. If a toddler feels unstable with their strength and balance going down the stairs, they turn sideways with two hands on the wall/rail, scoot down the stairs on their bottom, or roll onto their bellies and creep downwards on hands and knees.

c.   **Facilitation:** The most important movement is to initially show the toddler how to first move their hands forward along the wall or hand rail before even taking a step up or down. Moving the hands first before the legs will put the toddler in a stronger position to negotiate the stairs. The next important movement involves making sure that the stronger leg leads the climb upward and that the opposite side hand gains support from the wall, rail, or caregiver. Going downward, the weaker leg leads the climb downward and the opposite hand holds the wall.

d. **Major Problems:** A child will creep up the stairs on hands and knees or constantly place their hands on the ground during a standing stair climb due to a lack of push-off from lower extremities and support from the upper extremities when walking up the stairs. A child will learn to scoot, walk sideways, and creep down the stairs due to a fear of falling down the stairs. These strategies will not be appropriate when stair climbing in public or participating in school activities.

e. **ASD Perspective:** The toddler may be diagnosed as having ASD at this time. It will be important for caregivers to continually give assistance to the child to learn how to star climb independently and be more aware of their body in space. Surprisingly, most of the children who have ASD are excellent stair climbers up/down. The danger of the environment forces the toddlers to fully pay attention to their surroundings to prevent a fall. The concept of stair climbing is very tangible because there is a purpose in moving up/down stairs; compared to abstract games such as catching & throwing a ball or jumping.

VII. Ball Playing

a. **Major Milestones:** 15–20 months—Kicking balls, throwing balls overhand & underhand, & catching balls.

b. **Fear:** During a kicking motion, a toddler may be hesitant to make a strong kick due to a fear of falling. Having good single-leg stance balance is required to make a strong kick with a good follow-through because the kicking leg will be off the ground for a longer period of time. During a game a catch, a toddler may be hesitant to catch a ball heading towards them for fear of getting hit by the ball. As a result, they will often close their eyes when attempting to catch a ball.

c. **Facilitation:** When practicing ball skills, it is essential that the toddlers throw or kick towards a target that can visually fall down. If kicking with the right leg, you must support the left hip during the weight shift and swing the strong right leg through the ball in a sweeping motion. If throwing with the right hand, it will be important to kneel behind the toddler to facilitate an overhand throwing motion toward a target.

d.   **Major Problems:** When kicking a ball, a toddler may learn to kick by walking through the ball because of a lack of balance to kick off one foot. Also, a toddler might also step directly onto the ball because taking a step downward means less time in single-leg stance. When learning to throw a ball, a toddler only learns to throw a ball with two hands, drops the ball in front of them, or hands the caregiver the ball. When attempting to catch, the toddler refuses to catch a ball by not putting up their hands or closes their eyes due to fear of the ball coming towards them.

e.   **ASD Perspective:** The toddler may be diagnosed as having ASD at this time. It will be important for caregivers to place a target when teaching their toddlers how to throw or kick a ball. Merely throwing a ball back or returning a ball kick is an abstract concept that may not be grasped by a child with ASD. By providing a target to knock down, the ball game becomes more concrete because the toddler can visually see that their ball throw or kick has knocked down a target. At this age, toddlers often take pleasure in knocking down or breaking things.

VIII. Jumping

a.   **Major Milestone:** 24–34 months—jumping up/down, jumping downward off a stool, jumping forward over a line, jumping upward over hurdles.

b.   **Fear:** The toddler showing delays in jumping can have a normal feeling of helplessness when lifting themselves with 2-feet off of the ground. It is safer for a toddler to perform a leaping jump; which is when the toddler will lead with 1-foot instead of jumping off 2-feet at the same time. This 1-foot jump shows itself especially when a toddler is asked to jump with direction over a line, over an obstacle, downward off a stool or step, downward off a chair, and over a hurdle. As the jumping challenge increases with difficulty, the more likely the toddler will leap with 1-foot unless they are transitioned slowly to increase their confidence to produce a jump without falling or hurting themselves.

c. **Facilitation:** The first motor movement to teach a toddler involves squatting down by bending their knees in order to get maximum power to produce a 2-foot jump. Without an adequate knee bend, a toddler with resort to leaping using a 1-foot jump because they will not have enough power to leave the ground. Before this age range of 24-34 months, the toddler has grown accustomed to using their upper extremities for activities. The facilitation techniques will need to teach the toddler to solely use their lower extremities to produce a jump. This involves progressing the facilitation and support for a 2-foot jump from under their underarms initially, to their forearms, to their hands, and then to their hips.

d. **Major Problems:** When asked to jump forward, downward, or upward, a toddler may get stuck with the habit of jumping by leaping with one foot due to fear or not having adequate knee bend before pushing-off. Jumping off 1-foot is easier to complete a jumping task, but this technique is not utilizing the full power of both feet and may delay the strength building of the lower extremities. Another problem to be aware of involves the landing of a jump. Often times, a toddler may learn to land a jump with both knees straight. Having both knees straight give the toddler more stability initially for a simple jump up/down. However, when asked to complete a bigger jump forward or downward, the toddler needs to be shown to also bend the knees upon landing to cushion the downward motion of the body towards the ground.

e. **ASD Perspective:** The toddler may be diagnosed as having ASD at this time. But unlike stair climbing, there may not be a clear purpose for the toddler with ASD to learn the jumping motion. To negotiate over an obstacle, one can merely step over. To step down a stool or stair step, one can merely step down. However, at this age range, it is important to teach the jumping techniques to jump over obstacles or to jump down from a step in order to develop their leg strength and body awareness for future milestones and to participate with activities with same aged peers.

The gross-motor development of a baby and toddler becomes an exciting time for the family. With each accomplished gross-motor milestone, a child's confidence begins to shine and they are better able to participate in play activities with same-aged peers and caregivers. However, when a child is diagnosed as having ASD, there is not an automatic delay in gross-motor skills. The difficulties with attention and social awareness may impact gross-motor development because the toddler may not have the desire to perform abstract concepts like running after a ball, walking backwards or sideways, ball playing, and jumping. By not participating in these activities, those muscles and motor planning skills do not become developed and may lead to other issues affecting participation in the community and school. But with the proper guidance from an early intervention physical therapist and provider team, many of these milestones can be accomplished to prepare a child for school and life.

63

YOGA AND MARTIAL ART THERAPIES FOR THE ASD CHILD

By Isauro Fernandez

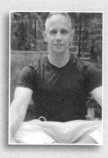

Isauro Fernandez, JD, E-RYT

info@kipowervinyasa.com

Born and raised in New York City, ki power vinyasa™ creator Isauro Fernandez practiced law for 20 years before experiencing the transformational effects of yoga. His commitment and passion for yoga began with martial arts, which he began studying at age six. He holds black belts in judo and tae kwon do. Isauro is an E-RYT (a Yoga Alliance Experienced Registered Yoga Teacher) and is also certified in Thai yoga massage bodywork. He created and trademarked ki power vinyasa,™ which fuses the movement and breath of vinyasa yoga with the grace, focus, and physical intensity of martial arts. Isauro has been featured on *Good Morning America*, and in several national magazines.

In each class, he challenges his students to embark on a journey of personal development to uncover their authenticity through a powerful blend of sweat, strength, and spirit. Isauro seeks to connect students with their ki—their life force, authentic self, and essential energies.

Isauro teaches private and semi-private classes around the city for children who are on the autistic spectrum. He also holds workshops and retreats nationally and internationally and is available for private, school based, and corporate individualized classes.

When Isauro is not busy helping yoga students with their physical and personal journeys, he remains deeply rooted in martial arts; he competes in national and international Judo Master Tournaments. Isauro continues to practice law and currently lives in New York City. For more information on ki power vinyasa and Isauro Fernandez, visit www.kipowervinyasa.com.

Yoga and martial art therapies can help the child on the autism spectrum develop effective, lifelong and life changing strategies that will empower them to live a better and fuller life. Through the practice of these ancient art forms, the ASD child will be introduced to basic mind body techniques that will help him feel peaceful, calm, and safe. The child will also be engaging in a physical practice that will strengthen, stretch, and tone the body, focus the mind, and awaken the spirit.

I. Yoga

The practice of yoga is both an art and a science. Yoga literally means "to yoke," a union. It is a union of mind, body, and spirit. It has been around for thousands of years and more recently all over the news as students, young and old, line up at yoga studios to practice. The foundation for yoga philosophy can be found in *The Yoga Sutras of Pantanjali,* which were written in approximately 200 AD. Pantanjali outlined an eight step blueprint or eight limbed path offering guidelines in personal development with the goal of achieving harmony in mind, body, and spirit.

The poses (asanas) and the breath (pranayama) are two of the eight limbs and a perfect and powerful place to start incorporating yoga into the child's life.

I. Asana

Asana is a physical practice, or pose/posture, of yoga. Asana means "seat," and it originally referred to a seated meditation position. The asanas are meant to create ease, flexibility, and strength in the body, allowing for future seated and still meditation.

The continuous practice of yoga asanas will strengthen and tone the child's muscles. It will also create more flexibility in the body. The postures will also improve the child's coordination and balance. In addition, and very important for the child on the spectrum, the practice of yoga will help in quieting and stilling the mind. The child is physically and mentally engaged while in the pose. He is focused on holding the pose and breathing into it. The racing thoughts that are prevalent amongst these children stop, and the child once again feels peaceful, calm, and safe.

Here are seven poses you can start with your child today. Please note that it doesn't matter how long he/she holds the pose or how many poses you introduce initially. All you need to start is one pose... one long inhale and one deep exhale.

1. Downward Facing Dog

Come to your hands and knees. Align your shoulders with your hands and your knees with your hips. Walk your hands a few inches away from you and curl your toes under. Push downward and forward with your hands and upward and backward through your pelvis. This two-way stretch will elongate your spine and flatten your shoulders. Spread your fingers evenly apart and squeeze your elbows towards each other. Drop your head. Breathe five deep, slow, and long breaths.

This pose increases blood flow to the brain, relieves fatigue, slows the heart rate, tones the arm and leg muscles, stretches the hamstrings, and is therapeutic for headaches.

2. Ragdoll—Standing Forward Bend

Separate your feet hips' width apart and hang your torso forward. Soften the knees, take opposite hand to opposite elbow and drop your head, letting it dangle in the space between the biceps. Hold for five breaths.

This pose slows the heart rate, refreshes spinal nerves, and calms the mind.

3. Warrior Two

Place your right foot forward and left foot back and flat on mat. Bend the right leg, straighten the left leg, and open hips and shoulders to face the side of the room. Extend your arms front to back, palms down and parallel to the floor. Press heels away from each other and relax your toes. Hold for five breaths. Gaze straight and softly over your right middle finger. (Repeat on left side.)

This pose strengthens the legs and arms, and helps with focus and body awareness.

4. Mountain Pose

Stand fully erect with feet together. Bring your belly button into your spine. Relax your shoulders and let both arms reach down by your sides. Press your feet into the floor and reach the crown of your head towards the ceiling. Keep gaze forward. Hold for five breaths.

This pose promotes skeletal alignment. It improves standing posture and corrects roundness in the upper back. It also increases alertness and calms the breath.

5. Child's Pose

Kneel down and separate your knees wide. Drop your sit bones towards your heels. Stretch your torso and arms forward. Keep your arms shoulders' width apart as you drop your forehead towards the floor. Rest your forehead and palms on the floor and take a minimum of five breaths.

This pose will calm the breath and center the mind. It relieves stress in the lumbar spine and facial muscles.

6. Tree Pose

Standing in mountain pose, you lift your right foot up to the left inner thigh. You can also drop the right foot to the floor and rest the right heel on the left ankle. Next, bring your hands to your heart's center. Relax your shoulders away from your ears and relax your face as you gaze forward. Take five breaths here and repeat on the other side.

This pose is a standing meditation. It is calming and rejuvenating, while it simultaneously engages the spine, thighs, calves, and ankles.

7. Locust Pose

Lie on your belly and bring your arms by your sides. Extend your legs straight behind you and rest your forehead on the floor. As you inhale, lift your chest off the mat and keep your chin tucked in. Lift your legs off the floor as you press your feet away from you. Squeeze your shoulder blades together but keep your chin tucked in. Hold for five breaths.

This pose aids in digestion and tones the bladder. It increases blood flow to the abdomen, stimulating the digestive organs.

II. Pranayama

This refers to yogic breathing. Pranayama will guide the child to pay attention to his breathing. It is gently focused and deliberate breathing that creates a calming effect on all who practice. One such breath technique is called ujjayi. Ujjayi is a sanscrit word that means "to expand success."

This breathing is done with the mouth closed and the inhales and exhales flowing from the nostrils. The breath is an audible oceanic breath. A *Star Wars* Darth Vader breath might paint a clearer picture for the child. Each inhale should be long, and each exhale should be full. This breath has 4 parts: 1) the long inhale, 2) a pause in breath, 3) full exhale, and 4) another pause.

The breath is the key to calming the mind, and, when linked to holding the poses, will create a sense of well-being that the child will sense—although perhaps not be able to express.

A simple, effective, and immediate technique to help the child find the peace, calm, and safe state of being he needs is the seated meditation.

Seated Breath Meditation

Practice with your child by finding a comfortable seat or crossed legged seated position. Lengthen your spine and relax your shoulders and facial muscles. Close your eyes and breathe, inhaling and exhaling through the nostrils. Let every inhale be long and every exhale be full.

You can incorporate positive affirmations or mantras (words of power) into the breath work. For example, inhale peace, exhale calm, inhale love, exhale safe, inhale relaxed, exhale happy, etc.

Like the poses themselves, don't be concerned about the duration of this breath meditation. Slowly incorporate it into the child's day, be it for 10 seconds or 10 minutes. The key is to start.

Martial Arts

Similar to Yoga, the martial arts also developed thousands of years ago. Martial arts started as a combat and fighting discipline, but slowly evolved in a way of life or Budo, way of the warrior. The fighting arts became more of a personal development program that had the added benefit of teaching self defense.

All martial arts, regardless of style, have two components to their system: the forms (katas) and the sparring (randori). The dojo or school structure in training is routine, systematic, and constant. It's this consistency, structure, and routine within the martial arts that helps the child on the autistic spectrum concentrate and learn how to focus.

Through the practice of martial arts, the ASD child will not only develop strength, stamina, flexibility, and body awareness, but also the martial arts will help the child emotionally by building self-esteem and teaching self-control. Children with ASD love structure and routine, and that is why martial arts should always be considered when looking for alternative therapies for your child.

At its core, the martial arts are more than kicks and punches, flips and blocks. The martial arts offer the child effective and proven strategies to navigate the world feeling calm, peaceful, and safe.

7 Top Reasons for Incorporating a Martial Arts Regimen into Your Child's Therapies:

1. Improve balance, motor skills, and coordination
2. Build body awareness
3. Maintain calm
4. Develop focus
5. Build confidence
6. Learn self defense
7. Make friends/socialize

The martial art itself will teach the child to focus, relax, and communicate more effectively. Through practice, the child becomes self-aware and starts to integrate the mind and body holistically. Through repetition, the child learns to control both the body and emotions.

In addition, through the martial arts you can train and teach the child strategies in behavior management as they grapple with many of the emotional components of ASD such as fear, anger and anxiety.

In the yoga studio, karate dojo, at school or at home, yogic and martial art therapies can effectively empower your special child to live life centered, at peace, calm and focused.

SENSORY

THE LISTENING PROGRAM®: AN EFFECTIVE TREATMENT FOR AUTISM

By Alex Doman

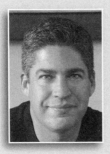

Alex Doman

Advanced Brain Technologies
5748 South Adams Avenue Parkway
Ogden, Utah 84405
801.622.5676
advancedbrain.com
info@advancedbrain.com

Alex Doman is founder and CEO of Advanced Brain Technologies, creators of The Listening Program®, and the bestselling co-author of *Healing at the Speed of Sound®*.

The third generation in a family of pioneers in the field of child and human brain development, Alex has focused his career on sound, music, and technology and their capacity to improve brain health and performance. He heads product development at Advanced Brain Technologies with credits including co-producer of *Music for Healing at the Speed of Sound™*, *Music for Babies™*, executive producer, creator, or collaborator on numerous other music albums, products, and technologies including; *Spatial Surround®*, *Sound Health®*, *Music for the Mind™*, *BrainBuilder®*, *The Listening Program®*, Waves™ multi-sensory audio system, and more.

Alex has been interviewed for NBC, CBS, ABC, MSNBC, *Today, NPR Marketplace, Wall Street Journal, Self, Women's Health, Men's Health, CBS Moneywatch*, LiveStrong.com, Health Radio with Dr. Mike Roizen, Dennis Prager, *Pia Lindstrom Presents*, Blog Talk Radio, ESPN Radio, *Hearing Health Magazine,* among others. He has written for publications including *SI Focus Magazine, Autism Asperger's Digest*, and *Autism Science Digest*. Doman is the host of The Listening Program Radio and blogs at alexdoman.com which is featured on Alltop Neuroscience.

He lectures internationally and has trained thousands of allied health, education and music professionals in brain based applications of sound and music; and serves as an advisor to Sanoson, NeuroPop, Sleep Genius, Aurora Schools, Autism Brain Storm, Autism Hope Alliance, and Concord Music Group.

Alex lives with his family in Ogden, Utah.

Children with autism spectrum disorders (ASDs) experience difficulties with social interaction, communication, attention, motor skills, sensory processing, sleep, and anxiety; they also have a tendency to engage in repetitive behaviors. These symptoms and their severity vary widely with each child and are often accompanied by challenges with immune dysfunction, allergies, GI issues, seizures, and other medical conditions.

Parents face a daunting array of treatment options to help their children attain their fullest potential. Each child is unique and as such, their autism intervention should be holistic and adapted to meet their individual needs and goals.

The Listening Program® (TLP) by Advanced Brain Technologies is an easy, personalized, and effective method of music listening therapy for improving brain health and performance.[1] TLP has a global effect on the brain influencing the central, and peripheral nervous systems, influencing: auditory, vestibular, visual, motor, cognitive, emotional and arousal systems and their function. It is a safe and enjoyable way to exercise the brain while also helping to regulate stress. This makes TLP an ideal approach for helping children with autism, which integrates well with behavioral therapies, neurodevelopmental programs, sensory-based approaches, educational treatment modalities, social skills training, biomedical treatments, neurofeedback, occupational therapy, and speech & language therapy.

The Musical Brain

One may ask how The Listening Program® can have such global effects. The answer lies deep within each of us. The brain is musical; neuroscience has established through functional brain imaging that when we listen to music, virtually the whole brain is involved.

Music listening not only involves the auditory areas of the brain, but also engages large-scale neural networks including; prefrontal cortex, motor cortex, sensory cortex, auditory cortex, visual cortex, cerebellum, hippocampus, amygdala, nucleus accumbens, corpus callosum, vestibular system, and peripheral nervous system.

TLP helps conduct the neural symphony, connecting the most ancient parts of the brain to the most advanced. The areas of brain focus The Listening Program is designed to help improve include:

- **Executive Function**

  Executive function is an umbrella term for a set of high-level mental processes that control and regulate other abilities and behaviors. They include the ability to initiate and stop actions, to monitor and change behavior as needed, and to plan future behavior when faced with novel tasks and situations. Executive functions allow us to anticipate outcomes and adapt to changing situations.

- **Communication**

  Communication is your ability to exchange information, thoughts, and opinions through verbal and written expression including speech, language, voice and writing; as well as non verbal expression such as gesture, facial expressions, and body language.

- **Auditory Processing**
  Auditory processing is your ability to understand and make sense of what you hear. Difficulty processing auditory information can have a negative impact on learning, thinking, communication and relationships.

- **Social & Emotional**
  Your ability to relate to others, manage emotions, resolve conflicts, understand and respond to social situations is impacted by your social skills and emotional intelligence.

- **Stress Response**
  Your body and brain is hard-wired to react to stress to protect you against threats, whether real or imagined. But, if your mind and body are constantly on edge because of excessive stress in your life, you may face serious health problems. That's because your body's "fight-or-flight reaction"—its natural alarm system—is constantly on.

- **Motor Coordination**
  Motor coordination is the harmonious functioning of body parts that involve movement including: gross motor skills such as walking, skipping, running and throwing; fine motor movement such as handwriting, buttoning a shirt, and key-boarding; and motor planning, the ability of the brain to conceive, organize and carry out purposeful movements.

- **Creative Expression**
  Your ability to express yourself creatively involves original and open thinking, imagination, problem solving, and movement to create something new and/or respond to opportunities.[2]

Auditory Hypersensitivity: An Emotional Response

One of the most commonly reported challenges for people with autism spectrum disorders is hypersensitivity to sound.[3] Auditory hypersensitivity involves a brain network called the non-classical auditory system and is an emotional response to sound rather than an auditory response.[4] Children described as being hypersensitive to sound have negative emotional reactions to sound and situations in which the sounds are present. A toilet flushing, vacuum, or loud restaurant are examples of commonly reported sounds or situations in which a child may have an autonomic nervous system reaction, which typically involves fight or flight responses. For example, in anticipation of the frightening sound a child may lose control of their behavior and try to run away (flight); they may put up a strong, negative, emotional fight to avoid the sounds (fight); or they may retreat into themselves seeking calm through behaviors such as covering their ears and rocking. A hypersensitive reaction can occur in anticipation of a sound, even if the sound itself is absent. It is possible to desensitize these negative emotional reactions and reprogram the emotional memory system so that children are no longer frightened by sounds.[5]

A series was developed for The Listening Program® called SPECTRUM that involves a gentle method to desensitize the limbic system and reprogram the emotional memory system, with the aim of making sounds something one desires to listen to rather than avoid. It is comprised of High Definition recordings of classical music presented in Spatial Surround® sound through multi-sensory headphones, called Waves™, which provide an immersive listening experience including both air conducted sound, and gentle, calming vibrations throughout the body, or bone conduction.[6] This highly specialized music is listened to once or twice daily for fifteen minutes, 5 days per week for a total of 200 sessions done over the period of several months. The music is recorded then acoustically modified to lead the child to react less negatively to sounds and, thus, reduce the child's hypersensitivity. A trained provider, usually a professional such as an occupational therapist or speech-language pathologist, monitors the TLP training. The provider typically establishes the actual program and protocol based on the individual child's needs and parents carry out the training in the home or it is offered at school.

When listening to TLP SPECTRUM, it is thought that the sound signal travels along both the classical and non-classical auditory pathways. Likely confirming this assumption, one of the first outcomes that parents, educators, and professionals often see in children undergoing TLP training is that the children are calmer. This is a good indicator that the listening has tapped into the emotional areas of the limbic system via the non-classical auditory pathways. Over the course of training, children often are also reported to be more attentive to sounds, better able to detect sounds they hear, and more communicative when communication is verbal, likely because they are more open to listening. As the training proceeds, the child continues to relax and become calmer when listening. We hypothesize that this is because a reprogramming of emotional memory in the amygdala is occurring. The training reprograms listening and sounds as positive experiences. When the child then finds him- or herself in a real-world situation and hears sounds that may have been frightening or annoying in the past, the training allows the child to process the sounds in more neutral manner.[7]

TLP SPECTRUM[8] is available through trained providers on an iPod preloaded with the acoustically modified music programs, including with the Waves multi-sensory audio system, or high quality headphones. It is also available through online audio streaming to most web connected devices (computers, tablets, mobile phones) on The Listening Program Online[9] platform.

Toilet Training

Toilet training can be challenging for children with autism spectrum disorders. A number of common problems can make toileting hard including, physical, language, dressing, fears, body cues, and need for sameness.[10] Competent toileting is a critical life skill.[11] It is an important step in personal independence, and incontinence is a significant barrier to quality of life.

Over the course of many years we heard frequent anecdotal reports from parents and therapists that The Listening Program® led to spontaneous remission of bedwetting, and helped children become toilet trained. Previous research involving TLP reported improvements in many areas including auditory skills[12], speech and learning, but none had looked specifically at toilet training outcomes. A nurse and continence expert in the United Kingdom named June Rogers conducted a pilot investigation funded by the National Health Service to look specifically at the effects of The Listening Program, including air and bone conduction sound delivery, in improving toilet training outcomes for children with autism, developmental, and learning difficulties. The results from the pilot project exceeded all expectations. The hope was at the end of the 12 week study the children would at the very least be relaxed enough to sit on the toilet and potty and cooperate with a toilet training program. The fact that 7 of the 11 children who completed TLP became toilet trained was very encouraging. And the 4 who did not become toilet trained in the time, each made improvements, very positive considering all previous attempts at toilet training lead to no real progress. The results of this research were presented at the European Society for Paediatric Urology (ESPU) conference in Turkey in April 2010 when it was awarded the best Nurse Research Paper Presentation.[13]

While this was a small study it has laid the groundwork for larger scale clinical trials to be carried out, and has given parents and therapists the confidence to utilize TLP to improve quality of life for children with autism as part of a successful toilet training strategy.

Sleep Matters

Sleep is precious, and most of us don't get enough of it. In fact the Centers for Disease Control and Prevention stated that insufficient sleep is a public health epidemic.[14]Over 70 million Americans are not getting sufficient sleep, and our children are among them.

Children with autism may sleep less each night due to disturbed sleep than typically developing children and those with other developmental disabilities according to a new study. While the study only showed an association between autism and sleep disturbance, researchers noted that the findings do suggest there is some sort of "shared neuropathological basis" between autism and biological clock disturbances.[15]

"There are increasing biochemical and genetic data to support the existence of fundamental disturbances in circadian melatonin production in some children with autism, which may partly explain these findings," the authors wrote. "Children with ASD are reported to have reduced levels of circulating melatonin and disrupted circadian rhythms, and links have been identified between genes involved in melatonin synthesis and ASD, which could help explain the disturbed sleep patterns observed in children with ASD."[16]

The most commonly reported sleep disturbances in autism are increased sleep latency, and frequent night waking which result in reduced sleep duration. Sleep matters and lack of sleep comes with a high cost to our ability to learn, our health and safety, behavior, and quality of life. In the short term, a lack of adequate sleep can affect judgment, mood, ability to learn and retain information, and may increase the risk of serious accidents and injury. In the long term, chronic sleep deprivation may lead to a host of health problems including, diabetes, cardiovascular disease, depression, obesity, and Alzheimer's disease.

Advanced Brain Technologies has developed a new and highly effective auditory sleep aid that is used when going to sleep called The Listening Program® SLEEP (TLP SLEEP).

The technology behind TLP SLEEP is based in part on over fifteen years of research in hearing, balance, and sleep by neuroscientist Seth Horowitz. It is a new approach to helping people of any age go to sleep more quickly and stay asleep longer. TLP SLEEP uses three kinds of sound that work directly on the brain's global sleep network in different ways.

1. Very low frequency sounds activate the vestibular system to trigger Sopite syndrome, the motion-induced sleepiness that babies experience while being rocked and that most people feel while riding as a passenger in a car or on a train.

2. Quiet "pink" noise shaped to match the sound signatures of heartbeats and breathing reduces activity in the brain's arousal centers to encourage relaxation.

3. Binaural beats—slightly different sound frequencies delivered to each ear to trigger frequency-following response between the brain's hemispheres—help the brain match the waveforms that characterize the stages of sleep.

The sleep-inducing technology embedded within the acoustically modified music created for TLP SLEEP uses all three methodologies. These music programs were composed, arranged, and recorded specifically for aiding sleep. They were created by Advanced Brain Technologies and an international team of experts, leaders in music effects research and production, psychoacoustics, and neuroscience.[17]

Each of the three music programs which are provided on an iPod Shuffle and are played through Sleep Phones (a sleep safe headband with speakers) provides soothing, unobtrusive, instrumental music with subtle sounds of nature, and ambient music that entrains the brain to improve sleep regulation. Embedded within these beautiful recordings are proprietary neurosensory algorithms that produce sleepiness. The result is that TLP SLEEP helps retrain the brain's sleep rhythms so that people naturally go to sleep faster, have less night waking, with improved sleep quality and duration.

Will The Listening Program Be Helpful for Your Child?

More than fifteen years of clinical evidence, studies, and case reports indicate that children with autism benefit from The Listening Program®.[18] Thousands of therapists and other professionals working in leading autism organizations, hospitals, clinics, schools, and in private practice worldwide have helped families affected by autism with TLP and have not observed any significant negative responses to listening. Some children do have temporary adjustment symptoms as their brains begin to reorganize in response to the music, but this usually resolves within a few days. Listening schedules can be adjusted to accommodate more sensitive children. Although TLP can take a few months to make lasting changes it will often make a positive impact in the life of the child within weeks. Awarded Best Autism Product by Autism One, TLP is also Autism Approved by Autism Hope Alliance, and is offered as part of the Generation Rescue *Rescue Family Grant*. The Listening Program is a safe, effective, and complementary approach that should be considered as a foundational treatment for children with autism.

NACD'S TARGETED NEURODEVELOPMENTAL INTERVENTION: PERSPECTIVES AND INTERVENTIONS FOR THOSE ON THE AUTISM SPECTRUM

By Bob Doman

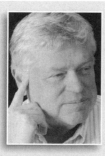

Bob Doman

Founder and Director
National Association for Child Development, Inc.®

Bob Doman has been working with autism since the late 1960s. He was part of the team that first discovered the connection between sensory dysfunction and autism. Bob has been instrumental in establishing the foundation for today's understanding of neurodevelopment and those within the autism spectrum. He has worked with families, organizations, and government agencies internationally. Having created new methodologies, model programs, tools, and understanding of the full range of developmental and educational issues, Bob established the National Association for Child Development (NACD®) and the NACD Foundation® in 1979. In 2004 Bob and the NACD Foundation created the Simply Smarter Project, an international effort to raise the awareness of and provide the tools to increase the processing/working memory of everyone on the planet. Since that time Bob and NACD's work has been disseminated and incorporated into many of the programs being utilized within the United States and the world. Bob and NACD continue to have an international influence on child development and education and continue to find more answers as they follow the philosophy of always seeking ways to help children faster and better and to help them all realize their innate potential.

National Association for Child Development
Chapters around the United States, Europe, and India
www.nacd.org
on YouTube: www.youtube.com/user/NACDDOTORG
801-621-8606

Understanding and remediating the neurodevelopmental issues (i.e. brain-related) of those within the autism spectrum is critical if we are going to provide these children and adults with an opportunity to overcome their issues and to function at higher, "normal," or even "superior" levels. To understand NACD's TDI Targeted Developmental Intervention®, one must understand NACD's neurodevelopmental perspective on autism. NACD's TDI programs incorporate literally thousands of specific techniques, addressing all aspects of the child's development and function — including everything from sensory issues and development to cognition, motor function, language, academics, and social skills. It is important to understand that most neurodevelopmental issues will not just go away. Merely teaching new skills or applying aggressive medical or nutritional intervention without addressing the underlying neurodevelopmental issues may change some function; but if the neurodevelopmental foundation is not established, abnormal neural patterns and function are only going to perpetuate the underlying problems, and the results are going to be limited at best. The view held by many that children within the spectrum have only limited potential and cannot substantially overcome their issues reflects the overall misunderstanding of the problem. There is a lack of attention to the uniqueness of each individual and a general misperception that we are dealing with a specific disease, waiting for a pharmaceutical cure or single intervention or magic bullet. However autism is not polio or chickenpox; you can't catch it. It is neurologically based, regardless of the initial cause or causes. I am sure we will ultimately see that there are many causes, and like other developmental problems, that there is neither a single cause, a single solution, nor any two children who have exactly the same issues. The disease model is leading many parents, researchers, and practitioners in the wrong direction. Those within the spectrum are unique individuals. Yes, there is some commonality; but each individual has their own set of issues and underlying problems and associated hierarchy of needs and should not be perceived as having a disease. Again, I believe there are many causes of autism; but the perception of autism (or other developmental issues such as ADD, which some will include in the autism spectrum as well) as a disease is counterproductive.

Those who have issues that place them within the autism spectrum are aptly identified as having a pervasive developmental disorder. "Pervasive" correctly implies a whole or inclusive developmental problem affecting most or all aspects of the child's function. The implication of this perception, and the foundation of NACD's TDI programs, is that truly successful intervention and remediation requires not only a gestalt, or global, perspective of the associated developmental issues, but also must serve as the basis for prioritizing and approaching the issues as hierarchical. As an example, some of the hierarchical foundations of language include hearing, auditory tonal processing, auditory figure-ground processing, auditory sequential processing, auditory short-term and working memory, conceptual thought, executive function, general neurological organization, knowledge/experiential base, and, of course, need. If we are to look at a really complex function, such as social interaction, we need to address a plethora of neurodevelopmental issues in a balanced, targeted hierarchy of neurodevelopmental pieces. Merely wanting to produce a function, or asking for a function without establishing the foundation or focusing on one aspect of the dysfunction, is grossly inadequate.

At the foundation of NACD's TDI programs is the family. Successful implementation and remediation requires parental education. This goes beyond the simple application of specific methodologies. It also requires an understanding of the neurodevelopmental issues and addresses perhaps the most difficult aspect of remediation for these children—the need for an understanding and appreciation of their issues, as well as appropriate engagement for the majority of the child's waking day. NACD sees parents as not only a critical component in the application of specific program components in the TDI program, but also trains, coaches, supports, and guides the parents so they can supervise the involvement of physicians, therapists, schools, and caregivers as informed and empowered advocates for their child. Successful intervention requires coordinated, supervised, and targeted intervention. A small army of people each working on their own "pieces" of the child is not part of the NACD TDI program. NACD and the parents pilot the TDI program and everyone involved with the child's development and education.

Discovering, understanding, and learning how to address the unique underlying neurodevelopmental issues has been an effort of a lifetime and a dynamic process. NACD, which was established in 1979, has designed and supervised over 30 million hours of comprehensive developmental and educational intervention. This experience has afforded us the opportunity to gain numerous insights, opening more doors and assisting in the understanding of these unique minds and leading to better outcomes.

Although each child is unique, we have discovered some neurodevelopmental issues that are expressed in varying degrees in virtually every individual on the spectrum. Successful intervention necessitates an understanding of and attention to these fairly universal neurodevelopmental components and needs, including:

Interrelationship of neurology and physiology

That which impacts the child's physical function impacts their neurological function. Most children on the spectrum are extremely physiologically sensitive. Diets, medications, supplements, and interventions need to be applied with a gentle scientific hand, measuring and evaluating the effects of each specific component with an understanding that generally many interrelated aspects of physiological function are involved. Aggressive intervention often interferes with efforts to trigger positive neuroplasticity, which creates additional problems. Also, as the neurological function improves, so does the physiology. The child becomes healthier and less physiologically sensitive. Intervention needs to be applied gently, with the goal of producing overall health and wellness. NACD educates, advises, councils, and assists the family in the pursuit of health and physical wellbeing.

The need to address DSAs (debilitating sensory addictions)

I coined the term "DSA" a number of years ago in appreciation of what I realized was the developmentally negative and addictive nature of what are commonly called "stims" or "stimming" in this population. Back in the early seventies we realized that the behaviors exhibited by many autistic children were very similar to what were called "blindisims" and "deafisims" in the blind and deaf communities. These ritualistic behaviors were simply the child playing with their underdeveloped or broken sensory channels. For the autistic child, their stims (such as rocking, using echolalic speech, stimulating their peripheral vision, etc.), which can involve any of their sensory channels or combinations of channels, reinforce what is wrong with that channel and trigger what is called "negative neuroplasticity." (Although there can't truly be positive or negative neuroplasticity, there certainly are negative and positive outcomes. Therefore, using the term in this way helps people understand the issues more accurately.) I include "debilitating" in the term because triggering negative neuroplasticity is in fact debilitating, and it impairs normal sensory function and development. It is addictive because the brain appears to react to such stimuli as it would any other addiction. The more you do it, the more you want and need it. Some DSAs are obvious; many more are subtle and often ignored; but all are neurologically and developmentally harmful and debilitating. NACD identifies the DSAs, educates the parents about them, and develops strategies to appropriately engage and redirect the child, while working to normalize the sensory channels and eliminate the addictions.

Normalization of sensory function

The brain develops based on the perception of the input it receives through the sensory channels. How we hear, see, feel, taste, and smell defines our world. *All neurodevelopment is based upon brain plasticity.* Simply stated, this means that all perceived input and brain activity affects, develops, and reinforces the wiring of the brain. Brain function is based on patterns and associations; specific sensory input, as it is perceived, stimulates the brain and triggers neural growth/connections/networks that physically change the brain and its function, be it for the good or bad. This process is called neuroplasticity. In autism the foundational issue in the hierarchical list of concerns and treatment is normalizing sensory dysfunction. If the brain does not correctly process sensory input (thus interfering with the typical neurodevelopment and triggering what is now being referred to as negative plasticity), typical development goes awry. In the computer world they refer to "garbage in, garbage out." Function determines structure; how you use your brain determines how it develops. Normalization of all these sensory channels establishes the foundation upon which neurodevelopment can occur. Most children within the spectrum have a variety of sensory issues affecting most, if not all, sensory channels. Normalization of sensory issues involves providing the child with very specific targeted interventions, creation of a controlled sensory environment, elimination of DSAs, and creation of activities that foster sensory normalization. An hour of appropriate sensory normalization therapy can be undone with five minutes of negative sensory immersion, whether self-initiated or environmentally based. NACD uses and has developed or assisted in the development of many hundreds of specific targeted sensory treatment techniques and methodologies. Our TSI-Targeted Sound Intervention® programs include Focused Attention, Boost, and Individualized for Frequency Normalization (tsi.nacd.org). We also initiated the development of programs such as The Listening Program® (www.nacd.org/speech_sound/the_listening_program.php) and the Sound Health Series (www.nacdstore.com/collections/music-programs/products/sound-health-series-complete-set), both of which are now produced by Advanced Brain Technologies. As NACD develops greater understandings of the pieces involved in neurodevelopment, we will continue to identify more and more needs and to develop new tools when what is needed does not exist. TDI programs include very specific targeted treatment techniques and environmental recommendations to normalize sensory function.

Development of the foundation of language, thought, and global maturity

There is a progression in the development of thought. I refer to this as the "cognitive hierarchy." The components of the cognitive hierarchy, including sequential processing, short-term memory, working memory, complexity of thought, receptive and expressive language, conceptual thought, long-term memory, and global neurological and developmental maturity, are critically linked. For those within the spectrum, the issues produced from sensory dysfunction have a negative impact on this cognitive hierarchy that is in direct proportion to the degree of sensory dysfunction. Addressing and developing this cognitive hierarchy has been the focus of NACD for decades. NACD developed the first "brain software" in the early eighties and through the decades has developed hundreds of 1:1 activities, online programs (www.nacdtheproject.com, www.simplysmarter.org) and apps to help develop these critical functions (see Simply Smarter Kids-Memory® in the Apple store). The NACD staff receives extensive ongoing training to help determine which of these specific techniques are appropriate given the individual child's issues and placement in the cognitive hierarchy.

Correcting imbalances between visualization and conceptualization

One of the more pervasive problems with those in the spectrum is the difficulty in being cognitively "present," which is a reflection of the more significant underlying problem—the poor conceptual thought and typically exceptional visualization. I use the term "conceptualization" to refer to thinking in words as opposed to pictures. The vast majority of autistic children are very strong visualizers and poor conceptualizers. This imbalance exists because the typical cognitive hierarchy gets obstructed. All children beginning life without the ability to process language start off as visual learners and visual thinkers, or visualizers. In typical development, language processing starts kicking in within months, and the child generally develops a good balance between visualization (thinking in pictures) and conceptualization (thinking in words). Following this normal cognitive hierarchy produces an individual who can use both skills when and as needed. Disruption of this normal progression creates individuals who are too good at visualization, who do not process words well, who do not think in words well, and who therefore cannot use words well. They tend to go off into their own worlds, reliving videos or situations over and over, creating another form of perseverative DSA. One cannot develop typical language or social skills if one cannot adequately process language, understand concepts, and communicate. Remediating this imbalance necessitates the implementation of many targeted activities. It also requires that the parents understand those things that feed the visualization and perseverative DSAs, and that they apply the necessary environmental controls and restrictions. NACD's TDI programs address and work to normalize the balance between visualization and conceptualization, and help to develop conceptual thought and social function.

Education and behavior management

Effective and efficient education and behavioral management require a thorough understanding of the child. To educate or simply manage an autistic child, it is imperative that you first understand the uniqueness of the child, where they are on the cognitive hierarchy, how they process information, how they think, and what they know. Then based upon this collective perspective, a totally individualized educational and behavioral management program needs to be created. NACD's TDI programs involve the creation and constant modification of behavioral and educational programs.

We have heard it said that if your only tool is a hammer, then every problem looks like a nail. For over forty years of involvement with autism, our NACD staff and I have been on a quest to understand autism and to find and develop tools to address the associated problems. We presently utilize over 3,000 different tools and are creating and often replacing tools weekly. One of our constant issues is helping families prioritize, coordinate, balance and sift through all of the programs and options "out there." There are many options, and part of NACD's role is to evaluate and determine which options or tools are most appropriate and when to implement them. Together with the family, NACD establishes the goals, determines the destination, and pilots the ship. NACD is not vested in specific tools; it's vested in children.

A comprehensive and coordinated treatment approach for children with autism involves educating the parents and creating specific neurodevelopmental programs for each child. These programs and treatment protocols must address health and wellness, sensory issues (visual, tactile, auditory, olfactory, and taste), processing problems (auditory and visual), lack of development of and imbalance in visualization and conceptualization, fine and gross motor function, cognitive and academic function, and speech and language, as well as behavioral and social issues. We tackle these issues by designing a very child-specific, holistic, coordinated program (TDI Targeted Developmental Intervention). A TDI program is created after we thoroughly review the child's history, interview the parents (those who know the child best), conduct a developmental and educational assessment, create a developmental profile to help identify priorities, and discuss resources, manpower, and time with the parents.

NACD respects those with autism for who they are. We believe that they, like any child, are capable of attaining their innate potential and that they deserve the opportunity to do so. NACD can only help a child through the parent. NACD trains, educates, supports, and coaches the parent in the implementation of their child's program. Families come to one of our chapters around the country, in Europe, or India (www.nacd.org/get_started/where_to_go.php) or through Skype every three months and have their child re-evaluated and their program modified. During the intervening three months, the family is supported through daily contact with NACD coaches and evaluators. Successful outcomes require constant and ongoing communication between NACD and our families. Working together as a team, we can significantly change the lives of individuals with autism and their families.

ANIMALS IN THE LIVES OF PERSONS WITH AUTISTIC SPECTRUM DISORDER (ASD): COMPANIONS TO CO-THERAPISTS

By Dr. Aubrey H. Fine

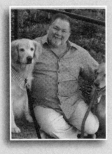

Aubrey H. Fine, EdD

Professor
Department of Education
CA Poly University
3801 W. Temple Ave.
Pomona, CA 91768
ahfine@csupomona.edu

Psychologist Dr. Aubrey Fine has been in the field of Animal-Assisted Therapy (AAT) for over twenty-five years. He is the editor of the most widely accepted book on the subject, *The Handbook on Animal-Assisted Therapy*, has had a featured monthly column in *Dog Fancy* magazine on the human-animal bond entitled "The Loving Bond." He has also been a guest on numerous national TV and radio shows, including on programs on ABC, Animal Planet, KTLA, and CNN. His newest book, *Afternoons with Puppy*, released by Purdue University in December 2007, is a heartwarming account about the evolving relationships and outcomes among a therapist, his therapy animals, and his patients over the course of over two decades. Over this period, he has applied AAT with a variety of children with diverse forms of etiology and has witnessed many moving outcomes as a result of incorporating animals as therapeutic agents. An active faculty member at California State Polytechnic University since 1981, he was awarded the prestigious Wang Award in 2001 for exceptional commitment, dedication, and exemplary contributions within the areas of education and applied sciences.

A special thanks is given to Karina Grasso who helped in the research for this chapter. Your efforts are greatly appreciated.

*H*is mother always wanted him to have a dog, but she wasn't quite sure how react that is when I got the call. I decided that Magic would be his best match ... is a very gentle, calm and attentive four- year old golden retriever, who seems very comfortable working with all children. She always approaches very slowly, giving all those she interacts with ample time to get acclimated.

When they first met, Bob was apprehensive and used poor eye contact. He also mumbled his speech and spoke with a pedantic flair. That didn't seem to be an obstacle for Magic. She moved closely next to Bob, waiting for him to pet her. Their relationship was just beginning. Over the following weeks not only did he become more comfortable with her presence, he also began to speak up and with more clarity. Puppy love and companionship may have been the initial goal, but Bob's family would quickly learn, that animal assisted interventions could have much more to offer.

Introduction

The unique bond between humans and animals and its powerful impact on human well-being has been documented over hundreds of years (Wells, 2009). It is amazing to recognize the growth of animals living in our homes. According to the 2011- 2012 American Pet Products Association (APPA) National Pet Owner Survey, 62% of households own a pet, which equates to about 72.9 million homes. It is apparent that in most cases, pets fill a void in most owners' lives. Instead of coming home to an empty house, people come home to the greetings of happy loving animals such as dogs or cats. Our pets provide companionship and unconditional love as well as providing friendship to those who may lack social contact.

Within this chapter, attention will be given to explain the value of the human animal bond and describe how animal assisted interventions including equine assisted therapy and pet companionship can be a viable alternative to persons with any autistic spectrum disorder (ASD). Over the past five years, there has been more attention given to the value of services animals and animal assisted interventions for persons with Autism. For example, O'Haire (2013) in a recent paper reviewing the literature pointed out that eleven new studies have been published highlighting the research community 's interest in regards to the value of animals in the lives of children with autism.

Before specifically discussing the roles that animals can have with people who have ASD, attention will begin with explaining the value of the human- animal bond and the field of animal assisted interventions (AAI).

Understanding the Human- Animal Bond

It was in 1979 that the term human-animal bond was used for the first time at a conference in Dundee Scotland. The term was borrowed from the warm hearted/loving relationship that exists between parents and their infants. Many believed that the qualities that are witnessed in that relationship also existed in our relationship with companion animals. In my new book Our Faithful Companions (2014: Alpine Publisher) I discuss the evolution of the definition and so many of the qualities that I have witnessed in this relationship. Perhaps the most unique element that I have witnessed in this relationship is the mutual expression of familial love that is often displayed. It is amazing when you talk to various pet owners that they share the tremendous devotion they have with their pet.

The sense of being needed and having a purpose in life has been researched by numerous scholars as one of the number of reasons why the bond between animals and people is established. Some also believe that our relationships with animals provide social supports in vulnerable times as well as opportunities for healthy interaction. For example, I think of one young man with autism whose best friend was a Labrador that he got on his 10th birthday. Alex always loved dogs. His parents recognized this when he was much younger. They noticed how much he enjoyed being around animals and his connection with them. The animals didn't appear to be as judgmental of his developmental differences and seemed to be accepting of his kindness and attention. It seemed logical for the family to get him a dog of his own. At first, there were challenges, especially when introducing any puppy in a family. Nevertheless the early hardship of training and cementing a bond between the two was outweighed by their evolving friendship. His beloved Dreamer , his dog, was always eager to see him, especially when he came home from school. At school, he was shunned by peers and at times was the brunt of their jokes and avoidance. When he returned home, that wasn't the case. He and Dreamer would frolic and play with each other for hours. Most of the time, Dreamer just sat by him vigilantly, waiting for their next adventure together. Alan (fictional name) seemed to cherish his friendship with Dreamer and through touch and in times in total silence they seemed to communicate well. The presence of his pet acted as a safe refuge and provided him with what we all would have considered unconditional love.

McNicholas and Colis (2000 and 2006) suggest that animals maybe more forgiving than their human counterparts and are more accepting than fellow humans of those who may have awkward social and communication skills. This would seem to be the case with Alan and Dreamer. She seemed to respond differently to Alan and seemed more patient with his developmental differences.

Numerous research studies and papers have also been written over the past few decades that illustrate the unique physiological benefits that animals' foster. The roots of these findings go back to the pioneer works of Friedmann, Katcher and Lynch (Friedmann et al, 1990) who have demonstrated the value of caressing an animal on cardiovascular health and decreased anxiety because of the physical contact of the pet. Since that time, there have been other researchers who have unearthed other specific physiological outcomes that have been enhanced due to the bond such as an increase in oxytocin and other healthy neurotransmitters as a consequence of gently stoking and petting dogs (Odenthal and Meintjes, 2003; and Dayton, 2010). The researchers have also found that petting and interacting with the dogs also caused a decrease in the cortisol levels (stress hormones). In essence, the research (Wells, 2009 has an outstanding review of the literature) leaves us with an understanding that interacting with animals may be similar to a welcoming spa treatment that promotes a relaxed state. In fact, two researchers named Headey and Grabka (cited in Dayton, 2010) attempted to quantify the health correlates of pet ownership using national survey data in Australia, Germany and China. Their results suggested that compared with people who didn't have pets, those who live with other species seem to benefit from better overall health, get more exercise, sleep better, take fewer days off work and see their doctor less. Although these finding are interesting, little is still known on how interactions with animals impact some of these variables with persons with ASD. Attention to some of the findings and practical solutions will be given later in the chapter.

Defining Animal Assisted Interventions

The reputation of AAI has blossomed in the past several decades ever since Boris Levinson coined the term pet therapy (Levinson, 1969). As a clinician, Levinson suggested that animals could provide a calming effect in therapy. Ever since that time, numerous terms have been used to explain the therapeutic use of animals. Terms such as "pet therapy," "animal-facilitated counseling," "animal assisted therapy and activities," "pet-mediated therapy," and "pet psychotherapy" have been commonly used interchangeably as descriptive terms. Nevertheless, the two most widely utilized terms are "animal assisted therapy" and "animal assisted activities." Both of these alternatives could be classified under the rubric of animal assisted interventions.

The Pet Partner's (previously Delta Society) Standards of Practice for Animal Assisted Therapy (1996) defines animal assisted therapy (AAT) as an intervention with specified goals and objectives delivered by a health or human service professional with specialized expertise in using an animal as an integral part of treatment. On the other hand, but equally valuable, animal assisted activities (AAA) occur when specially trained professionals, paraprofessionals or volunteers accompanied by animals interact with people in a variety of environments (Delta Society, 1996). In AAA, the same activity can be repeated for many different people or groups of people, the interventions are not part of a specific treatment plan and are not designed to address a specific emotional or medical condition, and detailed documentation does not occur.

On the other hand, equine assisted therapy has also had a long history in supporting diverse groups of people including persons with autism. Although not a household pet, horses have been found to be extremely helpful to children with autism, especially because of the added benefit of being in the outdoors. Horses also appear to be quite capable of perceiving human emotions. This ability is an asset to their interactions with people. Children eventually learn that calmer behavior usually gets the horses to feel more comfortable around them. Rupert Isaacson, the author of **Horseboy**, and father of a child with autism has had positive experiences with horse riding with many children with ASD. In a recent interview on January 19, 2011, Isaacson pointed out that he believed the best horses to utilize in therapy seemed to be alpha mares. He believes that these horses often are more confident and are not afraid of new challenges. They also seem to take on more caring and giving roles in their herds. For example, it is not uncommon in the wild to see alpha mares take on the maternal responsibilities of juveniles who have been abandoned or separated from their mothers. We will discuss this point a bit more, later in this chapter.

Therapeutic horseback riding has been used to help people with their balance and posture while taking advantage of the bond between the horse and the individual. Some believe that the effectiveness of horse riding stems from the kinesthetic stimulation that occurs during riding. Originally, therapeutic riding was given attention by some Germans who in the early 60's believed that riding horses could be a viable treatment for people with compromised motor control and neurological disorders (Frewin & Gardiner, 2005). They called the process Hippotherapy, utilizing the Greek word Hippos, which means horse. The term hippotherapy actually means providing treatment with the help of a horse. The primary focus of the intervention pertains to the movement of the horse.

In the US, The North American Riding for the Handicapped Association (NARHA) was formed in 1969 with the mission of promoting equine assisted therapies and activities for people with special needs. It was at this time that hippotherapy began to attract more attention in this country. As years progressed, the use of horses within therapy has grown beyond its use for physiological benefits and attention is now given to the psychological benefits that include our interacting with the horses and taking care of their needs (husbandry). Responsitbility for another or someone else may be an important factor in the bonding process. Equine psychotherapy was formally started in the late 1990s. In 1999, the Equine Assisted Growth and Learning Association (EAGALA) was established. EAGALA is also devoted to the development of high standards and professionalism in the field of EFT. Both organizations offer training programs, which include conferences, continuing education, and support groups.

In a recent study reported by Gabriels' and her colleagues in Colorado (2012), they found significant benefits for children with autism who were engaged in a therapeutic riding program. As a consequence of being involved in a ten week program, the results showed significant improvement in self regulation skills.

Understanding the Underlying Mechanisms of Animal Assisted Interventions

The author, in numerous articles has identified several tenets that he believes are some of the major purposes of incorporating animals as an aspect of therapy. Briefly two of the tenets are as follows:

Tenet 1: Animals acting as a social lubricant

As stated earlier, this tenet has been the primary force behind AAI including equine assisted therapy. The animals act as a social lubricant and ease the stress of therapy by being comforting. The animals also act as a link in conversation between clinician and client, and help establish trust and rapport between patient and clinician. The mere presence of an animal can also give clients a sense of comfort, which further promotes rapport in the therapeutic relationship. In regards to persons with ASD, the literature does suggest a similar outcome. For example, Martin and Farnum (2002) noted several improvements in children with ASD when they interacted with therapy dogs. It appears that the animals in therapy promoted more playful moods and better attentiveness in the youngsters who participated in the project. Martin and Farnum concluded that these changes in their behavior were a direct consequence of being around the dogs. They also explained that "animals are believed to act as transitional objects, allowing children to first establish bonds with them and then extend these bonds to humans" (Martin and Farnum, 2002).

Tenet 2: Animals as teachers

Perhaps one of the strongest outlets for applying AAI is how clinicians have often utilized animals for teaching as well as role models. This is one of the greatest advantages of incorporating animals into therapy. Teaching animals and supporting their growth can also have therapeutic benefits for the clients. There have been many clinicians who have used the bonding relationship with the animal as a method to enhance developmental skills. For example, in a study with a child with Autism, Barol (2006) used the relaxed atmosphere that the dog promoted to teach skills that were normally avoided by the young boy. Prior to the onset of her study, Barol met with the therapeutic team to discuss what sorts of activities they would offer the child using the therapy dog as a motivational tool. For example, traditionally when asked to cut things in occupational therapy, the boy would often be uncooperative, squeal and whine. However, when asked to do a similar task when cutting up bacon-like dog treats, he seemed more willing to cooperate. In addition, the speech and language therapist worked with the child to say "Here Henry" when he gave the dog the treat. In essence, the responsibility of taking care of the animal seemed to be the impetus for his actions.

Pet Companionship and AAI: Suggestions for Applications

It is clear that there has been a recent interest in the roles that animals have in the lives of persons with ASD. Before I actually cover the therapeutic benefits of animals, I want to stress that companion animals can be wonderful in the lives of all children including children with ASD. Silva and his associates (2011) found that a friendly dog could enhance the moods of children wit ASD. Perhaps one of the additional benefits of having animals around children with ASD is their impact on reducing anxiety. One of the symptoms that children with ASD experience is a higher rate of anxiety. In one study, the data suggested that children with ASD had lover levels of salivary cortisol after being introduced to their service animals (Silva et al, 2011).

Depending on the needs of the child, adjustments will be needed in selecting the best pet for a specific child. For example, some children will enjoy the companionship of more slow moving animals while others may need pets that are more engaging and will seek out more interaction. Ming-Lee Yeh (2008) suggested several interesting outcomes from her three years of research on evaluating a canine animal assisted therapy (AAT) treatment for children with ASD in Taiwan. She reported significant improvements for the children on the social skills subscale and total score on the VABS (The Vineland Adaptive Behavior Scale -VABS, Chinese version). She also reported that after interacting with dogs, children revealed significant improvements in various dimensions of communication and language as well as increasing their on-task behavior.

Grandin, Fine and Bowers (2010) have suggested several reasons why AAI may be more appropriate for some people with ASD, while others may react indifferently. One argument that was made pertains to the fact the some people may respond negatively to their interactions due to their sensory oversensitivity. For example, a person with ASD may not be able to tolerate the smell of a dog. Another may have auditory oversensitivity and the sound of a dog barking may not be able to tolerate the sounds. The impact of sensory oversensitivity is extremely variable and can have a very strong effect on an interaction. For instance, when Bob first met Magic, he seemed very conscious of how she smelled. Attention was given to bath her right before his visits with a very neutral smelling shampoo. On the other hand, a barking dog or a squawking bird may not bother some, while others will find it extremely aversive and offensive. Simply put, some people with various levels of ASD may avoid animals because they have extreme sensitivity to either sound or smell (it may not have anything to do with the animal specifically). One needs to carefully consider this point prior to introducing an animal.

Some believe that persons with ASD may respond differently to animals due to their differences in cognitive problem solving. For example, Grandin and Johnson (2005) hypothesize that one of the reasons why some children and adults with ASD relate really well to animals is due to sensory based thinking. They suggest that there may be some similarities in the way that both people with ASD and perhaps companion animal's process information. In essence, animals do not think in words. They believe that dogs' cognitions are filled with detailed sensory information and their world is filled with pictures, smells, sounds and physical sensations. Grandin et al (2010) summarized their impressions about some of the safeguards to consider when utilizing animals in therapy with the following conclusions. Table 1 summarizes these perceptions.

Table 1

Guidelines to consider when applying AAI with persons with ASD	
1.	Children and adults with ASD may relate better with companion animals because they both use sensory-based thinking.
2.	Sensory oversensitivity may have a tremendous impact on the outcome and is extremely variable. This means that some people may not be able to tolerate smells or sudden sounds from an animal. On the other hand, some will have no sensory problems with animals and will be attracted to them.
3.	Animals, specifically dogs, may communicate their behavioral intentions more easily to persons with ASD especially because their relationships are simpler.

Additionally, AAI can also be applied with individuals who have a milder version of ASD. Perhaps one of the greatest benefits has been how the animals have supported companionship and friendship in the lives of people who have felt very isolated and lonely. Fine and Eisen (2008) in Afternoons with Puppy, discussed several cases of youth with Autism and the roles that animals had in their lives. One case that clearly stands out was about a teen-age boy diagnosed with high functioning autism who had tremendous social skill difficulties. Unfortunately, the boy led a very isolated life until he developed an interest in the birds in my office. Eventually he adopted a bird and it provided him with compassion and joy. He often would sit next to the bird when he was anxious and upset. The bird seemed to provide him with a blanket of warmth that helped him regulate his anxiety. He also realized the importance of handling the bird gently. They seemed to become protective of each other and enjoyed each other's company. Grandin (2011) agrees with this point of view and believes that one of the strongest benefits of having a pet for a person with ASD is for companionship. The animal can also act as a social lubricant and help the individual feel wanted.

How Horses Can Help

"Because she listens to me". Five words said it all! This simple phrase was volunteered by an eight-year -old boy with autism named Stan when describing his love for his new equine friend named Lady and his perceptions of therapeutic horseback riding.

Stan's story with horses starts about three years earlier when his parents decided to look for another option to help him in his development. He was diagnosed when he was three and continues to be vey uncommunicative and distractible. When Stan started at the Queen of Hearts Therapeutic Riding Center program, his progress was somewhat uneventful with a 27-year-old horse named Buddy. His sessions primarily consisted of being lead on a horse by three instructors—one on each side of him and an instructor leading. Although Stan seemed to enjoy the interaction, the gains hoped for didn't materialize. It was after about a year, that Robin Kilcoyne, the Executive Director, decided to alter his program. That's when the lights turned on for Sam and things began to change. Stan was introduced to a new horse named Lady and there was an immediate connection. The activities were altered and Stan was taught to western ride so more creative activities could be implemented while he was riding. For example, he went on letter searches around the ring or had the opportunity to direct Lady to various spots around the ring where he was able to drop a ball in a basket. Stan also was taught to use simple words to get Lady to respond to him, such as whoa, walk on and trot. To Sam's initial amazement, Lady followed his lead. Ultimately, it was the friendship between the two that cemented their bond. Stan often found himself coming early and staying later to interact and talk with his new four-legged friend. Lady often responds with a bowed head and a wiggling nose nudging his cheek. Stan doesn't even bribe her to come his way. She seems attuned to his presence.

Although Stan continues to have his challenges, his friendship with Lady is still flourishing. He now rides her more independently and is often seen trotting around the ring. His early comment about his friend was accurate. Lady does listen and follow his direction. More importantly, she is his beloved friend!

It seems that the greatest benefit derived in therapeutic riding comes from the movement of the horse (because of the multisensory benefits derived from the interaction). However, therapeutic riding may also assist in enhancing communication and social behavior (Foxall, 2002; and Mason, 2004). For example, Rupert Isaacson, (personal communication, January 19, 2011) agrees that one advantage of using horses is that a child can teach a horse to do tricks using very limited words and vocabulary. Children can use one-word phrases to possibly get the horse to bow, smile or even lay down

(very similar to what was done with Stan). This can be very empowering and reinforcing to a child especially when the horse responds. The interaction between them
seems to act as a social catalyst similar to the other animals discussed earlier. In our
discussion, Isaacson also noted an approach he called "Back Riding" which is when an
adult and child riding together. He believes that this technique is extremely useful for
promoting communication. He believes that the combination of deep pressure (holding
the child), speaking into the child's ear (not face to face speaking which may agitate the
child), and the movement of the horse all combine to create an optimum opportunity
for the child to receive and retain information. Perhaps it is the movement of the horse
that causes a neurological awakening, and makes the child more capable of interacting
with the external world.

However, just like any animal assisted intervention, a child needs to be receptive
to the interaction. S/he needs to be ready for the process and sometimes that means
one has to be patient and adjust. Over the years I have experienced this dilemma and
I have learned that sometimes just giving the process time to simmer, actually can be
extremely effective. This principle reminds me of the old proverb that should be seriously taken into consideration. In essence we have to appreciate that "when the mind
is ready the teacher comes". In the case of equines and therapeutic riding, it sometimes
may mean that you must bring the horse into the child's orbit and be patient with the
outcomes. It sometimes may mean that a lesson may not even include riding for the
day, but just being in the environment and nearby the horse.

In regards to therapeutic riding, trainers including Isaacson, believe that training
a horse in the skill of collection is extremely valuable in supporting children with ASD.
In essence, collection is when a horse carries more weight on his/her hind legs than the
front legs. The movement makes it easier for the horses to change direction quickly.
When horses are capable of moving with collection it enhances their power and causes
more of a rocking motion. It is this rocking motion that seems to cause a euphoric
response in children with autism.

Therapeutic riding requires that the person with ASD work on his/her balance.
Some believe that the horse's gait simulates the pace at which a human walks, making
the pelvic position and swaying while riding a horse very similar to the sway one experiences when walking (Reide, 1988). Even though the horse has a smooth gait at the
walk, the horse's stride is quite long which requires one to work on balance and posture
while riding. OTs often use horses to deliver controlled sensory input to an individual.
For example, this occurs while one manipulates the movement of the horse, its speed
and gait. The process can also be altered by using different horses, whose physical size
and make-up may cause a different response for an individual. For example one may
select a horse with increased movements for a person who is in need of more sensory

seeking (hypotonicity) while one may want to select a horse with more rhythmical movement for an individual who is more sensory avoidant or has hypertonicity.

According to Isaacson, smaller children relish periods of time where they lay full length on the horse's back. Some children seem to get great comfort from this, and he has observed that their self-stimming is often curbed during these opportunities. He feels that back riding is helpful because it is similar to laying on a big couch.

Finally, the research points out that the most effective sessions last for 20 minute intervals and that the riding arena should have limited distraction so that a child will not be over stimulated. Once the 20-minute ride is completed, one could have the person engage in another activity. Grandin, Fine and Bowers (2010) note that depending on the functional skills of the person with ASD, the individual may also be encouraged to engage in many other chores including grooming the horse, leading it to and from its stall, perhaps help in feeding or giving the horse treats, or even saddling the horse before they ride. This additional contact with the horse may provide many of the same therapeutic benefits offered through interaction with more traditional therapy animals such as dogs. After the break, the child could get back on the horse for another 20-minute session of riding (Grandin, et al, 2010).

Concluding Remarks:

George Eliot (1857) in his book **Mr. Gilfil's Love Story, Scenes of Clerical Life,** once stated that *"animals are such agreeable friends - they ask no questions, they pass no criticisms"*. His comments seem very après pros in our concluding remarks for this paper. The love and unconditional regard received from a pet or a therapy animal may represent a catalyst for emotional and psychological growth. A well-trained therapy animal working alongside a seasoned therapist may be a viable team used to promote various developmental and functional skills. On the other hand, families may want to consider adopting an animal for companionship. However, one must realize the importance of selecting a compatible pet, and the need for effective training. Provisions need to be thought through to support not only the welfare of the person but also the animal. Although AAI shouldn't be unrealistically viewed as a panacea, one should not overlook the power of our connection to animals. We may find some significant benefits derived from this relationship.

ARCHITECTURE AND AUTISM: CREATING A TOXIC-REDUCED ENVIRONMENT FOR YOUR AUTISTIC CHILD

By Catherine Purple Cherry

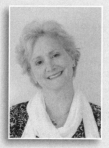

Catherine Purple Cherry, AIA, LEED AP

Purple Cherry Architects
One Melvin Ave.
Annapolis, MD 21401
410-990-1700
info@purplecherry.com
www.purplecherry.com

Cathy Purple Cherry, principal, Purposeful Architecture and Purple Cherry Architects, is a leader in the design of environments for children and adults with special needs. As a special needs architect, Mrs. Cherry creates spaces that foster thoughtful living and learning environments and inspire creativity, individuality and independence. She is personally connected to the special needs community by her life experiences with her autistic son and disabled brother and strives to connect these experiences with the incredible design skills of her firm. Mrs. Cherry currently works as a Special Needs Architect on many projects being designed and constructed nationally to better serve our special needs population.

Mrs. Cherry has presented to the Autism Society of America national conference, the AutismOne national conference, the National Association of Private Special Education Centers (NAPSEC) members conference, and the Association of School Board Officials. Mrs. Cherry has written several articles on home and school environments for children and adults with special needs, as well as other topics of interest for parents, which have appeared in *The Autism File*, *Autism Science Digest*, *School Planning and Management*, *Parenting Special Needs*, *Autism Advocate*, and *Autism & Aspergers Digest*.

This article is founded on the precautionary principle: "When human activities may lead to morally unacceptable harm that is scientifically plausible but uncertain, actions shall be taken to avoid or diminish that harm." United Nations Educational, Scientific and Cultural Organization, The Precautionary Principle World Commission on the Ethics of Scientific Knowledge and Technology (COMEST), http://unesdoc.unesco.org/images/0013/001395/139578e.pdf.

As parents, we desire a healthy and safe environment for our children, whether young or old, neurotypical or special needs. As intense research continues to explore the causes of autism, it is becoming apparent that a common contributing element to the explosion of ASD is the impact of toxins on our environment. This knowledge is beginning to shape the physical environments that support our kids on the spectrum. Fortunately, due largely to the green building movement, the building industry is already addressing several of the harmful toxins that have historically been used in construction materials. In my professional opinion as both a mother of a child on the spectrum and a principal of an architectural firm that designs spaces for special needs individuals, there are three strong components—beyond building material content—to making healthy and safe environments for those on the spectrum. The three components are as follows:

1.   Reducing or eliminating toxic elements
2.   Implementing physical safety elements
3.   Developing spaces and spatial arrangements for individuals with autism that support good choices, address unique behavioral issues, and support successful behavioral models

This chapter will explore the first component—**reducing or eliminating or toxic elements**—and is a living document that reflects available information as of the date shown. There is still much be learned with reference to the impacts of the environment on children and adults with autism.

Eliminating or Reducing Toxic Elements

Extensive research over the years has shown general health risks from harmful chemicals used in many building products and practices. On a daily basis, our world is exposed to a broad array of contaminants and impurities, ranging from irritants to potentially harmful chemicals. There is growing medical evidence that even limited exposures to some of these chemicals may have serious health impacts on certain people. These impacts can include respiratory problems, immune system dysfunction, damage to the kidneys and GI tract, neurological damage and related developmental problems, and, in some cases, cancer. Extensive research remains to be done, but current published studies seem to suggest a possible link between environmental exposure to certain toxins and the growing rates of autism in our population.

Toxic Body Burden

To further understand the link between autism and toxicity, you need to understand how your body processes toxins. The term "body burden" is used to describe the total quantity of toxic chemicals that are present at any selected time in the human body. Roughly 80,000 different kinds of chemicals are used in the United States. Some are naturally occurring and others are man-made and build up in the environment due to releases during production, industrial, and consumer use. These toxins end up in many places, including in our bodies. We come into direct contact with such toxins in a variety of ways. We might inhale them, swallow them in food or water, or absorb them through the skin. Sometimes body burden can be examined in terms of a specific, single chemical like lead or mercury. Studies show that every one of us contains dozens of chemicals in our bodies. In some cases, several hundred have been reported to be measured in select people.

Toxins and Autism

Many of these toxins are more prevalent today than they were in past decades. Those with or at risk for ASD or other chronic diseases may be especially vulnerable to some toxins. Many children (who are in-vitro or at-risk for developing autism) suffer from an impairment that reduces the body's normal ability to get rid of toxins and heavy metals. Research has shown that the buildup of such toxins in the body can lead to nervous system damage and developmental delays. Some individuals with autism are extremely sensitive and reactive to noxious substances. Research dollars have only recently started to support a more systematic evaluation of environmental toxins as possible risk factors for ASD. No "single cause" has emerged at the time of this publication for the trigger of autism. In fact, there appears to be a blend of environmental and genetic risks in which many potential contributors to autism can have similar effects. Thus, there is a need to take seriously the harm caused by various combinations of factors and to develop more sophisticated knowledge, awareness, and precautionary steps to minimize exposure to these health risks.

Summary

Children and adults with autism spectrum disorder (ASD) and other special needs may be characterized by repetitive or severely restricted activities and interests, impaired social interaction, and problems with verbal and nonverbal communication, as well as other possible impairments. Limited scientific advances have been made regarding the causes of autism. Overall, there appears to be general agreement amongst many medical professionals that both genetic and environmental factors contribute to the occurrence of autism.

The current science indicates that cellular level dysfunction is found in children with ASD:

Science Daily *(Nov. 30, 2010)—Children with autism are far more likely to have deficits in their ability to produce cellular energy than are typically developing children, a new study by researchers at UC Davis has found. The study, published in the* Journal of the American Medical Association (JAMA)*, found that cumulative damage and oxidative stress in mitochondria, the cell's energy producer, could influence both the onset and severity of autism, suggesting a strong link between autism and mitochondrial defects.*

Overview of Possible Reported Health Risks For Children and Adults with ASD and Other Special Needs

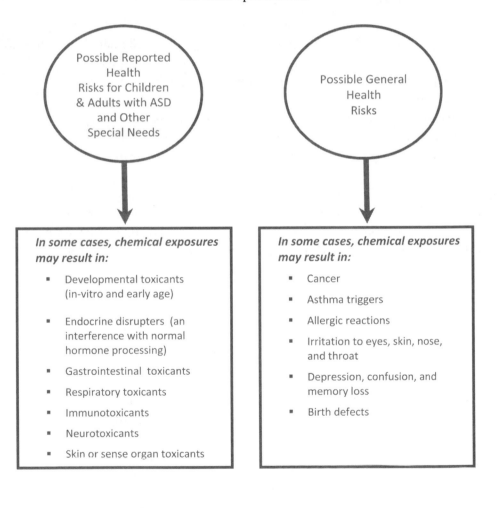

Possible Reported Health Risks for Children & Adults with ASD and Other Special Needs

Possible General Health Risks

In some cases, chemical exposures may result in:

- Developmental toxicants (in-vitro and early age)

- Endocrine disrupters (an interference with normal hormone processing)

- Gastrointestinal toxicants

- Respiratory toxicants

- Immunotoxicants

- Neurotoxicants

- Skin or sense organ toxicants

In some cases, chemical exposures may result in:

- Cancer

- Asthma triggers

- Allergic reactions

- Irritation to eyes, skin, nose, and throat

- Depression, confusion, and memory loss

- Birth defects

Research has shown that exposure to harmful chemicals could possibly lead to neural, gastrointestinal, respiratory, and/or immune dysfunction in individuals. Ongoing exposure to toxic chemicals may exacerbate these health issues. In understanding our surroundings, the chemical elements contained within them, and the impact of those elements on our physical and mental health, we can begin to help improve the toxic levels within the built environments for our ASD children and adults.

Overview of Potentially Unhealthy Building Products for ASD individuals

In some cases, man-made chemicals used in some building-related products have been linked to health risks for children and adults with ASD and other special needs. Some, not all, of these known and suspected health risks are summarized in the following **General Guidelines** chart. The chart identifies areas of risk within a building application, recommends strategies, provides examples of products to avoid, and notes potential health impacts. The applications and products indicated to avoid have been identified in various reports as potential contributors to health risks for individuals with autism and other special needs. The guide is a draft compilation of information from various sources and is not intended to be comprehensive. Applications and products that may contribute to health risks for children and adults with ASD and other special needs are shown in bold. More general health risks are shown in normal type. *Known* health risks are shown with an asterisk (*). All other health risks shown in this table are *suspected* (i.e., have not been scientifically documented, but have been flagged as chemicals of concern by various reputable organizations).

General Guidance on Healthy Environments for Residential, Educational and Vocational Facilities for Individuals with ASD and Other Special Needs

Building System	Application	Recommended Strategy	Example Products to Avoid	Potential Health Impacts
Site Construction	Radon Mitigation	Minimize exposure to radon and other harmful soil gases	Building is located in EPA's moderate or high risk areas (Radon Zone 1 and 2)	Lung Cancer* (Ref: 3, 4)
Metal, Wood, and Plastics	Adhesives	Use non-toxic alternatives	Bisphenol (BPA)	Endocrine Disrupter,* Developmental Toxicant* (Ref: 1, 2, 4)
		Use low emission alternatives	Volatile Organic Compounds (VOCs), e.g., Benzene, Toluene	Varies by Chemical, Development Toxicant, Asthma Trigger, Carcinogen (Ref: 1, 2, 4)
	Metal Materials and Coatings	Use non-toxic alternatives (e.g., stainless, galvanized)	Cadmium, Chromium, Lead, Mercury	Varies with Metal, Developmental Toxicant,* Carcinogen (Ref: 1, 2, 4)
	Wood Treatment	Use non-toxic alternatives (e.g., borate)	Arsenic, Creosote, Pentachlorophenol	Developmental Toxicant,* Carcinogen (Ref: 1, 2, 4)
	Plastic	Use non-toxic plastic products	Bisphenol (BPA), Phthalates	Endocrine Disrupter,* Carcinogen (Ref: 1, 2, 4)
Envelope	Insulation	Use non-toxic insulation (e.g., Bio-Based Foam, Icynene, Cellulose)	Formaldehyde,* Spray Polyurethane Foam (SPF)	Cancer,* Respiratory Irritant, Asthma Trigger (Ref: 1, 2, 4)
	Sealants	Use non-toxic sealants	Volatile Organic Compounds (VOCs)	Varies by Chemical, Development Toxicant, Asthma Trigger, Carcinogen (Ref: 1, 2, 4)

Category	Subcategory	Recommendation	Substance	Health Effects
Finishes	Gypsum Board	Use non-toxic drywall (avoid harmful sulfur gases)	Drywall manufactured in China	Allergic Reactions, Asthma Attacks, and Irritation to Eyes, Skin, Nose, and Throat
	Carpet	Use non-toxic carpeting, and padding	Volatile Organic Compounds (see also PBDE Fire Retardants)	**Varies by Chemical, Development Toxicant, Asthma Trigger,** Carcinogen (Ref: 1, 2, 4)
	Painting	Use paints that are free of heavy metals	Arsenic, Cadmium, Lead, Mercury	**Developmental Toxicant,* Gastrointestinal and Neurotoxicant,** and Cancer (Ref: 1, 2)
		Use non-toxic paints	Bisphenol (BPA)	**Developmental Toxicant,* Endocrine Disrupter*** (Ref: 1, 2)
		Use low emission paints	Volatile Organic Compound (VOCs)	**Varies by Chemical, Development Toxicant, Asthma Trigger,** Carcinogen (Ref: 1, 2, 4)
	Fire Protection Specialties	Minimize use of toxic flame retardants	Bromine, Chlorine, Halon, PolyBrominated Diphenyl Ethers (PBDEs)	**Adversely affects brain development, weakens immune system*** (Ref: 1, 2)
Equipment And Furnishings	Cabinets	Use non-toxic wood cabinets	Formaldehyde	Cancer,* Irritation to Eyes, Skin, Nose, Throat (Ref: 1, 2, 4)
	Fabrics and Furniture	Minimize exposure to toxins used in fabric/carpet protectors	Perfluorinated Compounds (PFCs), including Scotchgard	**Links to Developmental Toxicity,** and Cancer (Ref: 6)
		Use non-toxic flame retardants (e.g., argon)	Brominated Flames Retardants (BFRs, PBDEs)	**Neurodevelopmental Toxicity, Hormone Disrupter** (Ref: 4)

Continued...

General Guidance on Healthy Environments for Residential, Educational and
Vocational Facilities for Individuals with ASD and Other Special Needs, Continued

Building System	Application	Recommended Strategy	Example Products to Avoid	Potential Health Impacts
Special Construction	Pest Control	Minimize use of toxic pest controls, herbicides, & fungicides	Various	**Varies with Chemical, Endocrine Disrupters,** Carcinogens (Ref: 4)
Mechanical	Plumbing	Use non-toxic water piping, especially for drinking water	Polyvinyl Chloride (PVC), often includes Phthalates	**Endocrine Toxicant, Gastrointestinal or Liver Toxicant** (Ref: 4)
	Heating and Cooling	Minimize exposure to combustion gases	Carbon Monoxide (CO)	Chronic exposure to low levels of carbon monoxide can lead to depression, confusion, and memory loss (Ref: 4)
		Use non-toxic refrigerants	CFCs	**Weakening of Immune System** (Ref: 4)
	Humidity Control	Minimize exposure to high indoor humidity levels	Molds and Mildews	**Allergic Reactions, Asthma Attacks, and Irritation to Eyes, Skin, Nose, Throat, and Lungs** (Ref: 5)
	Air Distribution	Minimize exposure to dust and pollen in the home's air supply	Small particulate matter (trapped in carpets and air-duct system)	**Changes in Lung Function and Respiratory Illness, Asthma Trigger** (Ref: 4)

Electrical	Base Electrical Materials	Use non-toxic electronic sheathing (e.g., PET)	Bisphenol (BPA), Chlorinated Polyethylene	Endocrine Disrupter,* Developmental Toxicant* (Ref: 1, 2, 4)
		Use non-toxic solder, and cable jacketing	Lead	Developmental Toxicant,* Neurotoxicant, Cancer (Ref: 1, 2, 4)
	Lighting	Use non-toxic lamps	Mercury	Developmental Toxicant,* Neurotoxicant (Ref: 1, 2, 4)
	Controls	Use non-toxic HVAC controls, switches and relays	Mercury	Developmental Toxicant,* Neurotoxicant (Ref: 1, 2, 4)
Operations and Maintenance	Cleaning	Use household products free of toxic chemicals (e.g. cleaners, spot removers, paint, pressed wood)	Volatile organic compounds (VOCs), e.g., Benzene, Toluene	Varies by Chemical, Development Toxicant, Asthma Trigger, Carcinogen (Ref: 1, 2, 4)
	Personal Care	Minimize use of harmful chemicals in personal care products	Acetone, BHA/BHT, Parabens, Phthalates, Lanolin (contaminated by agricultural chemicals)	Neurotoxic Agent, Endocrine Disruption, Carcinogen (Ref: 1, 2, 4)
	Cooking	Minimize exposure to toxins used in non-slip coatings, and food-wrap coatings	PFOAs and PFCs, included in products like Teflon, and Oil Resistant Coatings	Links to Developmental Toxicity, and Cancer (Ref: 6)

ART THERAPY APPROACHES TO TREATING AUTISM

By Nicole Martin and Dr. Donna Betts

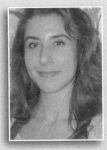

Nicole Martin, MAAT, LPC, ATR

Sky's The Limit Studio, LLC
Lawrence, KS 66044
785-424-0739
arttherapyandautism@yahoo.com
arttherapyandautism.com

Sky's The Limit was founded in 2007 by Nicole Martin, a registered art therapist, licensed professional counselor, and artist living in Lawrence, Kansas. As the big sister of a brother with autism, she is dedicated to improving public access to creative arts therapy services tailored specifically to the needs of people on the spectrum. STL's treatment model is a synthesis of her many years of experience working in developmental/behavioral art therapy, applied behavior analysis, and recreational arts and disabilities programs. She is the author of *Art as an Early Intervention Tool for Children with Autism* (2009) and various articles, and received her training at the School of the Art Institute of Chicago.

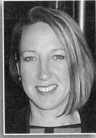

Donna Betts, PhD, ATR-BC

Art Therapy Program
The George Washington University
1925 Ballenger Avenue, Suite 250
Alexandria, VA 22314
dbetts@gwu.edu
www.art-therapy.us
www.gwu.edu/~artx/

Dr. Betts is a registered and board-certified art therapist and assistant professor in the George Washington University graduate art therapy program. Dr. Betts serves on GW's Autism Initiative Committee, which is working toward the establishment of the GW Autism Research, Treatment & Policy Institute. Her own research addresses the clinical utility of art therapy approaches with individuals on the autism spectrum. Dr. Betts is also the author of the Face Stimulus Assessment (FSA), (Betts, 2003, 2009) a performance-based, nonverbal drawing instrument used primarily to identify strengths of people with autism and related disabilities, establish treatment goals, and determine progress in therapy. Ongoing research related to the reliability and validity of the FSA is another focus of Dr. Betts's work.

Art therapy is a mental health profession that uses the creative process of art-making to improve and enhance the physical, mental, and emotional well-being of individuals of all ages (AATA, 2009a). Art therapy is based on the belief that the creative process involved in artistic self-expression helps people to increase self-esteem and self-awareness, achieve insight, develop interpersonal skills, resolve conflicts and problems, manage behavior, and reduce stress.

Creative expression has been used for healing throughout history (AATA, 2009b). In the early 20th century, psychiatrists became interested in the artwork created by their patients with mental illness. Educators simultaneously discovered that children's art expressions reflected emotional, developmental, and cognitive growth. By midcentury, hospitals, clinics, and rehabilitation centers increasingly incorporated art therapy programs along with traditional therapies.

Today, art therapy integrates the fields of human development, visual art (drawing, painting, sculpture, and other art forms), and the creative process with models of counseling and psychotherapy (AATA, 2009a). Art therapy is used in a number of settings with individuals of all ages, and with a variety of mental and emotional problems and disorders, and physical, cognitive, and neurological problems.

Art therapy is an effective approach when working with individuals with autism spectrum disorder (ASD). Art therapy involves the application of techniques specifically designed to reduce the symptoms of autism and promote healthy self-expression. A number of clinical reports support the use of art therapy with ASD, as well as with individuals with developmental disabilities in general (Gilroy, 2006).

The art therapist is adept at facilitating therapeutic processes with the use of visual art media and modalities such as painting and drawing, sculpture, cartooning, clay modeling, animation, and puppetry. The sensory appeal of the art materials makes them desirable tools for self-regulation and self-soothing. Projects designed to tackle specific treatment goals are limitless and may include group murals (to work on collaboration, reciprocity, and flexibility skills), portrait drawing (to work on face processing and relationship skills), friendship boxes (to work on memory and relationship skills), and many more (Martin, 2009a).

Art therapy differs from art education due to the therapist's expertise in the psychological application of art techniques, master's-level training in child development, knowledge of autism spectrum disorders, and how to tailor projects accordingly. An art therapist working in this specialty should be fluent in developmental/behavioral art therapy approaches, have a solid understanding of early childhood artistic development, have experience in the use of current best practices in behavioral and communication supports for individuals with autism, and be a patient and enthusiastic coach. Improving artistic skills and striving for aesthetic beauty are desirable qualities and will help maintain the client's enthusiasm, but remain secondary to the focus on personal growth and reduction of symptoms.

No possible risks or side effects from art therapy with this population have been published to date; however, the risks that can arise from poorly selected art materials and their poorly supervised use must be carefully considered. Art therapists should know the toxicity level and ingredients of all their art supplies as well as the allergies, diet restrictions, and behavioral patterns of their clients, and pair them wisely. For example, a child on a gluten-free diet should avoid traditional playdough since it contains wheat flour, and a child who tends to throw objects should not use sharp tools without close supervision. Art therapists can start by offering a sensible variety of nontoxic materials and then increasing the variety, number, and quality as the child matures. Art materials should also be carefully matched to the child's symptoms and energy level; a poor match can aggravate or encourage symptomatic behavior, while a good match can soothe and create an appropriate outlet for symptoms (Martin, 2009a).

The wide range of symptoms experienced by people with ASD makes them very unique in presentation, so treatments must be tailored to a range of varying needs (Evans & Dubowski, 2001). It is especially important to offer a safe, predictable, and stable environment by providing therapy at the same time every week and setting up materials in an orderly fashion. By doing so, the art therapist establishes psychological continuity and a stable environment for the client (Stack, 1998). Treatment takes place within the professional therapeutic relationship between the art therapist and the client, in either private sessions or a group setting. Additionally, an art therapist can train the client's caregivers and teachers in the use of art therapy techniques in order to help generalize progress to the client's natural environment, such as home or school.

To begin, the art therapist assesses the individual's skills and interests in order to formulate individualized treatment goals. Using a combination of formal and informal assessment, the art therapist determines the client's capacity for imagination and socialization, artistic developmental level, the impact of different art materials on the client's senses and behavior, and the client's initial interests and personality, before developing appropriate treatment goals. Assessment tools such as the Face Stimulus Assessment (Betts, 2003, 2009) and the Portrait Drawing Assessment (Martin, 2008) can provide insight into the skills of clients with autism.

Art therapy helps clients with autism on many different levels. Major treatment goal areas include socialization, communication, and sensory regulation (Martin, 2009b). Martin (2009a) highlights six treatment goal areas that distinguish art therapy from other therapies used to treat autism: imagination/abstract thinking skills, sensory regulation and integration, emotional understanding and self-expression, artistic developmental growth, visual-spatial skills, and appropriate recreation/leisure skills.

Early intervention is crucial. Goals that a child with ASD might accomplish in art therapy include age-appropriate drawing or modeling skills, improved self-expression and reduced anxiety or frustration, independent or semi-independent use of art making as a coping skill or self-soothing tool, improved social skills such as project collaboration and flexibility, and age-appropriate imagination and ideation skills.

The art therapist's ability to troubleshoot possible hindrances to the client's interest in art—such as sensory discomfort, perfectionism, anxiety, difficulty translating or generating ideas, compulsive/impulsive behaviors, lack of personal relevancy, or past punitive experiences associated with art materials—and take corrective action, means that art therapy has the potential to benefit the majority of individuals with autism, not just those who demonstrate a precocious talent.

To illustrate with a case example, an individual with autism who is withdrawn may be approached through the objects and activities that he or she prefers (Kramer, 1979). By beginning with the familiar and progressively introducing the new, clients with ASD are more willing to accept the unfamiliar. For instance, Dr. Betts once worked with a student who was obsessed with his own wet saliva. The boy was fascinated with the patterns of movement he created with his spit, and this is what kept him engaged in the kinesthetic activity. Thus, Dr. Betts came up with a way to divert the boy away from his excessive interest in saliva by introducing a dry substance—sand. In his art therapy sessions, the boy was encouraged to play with sand and its containers in a tabletop box. As he learned about how to manipulate his environment through sand play, his obsession with the spit eventually disappeared. With Dr. Betts's continuous encouragement and praise for using the sand, contained within the boundaries of a box, the client progressed toward a more flexible and mature ego functioning. He therefore made gains that addressed his Individualized Education Program (IEP) goals related to cognitive, behavioral, and emotional growth.

Including art therapy as a component of early intervention treatment helps individuals with autism form good habits for a lifetime of using art as a vital means of expression. Appropriate art therapy goals and projects can be created for a person with ASD at any age, level of functioning, or initial interest level. All individuals with autism can benefit from learning how to express their thoughts, feelings, and interests in a creative, hands-on way, whether to ease and enhance communication, externalize feelings of anxiety, or simply realize their potential as imaginative, productive human beings.

Ongoing Research

Dr. Betts is currently engaged as a co-investigator in a George Washington University Medical Faculty Associates funded research project entitled "Assessing Medication

Responsiveness in Persons with Autism Spectrum Disorders (ASD)." Led by Principal Investigator Dr. Valerie Hu of GW's Department of Biochemistry and Molecular Biology, the primary purpose of this project is to gather and use validated responses to psychotropic medication in the autistic population in order to assess the range of responses to specific medications in the ASD population. This information will be used to reduce the heterogeneity of potential subjects for genetic and biological profiling studies. Successful identification of clearly positive responders to a specific type of medication will lead to submission of an NIH proposal to study this subgroup of individuals vs. non-responders using genotype, gene expression, and metabolomics analyses to identify genetic variants and biological pathways associated with the positive response. Indicators of medication responsiveness will be measured by a patient/parents/caregivers questionnaire, a clinician questionnaire and an art-based assessment designed and evaluated by Dr. Betts.

69

BERARD AUDITORY INTEGRATION TRAINING

By Sally Brockett

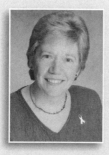

Sally Brockett, MS

Mrs. Brockett is the Director of the IDEA Training and Consultation Center in North Haven, Connecticut. She founded the center in 1992 to focus on interventions for developmental disabilities after 12 years as a special education teacher with all categories of disabilities. After training in France with Dr. Guy Berard, the Berard method of auditory integration training (AIT) and consultation became a special focus of her work. Mrs. Brockett has completed advanced training in AIT with Dr. Guy Berard and is approved by him as a certified International Professional Instructor in the Berard method. Mrs. Brockett founded the Berard AIT International Society and has served on the Board of Directors since its beginning. She and Dr. Berard have co-authored *Hearing Equals Behavior: Updated and Expanded*, the newest edition of Dr. Berard's book about his method of auditory integration training.

Introduction

Dr. Guy Berard, a French ENT physician, developed a listening program that was used primarily to assist in certain cases of hearing impairment. However, he quickly discovered that learning-related skills and abilities, such as attentive listening, concentration, auditory discrimination and memory skills often improved following the training program. Berard's auditory integration training (AIT) program requires that individuals passively listen to processed music through headphones for a total of 10 hours (half hour sessions usually over 10-12 days). The Berard program is now noted for its use as an educationally related intervention and is provided by Berard AIT practitioners in many countries throughout the world.

Interest in Berard's Program Expands

Dr. Berard meticulously describes his understanding of the auditory imbalances that interfere with efficient listening and learning in his book, *Audition Égale Comportement* published in French in 1982, followed by the English translation in 1993, and most recently published in English as *Hearing Equals Behavior: Updated and Expanded*. Professionals and parents were introduced to the concept that **how** we hear plays a very significant role in *how* we behave and learn. Unfortunately, even today, there are professionals who are not aware that many individuals who are struggling with academics and behavioral problems have inefficient auditory skills that interfere with effective listening and processing which puts them at a great disadvantage in the classroom and workplace.

By 1991, public awareness and interest in the Berard method grew and Dr. Berard expanded his training of new practitioners through seminars offered in the U.S. as well as in France. The program began to receive recognition as an intervention for behavior and learning difficulties, in addition to its use for auditory hypersensitivity. Parents, especially those with children on the autism spectrum, began seeking this intervention for their children and professionals began to include the program in their services.

Research on the Berard Method of AIT

Dr. Bernard Rimland and Stephen M. Edelson, from the Autism Research Institute, organized research studies to document the effectiveness of the method. They had heard many anecdotal reports from parents about the success of this intervention and wanted to document its efficacy. These studies focused on the autism population, but later studies by other researchers included subjects with attention deficit disorder (ADD), central auditory processing disorder (CAPD), and other disabilities. By 1998 there were 28 studies completed and 82% demonstrated positive effects from AIT.

Dr. Rimland recommended the term "auditory integration training" be used to refer to the Berard method of training. This term was agreed upon because it took into account the "integration" of the senses and processing that occurs with Berard AIT. Unfortunately, "auditory integration training" or AIT was not trademarked and new types of listening programs have also used the term AIT. In order to help distinguish Dr. Berard's method from these others, Berard Practitioners now use "Berard AIT" instead of just AIT. However, it is still confusing for parents who may not realize that all AIT is not the same, and the research that applies to the Berard method does not apply to other methods.

Berard AIT in the 21st Century

Berard AIT has expanded to more than 30 countries around the world and continues to spread to new regions. Currently, there are Berard AIT Instructors in 7 countries and seminars for professionals are provided in several different languages. New research continues to document the benefits derived from this method, which currently is available for those as young as 3 years of age. There is no upper age limit since the brain is capable of reorganizing through neural plasticity until death.

The Berard method continues to be studied in order to gain deeper understanding about the process. Technology is available today that was not available during the period that Dr. Berard actively developed his program. The Cognitive Neuroscience Lab at the University of Louisville, KY, is investigating changes in the individual's auditory response pattern such as auditory evoked potentials (AEP) and event-related potentials (ERP) using electroencephalographic (EEG) responses prior to AIT and post-AIT.

As new understanding of the brain emerges, and new technologies develop, there may be changes in the Berard AIT protocol. New equipment may become available and adjustments may be made in the program. However, any changes must first undergo high quality, scientific study to measure whether the suggested change actually provides equal or greater benefit in terms of functional performance of the clients.

Who May Benefit from the Program?

Berard practitioners consider the presenting concerns reported by parents, teachers and therapists rather than simply making a decision about eligibility based on diagnostic labels. If the presenting concerns focus on skills and abilities in developmental or academic areas that have been shown to respond to the training program, then it is quite possible that the individual will show positive responses in functional performance. Individuals with one or more of the following concerns may benefit from Berard AIT:

- poor attention
- difficulty listening, understanding, and remembering
- low tolerance for distractions
- poor ability to modulate sensory experiences
- over- or under reactive emotional responses
- slower thinking and processing
- brain "traffic jams" when processing information
- difficulty putting ideas in sequence
- sound hypersensitivity and hyposensitivity (tuned out)
- sensory seeking/avoidance behaviors
- misunderstanding directions.

The Berard AIT Procedure

The Berard AIT program requires ten hours of listening. Each day consists of two 30-minute sessions separated by a minimum of a three hour break (go to the park, relax, or do other activities of interest). Preferably the ten days are consecutive, running through weekends, although many practitioners may provide the training with a weekend break in the middle, which is acceptable.

Participants listen with headphones to music specially modulated through an instrument approved for Berard AIT called an Earducator™ (or the Audiokinetron) during the training sessions. The Berard AIT device modulates the music during all sessions which provides random dampening and amplification of high and low frequencies. The process is non-intrusive with the volume adjusted to be comfortably loud, below an average of 85 dB.

An audio test, according to the Berard protocol, is given to participants who are able to cooperate with this evaluation. This shows how the participant hears across all the frequencies and helps to identify conditions that may cause disruption in the auditory system. This information is used to determine if any narrow-band filters will be used during the training sessions. When the audio tests can be obtained, this evaluation is repeated after 5 days of training, and again at the end of the 10 day training period to see how the listening pattern is responding.

There are many young children and those with disabilities who cannot cooperate with the audio test protocol due to inability to focus on the tones and spontaneously communicate when they do hear the tones. Research with subjects with autism spectrum disorder showed that even when the audio test cannot be obtained, the training can still be done and significant benefits achieved.

How Does Berard AIT Compare with Other Similar Approaches?

The Berard method is provided under direct supervision by trained professionals and requires only 10 hours of listening while most sound-based intervention programs require 40 or more hours. Due to the nature of the stimulation provided by the Berard AIT device, the changes usually occur more quickly and include a broad area of response. Parent observations of improvements in language, social skills, sensory modulation, cognition, fine motor skills and reduction of challenging behaviors and sound sensitivity are supported by data obtained through research studies and clinical observations. It is easier to monitor results from Berard AIT since there is a definitive ending of the training after 10 days. Typically, the majority of change occurs within the first 3 months after the program is completed, and the benefit is usually permanent. The Berard method is also well-researched and statistically significant results are documented. Professionally trained practitioners achieve similar results around the world when using the approved equipment and following the protocol. Berard AIT is not offered as a home program through the use of CDs.

Results Achieved with Berard AIT

There are results from research studies and anecdotal reports of success with Berard AIT that document behavioral and learning improvements following the 10 hours of training. The largest study to date was completed by the Autism Research Institute and included 445 subjects on the autism spectrum with an age range from 4 to 41 years. A significant reduction of sound sensitivity and a sharp reduction in problem behaviors occurred and was maintained through 9 months of post-AIT evaluations. A pilot study of the effect of Berard AIT on sensory processing problems was conducted by IDEA Training Center by Sally Brockett, Director. The median change was a 79% reduction of sensory problems 6 months after AIT. A long-term study with students in Sweden by Lars Persson, Director of the Berard's Method Center, documents that at 21 months after AIT, 38% of those students who received AIT were returned to regular education classes, while only 5.6% of students in the control group were returned to regular education classes. A summary of studies on AIT is posted at http://www.berardaitwebsite.com/sait/aitsummary.html. There are also pre and post AIT results at http://www.ideatrainingcenter.com/ait-results.shtml and http://www.ideatrainingcenter.com/stories.shtml which show the types of responses participants may achieve with Berard AIT.

This figure is an example of the type of change documented following a 10 day program of Berard AIT. The Attention Deficit Disorders Evaluation Scale was completed to obtain a baseline and then completed at 3 months after the training. The change shown is the median percent gain for 48 subjects.

Berard AIT balances the hearing and eliminates sound sensitivity and distortions for most participants. The changes in the auditory system also impact on the vestibular system which regulates many aspects of sensory processing. As the sensory problems diminish, the individual may feel more relaxed, less hypervigilant and defensive. There is typically a reduction in challenging behaviors and they can then focus their attention on other things, such as communication, socialization, and learning. Many participants seem to progress from the "bottom up". As the hearing distortions and misperceptions, and sensitivity if it is present, are reduced or eliminated, they show progress with other areas of development and behavior. This may include:

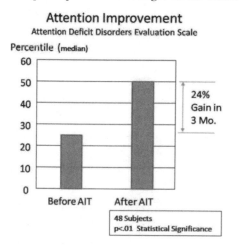

- sensory modulation
- receptive and expressive communication,
- articulation
- self-confidence,
- social and emotional relatedness,
- faster and higher level cognitive processing.

Many also show progress with gross and fine motor skills due to the changes in the vestibular system and most likely, the cerebellum, which regulates many aspects of motor function.

To learn more about this intervention, visit the official Berard AIT website at www.berardaitwebsite.com. An international list of Berard Practitioners is available on the website as well as many articles that explain more details about the program. Professionals interested in becoming a practitioner will find a list of approved Berard Instructors. *Hearing Equals Behavior: Expanded and Updated* is now available. This edition, co-authored by Dr. Berard and Sally Brockett, explains the concepts underlying Dr. Berard's method and how he developed his retraining program through years of detailed clinical observations. This book is also available in e-book formats, including the Spanish translation, *Audición Igual A Comportamiento: Revisado y ampliado*. Readers will learn how listening and learning can "switch on" when the auditory system is rebalanced and functioning effectively. The comprehensive information focuses on auditory processing problems and associated learning and behavior difficulties and is an important addition to the small collection of resource books available on this topic.

70

OCCUPATIONAL THERAPY AND SENSORY INTEGRATION

By Markus Jarrow

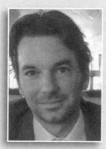

Markus Jarrow, OTR/L, C/NDT

Clinical Director
The SMILE Center | The Sensory Motor Integration + Language
Enrichment Center
171 Madison Avenue 5th Floor
New York, NY 10016
212-400-0383
markus@smileny.org
www.smileny.org

Markus Jarrow received his BA in Occupational Therapy from Sargent College of Boston University in 1997. Markus has more than twelve years of experience in pediatrics, specializing in the evaluation and treatment of children with autism spectrum disorders, sensory integration dysfunction, and neuromuscular disorders. Markus has extensive training in sensory integration, neurodevelopmental treatment, and DIR/floortime methodologies. His approach to treatment draws from the fundamentals of these three models in a comprehensive style that addresses the whole child. Markus co-founded the SMILE Center | the Sensory Motor Integration and Language Enrichment Center in 2009, a state-of-the-art pediatric treatment facility in New York City.

W hy does my child like to spin so much? Why does she refuse so many foods? Why does he scream each time I change his diaper or give him a bath? Why does my daughter make strange sounds and look out of the corner of her eyes? Why does he seem to shut down or go into a panic when we go to a restaurant or a party?

Occupational therapists can provide valuable insight to help families better understand many of the questions they struggle with when raising a child with an autism spectrum disorder. Occupational therapy and a sensory integration (SI) treatment approach can be very effective in addressing many of the root challenges that children with ASD face. In order to understand how sensory integrative treatment can be effective, it is important to understand the basics of sensory integration theory and dysfunction. This chapter will provide you with a brief overview.

What Is Occupational Therapy?

Occupational therapy is a broad profession that shares a common goal of utilizing functional and purposeful activities, or occupations, to increase an individual's functional independence. In the scope of treatment of children with autism spectrum disorders, occupational therapy can be very effective in improving functional fine and gross motor skills, postural control and movement patterns, motor planning, self-help skills, hand-eye coordination, and visual perceptual and spatial skills. However, perhaps most significant is the impact that a sensory integration treatment approach can have on a child's sensory processing skills. After all, if a child cannot maintain an optimal level of arousal and appropriately integrate sensory information, his or her ability to learn, acquire new skills, and interact with his or her environment will be greatly compromised. A child who relies of self-stimulatory or self-regulatory behaviors to control his or her arousal level or tune out adverse stimuli, is a child less available for engagement, learning, and skill acquisition. Therefore, with this population in particular, sensory integration is one of the primary frames of reference utilized by occupational therapists.

History of Sensory Integration

Sensory integration is a theory and treatment approach originally developed by the late occupational therapist, Dr. A. Jean Ayres, PhD, OTR, in the 1960s. She defined sensory integration as the ability to organize sensory information for use by the many parts of the nervous system in order to work together to promote effective interactions with the environment. Sensory integration had evolved over the years, but much of the original theory remains. It is a dynamic and child-directed treatment approach based on specific principles, treatment techniques, and equipment. It is a problem solving and individualized approach that requires ongoing analysis and assessment in order to monitor changes in the child and adapt the treatment accordingly. A trained occupational therapist utilizes a wide range of techniques and strategies in order to help a child achieve and maintain an optimal level of arousal. It is in this state that adaptive responses can be made to incoming sensory information, enabling learning and development. This in turn enables them to become more confident, successful, and interactive explorers of their worlds.

Dr. Ayers' treatment and research pertained primarily to the vestibular, proprioceptive and tactile systems. Toward the end of her life, she began to look more closely at the important roles of the auditory and visual systems. Unfortunately for all of us, her work was cut short, as she lost her life to cancer. Since that time, occupational therapists have continued to research and build on the treatment vision of sensory integration and make great strides in further identifying the important roles of the auditory and visual systems. Although considered by some to be outside the scope of traditional, child-directed sensory integration, multiple effective treatment modalities have become widely used today that more specifically address the auditory and visual systems.

What to Expect

Typically, a child will first be evaluated by an occupational therapist trained in sensory integration. This process will likely consist of an interview with caregivers and a variety of questionnaires, clinical observations, and standardized testing, potentially including the Sensory Integration and Praxis Test (SIPT). The entire process may take anywhere from a few hours to several lengthy visits. Following a thorough assessment, a treatment plan will be formulated and a recommendation will be made regarding the frequency and duration of the child's treatment.

Sensory integrative treatment is best implemented in a therapy gym outfitted with a wide variety of specific equipment and adaptable environments. These treatment facilities are referred to as sensory gyms. Therapists, however, have found creative solutions to providing treatment with limited space and materials, such as in schools and in the home. Treatment should only be carried out by a clinician trained in sensory integration and should always involve the parents/caregivers, as carryover into the home is critical. No matter how effective the clinician, he or she will likely have a maximum of an hour or two per week with the child. It is therefore essential that a home program be implemented to provide the child with the consistency needed to make significant change. This may include simple modifications to the home, adaptations to the child's routines, toys, clothing, etc., and most importantly, individualized treatment strategies to be carried out in the home and/or school. This is referred to as a sensory diet. This piece is critical in ensuring optimal progress.

In treatment, you may see your child flying and spinning through the air on swings suspended from the ceiling. You may see her climbing over or under enormous padded obstacles, up rope ladders, or through suspended tunnels that challenge her every move. She may zip by you on a scooter board, holding tightly to a bungee cord, coordinating rhythmical movements of her arms with activation of deep core muscles to keep her body stable. She may climb a rock wall and jump from a platform into a crash mat or ball pit. She may appear surprisingly organized and engaged.

Treatment with another child may appear completely different... at least initially. You may see him sitting with the clinician in an enclosed play tent, covered in heavy blankets, playing with a new toy. You may see him in a dimly lit room, gently rocking on a platform swing with the clinician cradling him from behind, as he reaches out to rhythmically drop beanbags in a target. He may be slowly rolling across a room of soft, foam-filled cushions, to the soothing hum of the therapist, to gather pieces of a desired game. He may smile and appear surprisingly comfortable and regulated.

SI treatment can appear very different from one child to the next, as it is individualized to each child. While an experienced clinician can make treatment simply look fun and playful, rest assured careful clinical reasoning is behind every move.

The cost of an evaluation can range from a couple hundred dollars to a couple thousand dollars. Private treatment ranges greatly; depending on your location, the cost may be less than one hundred to two hundred dollars or more per one-hour session. Sessions can be as short as thirty minutes; however, the nature of the treatment tends to lend itself to longer sessions of forty-five minutes or an hour. Occupational therapy evaluations and treatment are typically covered, to some extent, by local school systems as well as Early Intervention programs for children less than three years of age. Therapists more experienced with sensory integration are often affiliated with independent clinics or sensory gyms and may or may not accept public funding. In some cases, private insurance can cover some or all of the out-of-pocket costs for treatment.

Occupational therapists can work with children with ASD in a variety of settings. In schools, treatment often carries over to the classroom, as the primary focus is improving function in school-related tasks and environments. School settings do not typically have extensive treatment rooms and equipment. For children three years of age and under, treatment often takes place in the home through the local Early Intervention program. At an early age, this can be very effective in meeting the needs of the child and family and in making helpful modifications to the home environment and routine to best support the child. However, treatment strategies are generally limited to a creative imagination with what is in the home and what the clinical can carry with them to the home. In a private practice, sensory gym, or outpatient setting, the OT typically has access to more therapy equipment and can more precisely address all of a child's sensory needs.

What Is Sensory Integration and Sensory Integration Dysfunction?

In order for a child to appropriately move through space and interact with their world in an alert, regulated, and effective manner, they must take in an extraordinary amount of sensory information, unconsciously interpret it, and then make appropriate adaptive responses on a rapid and continuous basis. This is an incredibly complex process that relies on an intricate network of sensory systems functioning appropriately and simultaneously. It is called sensory integration. It's an amazing process that most of us take for granted; it just happens and we never think twice about it. However, for many of the children with ASD, this is not the case.

For a child with sensory integration dysfunction, the seemingly simple task of walking across a classroom, putting on a t-shirt, finding a toy in a closet, listening to mom on a busy street corner, walking barefoot on a beach, skipping down the sidewalk, or playing in a swing in the park may be perceived as overly challenging, seemingly impossible, or even terrifying. Sensory integration dysfunction can impact every aspect of development including: social-emotional, behavioral, attention and regulation, gross and fine motor, postural, adaptive and self-help, visual motor, visual spatial/perceptual, speech and language, and learning. Our ability to appropriately meet the many challenges faced in our daily lives is a result of the integration and proper "wiring" of five major sensory systems: vestibular, proprioceptive, tactile, auditory, and visual.

The vestibular system is located in the inner ear and is the integral system that responds to gravitational forces and changes in the head's position in space and plays a key role in regulation. It is the sense that tells you when you're right side up or upside down, and is responsible for helping with balance and spatial orientation. The vestibular system is also responsible for proving a stable basis for visual function, even when the head is moving through space. Also, for example, when an object is getting larger in your visual field, your vestibular confirms that you are not moving, thus indicating that the object is coming toward you. The appropriate response can then be made, whether it's to move out of the way, catch it, etc.

Movement is a component of almost everything that we do; so vestibular function applies to almost every interaction we have with the world. It's the sense that, when overstimulated, makes one feel seasick and carsick. It's the sense that thrill seekers try to satiate with roller coasters, bungee jumping, and skydiving. Because of its role in movement and space, it works hand in hand with the auditory and visual systems in order to provide us with a sense of our three dimensional spatial envelope, compelling us to move, explore, and understand. This collaborative system is referred to as the vestibular-visual-auditory triad.

Without this functioning triad, it would be impossible to appropriately process movement, space, time, and sequencing. When we enter a new restaurant for the first time, we immediately take in a sense of the room's size, relative shape, and arrangement of its contents. After navigating the delicate environment and taking a seat, we understand the quiet clinging of pots is coming from the open kitchen behind us and to the left, the gentle humming sound is coming from over-head ceiling fans, and the waitress walking slowly from across the room will be within a respectful distance in seven to eight seconds to kindly request a glass of water in a suitable volume level for the environment. None of these seemingly simple processes that we take for granted would have been possible without appropriate integration of the vestibular-visual-auditory triad. This same analysis can be reapplied to countless scenarios, in countless environments, on countless different levels.

> "Without a properly functioning vestibular system, sights and sounds in the environment do not make sense—they are only isolated pieces of information disconnected from the meaningful whole. It is the integration of the sensory information that holds the key for finding the meaning in the world. Because movement is part of everything we do in life, it could be said that the vestibular system supports all behavior and acquisition of skills, as well as helping to balance the stream of sensory information that constantly bombards the system." (*Astronaut Training: A Sound Activated Vestibular-Visual Protocol for Moving, Looking and Listening*; Kawar, Frick & Frick, 2005)

While the vestibular system is primarily involved in movement and spatial processes, it works closely with the proprioceptive system in connecting spatial information and movement back to the body. The proprioceptive system is made up of a network of sensors throughout our muscles and joints that work together to create an internal body map. It is through proprioceptive awareness that we know the position of our body, without having to see it. If someone was to close your eyes and position your right arm, hand, and fingers in any position, you could replicate the position with the left without looking. It is through intact proprioception that we can execute the "touch your nose" test by extending an arm out straight to the side and then bending at the elbow and accurately touching the tip of our finger to our nose. It is the sense that allows us to reach and grab an object on our desk behind us, without looking. It is also the sense that grades our pressure, allowing us to use the appropriate force when picking up a brick versus a thin paper cup of water. It allows us know the position of our body at all times and helps to appropriately grade quality and force of movement. It is understandable how a child with decreased proprioceptive processing could face many challenges.

Input to the proprioceptive system through passive deep pressure, and much more significantly, resistive muscle activation or "heavy work," enhances serotonin release and can be very grounding, organizing, or even alerting depending on the circumstance and sensory profile of the child. This is the reason why a hug can feel so good. This is why some people stomp their feet or clench their fists when they are angry or overwhelmed. Have you ever seen a boxer or other athlete jump up and down, shake their head, or even hit themselves in order to get "revved" up before entering the game or boxing round? This is why some adults chew on pen caps when the coffee wears off and their attention wanes in a lecture.

It is difficult to feel secure in oneself, and therefore in one's environment, without a secure sense of body schema. For this, the proprioceptive system collaborates extensively with the closely associated tactile system. Together, they provide us with the critical sense of body awareness, or somatosensory awareness.

The tactile system is made up of the largest organ of our body, the skin. It is the system that provides us with the sense of touch for pleasure, pain, discrimination, and protection. Being that the tactile system is our exterior boundary, it is critical that it appropriately processes the wide variety of elements and touch sensations that surround us. If dysfunctional, pleasurable touch can be misinterpreted as noxious, or potentially dangerous sensations can go unregistered and can be damaging. It is a critical sense in the early stages of attachment and for nurturing throughout life. If a mother's gentle touch is perceived as painful or frightening by the baby and/or child, the bond will be challenged, and typical, maternal efforts to calm and nurture may only make matters worse.

Each of these systems must function properly and collaboratively in order to support appropriate sensory integration. A typical sensory system processes a wide variety and range of intensity of information and makes the necessary filtrations in order for a person to function comfortably and without conscious effort. However, with many children with autism spectrum disorders, we find that one or more of these systems does not function properly. Any of the sensory systems can be hyper-responsive (sensory avoiding) or hypo-responsive (sensory seeking) to incoming information.

This can be easily demonstrated with an example of the tactile system. A hyper-responsive tactile system (sensory avoiding) is generally associated with a high level of arousal. This child is typically always in varying states of fight or flight and is therefore less available for engagement and learning. She may avoid messy play and unfamiliar textures at all cost; she may hold objects in her fingertips, avoiding contact with palms; or, she may need to remove tags from shirts and only wear soft old clothes. In fear of the unpredictable touch, she may avoid standing close to her peers in school or at the playground, may avoid interactions all together, and may resist cuddling and affection even from parents and family members. Her tactile issues may also result in poor body awareness, stiff movement patterns, delayed motor planning, and difficulty with fine motor skills. This girl may tend to be inflexible emotionally and rigid in her play, routines, and ways in an effort to attempt to compensate and control a world that she perceives as threatening and out of control.

A hypo-responsive tactile system (sensory seeking) is generally associated with a low level of arousal. This child may typically appear "tuned out" and is therefore also less available. In order to obtain input to raise his arousal level, he may gravitate to messy and unfamiliar textures in an effort to better process his body and the things around him, may not seem to notice or mind when socks or clothing are twisted in uncomfortable ways or when sticky food is on his hands or face, may frequently bump into others or play excessively rough without ill intentions, and may present with poor body awareness and poorly graded, ballistic movement patterns, delayed motor planning, and difficulty with fine motor skills. This boy may tend to be disorganized in his ways, as he has difficulty accurately making sense of his body and thus making sense of his world.

The cases presented about the tactile system above can be applied to all five major sensory systems with different, but equally challenging, issues posed by hyper- and hypo-responsiveness of each.

Sensory issues can often be mistaken for behavioral problems. If a child has vestibular and proprioceptive issues, he may have great difficulty sitting in a chair without squirming and falling from time to time. He may fidget or get out of his seat often in order to provide himself with alerting input better process his body. He in turn, will present as a child who "won't" stay seated. Another child with severe tactile defensiveness may be terrified to stand in line next to his peers due to the fear of being touched. To protect himself, he stands away from the group with his back against the wall or casually wanders out of reach. He, again, will present like a child who "won't" stay in line. With children with sensory integration dysfunction, it is important to remember that these behaviors may be nothing more than effective coping mechanisms. When the underlying sensory issues are addressed, the behavior may disappear all together.

What Is Sensory Integration Therapy?

Sensory integration is a complex treatment approach. A breakdown of a few of the basic principles can help to provide a general understanding. We as humans need a wide variety of sensory and motor experiences to develop and sustain typical nervous system function, much like plants need a full spectrum of light to grow and flower to full potential. We respond strongly to sensory information. Consider the devastating effects of prolonged sensory deprivation. Consider the positive effects of gently rocking a baby or tightly hugging a friend in need. Within the range of typically functioning systems, we find some variance. One "typical" adult make it a point to try to ride roller coasters at the local amusement park every Saturday afternoon. Another may gasp at the sight of one. With a little encouragement, perhaps, she hops on and keeps her eyes closed. These two people are quite different, yet fall within a range where they experience a variety of rich sensory movement experiences. Children with ASD sometimes present with a much greater range. For whatever reason, their nervous systems are wired differently.

Children inherently attempt to provide themselves with what they need and avoid what they are frightened of. They constantly listen to their bodies and try to regulate themselves. By listening to what a child's body is telling us, we can help them to make a great deal of positive change. A therapist can provide them with calculated input that is stronger and more effective in reaching the threshold of the system the child is trying to stimulate. In turn, the child may begin to process the input more appropriately and therefore need less of it over time, demonstrating fewer sensory seeking or self-stimulatory behaviors. Children demonstrate self-stimulating behaviors for a reason. It is our responsibility to determine why and to address the root of the issue.

Children who avoid sensory input face another challenge. They develop compensatory strategies to protect themselves and seldom subject themselves to the sensory information. Therapists utilize various strategies to help desensitize these children. This should never be done solely through repeated exposure of the noxious experience. It often involves looking carefully at the stimuli and the relationships of the supporting sensory systems. Clinicians can then systematically address all the systems involved in order to support sensory integration. For example, a defensive tactile system may better process information following deep pressure touch and organizing input to the proprioceptive system. A defensive vestibular system may better process movement following appropriate input to the auditory or proprioceptive system.

Consider This Example:

One young girl may spin around for hours and never appear to get dizzy. Another young boy may fearfully cling to his mother when she tries to put him in a bucket swing at the park, or even just picks him up. These ranges pose a problem. The first child appears hypo-responsive (sensory seeking) and unable to provide herself with strong enough movement input to satiate her vestibular system. This compels her to spin, climb, run, jump, and crash. After all, if you were hungry, wouldn't you eat something? The second child, on the other hand, appears hyper-responsive (sensory avoiding) and avoids movement at all cost. If you were scared of spiders, would you sit next to a tarantula? This particular sensory dysfunction leaves the child in a heightened sense of arousal and typically in some degree of fight or flight. His vestibular system, however, still requires and craves input despite his interpreted fear. So he may compensate for his inability to tolerate dynamic movement activities and in turn provide himself with continual, "safe" doses of movement that he is comfortable with. He may appear to be in constant motion. This may present as steady pacing, walking around the perimeter of rooms, rocking, spinning, etc. Almost instinctually, some children quickly discover that by looking out of the far corners of their eyes, by looking at spinning objects, or by closely looking along linear edges, they can provide themselves with a vestibular-like experience, or even disorientation, through the visual system.

These two children are significantly impacted by this relatively simple sensory dysfunction and have developed effective coping mechanisms. However, the vestibular system works closely together with other systems to support many functions, so the ramifications may increase and broaden over time if left unaddressed. Both of these children are less available for engagement and learning.

The first child can only provide herself with so much dynamic movement input due to human limitation. A trained therapist, on the other hand, can make informed clinical decisions after assessment and assist the child in obtaining calculated vestibular experiences in all planes of movement, providing strong and organizing input to every receptor of the vestibular system. By actively propelling herself through space on a variety of pieces of equipment and swings, her vestibular system will receive powerful stimulation while her core and proprioceptive system are activated, further anchoring the movement to her body and promoting regulation. This may be followed with additional resistive activities that further activate her core muscles to provide additional grounding and organizing information. The movements can help her vestibular system to reach its threshold, perhaps for the first time, thus facilitating regulation and organization. Vestibular input can having lasting impacts up to six hours or more, resulting in a substantial period of time to follow in which she may seek less movement and therefore be more available to the world around her. With steady sources of input through treatment and a sensory diet, these windows of time will allow her to be more consistently regulated, engaged, and set up for learning and skill development. Due to the plasticity of her nervous system, she will likely need less input over time. As her system becomes more integrated, the regulation, engagement, and skills that she develops will provide her with a new foundation to continually build upon.

Based on the presentation of the second child, there is likely to be involvement of the tactile and proprioceptive systems. In order for a child to appropriately process vestibular input and feel comfortable in space, the proprioceptive and tactile systems need to function properly. Dysfunction in one of these two systems, as described earlier, typically results in decreased body awareness, which can result in a fear of moving through space. If this child does not perceive his body properly when seated or walking, he most certainly will not feel safe when placed in a swing and pushed three feet off of the ground. A trained therapist will identify these patterns and recognize the need to address his tactile and proprioceptive systems, despite the fact that the initial red flag went off when his mom reported an issue that appear to be related solely to his vestibular system. All involved systems will be addressed in treatment.

Specific brushing/deep pressure strategies and resistive activities that provide him with powerful doses of feedback from his body and help connect him to the support surface can be very effective in improving body awareness. Children need to feel connected to the ground before they can feel free in space. Core muscle activation can improve alignment and postural control and help lay the foundation for the introduction of new, controlled movement experiences. A careful sequence of movement may now be explored, paired with continued body awareness work. All activities are paired with his passions and interests, enabling motivated play, exploration, and regulation that he can take ownership of. He ideally gains a level of mastery of his body and movement through space, and begins to freely explore on his own. The previously timid, fearful child can now become a confident explorer.

This example provides a little insight into the sensory integration treatment approach. The examples provided outline approaches to particular sensory dysfunctions. The same principles can be applied to the multitude of issues involving all of the sensory systems that children present with today. Sensory integrative treatment can effectively help to change a child's "wiring." It is the clinician's goal to provide children with the tools necessary to create their own ideas and develop more naturally and spontaneously in a world that they can make sense of and feel safe in.

71

THE DAVIS MODEL OF SOUND INTERVENTION^{SM}

By Dorinne Davis

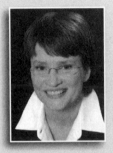

Dorinne Davis, MA, CCC-A, FAAA, RCTC, BARA

The Davis Center
19 State Rt 10 E., Ste 25
Succasunna, NJ 07876
862-251-4637
info@thedaviscenter.com
www.thedaviscenter.com
www.dorinnedavis.com

Ms. Davis is President/Founder of The Davis Center, the world's premier sound therapy center in Succasunna, NJ. She is author of 5 books including her 2012 award winning book, *The Cycle of Sound: A Missing Energetic Link,* the primer on sound-based therapy, "Sound Bodies through Sound Therapy" and "Every Day A Miracle: Success Stories through Sound Therapy". She established "The Davis Addendum to the Tomatis Effect" and designed *The Tree of Sound Enhancement Therapy®* and *The Diagnostic Evaluation for Therapy Protocol (DETP®).* She has introduced a previously unknown subtle energy system called *The Voice-Ear-Brain Connection.* Her 2 radio shows called *Sound Effects with Dorinne Davis*: weekly on cbs radio at www.newskyradio.com and monthly on www.AutismOne.org have a large following. She has a patent pending on her Ototoner^{SM} device and she is recognized as a pioneer in advancing the concepts of sound-based therapies.

The Davis Model of Sound Intervention^{SM} is a new process that developed from years of evaluating how the many different sound-based therapies support change for people by using the vibrational energy of sound. Some readers may assume that sound only involves a hearing sensory process. Other readers may assume that sound is only music. Most people don't immediately think of sound as energy. Within the field of energy medicine, sound is vibration or the frequency of specific energetic movements at the person's core—meaning at their atomic, quantum or cellular level. We each resonate at our own frequencies and as such, The Davis Model of Sound Intervention^{SM} works to tune-up or balance those frequencies thereby making the approach an holistic approach for change. Each autistic child, or any person whose frequency energies are off-balance, can be supported towards self-healing with issues associated with learning, development and wellness by using specific individualized protocols of sound-based therapies.

Sound-based therapies are defined as using the vibrational energy of sound to make change with learning, development and wellness challenges through the use of special equipment, specific programs, modified music, and/or specific tones/beats, the need for which is identified with testing. Many individual sound-based therapies have been demonstrated as helpful to autistic individuals and within The Davis Model of Sound Intervention ˢᵐ these therapies need to follow a specific order defined by the testing to make maximum change.

*The Davis Model of Sound Intervention*ˢᵐ utilizes the analogy of a tree, *The Tree of Sound Enhancement Therapy*®, for discussing how the many therapies make change for each person. Originally The Tree analogy was introduced with 4 parts. In 2012 a 6 part Tree analogy was introduced for more defined interpretation.[1] *The Seed* addresses one's core body rhythms. The *Root System* Therapies address the sense of hearing. *Trunk* Therapies address the ability to process all basic sound stimulation. The *Lower Leaves and Branches* Therapies address specific auditory processing issues. The *Upper Leaves and Branches* addresses communication and academic skills. The *Head* surrounding the Tree portion addresses general wellness with information and use of one's voice. All of the therapies use the vibrational energy of sound to make change for the specified processes.

The background for *The Tree of Sound Enhancement Therapy*®'s successful flow of therapy progression is inherent in the 3 key concepts of The Davis Model of Sound Intervention ˢᵐ: 1) There is a subtle energy system between the voice, the ear, and the brain supported by 5 laws known as The Tomatis Effect and The Davis Addendum to The Tomatis Effect., 2) Every cell in your body resonates sound, and 3) Your ear helps stimulate all of your senses by sound vibration, not just hearing.

The *Diagnostic Evaluation for Therapy Protocol (DETP*®) evaluates each person's responses for the various levels of the Tree analogy and determines if, when, how long, and in what order any or all of the many different sound-based therapies should be appropriately applied. This battery of tests is key for determining how to best use any sound-based therapy. Assuming that each person starts with *The Root System* therapy is incorrect. Not everyone needs every therapy. The test battery takes the guesswork out of determining if a sound-based therapy is appropriate and provides the order for the correct administration of a sequence of therapies. Currently the assessment can only be obtained at www.thedaviscenter.com, but there are plans on developing this assessment

---

1 For a visual understanding of this Tree analogy in 6 parts, visit http://www.thedaviscenter.com/the-tree-of-sound-enhancement-therapyreg.html

into an easier format so that others can begin to use this modified assessment and programming within the next 2 years.

Sound is powerful! Sound energy is all around you. While your ear supports hearing as a sensory response, sound in the form of energetic movement at the minutest vibrational frequency is more a response that your brain interprets and understands. Therefore, it is important to know how sound impacts your whole body, not just the symptoms demonstrated by the body.

Any sound-based therapy can make change! The Davis Model of Sound Intervention℠ introduces the various sound-based therapies from the needs of the whole body to make sure the changes happen energetically, not just eliminate them symptomatically.

As quantum physics took hold in the twentieth century, it became apparent that the world's and the body's energy interact with each other. Einstein's E=mc2 provided the foundation for considering the body as an energy system. The fields of our body energy system could be manipulated, thereby balancing our internal and external cellular, atomic, and most likely quark movement vibrational patterns. Within the context of energy medicine, when a disturbance is created in the body's energy field, whether internal or external to the body, the disturbance is felt throughout the body. For most, this disturbance is so minute that the impact is not consciously felt in the body, but the brain would be able to interpret this disturbance. The cells interpret the disturbances from the brain and begin a self-correcting or self-healing process in the body. Our bodies are constantly working at this balancing process. And energy medicine techniques attempt to change the person by changing and balancing their cellular energy. Sound-based therapies attempt to change the person by changing their frequencies or sound energy.

The DETP® becomes the important tool for determining if, when, how long and in what order any or all of the many different sound-based therapies should be appropriately applied. For it may not be 'the specific method' or 'program' that makes the most significant change; rather it should be the order of the correct supportive methods or programs that will make the most foundational, long-lasting change. Because sound-based therapies begin to make change from the internal core of each person, an overall self-healing process is started from the inside outward.

The Tree of Sound Enhancement Therapy®introduces the various therapies as follows:

1.   The *Seed* therapies all make a change with body rhythmical patterns. Our body has many rhythms and patterns such as our heart rate and breath stream. Currently two therapies exist at this level: REI® and Cymatherapy®.

     a.   REI was developed by Jeff Strong and uses rhythmical drum patterns to stimulate and repair the nervous system. A pair of custom made CD's are created and used for a 10 week period.

Symptoms helped: inability to 'fit in' with the rhythms of those around them, significant sensory processing issues, self-stimulatory behaviors, attention span, sleep, aggression and more.

Testimonials from parents of autistic children:

1. My child fell asleep faster and more calmly.
2. My child became less aggressive.
3. My child became less impulsive.
4. My child attended better with the music on.

www.reiinstitute.com

b. Cymatherapy represents the work of Dr. Guy Peter Manners who explored sound as a healing modality. This approach uses sound frequency stimulation on different parts of the body working to balance the body's energy patterns. The current devices are called the AMI1000® and AMI750®.

Symptoms helped: issues with attention, behavior, social connections, cognition and much more.

Testimonials from parents of autistic children:

1. My child waited and listened for instructions.
2. My child waited his turn better.
3. My child wanted to be around his family more.
4. My child wanted to listen to his sounds every day.

www.cymatechnologies.com

2. The *Root System* therapies are called "Auditory Integration Training". The originator of this type of therapy is Dr. Guy Berard, a French physician, who wanted to establish a program that would create a kind of physical therapy for the ear, which has been demonstrated with this author's research on the acoustic reflex muscle of the middle ear. His method is now known as Berard Auditory Integration Training. The equipment used in his method is either an Audiokinetron or an Earducator®. His method can only be applied in a practitioner's office. There are other applications within the generalized term "Auditory Integration Training" that can be used at home. The available equipment applicable for home programs are FST and DAA, which do a similar type of physical retraining of the acoustic reflex muscle. Each of these programs is modeled after Dr. Berard's work. All "Auditory Integration Training" programs address the person's 'sense of hearing'. The programs last for 10 days and the person listens for ½ hour in the morning and afternoon to specially chosen music played through the appropriate device. While listening, little or no sensory stimulation should occur because it is possible to negate the positive effects of retraining the acoustic reflex muscle.

Symptoms helped: one type of hearing hypersensitivity, lack of sound awareness, inability to discriminate sound differences, sense of self, body movement/rhythm, eye contact, awareness of the world around them, motor skills and more.

Testimonials from parents of autistic children:

a. My child no longer covers his ears in uncomfortable listening situations.

b. My child no longer reacts to fluorescent lighting.

c. My child responds immediately when his name is called.

d. My child spoke his first word on day 2.

e. My child participated in an assembly program and loved it.

www.berardaitwebsite.com and www.AITinstitute.org

3 The *Trunk* therapies are called "Listening Training Programs" and are modeled after the work of Dr. Alfred Tomatis, the founder of all sound-based therapies. The therapies at this level are 'core' therapies because they incorporate one of the main points behind The Davis Model of Sound Intervention—the connection between the voice, the ear and the brain. Dr. Tomatis was the first to discover that the voice produces what the ear hears and when the distorted frequencies are reintroduced to the ear, the voice regains coherence or stability. This became known as The Tomatis Effect and he incorporated this process into The Tomatis® Method. He differentiated between hearing and listening. Hearing is the passive reception of sound and we hear without thinking about it. But listening involves mentally thinking about what is heard. We must tune into what is heard. By doing so, we cortically 'recharge' the brain. When recharging the brain, the body's full response to sound must be stimulated. Every cell of the body must be stimulated. Every sense will be stimulated. Every way that the body responds to sound must be stimulated. Listening Training Programs must include air conduction vibration of sound, bone conduction vibration of sound, filtered and gated music, specific sound delays, and actively incorporating one's speaking and/or singing voice in the programming. All programs must be individualized at this level of The Tree, not generic.

The programs are brain intensive, meaning that the program lasts for many days in order to make sufficient change at the cortical level. Practitioners should incorporate activities that address the person's whole body response to sound, not just one type of skill such as academics or sensory integration as the full ability to balance the person's skills will not be met. Basic programs last for 60 hours, often applied with a break after 30 hours. Listening occurs for 2 hours per day for 15 days, then a 3-6 week break, followed by another 15 days of 2 hours per day. Some centers administer the second set in 8 and 7 days with another break in between. For people with autism, this basic program is typically not enough stimulation to establish sufficient skills for communication, so additional sessions are encouraged depending upon each person's needs. Follow up sessions should be determined by a proprietary Listening Test which shows the levels of progress. Each person's voice should begin to show a change in its tonal quality as progress occurs.

a.   The Tomatis Method® was established by Dr. Alfred Tomatis. He felt that a good listener was a good learner and by training a person to listen well provided them to opportunity to reach their full potential. He identified the benefit of a dominant right ear, supporting the most direct pathway to the language center in the brain. His method supports learning how to filter out irrelevant information and supports capturing the energizing frequencies of the speech sound spectrum. He uses all of the connections between the voice, the ear and the brain by stimulating the weaker body processes in order to advance overall skill levels resulting in improved listening and enhancement of body sensory needs and communication needs.

Symptoms helped: some hypersensitivities to sound, hyposensitivity to sound, sensory processing issues, oral motor issues, social/emotional connectedness, expressive/receptive language skills, sense of self, inappropriate behaviors, fluency of speech, vestibular imbalances, movement and rhythm, fine/gross motor skills, posture and more.

Testimonials from parents of autistic children:

1.   Within two years following The Tomatis Method, my child was declassified.
2.   My child began eating different foods and trying different textures of food.
3.   My child's high pitched voice disappeared.
4   My child's reading skills jumped 3 years growth in 6 months time.
5.   My child began using full sentences to express his thoughts.
6.   My child's anxiety to large groups practically disappeared.
7.   My child began to develop self-awareness and eventually self-confidence.
www.tomatis.com

b.   EnListen® was developed by Drs. Billie and Kirk Thompson and modeled from the concepts established by Dr. Tomatis. Their proprietary software program provides stimulation with air conduction, bone conduction, sound delays and filters, and active voice work for developing targeted learning skills and fit all the requirements for a Listening Training Program. This process stimulates growth of new and underutilized neural pathways.

Symptoms helped: weak receptive/expressive language skills, weak motor skills, poor communication skills, sense of self, poor social skills, disorganization, poor reading skills, singing abilities, phonics skills and more.

Testimonials from parents of autistic children:

1. My child began trying to connect socially with other children around him.
2. My child began combining 3-4 words in utterances.
3. My child no longer craved spinning.
4. My child began tasting new and different foods.
5. I was able to leave my child playing independently for up to ½ hour at a time.
6. My child's stammer disappeared.
7. My child's reading scores increased 3 grade levels in 1 year.

www.enlisten.com

3a. Some sound-based therapies are modeled after the work of Dr. Tomatis but do not include ALL of the requirements for a Listening Training Program at The *Trunk* level of *The Tree*. However, they can be inserted at the Upper Trunk/Lower Leaves and Branches of The Tree analogy because they offer more higher functioning changes. Some of these programs are:

a. The Listening Program® was developed by Advanced Brain Technologies as a music-based sound stimulation program designed to enhance listening skills and remediate auditory perceptual skills. The basic program included 8 CD's that incorporated music and nature sounds to create a balance of exercises for the middle ear muscles. A filtration system and a gating technique is also utilized supporting a full spectrum of sound frequencies. These CD's are listened to for ½ hour per day, 5 days per week for 8 weeks typically. Extended sessions are sometimes needed and the program has different levels now. A bone conduction segment has been added with practitioner supervision. The concept is for the brain to receive, process, store and retrieve the information from a person's surrounding sound environment.

Symptoms helped: learning challenges, attention/focus weaknesses, reading challenges, sense of self, communication weaknesses, sensory processing issues, self-regulation and more.

Testimonials from parents of autistic children:

1. My child began to have an interest in socially interacting with his peers.
2. My child began drawing clearly and writing legibly.
3. My child began to verbally label his drawings.

www.advancedbrain.com

b. The Samonas™ method was developed by Ingo Steinbach. SAMONAS stands for "spectrally activated music of optimum natural structure". By using his SONAS system, he was able to create a system for recording music where the therapeutic value of the music and the effectiveness of the musical recording could be maintained. This new system could only be produced on compact discs. He created CD's that emphasized high frequency listening, presented the sensation of being in the location of the music, created a calming effect on the body, while monitoring the overtone effects of most musical selections. The concept is to experience the energizing effects of sound through the expression of the overtones within the music. The Samonas CD's are generic in nature and no specific 'therapy' regimen is currently established for any one type of challenge.

Symptoms helped: vitality, stress, limited concentration, vestibular imbalances, lack of creativity and more.

Testimonials from parents of autistic children:

1. My child immediately began to notice everything going on around him.
2. My child could focus on an activity for a longer period of time.
3. My child decreased his need to spin constantly.

www.samonas.com

4. The *Lower Leaves and Branches* of *The Tree of Sound Enhancement Therapy*® reflect auditory processing skills like memory, discrimination and sequencing skills. These skills are higher functioning skills than basic sound awareness and utilization. These are skills inherent for our understanding of the communication process, including reading. However, these skills need the support of the more foundational skills established in *The Root System, The Seed,* and *The Trunk* of *The Tree* analogy in order for the reception, expression and interpretation of these skills to be well embedded for each person. Without the foundational skills well established, these skills simply become 'splinter skills' and testing can show that these skills have improved; but skill testing doesn't show how the body is fully integrating the skills. The Davis Model of Sound Intervention® encourages the full integration of all skills to maximize learning and developmental changes. A few of these therapies are:

a. Fast ForWord® is a series of programs that use an interactive computer training system to retrain language, reading and learning skills. The initial program targeted receptive language skills and retrained the skill of temporal sequencing—a skill necessary for auditory discrimination, auditory figure ground, and auditory sequential memory. By retraining how the brain comprehends and uses speech information, the person is better able to distinguish the many different components of speech sounds. The basic program still retrains temporal sequencing although the Fast ForWord series of programs now heavily emphasizes skills for reading. The basic program averages between 6 to 8 weeks for approximately 1 to 2 hours per day, a year license is required. Advancement to other programs that support reading and comprehension is very easy and helps overall development throughout the year license.

Symptoms helped: listening comprehension, phonological awareness, specific language structures, oral language skills, and more.

Testimonials from parents of autistic children:

1.   My child wants to listen on the telephone now to his grandparents.
2.   My child is able to go shopping with me at the mall now without covering his ears.
3.   My child is understanding more of what is being said to him.

www.scilearn.com

b.   Interactive Metronome® was developed by James Cassily who thought that learning, cognition and social skills were influenced by the ability to plan and sequence motoric actions. These actions are processed through the sensation of vibration through the ear and are therefore at this level of *The Tree* analogy. Mr. Cassily's theory was that man's intelligence is connected with the ability to process rapid movements and developed a computer-based interactive version of the musical metronome. The purpose of the program is to develop precise control over basic mental functions through the use of body movements. Interactive Metronome® is a technology-based therapy program that promotes change with motor planning and sequencing. The average program is composed of 15 one-hour sessions over a period of 3-5 weeks.

Symptoms helped: attention, motor control, reading, language processing, regulation of behavior and more.

Testimonials from parents of autistic children:

1.   My child began to talk more and became more engaged with those she was communicating with.
2.   My child's sleeping patterns improved.
3.   My child became less tactilely defensive.

www.interactivemetronome.com

5.   The *Head* surrounding *The Tree of Sound Enhancement Therapy* brings the connection between the voice, the ear and the brain full circle and demonstrates the laws within *The Davis Addendum™ to the Tomatis Effect* as making an important contribution to the full effect of how sound-based therapies make change in learning, development and wellness. Whereas The Tomatis Effect suggests that the voice produces what the ear hears, The Davis Addendum to the Tomatis Effect suggests that the ear also emits (yes, the ear gives out a sound) the same stressed frequencies as the voice and once the imbalanced frequencies are returned to the ear, the voice regains stability or coherence. *The Head* then represents the wellness piece of how sound impacts the entire body. The Voice is the

key component for *The Head*. There are two ways that the voice supports change at this portion of *The Tree*.

First, the science of BioAcoustics™ is used to help identify how well the body is able to support the changes possible with the other portions of *The Tree* analogy. For some people, this must be the starting place to begin a sound-based therapy protocol; for others BioAcoustics is the last piece of the protocol because the individualized tonal frequencies are established to help maintain and enhance the learning and developmental changes obtained with the other programs. Human BioAcoustics was developed by Sharry Edwards and after many years of research, the idea of vocal profiling has supported the idea that the body is a mathematical matrix of predictable frequency relationships. Every cell is the body vibrates and emits its own sound frequency. These cellular frequencies must stay 'in tune' in order for the body to maintain its wellness. For the autistic person, this piece is often the key for determining if the other many different sound-based therapies will make a change and more importantly maintain any changes.

Second, use of each person's own voice with the technique called Ototoning, an ear toning technique that supplies the sound/tone that the body says it most needs to promote self-healing at that moment in time. In the near future, a device called the Ototoner^{sm} will provide the needed sound to vocalize. This technique is best used once the other parts of the protocol are accomplished.

Symptoms helped: anything related to the body and wellness

Testimonials from parents of autistic children:

1. My child's sound sensitivities decreased dramatically.
2. My child can maintain his focus so much better.
3. My doctor likes supporting my child's detoxing with BioAcoustics.
4. My child did not go on 'sensory overload' as easily.

www.soundhealthinc.com

Overview:

The Davis Model of Sound Intervention^{sm} incorporates all of the many different sound-based therapies only after appropriately using The Diagnostic Evaluation for Therapy Protocol (DETP®) to determine if the therapies are needed, and if so, in the correct order. There are many stories of people using one or another of the therapies with limited or no success, or losing the effects after a period of time. Some people do need more than one therapy and some may need 'tune ups' periodically if their body doesn't maintain the support well enough.

Any sound-based therapy can produce change but for some, the change may take place over an extended period of time as the body integrates the changes so that higher ordered skills can develop. To date, most research on these methods have measured skill changes but the responses of sound go further into the body at the cellular and brain level, and researchers are beginning to recognize this fact.

Can there be side-effects to this approach? Sound-based therapies can produce skill changes, but the main change goes more deeply to core body needs. Picture the peeling of an onion—each layer represents a layer of development. For some children, many layers need to be removed to get to the heart of their issues and these main issues need to be repatterned so that movement forward can occur. Some people consider this as regression but in reality this repatterning is movement forward—a positive change. It is important not to get 'stuck' at this lower functioning level, though, so for many, movement up *The Tree* is necessary to help the person move toward higher progressive levels.

The Davis Model of Sound Intervention[sm] offers an alternative approach for addressing the learning, developmental, and wellness challenges associated with autism from a holistic paradigm.

©Davis2013

VISION THERAPY

By Dr. Jeffrey Becker

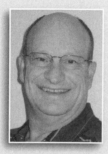

Jeffrey Becker, OD

NeuroSensory Center of Eastern Pennsylvania
250 Pierce Street, Suite 317
Kingston, Pennsylvania 18704
570-763-0054
Jbecker@Keystonensc.com
www.Keystonensc.com

Dr. Becker is a neurodevelopmental/behavioral optometrist with board certification and specialty training in neurosensory disorders. Dr. Becker is a Defeat Autism Now! (DAN!)–certified clinician. He is the director of Vision Rehabilitation Services for the Neurosensory Center of Eastern Pennsylvania. He has participated in multiple research projects involving neurologically impaired individuals. He has spoken about vision and learning at national and international autism conferences. He most recently published an article in *Autism File,* titled "Vision Therapy Can Help Children with Spectrum Disorders." Dr. Becker is also an adjunct faculty member of Misercordia University, Dallas, Pennsylvania, where he teaches vision rehabilitation courses to master's-level occupational and physical therapy students. In more than twenty-seven years of clinical and research experience, Dr. Becker has examined and treated over 3,000 patients who are neurologically impaired with neurosensory disorders.

"Vision" refers to how the visual system coordinates function between the two eyes and the brain. (Cohen, et al., 1988) We ask questions like: Do both eyes perceive the same image at the same time? Do both eyes move in unison? Do both eyes have equal focusing power? Do both eyes fulfill all these visual requirements easily, fluidly, and for an extended length of time? If the answer to any of these questions is no, then vision therapy may be indicated. Vision therapy is done in a sequential manner that mirrors normal developmental processes. This allows the child to most readily relearn the visual skills that were lost, or to learn those that were never developed. It is therefore necessary to start with very easy tasks and work toward more difficult tasks. The Piagetian approach to development indicates that this is the best way to remediate vision-related problems.

The therapy has been used by optometrists for years in the general population in those who have visual functioning disorders, and now it can be adapted to autistic spectrum disorder (ASD) individuals by developmental/behavioral optometrists

(Trachman et al., 2008). It is important that these clinicians have specific training with these disorders through DAN! and other agencies, such as Autism Research Institute (ARI).

Fifty-three percent of children who are poor readers have some form of visual functioning disorder, and it has been estimated that up to 80 percent of children with special needs have significant visual functioning disorders that affect the learning and developmental process (Cohen, et al., 1988).

Success is based on visual, subjective, and functional findings. Success rates vary depending on the initial functional loss. Studies indicate that success rates range from 63 percent to as high as 89 percent. This depends on the frequency and number of sessions completed (Cohen, et al., 1988).

DG, an eight-year-old boy, sat in my examination chair after his mother had completed all the appropriate intake forms as recommended by the Defeat Autism Now! protocol. She tried to control her son as he attempted to touch the bright instruments in my examination room. The paperwork indicated that DG had been diagnosed with ASD at two years of age. He was in and out of different programs and, at one time, was labeled as dyslexic. The interview proceeded typically, but his mother was not quite sure why she was here with her son, even though an observant occupational therapist had suggested she make an appointment with me. She said, "I've had my son's eyes checked before every school year, and he has always had 20/20 vision." My comprehensive neurosensory examination, along with the functional and developmental vision examination, indicated that the other eye care specialists were correct. DG did have 20/20 visual acuity in both eyes. But they had apparently not assessed another aspect of vision, which is very important (Holmes, et al., 2008). DG had significant eye tracking and eye focusing problems, reduced convergence difficulty with depth perception, and vestibular inaccuracies.

At this point, I explained to DG's mother the difference between sight (acuity) and vision. Sight is the ability to see a certain size object at a certain distance. The standard means to assess acuity was conceived by Herman Snellen in 1862, and since that time we have referred to normal sight as 20/20. The top number indicates the distance of the observer from the acuity chart, and the bottom number is the size of the letter being viewed. All this really means is that a person can see a certain size letter at a certain distance. This terminology is, of course, important for many aspects of our lives. However, even more important to our children with ASD, like DG, is functional/behavioral vision. Deficits with their visual systems can be very disabling.

Children with ASD, like DG, appear more likely to have visual functioning disorders than the general population (Taub, 2007). When doing the intake form for DG, it was noted that he disliked doing any near point tasks. He preferred to run randomly around the room, picking up items along the way. He would briefly look at them and then put them down quickly when he saw another item to view, examining the new item for a very short period of time. This behavior was repeated consistently. His mother noted that she felt DG was very smart because he could easily memorize songs and verses. (My experience has been that ASD children are very smart but are unable to utilize their intelligence in the positive and productive manner that we all expect.) He would not engage in eye contact and would attend to objects out of the corner of his eyes. Instead of moving his eyes, he turned his head to see objects.

DG's evaluation, which took over two hours, indicated visual functional deficits that needed to be remediated in order for DG to be able to function visually in the world. This two-hour evaluation included tests with the Sensory View diagnostic system (NeuroSensory Centers of America, 2009). This system assists in the evaluation of myelin health, eye movements, balance, proprioception, and dynamic visual acuity. After these tests are done, an additional evaluation is done to assess depth perception, visual suppressions, visual focusing, ocular health, and the ability of the eyes to work together. These tests, which are done by an eye care specialist trained in these procedures, need to be done without the use of the phoroptor, an instrument normally utilized in routine eye examinations.

Vision therapy can be done in an office by a trained therapist, in an outpatient rehabilitation center, or at home. Vision rehabilitation to correct most oculomotor, eye focusing, and eye deviation deficits typically continues for six to eight months when done two or three times per week. Treatment also requires home participation for thirty to forty-five minutes per day for five days per week on an outpatient basis. This does not mean that the rehabilitation cannot be concluded earlier (or later) than this prescribed time. Program length is dependent on the child's participation level and attendance.

Due to DG's particular needs, I began his therapy program in my office. The eye movement exercises I prescribed consisted of computer-based therapy, as well as hand-held therapy techniques. Both techniques have the same end result, but I have found that the computer techniques seem to work more quickly, and the results are more consistent in nature than those using the handheld therapies. The disadvantage of the computer therapies is that many children with ASD have difficulties sitting at the computer for any length of time, thus making the sessions more frustrating for them. Therefore, we incorporated both therapy techniques into DG's treatment program.

The computer programs we have had success with come from a company in Gold Canyon, Arizona (HTS, 2009). The programs can be tailored for each child and his or her skill level. We can incorporate therapies for all visual deficits, including gross motor, fine motor, vestibular, and focusing issues, into this program. The computer programs allow easy progression for each child and can be modified when a child has difficulty with certain tasks. I review progress at least two times per month but usually more frequently, making sure that the child is meeting the proper goals.

Case Example

DG's mother was completely amazed at her son's progress. His eye contact improved, his visual stimming significantly decreased, and his school performance accelerated. His teachers wanted to know what his mother had done to get him this far. He was a

---

WHAT IS VISUAL STIMMING?

Many parents ask, "Why does my child do this?"

There are many theories about the function of visual stimming and peripheral viewing, and the reasons for its increased incidence in those on the autism spectrum. The biomedical approach states that visual stimming can be a result of yeast over growth. For hyposensitive people, it may provide needed nervous system arousal, releasing beta-endorphins. For hypersensitive people, it may provide a "norming" effect, allowing the person to control a specific sense, and is thus a soothing behavior. Visual stimming can be demonstrated as flapping hands, blinking and/or moving fingers in front of eyes, and staring repetitively at a light (http://autism.wikia.com/wiki/Stimming).

Besides yeast overgrowth, there are many other reasons why visual stimming and peripheral viewing occur. If a person has visual misalignment, then visual stimming can be the product of this visual condition, and the person feels better by performing this activity. Another reason is that these individuals have either an intermittent and/or alternating visual suppression. The brain only sees images out of alternating eyes and the person then visually stims, trying to understand and/or perceive images out of the other eye. When a child visually stims under stress or under new environmental conditions, this should be considered a visual breakdown due to the stress of the new environment. Again, the brain is not simultaneously processing images from each eye.

Visual stimming first needs to be evaluated by a qualified doctor who understands these conditions. The best form of treatment is visual therapy procedures to correct this disorder and sometimes, specialized prisms may be used with the therapy and with other therapies to improve the ability of the eyes to work together. My experience has been that in most cases, the therapy works better than using prisms alone, although many times, using both systems of treatment jointly may be indicated.

more pleasant child, according to what others told DG's mother. Most importantly, DG now knows that he can do these tasks and has improved self-esteem.

Once the in-office rehabilitation program is completed, a reduction in rehabilitation time is given to the child, and a phase-out program is begun for several months. This is done to monitor and maintain all visual skills that are learned and to make sure the child has adapted adequately to the new visual functioning environment.

As a final step, DG was given a home maintenance program to follow and is checked every three months in the office to confirm that he has not regressed. The home maintenance program can be a computer-based program (HTS) or the procedures that are outlined in the next section. It is very important to do this program with the understanding that these visual skills have been learned and can easily be unlearned, if not reinforced on a routine basis at home (Becker et al., 2009).

Checklist for possible developmental visual deficits related to ASD. If you can answer yes to two or more of these signs, your child should engage in a complete neurosensory and developmental vision evaluation:

1. Child likes to look out of the corners if his/her eyes when doing either near point or distance viewing.
2. Child only does near tasks for short periods of time, then goes back to task after a few short minutes.
3. Child turns head to the left or right to view distant or near objects.
4. Child bends head to either shoulder when viewing distant or near objects.
5. Child covers or closes an eye when looking at near point tasks.
6. Child likes to visually stim with his hands in front of one eye or another.
7. Child moves closer and closer to near point tasks over a short period of time.
8. Child rubs eyes frequently.
9. Child's eyes tend to water when doing near point tasks.
10. Child likes to turn head up or down and moves head in strange positions to do near point tasks.

How to Find a Qualified Eye Care Specialist

To locate a neurodevelopmental optometrist in your area, log onto www.nora.cc (Neuro-Optometric Rehabilitation Association). When making an appointment, ask the following questions:

1. How frequently does the doctor examine children with autism spectrum disorders?
2. Does the doctor do functional vision testing, not just acuity testing?
3. Does the doctor prescribe vision therapy, and who carries out the therapy?

4. How long is the examination process with the doctor? (It should last at least sixty to ninety minutes to get a good understanding of the child's deficits.)
5. Will the doctor write and correspond with the school and/or other professionals?

Yoked Prisms and New iPad Vision Therapy Programs

Prisms are specially made lenses that shift targets to different parts of the visual system. Yoked prisms are used to alter a person's spatial awareness and to change the person's perception of his/her midline and can be used to alter both fine and gross motor control. They are used during therapy to help embed the visual learning process and have proven very successful with children who have ASD. Yoked prisms should only be used under the direction of a developmental/behavioral optometrist who is well versed in their use.

There are new iPad programs available directly through developmental/behavioral optometrists that can be individually customized for each patient. These programs are unique because they can be monitored by the prescribing doctor and changes can be made from the doctor's own iPad while the therapy is taking place. The newest Ocular Motor Therapy (OMT) for the iPad has games that develop skills for visual motor deficits, visual motor integration, visual tracking, visual pursuits, visual memory, visual scanning, visual fixations, visual stimming, 3-D perception, and fine and gross motor control.

Does the Vestibular System Influence the Visual System?

The vestibular system helps us understand the position of our head and body in space. It helps us with balance, spatial orientation, and maintaining a stable visual image while in motion.

The vestibular system teams up with the auditory and visual systems to perform many functions that involve moving, looking, and listening. Without reliable information coming in from the vestibular system, sights and sounds in the environment do not make sense.

All components of the Vestibular-Auditory-Visual Triad are needed to successfully function throughout life. Astronaut training activities can provide the sensory input needed to achieve optimal vestibular / visual input.

Astronaut therapy is now used in conjunction with vision therapy to give the patient improvements in gross motor and fine motor control

BELOW ARE SOME GUIDELINES FOR INCORPORATING VESTIBULAR THERAPY WITH VISION:

- Can be used at the beginning of treatment to jump start the system and optimize the therapeutic benefits of activities that follow.
- Activities should be functional and include proprioceptive activation to help regulate the system and integrate changes.
- Can be done with all ages
- Must receive solid support from a medical professional if the client has a history of seizures.
- All five vestibular receptors should be activated during each treatment session.
- Two times a day may increase tolerance and speed the process of integration
- Gradually increase input to the patient's tolerance level
- Gradually decrease frequency as gains are maintained
- Use the program as long as the client makes observable progress
- If there is regression after protocol is discontinued, return to the protocol for a boost
- Can be part of the client's maintenance program indefinitely

We have been using this program in conjunction with vision therapy and have seen more rapid improvements with our patients. Also, once the patients start using it, they feel very comfortable with the sensations.

AFTERWORD

By Teri Arranga

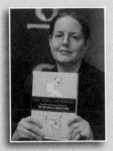

Teri Arranga

714-732-0704
tarranga@autismone.org
www.autismone.org

Teri Arranga is the executive director of AutismOne (www.autismone.org), the vice president of the Global Autism Collaboration (www.autism.org), and the secretary of Strategic Autism Initiative. She has served as the editor-in-chief of *Autism Science Digest* and as editor of the US/Canada edition of *Autism File* magazine. Teri is co-editor of the book *Bugs, Bowels, and Behavior: The Groundbreaking Story of the Gut-Brain Connection,* and she is editor of Dr. William Walsh's book *Nutrient Power* and Dr. Andrew Wakefield's books *Callous Disregard: Autism and Vaccines—The Truth Behind a Tragedy* and *Waging War on the Autistic Child: The Arizona 5 and the Legacy of Baron von Munchausen,* all of which were published by Skyhorse Publishing. Additionally, Teri has contributed to and provided editing for all annual editions of Skyhorse Publishing's *Cutting-Edge Therapies for Autism* series. Teri is the host of the radio program *Autism One: A Conversation of Hope* on the VoiceAmerica Health and Wellness Channel (www.health.voiceamerica.com), and she has been involved with a number of media projects.

Advances in Help Mean Advances in Hope

We have been trying to catch a bouncing ball. For children born in the late 20th century, the larger subset of children with autism had regressive autism—with evidence of normal development followed by a regression in the developmental trajectory—having been exposed to certain patterns of toxic or pathological insult. Objective laboratory and other diagnostic testing corresponding with clinical presentation give credence to this. In time, the pattern of external toxic insult changed. Additionally, more subtle factors also came to the fore, with food adulteration now being said to set up a trigger to loss of gut integrity and, therefore, a susceptibility to autism. Whatever the poison, pathogen, pesticide, or mechanism—as the gut goes, so goes the body—especially during a critical neurodevelopmental window like early childhood. The systems of the body do not exist in a vacuum. We are not disembodied heads. Gut pathology causes adverse consequences in the immune system that cause negative effects in the nervous system—like autism.

The evolving onslaughts of impurities, sometimes combined with an individual's own genetic profile, may be why we see different phenotypic presentations of autism. A note on "an individual's own genetic profile": With regard to younger children, they are dealing with the toxic soup to which their parents, grandparents, and great-grand-parents were exposed. There are contaminants that have genotoxic potential. So, I don't blame genetics. I don't blame the parents. I want to know what was in the environment that hurt people, whether with direct, dramatic, and relatively swift deleterious effects to the individual or by causing aberrant gene expression or by familial genotoxicity.

There are excellent researchers who have figured out aspects of autism causa-tion in subsets of individuals. Most hopeful is that there are excellent researchers and clinicians who are providing practical help to individuals who are already affected. I am fortunate to be writing this afterword close on the heels of the publication of a landmark paper by Drs. Bradstreet, Pacini, and Ruggiero. The study titled "A new methodology of viewing extra-axial fluid and cortical abnormalities in children with autism via transcranial ultrasonography" can be found in *Frontiers in Human Neurosci-ence*. This discovery is a milestone. Scientists now have a real-time window into the brain, which, to my mind, has profound implications for prediction, prevention, and remediation.

Another window into the mind, also in the toolbox of Dr. James Jeffrey Brad-street, is magnetic resonant therapy (MRT). A pre-treatment electroencephalogram (EEG) allows the MRT technician to provide individualized therapy to a client's brain-waves. Improvement can be seen in a follow-up EEG. The most exciting thing about this is that, once the brainwaves are remediated, rehabilitation—learning of deficit skill sets—can occur. Pioneers in this field in addition to Dr. Bradstreet include Dr. Yi Jin and Dr. Manuel Casanova.

Another recent pair of advances that I would signal as exciting, also brought to the fore by the team of Ruggiero, Pacini, and Bradstreet, concerns GcMAF (Gc macro-phage activating factor) and a related intervention called GOleic (a supplement: oleic acid stabilized by its physiological binding protein).

For more information on TUS, MRT, and GcMAF, please see Dr. Bradstreet's chapters and foreword in this book.

As of November 2013, the CD Autism protocol developed by Kerri Rivera, which includes a parasite protocol by Dr. Andreas Kalcker, has spread to more than 5000 fam-ilies in 57 countries. Upon review of quarterly ATEC scores submitted by the parents of 163 children (ages 2-17) who had been on the protocol for over one year, over 94% had shown a reduction in their ATEC scores, and, using this measure, over 100 have recovered. (Please see Kerri Rivera's chapter.)

Finally, states' laws are now opening up to the use of medical cannabis. There are cannabinoid receptors in many parts and systems of the body. (Please see the chapter by Nathan Coombs in this book.) Many people have talked about the use of medical cannabis for some mechanisms (e.g., inflammation) and conditions "comorbid" to autism, including, importantly, seizures. In the case of epilepsy, always obtain appropriate professional medical advice. And always follow the laws where you are, and obtain necessary authorization before undertaking use of medical cannabis.

Information about all of the interventions just mentioned, as well as many others in this book, will be presented at the AutismOne 2014 Conference, which is held annually in May (www.autismone.org). There are other worthwhile therapies too numerous to be contained in this afterword. For example, Homeopathy Center of Houston reports more than 100 recoveries (see Griffin/Lanham chapter in this book).

When beginning or changing any biological therapy, please consult with a qualified healthcare provider.

The autism epidemic was not caused by genetics, and autism is not a hopeless, hard-wired, genetic, psychological condition. Preconception, prenatal, and postnatal purity and nutrition can all help stave off an autism diagnosis. If an autism diagnosis does occur, then there are brilliant and sincere people working hard every day to turn the tide for your child, your family, and the children of the world.

"Thank you" to Tony Lyons, Joseph Sverchek, Ken Siri, and the team at Skyhorse Publishing for another courageous venture into the world of autism information. And "thank you" to the reader—your digging for the truth shows that there is hope for your child, just as so many other children have improved dramatically or recovered from the diagnostic label of autism. Take joy in your child.

AUTISM ORGANIZATIONS

NATIONAL

ACT Today!
Autism Care & Treatment Today!
19019 Ventura Blvd. Suite 200
Tarzana, CA 91356
818-705-1625
Info@act-today.org

ACT Today! is a nonprofit organization whose mission is to provide funding and support to families that cannot afford the treatments their autistic children need to achieve their full potential.

Advancing Futures for Adults with Autism (AFAA)
917-475-5059
AFAA@autismspeaks.org
www.afaa-us.org

AFAA was created to inform adolescents and adults with autism about living options and new developments, and promote active community involvement from adults with autism.

Global Autism Collaboration
4182 Adams Avenue
San Diego, CA 92116
619-281-7165
www.autismwebsite.com/gac

The Global Autism Collaboration brings together the most experienced autism advocacy organizations in an effort dedicated to advancing autism research in the interest of all individuals living with autism today and their families.

The Autism Hope Alliance
752 Tamiami Trail
Port Charlotte, FL 33953
888-918-1118
info@autismhopealliance.org

Dedicated to the recovery of children and adults from autism, the Autism Hope Alliance ignites hope for families facing the diagnosis through education and funding to promote progress in the present moment.

AutismOne
1816 W. Houston Avenue
Fullerton, CA 92833
714-680-0792
earranga@autismone.org
www.autismone.org

AutismOne is a nonprofit, charity organization educating more than 100,000 families every year about prevention, recovery, safety, and change.

Autism Research Institute
4182 Adams Avenue
San Diego, CA 92116
619-281-7165
Media Contact: Matt Kabler
matt@autism.com
www.autism.com

ARI is devoted to conducting research and to disseminating the results of research on the triggers of autism and on methods of diagnosing and treating autism.

Autism Science Digest
1816 W. Houston Ave.
Fullerton, CA 92833
714-680-0792
Contact: Teri Arranga, Editor in Chief
tarranga@autismone.org
www.autismsciencedigest.com

Autism Science Digest is the place for doctors, researchers, and expert mothers and fathers to get together to talk about research, treatment, and recovery. *Autism Science Digest* is the first Autism Approved™ publication of the globa lautism community. Dedicated to respecting the intelligence of parents, *Autism Science Digest* continues the philosophy of founding organization, AutismOne, featuring up-to-date biomedical information written for new and seasoned readers from clinicians and researchers you trust.

Autism Society
4340 East-West Hwy, Suite 350
Bethesda, MD 20814
www.autism-society.org
301-657-0881, 1-800-3AUTISM x 150
info@autism-society.org

The Autism Society exists to improve the lives of all affected by autism by increasing public awareness about the day-to-day issues faced by people on the spectrum, advocating for appropriate services for individuals across the lifespan, and providing the latest information regarding treatment, education, research and advocacy.

Autism Speaks
2 Park Avenue, 11th Floor
New York, NY 10016
212-252-8584
contactus@autismspeaks.org
www.autismspeaks.org

Autism Speaks is dedicated to funding autism research, disseminating information, and providing a voice for autistic people's needs.

The Canary Party
admin@canaryparty.org
Toll Free 855-711-5282
www.canaryparty.org
650-471-8897

The Canary Party is a movement created to stand up for the victims of medical injury, environmental toxins, and industrial foods by restoring balance to our free and civil society and empowering consumers to make health and nutrition decisions that promote wellness.

Generation Rescue
19528 Ventura Blvd. #117
Tarzana, CA 91356
1-877-98-AUTISM
www.generationrescue.org

Generation Rescue is Jenny McCarthy's autism organization dedicated to informing and assisting families touched by autism; it provides programs and services for personalized support, and Generation Rescue volunteers are researching causes and treatment for autism.

Helping Hand
1330 W. Schatz Lane
Nixa, MO 65714
877-NAA-AUTISM (877-622-2884)
naa@nationalautism.org
www.nationalautismassociation.org/helpinghand.php

Helping Hand is a program from the National Autism Association that provides financial assistance for autism families.

Kids Enjoy Exercise Now (KEEN)
1301 K Street, NW
Suite 600, East Tower
Washington, DC 20005
866-903-KEEN (5336) main
866-597-KEEN (5336) fax
info@keenusa.org

KEEN is a national, nonprofit volunteer-led organization that provides one-to-one recreational opportunities for children and young adults with developmental and physical disabilities at no cost to their families and caregivers. KEEN's mission is to foster the self-esteem, confidence, skills and talents of its athletes through non-competitive activities, allowing young people facing even the most significant challenges to meet their individual goals.

National Autism Association
1330 W. Schatz Lane
Nixa, MO 65714
877-622-2884
naa@nationalautism.org
www.nationalautism.org

NAA raises funds for autism research and support and also provides programs, such as Helping Hand, Family First, and FOUND, designed to aid specific needs for families dealing with autism.

National Autism Center
41 Pacella Park Drive
Randolph, Massachusetts 02368
Phone: 877-313-3833
Fax: 781-440 0401
Email: info@nationalautismcenter.org
www.nationalautismcenter.org

The National Autism Center is a nonprofit organization dedicated to serving children and adolescents with Autism Spectrum Disorders (ASD) by providing reliable information, promoting best practices, and offering comprehensive resources for families, practitioners, and communities.

Organization for Autism Research
2000 North 14th Street
Suite 710
Arlington, VA 22201
Tel: 703-243-9710
www.researchautism.org

The Organization for Autism Research (OAR) was created in December 2001—the product of the shared vision and unique life experiences of OAR's seven founders. Led by these parents and grandparents of children and adults on the autism spectrum, OAR set out to use applied science to answer questions that parents, families, individuals with autism, teachers and caregivers confront daily. No other autism organization has this singular focus.

SafeMinds
16033 Bolsa Chica St. #104-142
Huntington Beach, CA 92649
404-934-0777
www.safeminds.org

SafeMinds is an organization dedicated to research and awareness of mercury's involvement in such neurological disorders as autism, attention deficit disorder, and more.

Talk About Curing Autism (TACA)
3070 Bristol Street, Suite 340
Costa Mesa CA 92626
949-640-4401
www.tacanow.org

TACA provides medical, diet, and educational information geared toward autistic children, and the organization also has support, resources, and community events.

U.S. Autism and Asperger Association
P.O. Box 532
Draper, UT 84020-0532
888-9AUTISM, 801-649-5752
information@usautism.org
www.usautism.org

USAAA provides support, education, and resources for autistic individuals and those with Asperger's Syndrome.

Unlocking Autism
P.O. Box 208
Tyrone, GA 30290
866-366-3361
www.unlockingautism.org

Unlocking Autism was created to find information about autism and disseminate that information to families with autistic children; the organization also raises funds for research and awareness.

ONLINE

Age of Autism
www.ageofautism.com

Age of Autism is an online blog with daily news in the latest autism research, updates, and community happenings.

Foundation for Autism Information & Research, Inc.
1300 Jefferson Rd.
Hoffman Estates, IL 60169
info@autismmedia.org

F.A.I.R. Autism Media is a non-profit foundation creating original, up-to-date and comprehensive educational media (video documentaries) to inform the medical community and the public about the latest advances in research and biomedical & behavioral therapies for autism spectrum disorders.

Schafer Autism Report
9629 Old Placerville Road
Sacramento, CA 95827
edit@doitnow.com
www.sarnet.org

Schafer Autism Report is a publication to inform the public about autism-related issues; it can be found online.

STATE LEVEL

Alabama:

Autism Society of Alabama
4217 Dolly Ridge Road,
Birmingham, AL 35243
Jennifer Robertson, 1-877-4-AUTISM, info@autism-alabama.org
www.autism-alabama.org

ASA's mission is to improve the quality of life of persons with Autism Spectrum Disorders and their families through education and advocacy.

Alaska:

Alaska Autism Resource Center
3501 Denali Street, Suite 101
Anchorage, AK 99503-4039
866-301-7372
www.alaskaarc.org

AARC's mission is to increase understanding and support for Alaskans of all ages with autism spectrum disorder via collaboration with families, schools and communities throughout the state.

Arizona:

A.C.T. Today!
1620 N. 48th Street
Phoenix, AV 85008
602-275-1107
Fax: 602-275-1108
www.azacttoday.org

The ACT Today! Arizona chapter's mission is to support Arizona families impacted by autism by increasing their access to therapy and support. Our vision is that the quality of life for all Arizona children with autism has been improved through therapy and supports.

Southwest Autism Research & Resource Center (SARRC)
Vocational & Life Skills Academy
2225 N. 16th Street
Phoenix, AZ 85006
602-340-8717
sarrc@autismcenter.org
www.autismcenter.org

SARRC provides research and support as well as clinical and consultation programs for a widespread group of autistic individuals and their families.

Arkansas:

HEAR Helping Educate about Autism Recovery Arkansas Autism Resource & Outreach Center
2001 Pershing Circle, Suite 300
North Little Rock, AR 72114-1841
Telephone/TDD: 800-342-2923
Telephone: 501-682-9900
Dianna D. Varady, Parent Coordinator,
Partners for Inclusive Communities, UAMS
DDVarady@uams.edu
www.arkansasautism.org

We are a parent-run organization based in Little Rock, Arkansas, whose focus is to provide information and support to empower families, educate providers, and increase community awareness about autism spectrum disorders.

California:

ACT Today!
Autism Care & Treatment Today!
19019 Ventura Blvd. Suite 200
Tarzana, CA 91356
818-705-1625
Info@act-today.org

ACT Today! is a nonprofit 501(c)(3) organization whose mission is to provide funding and support to families that cannot afford the treatments their autistic children need to achieve their full potential.

Canine Companions for Independence
P.O. Box 446
Santa Rosa, CA 95402-0446
1-866-224-3647
www.cci.org

CCI provides support dogs for assistance to those with disabilities.

Center for Autism & Related Disorders, Inc. (CARD)
19019 Ventura Blvd
Suite 300
Tarzana CA, 91356
818-345-2345
info@centerforautism.com
www.centerforautism.com

The Center for Autism and Related Disorders, Inc. (CARD) diligently maintains a reputation as one of the world's largest and most experienced organizations effectively treating children with autism, Asperger's Syndrome, PDD-NOS, and related disorders. They follow the principles of Applied Behavior Analysis (ABA), and develop individualized treatment plans for each child.

For OC Kids Neurodevelopmental Center
1915 West Orangewood, Suite 200
Orange, CA 92868
714-939-6409
forockids@uci.edu
www.forockids.org

For OC Kids Neurodevelopmental Center provides education as well as treatment and support for children with developmental, behavioral, and learning issues ages 0–5.

Sensory Research Center
510 N. Prospect S-308
Redondo Beach, CA 90277
310-698-9008
Contact: Jennifer Hoffiz, Founder
Jhoffiz@sensorycenter.com
www.sensoryresearchcenter.org

Sensory Research Center researches treatments and provides services for children with sensory processing disorders and families without the means to participate in sensory therapy.

Colorado:

The SMART Foundation
PO Box 2181
Vail, Colorado 81658
970-476-7702
info@thesmartfoundation.org
www.thesmartfoundation.org

The SMART Foundation works to train professionals and provide a variety of resources and research for families dealing with autism.

Connecticut:

Autism Support Network
Box 1525
Fairfield, CT 06824
203-404-4929
info@AutismSupportNetwork.com
www.autismsupportnetwork.com

The Autism Support Network is a support community for individuals and groups who have dealt with autism.

Stamford Education 4 Autism, Inc.
1127 High Ridge Road PMB #315
Stamford, CT 06905
203-329-9310
stamforde4autism@aol.com
www.stamfordeducation4autism.org

Stamford Education 4 Autism is an organization to provide awareness and emotional support for autistic children and their families.

Delaware:

Autism Delaware
924 Harmony Road, Suite 201
Newark, DE 19713
302-224-6020
delautism@delautism.org
www.delautism.org

Autism Delaware provides support services, resources, and information for people with autism and their families.

Florida:

The Dan Marino Foundation
P.O. Box 267640
Weston, FL 33326
954-389-4445
www.danmarinofoundation.org

Healing Every Autistic Life
226-5 Solana Rd. #211
Ponte Vedra Beach, FL 32082
904-285-5651
info@healautismnow.org
www.healautismnow.org

The HEAL Foundation provides support for local autistic individuals through grants for organizations, information, and events.

Georgia:

Autism Society Of Northeast Georgia
PO Box 48366
Athens GA 30604-8366
706-208-0066
ga-northeastgeorgia@autismsocietyofamerica.org
http://negac-autsoc.tripod.com

The Autism Society of Northeast Georgia is a chapter of the Autism Society of America that provides support, information, and meetings for autism families in Georgia.

North Georgia Autism Center
PO Box 38
Cumming, GA 30028
770-844-8624
northgaautismcen@bellsouth.net
www.northgeorgiaautismcenter.com

NGAC's mission is to promote and provide intensive home, school, and center-based behavioral therapy to children, youth and families affected by Autism Spectrum Disorders.

Hawaii:

Pacific Autism Center
670 Auahi Street, Suite A-6
Honolulu, HI 96813
808-523-8188
laura@pacificautismcenter.com
http://pacificautismcenter.com

The mission of Pacific Autism Center is to use ABA and be a foundation for those individuals (and their families) within the autism spectrum, and to also provide access to high quality researched based services that support the individual in all areas of their life.

Idaho:

Idaho Center for Autism, LLC
5353 Franklin Road
Boise, ID 83705
208-342-0374
Jackie Mathias, jmathias@idahocenterforautism.com
www.idahocenterforautism.com

Idaho Center for Autism, LLC, is a small group of people who love the kids and families we work with and are committed to doing our best to help them understand that ASDs are complex disorders, with no easy answers and no guarantees, but we know that the lives of kids affected by autism can improve dramatically and are committed to working with families in order to determine and administer appropriate treatment.

Illinois:

Easter Seals Headquarters
233 S. Wacker Dr., Suite 2400
Chicago, IL 60606
1-800-221-6827 or 312-726-6200
www.easterseals.com

Easter Seals provides services and outreach for those with autism, including medical rehabilitation, employment, and recreation information.

Illinois Center for Autism
548 Ruby Lane
Fairview Heights, IL 62208
618-398-7500
info@illinoiscenterforautism.org
www.illinoiscenterforautism.org

The Illinois Center aims to prevent the unnecessary institutionalization of people with autism and to help people with autism achieve their highest level of independence within their home, school and community.

Indiana:

Hamilton County Autism Support Group
19215 Morrison Way
Noblesville, Indiana 46060
317-403-6705
Contact: Jane Grimes, President

janegrimes@hcasg.org
www.hcasg.org

Hamilton County Autism Support Group is a local support group that provides community awareness and resources for autistic individuals and families.

Iowa:

Eastern Central Iowa Autism Society
851 16th St SE
Cedar Rapids, IA 52403
319-431-9052
Sheri Grawe, Vice President: sherigrawe@aol.com
www.eciautismsociety.org

Eastern Central Iowa Autism Society strives to be an advocate for all those affected with Autism Spectrum Disorder—to advance their quality of life through biomedicine, education, community awareness, and therapies.

Kansas:

Autism Awareness Association Inc.
PO Box 780898
Wichita, KS 67278
316-771-7335
Email: tralanajones@autismawareassoc.org

Heartspring
8700 East 29th Street North
Wichita, KS 67218
316-634-8881, 1-800-835-1043
Contact: kbaker@heartspring.org
www.heartspring.org

Heartspring is a facility that supports special-needs children through a variety of clinical and support services.

Kentucky:

Kentucky Autism Training Center
College of Education and Human Development
Dean's Office
University of Louisville
Louisville, KY 40292
800-334-8635 ext. 852-4631
katc@louisville.edu
https://louisville.edu/education/kyautismtraining

The mission of the Kentucky Autism Training Center is to strengthen our state's systems of support for persons affected by autism by bridging research to practice and by providing training and resources to families and professionals.

Louisiana:

Unlocking Autism
PO Box 15388
Baton Rouge, LA 70895
866-366-3361
www.unlockingautism.org

UA's mission is constantly evolving to meet the ever-changing needs of families who are dealing with ASDs, and it includes bringing issues of autism from individual homes to the forefront of national dialogue, joining parents and professionals in one concerted effort to fight for these children who cannot lift their voices to the nation for help, and helping those on the autism spectrum reach their greatest potential in leading fulfilling and productive lives in relationships, society and employment.

Maine:

Association for Science in Autism Treatment (ASAT)
PO Box 7468
Portland, ME 04112-7468
207-253-6058
info@asatonline.org
www.asatonline.org

ASAT's mission is to disseminate accurate, scientifically sound information about autism and treatments for autism and to improve access to effective, science-based treatments for all people with autism, regardless of age, severity of condition, income or place of residence.

Maryland:

Autism Society
4340 East-West Hwy, Suite 350
Bethesda, MD 20814
www.autism-society.org

The Autism Society exists to improve the lives of all affected by autism by increasing public awareness about the day-to-day issues faced by people on the spectrum, advocating for appropriate services for individuals across the lifespan, and providing the latest information regarding treatment, education, research and advocacy.

Center for Autism and Developmental Disabilities Epidemiology (CADDE)
Department of Epidemiology
Johns Hopkins Bloomberg School of Public Health
615 N. Wolfe Street, Suite E6031
Baltimore, MD 21205

1-877-868-8014
cadde@jhsph.edu
www.jhsph.edu/cadde

The Center serves to foster communication, coordination, and collaboration among a multi-disciplinary team of researchers around the epidemiology of Autism Spectrum Disorders (ASD) and Developmental Disabilities (DD). We also strive to bring epidemiologic data and research to public health and educational practitioners, as well as to interested ASD and DD public constituencies.

Massachusetts:

Advocates for Autism of Massachusetts
217 South Street
Waltham, MA 02453
781-891-6270
Contact: Judy Zacek
zacek@AFAMaction.org
www.afamaction.org

AFAM is an advocacy organization dedicated to promoting rights and providing support for those with Autism and Asperger's Syndrome.

The Autism Research Foundation (TARF)
c/o Moss-Rosene Lab, W701
715 Albany Street
Boston, MA 02118
617-414-7012
tarf@ladders.org
www.ladders.org/pages/TARF.html

TARF is collection of researchers looking into the neurobiological effects of autism and similar disorders.

The Doug Flutie Jr. Foundation for Autism
PO Box 767
Framingham, MA 01701
508-270-8855
info@flutiefoundation.org
http://dougflutiejrfoundation.org/

The Doug Flutie Jr. Foundation for Autism is committed to supporting families by providing information, resources, and access to the most current autism news and events.

First Signs
P.O. Box 358
Merrimac, MA 01860
978-346-4380
info@firstsigns.org
www.firstsigns.org

First Signs is an organization to inform adults about the first warning signs of autism in children.

FRAXA Research Foundation
45 Pleasant St.,
Newburyport, MA 01950
978-462-1866
Contact: Katie Clapp, Executive Director
info@fraxa.org, mbudek@fraxa.org, kclapp@fraxa.org
www.fraxa.org

FRAXA's mission is to accelerate progress toward effective treatments and ultimately a cure for Fragile X, by directly funding the most promising research. It also supports families affected by Fragile X and raises awareness of this important but virtually unknown disease.

The Friendship Network for Children
100 Otis St. #4B
Northborough, MA 01532
508-393-0030
Contact: Nancy Swanberg, Executive Director
nancy@networkforchildren.org
www.networkforchildren.org

The Friendship Network for Children is dedicated to helping promote the use of creative activities, such as music and art, to reach children with communication-related disabilities, such as autism.

The Gottschall Autism Center
2 Brandt Island Road
P.O. Box 979
Mattapoisett, MA 02739
For information call:
Pam Ferro, RN, President
508-941-4791
Cheryl Gaudino, Executive Director
774-282-0293
email: info@gottschallcenter.com

The Gottschall Autism Center partners with families to provide children and adults with optimal health interventions, support services, educational enrichment and employment.

Greenlock Therapeutic Riding Center
55 Summer St.
Rehoboth, MA 02769
508-252-5814
www.greenlock.org
Laurel Welch, PT, HPCS, Intake Therapist
greenlocktrc@gmail.com

GTRC is a non-profit organization that utilizes equine-related activities for the therapy of individuals with physical, developmental, and emotional differences.

Learning and Developmental Disabilities Evaluation & Rehabilitation Services
1 Maguire Road
Lexington, MA 02421-3114
781-860-1700
info@ladders.org
www.ladders.org

LADDERS is a program that evaluates patients with a variety of disabilities, including autism, and provides individual and comprehensive treatment plans.

Michigan:

Michigan Autism Partnership
1601 Briarwood Circle, Suite 500
Ann Arbor, MI 48108
734-997-9088
office@aacenter.org
www.mapautism.org

The Michigan Autism Partnership's vision is to create a state-wide network of parents and professionals that supports and promotes intensive, developmental, play-based programming for young children with autistic spectrum disorders.

Minnesota:

Minnesota Autism Center
5710 Baker Road
Minnetonka, MN 55345
952-767-4200
info@mnautism.org
www.mnautism.org

The Minnesota Autism Center's Mission is to promote and provide intensive home, school and center-based behavioral therapy to children, youth and families affected by Autism Spectrum Disorder.

Mississippi:

TEAAM Together Enhancing Autism Awareness in Mississippi
P.O. Box 37
Mize, MS 39116
601-733-0090

takeaction@TEAAM.org
www.teaam.org

TEAAM is a non-profit organization dedicated to improving the lives of Mississippians with an Autism Spectrum Disorder by cultivating and enhancing family and community supports.

Missouri:

Family First
1330 W. Schatz Lane
Nixa, MO 65714
877-NAA-AUTISM (877-622-2884)
naa@nationalautism.org
www.nationalautismassociation.org/familyfirst.php

Family First is a program by the National Autism Association that provides marital support and promotes unity in autism families.

FOUND
1330 W. Schatz Lane
Nixa, MO 65714
877-NAA-AUTISM (877-622-2884)
naa@nationalautism.org
www.nationalautismassociation.org/found.php

Found is a National Autism Association program that raises funds to counter the rise of wandering-related deaths.

Touchpoint Autism Services
1101 Olivette Executive Pkwy.
St. Louis, MO 63132
314-432-6200
info@touchpointautism.org
www.touchpointautism.org

TouchPoint directly works with hundreds of children and adults with autism spectrum disorders (ASD). They also work with families, helping them learn the special skills they need to care for a family member with autism.

Nebraska:

Autism Action Partnership
14301 FNB Parkway, Suite 115
Omaha, Nebraska 68154
402-496-7200
info@autismaction.org
www.autismaction.org

AAP's mission is to improve the quality of life of persons on the Autism Spectrum and their families through education, advocacy and support, thereby enabling them to be an integral part of the community.

Nevada:

Autism Coalition of Nevada
1790 Vassar St
Reno, NV 89502
775-329-2268
acon@aconv.org
www.aconv.org

Our mission is to support legislation for screening, diagnosis and treatment clinics, and receive appropriations.

New Hampshire:

The Birchtree Center
2064 Woodbury Avenue, Suite 204
Newington, New Hampshire, 03801
603-433-4192
www.birchtreecenter.org

The Birchtree Center's mission is to improve the quality of life for children and youth with autism and their families through nurturing relationships, therapeutic programming and specialized education.

New Jersey:

The Daniel Jordan Fiddle Foundation
P.O. Box 1149
Ridgewood, New Jersey 07451-1149
877-444-1149
info@djfiddlefoundation.org
www.djfiddlefoundation.org

The DJ Fiddle Foundation was created to both develop and support programs for autistic individuals, as well as spread current information.

The Devereux New Jersey Comprehensive Community Resources (DNJCCR)
286 Mantua Grove Road, Bldg. #4
West Deptford, NJ 08066
856-599-6400

DNJCCR serves nearly 400 children, adolescents, adults, and their families with special needs. It also has a residential/educational center that serves individuals with autism spectrum disorders.

New Horizons in Autism
600 Essex Rd.
Neptune, NJ 07753
732-918-0850
Contact: Michele Goodman, Executive Director
goodman@nhautism.org
www.nhautism.org/default.asp

New Horizons in Autism is an organization that operates six homes, a vocational program, and after-school, voucher stipend and behavior therapy support options.

New York:

Autism United
100 West Nicholai Street
Hicksville, NY 11801
516-933-4050
www.autismunited.org

Autism United is a community for families and individuals with autism that supports the professional community of autism researchers.

Elizabeth Birt Center for Autism Law & Advocacy (EBCALA)
430 Henry Street, Suite 300
Brooklyn, NY 11231
347-709-5304
http://www.ebcala.org/

The purpose of EBCALA is to educate lawyers, advocates and parents about the legal challenges of autism. Formed in late 2008, EBCALA provides training, resources and a forum within which to advance legal and advocacy strategies to improve the lives of those with autism.

Foundation for Educating Children with Autism (FECA)
PO Box 813
Mount Kisco, NY 10549
914-941-FECA (3322)
questions@FECAinc.org
www.fecainc.org

FECA is a non-profit organization that provides educational opportunities for children with autism through the development of schools, inclusion and vocational programs, consumer advocacy and community outreach.

Special Needs Activity Center for Kids NYC (SNACK NYC)
220 E 86th Street (Lower Level)
New York, NY 10028
212-439-9996
info@snacknyc.com
www.snacknyc.com

SNACK is a New York-based activity center where children with special needs can socialize; it has after-school and weekend programs that include a variety of creative activities.

North Carolina:

Autism Services of Mecklenburg County, Inc.
2211-A Executive Street
Charlotte, NC 28208
704-392-9220
info@asmcinc.com
www.asmcinc.com/index.php

ASMC is a private, not-for-profit organizatio offering residential and support services for residents of North Carolina with Autism, Traumatic Brain Injuries and other developmental disabilties.

Autism Society of North Carolina
505 Oberlin Road, Suite 230
Raleigh, NC 27605
1-800-442-2762 (NC only), 919-743-0204
info@autismsociety-nc.org
www.autismsociety-nc.org

The Autism Society of North Carolina provides support services and resources for individuals, professionals, and families dealing with autism in North Carolina.

North Dakota:

North Dakota Autism Center
4733 Amber Valley Parkway, Suite 200
Fargo, ND 58104
701-277-8844
info@ndautismcenter.org
www.ndautismcenter.org

North Dakota Autism Center's mission is to help children affected by autism spectrum disorders to reach their full potential through excellence in care, therapy, instruction and support

Ohio:

4 Paws for Ability
253 Dayton Ave.
Xenia, Ohio 45385
937-374-0385
Contact: Karen Shirk
karen4paws@aol.com
www.4pawsforability.org
4 Paws provides service dogs for disabled people, and the company specializes in dogs that are specifically trained to work with autistic people.

Ohio Center for Autism and Low Incidence (OCALI)
470 Glenmont Ave
Columbus OH 43214
614-410-0321, 866-886-2254

ocali@ocali.org
www.ocali.org

OCALI's mission is to support, promote, and train individuals with autism and other low-incidence disorders to live fulfilling and successful lives.

Oklahoma:

Oklahoma Family Center for Autism
3901 Northwest 63rd St.
Oklahoma City, OK
405-842-9995
melinda@okautism-efca.org
www.okautism.org

The OFCA provides a way for organizations operating in the state of Oklahoma to share information and help each other advance the cause of families affected by autism. The OFCA is a resource and leadership forum for group leaders in Oklahoma who have a passion to serve their communities.

Oregon:

Autism Service Dogs of America
4248 Galewood St., Lake Oswego, Oregon 97035
info@autismservicedogsofamerica.com
http://autismservicedogsofamerica.com

Autism Service Dogs of America trains service dogs for autistic children.

Northwest Autism Foundation
519 Fifteenth Street
Oregon City , OR 97045
503-557-2111
www.autismnwaf.org

The Northwest Autism Foundation is a non-profit organization whose goal is to provide education and information for free or at a nominal cost to families, caregivers and professionals of autistic children.

Pennsylvania:

Advisory Board on Autism and Related Disorders (ABOARD)
35 Wilson Street, Suite 100
Pittsburgh, PA 15223
412-781-4116
support@aboard.org
www.aboard.org

ABOARD is a Pennsylvania-based support society for parents and autistic children, which provides both access to support groups and to a variety of autism information.

Autism Spectrum News
16 Cascade Drive
Effort, PA 18329
570-629-5960
Contact: Ira Minot, Executive Director
iraminot@mhnews.org
www.mhnews-autism.org/index.html

The Autism Spectrum News is a publication from Mental Health News Education, Inc. that informs the autism community about research, autism information, and current happenings.

Rhode Island:

About Families, CEDARR Family Center
203 Concord St., Suite 335
Pawtucket, RI 02860
401-365-6855
info@aboutfamilies.org
www.aboutfamilies.org

The About Families CEDARR Center is committed to supporting families of children who have autism spectrum disorders, mental health and substance abuse difficulties, and development, physical, and medical disabilities by providing state of the art information, evaluative, diagnostic, prescriptive, and support services that build on the strengths of the child, family, and community.

Advocates in Action
PO Box 41528
Providence, RI 02940-1528
401-785-2028
www.aina-ri.org

Together we work to help people understand information more clearly, learn about rights, participate in their communities and share their unique gifts with the rest of society.

Autism Project of RI
1516 Atwood Avenue
Johnston, RI 02919
401-785-2666
inquiries@riautism.org
www.riautism.org

Autism Project of RI was founded by parents intended to be a resource for other parents in the Rhode Island community who have members of their families who live with ASD.

Rhode Island Technical Assitance Project at the Department of Education
RIDE Office of Special Populations
255 Westminster St.
Providence, RI 02903

401-222-6030
Sue Constable sconstable@ritap.org
www.ritap.org

RITAP provides practitioners, parents, and policy-makers the knowledge and resources necessary to increase their capacity to provide comprehensive and coordinated services to all children including those with disabilities that result in improved educational performance and enhanced life-long outcomes.

South Carolina:

Autism Advocate Foundation
PO Box 7061
Myrtle Beach, SC 29572
843-213-0217
www.autismadvocatefoundation.com

To provide emotional, financial and therapeutic support for individuals with Autism Spectrum Disorders throughout their lifespan, while achieving their personal goals and dreams with integrity and distinction in their least restrictive environment.

National Autism Association
PO Box 1547
Marion, SC 29571
877-622-2884
naa@nationalautism.org
www.nationalautismassociation.org

The mission of the National Autism Association is to educate and empower families affected by autism and other neurological disorders, while advocating on behalf of those who cannot fight for their own rights.

Tennessee:

The Autism Solution Center, Inc.
9282 Cordova Park Road
Cordova, TN 38018
Phone: 901-758-8288
Fax: 901-758-1806
info@autismsolutioncenter.com

The Autism Solution Center, Inc. is a non-profit organization being developed to address an unmet, ongoing need within our communities for autism therapy, support services, research and other assistance.

Faces of Hope Children's Therapy Center
301 Hancock Street
Gallatin, Tennessee 37066
615-206-1176
Contact: Leslie Face, Executive Director

leslie@facesofhopetn.com
www.facesofhopetn.com

Faces of Hope provides speech, occupational, and physical therapies for autistic children in Tennessee and certain areas of Kentucky.

Texas:

ATC Rehabilitation Agency – Dallas
10610 Metric Dr., Suite 101
Dallas, TX 75243
214-221-4405

ATC Rehabilitation Agency – San Antonio
10615 Perrin-Beitel, Suite 801
San Antonio, TX 78247
210-599-7733

Autism Treatment Center – Dallas
10503 Metric Dr.
Dallas, TX 75243
972-644-2076
Anna P. Hundley, CEO

The mission of the Autism Treatment Center is to assist people with autism and related disorders throughout their lives as they learn, play, work and live in the community.

Autism Treatment Center – San Antonio
16111 Nacogdoches Road
San Antonio, TX 78247
210-590-2107
Anna P. Hundley, Executive Director

Vermont:

Howard Center
208 Flynn Avenue Suite 3J
Burlington, Vermont 05401
802-488-6000
Contact: Todd Centybear, Executive Director
www.howardcenter.org

Howard Center provides developmental, mental health, substance abuse, and child, youth, and family services through funding, support, and community programs.

Virginia:

Autism Learning Center
7600 Leesburg Pike #410
Falls Church, VA 22043
703-506-1930
autismlc@aol.com
www.autismlearningcenter.org

ALC emphasizes a positive and systematic approach to teaching skills and reducing problematic behaviors, taking a creative and flexible approach and capitalizing on the resources available for each child.

Organization for Autism Research
2000 North 14th Street, Suite 710
Arlington, VA 22201
703-243-9710
info@researchautism.org
www.researchautism.org

OAR's mission is to apply practical research that examines issues and challenges that children and adults with autism and their families face everyday to the treatment of individuals living with autism.

Washington:

Families for Effective Autism Treatment (FEAT) of Washington
14434 NE 8th St., Second Floor
Bellevue, WA 98007
206-763-3373
featwa@featwa.org
www.featwa.org

FEAT's mission is to provide families with hope and guidance to help their children with autism reach their full potential.

Washington, D.C.:

Autistic Self-Advocacy Network
1025 Vermont Avenue, NW, Suite 300
Washington, DC 20005
Contact: Ari Ne'eman, Founding President
aneeman@autisticadvocacy.org
www.autisticadvocacy.org

ASAN was created to encourage autistic individuals to seek rights and promote the positive aspects of a diverse community.

West Virginia:

Autism Services Center
The Keith Albee Building
929 4th Avenue, Second Floor
Huntington, WV 25701
304-525-8014

ASC is a nonprofit, licensed behavioral health care agency founded in 1979 by Ruth Christ Sullivan, PhD. Though specializing in autism, the agency provides comprehensive, community integrated services for individuals with all developmental disabilities, throughout their lifespan.

West Virginia Autism Training Center
Marshall University
One John Marshall Drive
Huntington, WV 25755
1-800-642-3463
www.marshall.edu/coe/atc

The mission of the Autism Training Center is to provide education, training and treatment programs for West Virginians who have Autism, Pervasive Developmental Disorder (NOS) or Asperger's Disorder and have been formally registered with the Center. This is done through appropriate education, training and support for professional personnel, family members or guardians and other important in the life of a person with autism.

Wisconsin:

Chileda Habilitation Institute
1825 Victory Street
La Crosse, WI 54601
Ruth Wiseman, President/CEO
608-782-6480 Ext. 237
www.chileda.org

Chileda is a nationally recognized and respected program for students with exceptional needs and exceptional potential. They serve children and young adults from ages 6 to 21.

Good Friend, Inc.
808 Cavalier Drive
Waukesha, WI 53186
414-510-0385, 262-391-1369
Contacts: Chelsea Budde and Denise Schamens, Founders
chelsea@goodfriendinc.com, denise@goodfriendinc.com
www.goodfriendinc.com

Good Friend, Inc. was created to spread awareness and understanding from regularly-developing children for autistic children; the organization offers information, events, and workshops.

Wyoming:

Casper Autism Society
750 West 58th Street
Casper, WY 82601
307-234-5838
cgarner@tribcsp.com
http://casperautismsociety.com/

The Casper Autism Society serves as a support group for all families affected by autism and for those on the Autism Spectrum (ASD). Monthly meetings are held and a free lending library is available.

INTERNATIONAL

Autism Canada Foundation
519-695-5858
www.autismcanada.org

The Autism Acceptance Project
P.O. Box 23030
Toronto, Ontario Canada M5N 3A8
Contact: Estée Klar-Wolfond, Founder and Executive Director
esteewolfond@mac.com
www.taaproject.com

TAAP is a site to promote public understanding and acceptance of autistic people. This site also has an online gallery with creations completely contributed by autistic artists.

The Autism File
PO Box 144
Hampton, TW12 2FF
England
020 8979 2525
info@autismfile.com
www.autismfile.com

The Autism File is a magazine covering autism spectrum disorders, providing information about biomedical research and treatments, education and therapies, advocacy issues, perspectives of individuals on the spectrum, and more.

The Autism Trust
Brackenwood
Hill View Road
Claygate
Surrey KT10 0TU
UNITED KINGDOM
020 8979 2525
info@theautismtrust.org.uk
www.autismtrust.com

The Autism Trust provides a variety of facilities and centers that assist autistic individuals by providing resources and support in health issues, residential needs, professional information, and more.

Child Early Intervention Medical Center, FZ LLC
Dubai Health Care City Al Razi Building, Block B,
Suite 2010
P.O. Box 505122 ,Dubai, UAE
Tel: +971 4 423 3667
Fax:+971 4 429 8474
Mobile: +971505512319
www.childeimc.com

Curando el Autismo
www.curandoelautismo.org

EmergenzAutismo (Italy)
www.emergenzautismo.org

MINDD Foundation
PO Box 151 Vaucluse
NSW 2030 Australia
+61 2 9337 3600
info@mindd.org
www.mindd.org

MINDD was created to inform and provide research findings on new and alternative treatments for disorders like autism, such as Chiropractic care, Chinese medicine, and holistic care.

Research Autism
Westbourne House
14-16 Westbourne Grove
London, W2 5RH020 8292 8900
UK
info@researchautism.net
www.researchautism.net

Research Autism is a UK-based charity dedicated to autism research, and is designed for anyone with an interest in autism.

Treating Autism
222 Bramhall Lane South
Bramhall, Stockport
Cheshire SK7 3AA UK
treatingautismuk@aol.com
www.treatingautism.co.uk

Treating Autism has a membership society that receives resources and newsletters, groups that meet for support, and conferences in the UK to inform about biomedical and therapeutic developments for autism.

SCHOOLS FOR PERSONS WITH AUTISM SPECTRUM DISORDERS

Alabama:

Glenwood

The Autism and Behavioral Health Center
150 Glenwood Lane
Birmingham, Alabama 35242-5700
Main Phone: 205-969-2880

Glenwood provides treatment and education services in a least restrictive setting, through a continuum of care, with the highest respect for individuals and families served.

Arizona:

Arizona Centers for Comprehensive Education and Life-Skills (ACCEL)

10251 North 35th Ave
Phoenix, AZ 85051
602-995-7366
Contact: Nancy Molder, Vice President of Educational Services.
nmolder@accel.org

ACCEL is a private, non-profit special education day school providing educational, behavioral and vocational services to students, ages 3-21, with cognitive, emotional, orthopedic, and/or behavioral challenges and Autism.

Chrysalis Academy

600 E. Baseline Rd., Ste. B6
Tempe, AZ 85283
480-839-6000
play.aba@gmail.com
www.play-aba.com

Chrysalis Academy is a private year-round school that serves children with autism and related disorders using ABA teaching methods.

Gateway Academy

7655 E. Gelding Drive
Suite #A-3
Scottsdale, AZ 85260
480-998-1071
www.gatewayacademy.us/index.htm

Gateway Academy is a private Preschool - 12th Grade day school specializing in students with Asperger's Syndrome, High Functioning Autism, and PDD-nos. It incorporates special techniques into the curriculum, such as puppy therapy, equine therapy, and music therapy.

New Way Academy

1300 North 77th Street
Scottsdale, Arizona 85257
480-946 9112
Contact: denise@newwayacademy.org
www.newwayacademy.org

New Way Learning Academy is Arizona's only non-profit, private K-12 day school specializing in children with learning differences.

Pieceful Solutions

6101 E. Virginia St.
Mesa, AZ 85215
480-309-4792
piecefulsolutions@yahoo.com
www.piecefulsolutions.com

Pieceful Solutions is an non-profit organization created specifically to offer children with autism and other developmental disabilities comprehensive schooling using innovative teaching techniques. We work cooperatively with students and parents to set, plan for and achieve goals that focus on academics, social, emotional development and life skills.

Arkansas:

The Allen School
824 N. Tyler St.
Little Rock, AR 72205
501-664-2961
Contact: Suzy Benham, Director
www.invitingarkansas.com/charity/allen-school.asp

Since 1958, The Allen School has enabled children birth to five, with developmental disabilities, such as cerebral palsy, autism, epilepsy, and mental retardation, to achieve their dreams, through treatment, nurturing, and education.

California:

Beacon Day School
24 Centerpointe Drive
La Palma, CA 90623
714-288-4200
Toll Free: 855-262-4755
Fax: 714-288-4204
Enrollment Information:
Edward S. Miguel
emiguel@beacondayschool.com

California Autism Foundation
4075 Lakeside Drive
Richmond, CA 94806
510-758-0433
contactcaf@calautism.org
www.calautism.org

The mission of the California Autism Foundation is to provide people with autism and other developmental disabilities the best possible opportunities for lifetime support, training and assistance in helping them reach their highest potential for independence, productivity and fulfillment.

Camphill Communities California
Soquel, California
http://www.camphillca.org

Camphill Communities California is a residential care community for adults with developmental disabilities. We're a community of about 25 people, 12 of whom have developmental disabilities. We're located near Monterey Bay, a region famous for its rich, social, cultural and recreational opportunities.

Volunteer opportunities are available at Camphill Communities California for both long and short term coworkers. Imagine a life where the qualities of patience, tolerance, flexibility and empathy are valued. Camphill offers volunteers a path of learning that nurtures personal growth and community involvement with people with special needs. We also offer opportunities for ongoing education and training. We welcome those with idealism who want to share their life with others.

The Help Group
13130 Burbank Blvd.
Sherman Oaks, CA 91401
877-994-3588

The Help Group is a large organization that offers education in seven day schools for preschool through high-school aged students with autism and similar disorders. The schools practice diagnostic teaching, therapies, and physical education.

New Vista School
23092 Mill Creek Drive
Laguna Hills, CA 92653
949-455-1270
office@newvistaschool.org
www.newvistaschool.org

New Vista School is a grade 6-12+ progressive educational center that provides a safe, structured educational environment serving the needs of students with Asperger Syndrome, high-functioning Autism, and language learning disabilities who may benefit from social and transitional skills development.

Orion Academy
350 Rheem Blvd
Moraga, CA 94556-1516
925-377-0789
office@orionacademy.org
www.orionacademy.org

Orion Academy provides a quality college-preparatory program for secondary students whose academic success is compromised by a neurocognitive disability such as Asperger's syndrome, or NLD (Non-verbal Learning Disorder).

Pacific Autism Center for Education (School and Administrative Offices)
1880 Pruneridge Ave.
Santa Clara, CA 95050
408-245-3400

Contact: Jack Brown, Office Manager
admin@pacificautism.org
www.pacificautism.org

PACE has a K-12 school with programs for autistic students; an adult day program; and residential homes. The school's curriculum is based on individual assessment and programs.

PACE (Early Intervention and Sunny Days Preschool)
897 Broadleaf Ln.
San Jose, CA 95128
408-551-0312
Contact: Gina Baldi, Early Intervention Director
ginabaldi@pacificautism.org
www.pacificautism.org/intervention.shtml

PACE's early intervention programs focus on intellectual development for children with ASD under 6 years of age through a variety of therapies and techniques.

Pioneer Day School
4764 Santa Monica Ave.
San Diego, CA 92107
619-758-9424
pioneeramber@sbcglobal.net
www.pioneerdayschool.org/Home.asp

Our award winning school has created a unique and innovative model to address underlying processing deficits for students with Autism Specturm Disorders (ASD) and other special needs. We also create individualized programs for privately placed students.

Pyramid Autism Center
2830 North Glassell
Orange, CA 92865
Grace Walker, Administrative Assistant
gwalker@pyramidautismcenter.com
www.pyramidautismcenter.com

The Pyramid Autism Center (PAC) is a not-for-profit organization dedicated to serving the Orange County autism community – with specific focus on children and their families. The PAC school utilizes the Pyramid Approach to Education developed by Dr. Andrew Bondy, a world-renowned leader in autism education and research.

Sophia Project
Oakland, California
http://www.sophiaproject.org

Springstone Middle School
1035 Carol Lane
Lafayette, CA 94549
925-962-9660
info@thespringstoneschool.org
http://thespringstoneschool.org

The Springstone School is an independent middle school that serves students with Asperger's Syndrome, Non-verbal Learning Disability and other executive function challenges. All instruction integrates pragmatic language, occupational therapy, organizational skills and life skills in the classroom and in the community.

Colorado:

Colorado Institute of Autism
P.O. Box 50254
Colorado Springs, Colorado 80949
719-593-7334

Colorado Institute of Autism is a newly established private organization dedicated to children on the autism spectrum. The institution will open its doors as the first school for children with autism, utilizing Applied Behavior Analysis principles, in the State of Colorado. Available services will include a school program, outreach, assessment, workshops, and service as a resource to the community.

The Joshua School
2303 E. Dartmouth Ave.
Englewood, CO 80113
303-758-7171
thejoshuaschool@yahoo.com
www.joshuaschool.org

The Joshua School serves children ages 2½ to 21 years. Our programming for learners often combines many research-validated methods (within ABA) into a comprehensive but highly individualized package.

Connecticut:

Connecticut Center for Child Development, Inc.
925 Bridgeport Ave.
Milford, CT 06460
203-882-8810
Peggy Fitzsimmons, Private School Program
info@cccdinc.org

The Connecticut Center for Child Development Inc. is a non-profit school that is dedicated to improving the lives of children with autism, Asperger's Syndrome and other pervasive developmental disorders.

Franklin Academy
106 River Road
East Haddam, CT 06423
860-873-2700
admission@fa-ct.org
www.fa-ct.org

Franklin Academy is a college preparatory school for grades 9 - 12, accredited by the New England Association of Schools and Colleges, specializing in serving students with Nonverbal Learning Differences (NLD or NVLD) and Asperger's Syndrome (AS).

The Glenholme School
81 Sabbaday Lane
Washington, CT 06793
860-868-7377
info@theglenholmeschool.org
www.theglenholmeschool.org/home.htm

The Glenholme School is a specialized boarding school that provides a therapeutic program and exceptional learning environment to address varying levels of academic, social and emotional development in boys and girls ages 10 to 18.

Greenwich Education and Prep
62 Main Street
New Canaan, CT 06840
203-594-9777
Contacts: Katja Krumpelbeck, Assistant Director; Kirsten DeConti Ziotas, Director
katja@greenwichedprep.com; kdeconti@greenwichedprep.com
www.greenwichedprep.com

K-12 school with specialized services including Applied Behavioral Analysis (ABA) methods that teaches current public– and private-school curricula for easy transitions.

Greenwich Education and Prep
49 River Road
Cos Cob, CT 06807
203-661-1609
Contacts: Victoria Newman, Executive Director; Meredith Hafer, Director; Stacy Smegal,Assistant Director
vnewman@greenwichedprep.com; meredith@greenwichedprep.com; stacy@greenwichedprep.com
www.greenwichedprep.com

K-12 school with specialized services including Applied Behavioral Analysis (ABA) methods that teaches current public– and private-school curricula for easy transitions.

Delaware:

Delaware Autism Program
Brennen School
144 Brennen Drive
Newark, DE 19713
302-454-2202
Fax: 302-454-5427

Florida:

The Chase Academy
700 Reed Canal Road
South Daytona, FL 32119
386-690-0893
Contact: Mimi Lundell, Executive Director
mtlundell@tcaofvolusia.org
www.tcaofvolusia.org

The Chase Academy, Inc., a private non-profit corporation located in Volusia County, Florida, was established in 2006 to provide educational services specifically tailored to meet the individualized needs of students with high-functioning Autism or any of the related Autism Spectrum Disorders (ASD) and to focus these services on maximizing the students' potential for inclusion into mainstream society.

Coral Rock Academy Operated By
Gersh Educational Development
11155 SW 112th Avenue
Miami, FL 33176
631-385-3342
www.coralrockacademy.org

The Gersh Academy's primary objective is to enable students to be emotionally available to learn. They provide customized educational services to students with neurobiological disorders. Coral Rock Academy educates students grades 4-12.

Florida Autism Center of Excellence
6400 E. Chelsea St.
Tampa, FL 33610
813-621-FACE (3223)
www.faceprogram.org

FACE serves students ages 3 to 22 with moderate to severe autism in pre-K through 12th grade and beyond. FACE is available to families in Hillsborough, Pinellas, Pasco, Polk, Manatee and Sarasota counties.

Jacksonville School for Autism
4000 Spring Park Rd.
Jacksonville, FL 32207
904-732-4343
info.jsa@comcast.net

JSA is a school for children on the autism spectrum, ages 3 to 18. The school uses a variety of curriculums based on each individual child.

The Jericho School
1351 Sprinkle Drive
Jacksonville, FL 32211
904-744-5110
jerichos@bellsouth.net
www.thejerichoschool.org

The Jericho School serves children with autism and developmental delays using ABA and verbal behavior treatments.

Palm Beach School for Autism
1199 W. Lantana Rd. #19
Lantana, Florida 33462
561-533-9917
contact@pbsfa.org
www.pbsfa.org

We serve children in our preschool program ages 3-5 years of age and children in our elementary program grades kindergarten through 5th grade.

Peace by Piece Learning Center
965 Pondella Rd.
North Fort Myers, FL 33903
239-652-4323
info@peacebypieceinc.com
www.peacebypieceinc.com/school.html

Here our mission is to employ our extensive education and experience, in combination with Applied Behavior Analysis, to provide evidence-based and compassionate services to individuals, families, schools and organizations.

Sydney's School for Autism
St. Patrick Catholic Church
4518 South Manhattan Avenue
Tampa, FL 33611
813-835-4591
Contacts: Kathy Swenson, Founder; Antia Maurer, Preschool Director
autisticangels@yahoo.com, anitam@sydneyschool.com
www.sydneysschoolhouse.com

Sydney's School for Autism serves autistic children and those with similar disorders for preschool, kindergarten, and first-grade students, based on ABA teaching methods.

Victory Center for Autism and Behavioral Challenges
18900 Northeast 25th Avenue
North Miami Beach, Florida 33180
Contact: Courtney Richel, Admission
office@thevictoryschool.org
www.thevictoryschool.org

Preschool, secondary school, and after-school program that uses Applied Behavioral Analysis (ABA) methods and one-on-one teaching in the education of children with autism and related disabilities.

Georgia:

Keystone Center for Children with Autism
1675-A Hembree Road
Alpharetta, GA 30009
404-496-4673

Keystone's mission is two-fold: first, we are dedicated to the educational and social development of children with Autism Spectrum Disorders, and second, we are committed to providing support and training to families affected by autism.

The Lionheart School
180 Academy Street
Alpharetta, Georgia 30004
770-772-4555

Lionheart's mission is to provide a developmentally appropriate program for children on the autism spectrum and other disorders of relating and communicating who need a specialized learning environment, therapeutic interventions, relationship building skills and the educational tools necessary to achieve their greatest potential.

Summit Learning Center
700 Holcomb Bridge Road
Suite 400
Roswell, Georgia 30076
Contacts: Jennifer Mitchell and Shauna Courtney, Directors
jennifer@summitlearningcenter.org, shauna@summitlearningcenter.org
www.summitlearningcenter.org/index.html

The Summit Learning Center aims to provide individualized, effective, and scientifically based treatment for children with autism and related disabilities that is not otherwise available in the state of Georgia. The Summit Learning Center provides effective treatment, based on the science of Applied Behavior Analysis (ABA).

Hawaii:

Loveland Academy Hawaii

1506 Piikoi Street
Honolulu, HI 96822
contact_information@lovelandacademyhawaii.com
808-524-4243

As a service provider in Honolulu, Oahu, Hawaii for children and young adults with autism, the mission is to provide an array of state of the art, research based, child and family centered, culturally sensitive therapeutic and educational services targeting the biological, psychological, educational, social and emotional needs of children.

Pacific Autism Center

670 Auahi St., Suite A-6
Honolulu, HI 96813
808-523-8188
laura@pacificautismcenter.com

The mission of Pacific Autism Center is to use ABA and be a foundation for those individuals (and their families) within the autism spectrum, and to also provide access to high quality researched based services that support the individual in all areas of their life.

Illinois:

Giant Steps Illinois

2500 Cabot Dr
Lisle, IL 60532
630-455-5730
Contact: Bridget O'Connor, Executive Director
boconnor@atc-gsi.org

Students in our private day school receive an intensive educational and therapeutic program based on the strengths and individual needs of the child. Using various methodologies such as ABA, repetition and practice, errorless learning, forward and backward chaining, visual supports, hands-on manipulatives, sensory strategies, etc. students focus on reading and language arts, vocabulary, functional mathematics, vocational life skills and more.

Illinois Center for Autism (Children's Special Day School Program)

548 Ruby Lane
Fairview Heights, IL 62208
618-398-7500
info@illinoiscenterforautism.org
www.illinoiscenterforautism.org/programs/dayschool.html

ICA serves students ages 3-21 who have been diagnosed as having autism, pervasive development disorder, Aspereger's Syndrome, and/or students who exhibit compatible characteristics of autism, such as severe communications disorders, severe behavioral disorders, uneven intellectual skills, and socially inappropriate behaviors.

Soaring Eagle Academy

PO Box 63
Riverside, IL 60546
312-683-5151
contact@soaringeagleacademy.org
www.soaringeagleacademy.org

Soaring Eagle's mission is to provide a social and academic learning environment for students with special needs supporting their individual strengths and learning styles while integrating learning and interaction within a Developmental Individual-Difference Relationship (DIR®) Based Approach.

Kansas:

HeartSpring School

8700 East 29th Street North
Wichita, KS 67226
316-634-8730 or 1-800-835-1043 (calls outside Wichita area)
admissions@heartspring.org
www.heartspring.org/school/index.php

The Heartspring School, a residential and day program, provides a warm, loving environment for children with developmental disabilities such as autism, and teams of specialists discover and develop the whole child using a multidisciplinary approach.

Rainbows United, Inc.

340 S. Broadway, Wichita, KS 67202
316-267-KIDS
www.rainbowsunited.org/services-child_care.php
info@rui.org

Kids' CoveSM and Kids' PointSM services include progressive plans for all children regardless of their skill levels to provide the most trusted educational opportunities for all children ages birth through 5.

Maine:

Merrymeeting Center for Child Development
2 Davenport Circle Suite 20
Bath, ME 04530
207-443-6200
Contact: karenz@mccdworks.org
www.mccdworks.org/index.html

Merrymeeting Center for Child Development is committed to ensuring that children with autism, Asperger's syndrome and pervasive developmental disorder (PDD) have access to education, treatment and care that is objectively and scientifically validated as effective, delivered by professionals with specific minimum methodological competencies.

Maryland:

The IvyMount School, Inc.
11614 Seven Locks Rd.
Rockville, MD 20854
301-469-0223
www.ivymount.org/index.cfm

Named twice by the U.S. Department of Education as a Blue Ribbon School of Excellence, Ivymount is a non-sectarian, non-public special education day school. Ivymount's integrated approach to learning includes educational programs and therapeutic services for over 200 students annually, ages 4-21.

Linwood Center
3421 Martha Bush Drive
Ellicott City, MD 21043
410-465-1352
admin@linwoodcenter.org
www.linwoodcenter.org

The Linwood Center serves autistic students ages 9 to 21 with residential and educational programs, and uses a variety of individualized techniques.

Massachusets:

Boston Higashi School
800 North Main Street
Randolph, MA 02368
781-961-0800
Contact: Deborah Donovan, President

donovan@bostonhigashi.org, admissions@bostonhigashi.org
www.bostonhigashi.org/index.php

Boston Higashi School, Inc. is the international program serving children and young adults with autism. Our philosophy is based upon the world-renowned tenets of Daily Life Therapy® developed by the late Dr. Kiyo Kitahara of Tokyo, Japan.

Eagleton School
446 Monterey Road
Great Barrington, MA 01230
413-528-4385
www.eagletonschool.com

Eagleton School serves boys with PDD and Asperger's, teaching and providing daily therapy with a mainly holistic approach. Students' ages range from 9 to 22.

Melmark New England
461 River Road
Andover, MA 01810
978-654-4300
www.melmarkne.org/index.html

Melmark New England specializes in serving those students within our clinical profiles who are currently unable to attend public school. For some children served, the goal is to return the child to the public school setting after the benefits of a Melmark New England education are achieved. For children ages 4 - 8, classroom teachers follow a theme-based curriculum into which individual goals and objectives for each student are carefully embedded

New England Center for Children
33 Turnpike Road
Southborough, Massachusetts 01772
508-481-1015
Contact: Cathy Welch, Director of Admissions
cwelch@neec.org
www.necc.org

NEEC provides individualized teaching methods for children with autism and related disorders, and the school provides a variety of extra-curricular activities and therapies.

Riverview School
551 Route 6A East Sandwich
Cape Cod, MA 02537
508-888-0489

admissions@riverviewschool.org
www.riverviewschool.org

Riverview School provides middle-school to post-secondary school education for students with learning disabilities, focusing on transitions, personal growth, and wellness.

Minnesota:

Camphill Village Minnesota
Sauk Centre, Minnesota
http://www.camphillvillage-minnesota.org

Camphill Village Minnesota is a spiritually striving intentional community of approximately 45 people, including adults with disabilities. Our Village is nestled among 470 acres of gently rolling hills and sparkling lakes and waterways in the beautiful Heartland of America, about 2 hours west of the city of Minneapolis. The life, work, and celebrations of our community are based on the strong belief that every individual, regardless of ability, is an independent spiritual being. Developmental disabilities are treated not as illnesses, but as a part of the fabric of human experience, and we believe that people with these disabilities are worthy of recognition, respect, and honor. Our community has a strong agricultural component with farming, gardening, and a small goatherd. Our craft shops include a bakery, weavery, woodworking shop, card shop, hemp jewelry shop, and a food processing and cheese-making kitchen. All members of the community are cared for within the context of healthy home environments and an active village life.

The Fraser School
2400 W. 64th St
Minneapolis, MN 55423
612-861-1688
school@fraser.org
www.fraser.org

Fraser's mission is to make a meaningful and lasting difference in the lives of children, adults and families with special needs. We accomplish this by providing education, healthcare and housing services.

Lionsgate Academy
3420 Nevada Ave N.
Crystal, MN 55427
763-486-5359
Contact: Elaine Campbell, Administrative Coordinator

ecampbell@lionsgateacademy.org
www.lionsgateacademy.org

Lionsgate Academy provides a transition-oriented and personalized learning program focused on secondary (grades 7-12) higher-functioning students on the autism spectrum that supports their full potential.

Missouri:

Oakwood
West Plains, Missouri
For information, contact:
ottow1@peoplepc.com

Ozark Center for Autism
3006 McClelland Boulevard
Joplin, Missouri 64804
417-347-7600
Contact: Paula Baker, Ozark Center CEO
pfbaker@freemanhealth.com
www.freemanhealth.com/ozarkcenterforautism

Ozark Center for Autism impacts lives daily through the use of Applied Behavior Analysis. Students attend school six hours a day, five days a week to minimize loss of skill.

New Jersey:

The Allegro School
125 Ridgedale Avenue
Cedar Knolls, NJ 07927
973-267-8060
www.allegroschool.org

The Allegro School is a non-profit school that provides quality education, keeps autistic children with their families, and prepares them for community living. The school serves approximately 105 students ages 3-21.

Alpine Learning Group
777 Paramus Road
Paramus, NJ 07652
201-612-7800
Bridget A. Taylor, Executive Director
btaylor@alpinelearninggroup.org
alpinelearninggroup.org/default.asp

The Alpine Learning Group is a non-profit education and treatment program facility for leraners 3 to 21 years of age that utilizes the Applied Behavior Analysis (ABA) treatment for autism.

Bancroft Schools
425 Kings Highway East, P.O. BOX 20
Haddonfield, NJ 08033
1-800-774-5516
Contact: Theresa Tolatta, Director of Admissions and Marketing
inquiry@bnh.org.
www.bancroft.org/ID_DD/IDDD_bancroftschool_home.html

The Bancroft School offers early education through secondary education for autistic students with a variety of techniques, including ABA, community-based instruction, and incidental learning.

Bright Beginnings Learning Center
1660 Stelton Road
Piscataway, NJ 08854
732-339-9331
Wendy Eaton, Principal
www.mcesc.k12.nj.us/special/bright.htm

The Bright Beginnings Learning Center provides specialized, classroom based instruction, based on the principles of Applied Behavior Analysis for students with autism or autistic-like behavior, ages 3 to 12.

Celebrate the Children School
345 South Main Street
Wharton , NJ 07885
973-989-4033
Contact: Monica G. Osgood, Director
info@celebratethechildren.org
www.celebratethechildren.org

Celebrate the Children School uses the developmental, individual, relationship-based model to teach autistic students ages 3 to 19 with a focus on a positive and social educational experience.

The Children's Institute
One Sunset Avenue
Verona, NJ 07044
973-509-3050
Bruce Ettinger, Ed.D., Superintendent/ CEO
webmaster@tcischool.org
www.tcischool.org/default.aspx

TCI uses a model alternative program in which each student's social/emotional and cognitive learning needs are addressed in a prescriptive Individualized Educational Plan (IEP).

Douglass Developmental Disabilities Center
151 Ryders Lane
New Brunswick, NJ 08901-8557
732-932-4500

Dr. Lara Delmolino, PhD, BCBA, Acting Director, Adult Services
www.dddc.rutgers.edu

The Douglass Developmental Disabilities Center (DDDC) was established by the Board of Governors of Rutgers, The State University of New Jersey in 1972 to meet the needs of people with autism spectrum disorders and their families and continues to do so by employing ABA-based therapies.

Garden Academy
P.O. Box 188
Maplewood, NJ 07040-0188
973-761-6140
info@gardenacademy.org
www.gardenacademy.org

Garden Academy will serve individuals with autism ages 3-21. Garden Academy uses scientific, data-based and accountable interventions to provide an individualized education to students with autism so that they may lead lives of the greatest possible independence.

The Midland School
94 Readington Road
PO Box 5026
North Branch, New Jersey 08876
908-722-8222
info@midlandschool.org
www.midlandschool.org/index.asp

The Midland School is a nationally recognized program approved by the New Jersey Deparment of Education that serves children with special needs.

New Beginnings
28 Dwight Place
Fairfield, NJ 07004
973-882-8822
www.nbnj.org

New Beginnings is dedicated to working with children ages three to 21 diagnosed on the autism spectrum. We use a variety of techniques and resources aimed at helping individuals reach their potential and live productively—increasing social, educational and employment opportunities through integration into all aspects of community life.

Reed Academy
85 Summit Ave.
Garfield, NJ 07026
973-772-1188

info@reedacademy.org
www.reedacademy.org

Reed Academy is a private, not-for-profit program for individuals with autism spectrum disorders ages 3-21 using ABA techniques. In addition to an individualized full day school program, we also provide family consultation services and parent training.

Somerset Hills Learning Institute
1810 Burnt Mills Road
Bedminster, NJ 07921
908-719-6400
info@somerset-hills.org
www.somerset-hills.org/home.html

With our reliance on education and treatment approaches derived from the science of applied behavior analysis, some of our students will graduate to traditional education settings. Others will graduate into the workforce and independent living. None will be relegated to a bleak and inhumane future.

Stepping Stone School
45 County Road 519
Bloomsbury, NJ 08804
908-995-1999
Frank Jiorle, Executive Director
frankji@ptd.net
www.sstoneschool.com/page1.html

Stepping Stone School serves Children and Adolescents with Emotional Disorders,Learning Disabilities, Asperger's Syndrome, ADD,ADHD. An individualized instructional and restorative counseling program is provided as an integral part of the school experience.

Y.A.L.E. School Atlantic
(Hamilton Township, NJ)
856-346-0007
www.yaleschool.com/schools/atlantic

This school provides year-round, full-day educational programming to children with autism or pervasive developmental disorder not otherwise specified (PDD-NOS), ages 3-7.

Y.A.L.E. School Southeast
1004 Laurel Oak Road
Voorhees, NJ 08043
856-346-0007
www.yaleschool.com/schools/southeast

This school provides year-round, full-day educational programming to children with autism or pervasive developmental disorder not otherwise specified (PDD-NOS). The program provides educational services to students ages 3 to 14 years.

Y.A.L.E. School Southeast II
856-346-0007
www.yaleschool.com/schools/southeasttwo

This school provides year-round, full-day educational programming to children with autism or pervasive developmental disorder not otherwise specified (PDD-NOS). The program provides educational services to students ages 14 to 21 within a public Jr/Sr high school in Audubon, NJ.

New York:

Anderson Center for Autism
4885 Route 9, P.O. Box 367
Staatsburg, New York 12580
845-889-4034
info@ACenterforAutism.org
www.andersoncenterforautism.org

The Anderson Center for Autism is a private center with residential and educational programs for both children and adults with autism, based on ABA treatment.

Ascent: A School for Individuals with Autism
819 Grand Boulevard
Deer Park NY 11729
631-254-6100
Nancy Shamow, PhD, Executive Director
NShamow@aol.com
www.ascentschool.org

Ascent is a private, non-profit school for children diagnosed with autism and atypical pervasive developmental disorders. It provides a full day, 12 month academic and behavioral treatment program to preschool and school age children ranging in age from 3 to 21 years.

Brooklyn Autism Center Academy
111 Remsen Street
Brooklyn, NY 11201
718-554-1027
info@brooklynautismcenter.org
www.brooklynautismcenter.org

The BAC is a non-profit school serving children with Autism Spectrum Disorders (ASD) in Brooklyn. Their philosophy is grounded in the

Applied Behavior Analysis (ABA) model, which is the educational standard and best practice for children with autism.

For Adults
Camphill Village U.S.A.
Copake, New York
http://www.camphillvillage.org

Camphill Village is a unique therapeutic residential community in Copake, New York, where dedicated volunteers and people with developmental disabilities share a full life together. Located in rural Columbia County 100 miles north of New York City, the Village comprises 600 acres of wooded hills, gardens and pastures. Villagers (adults with disabilities), coworkers and coworkers' children live together in extended family households and work together in a variety of craft shops and work areas. Crafts include candle making, stained glass, bookbinding, weaving, and woodworking. Land work includes a biodynamic dairy farm, vegetable gardens, a Healing Plant garden and workshop, and Turtle Tree Seed biodynamic seed workshop. The Village also has a medical care center, culture and arts center, bakery, Café and Gift Shop.

The Center for Developmental Disabilities
72 South Woods Road
Woodbury NY, 11797
516-921-7650
vprew@centerfor.com
www.centerfor.com

The Center for Developmental Disabilities has a residential program for autistic and developmentally disabled individuals ages 5 to 21, with educational programs, access to therapy, and clinical services.

Gersh Academy (multiple locations)
358 Hoffman Lane
Hauppauge, NY 11788
254-04 Union Turnpike
Glen Oaks, NY 10004
631-385-3342
www.gershacademy.org

The Gersh Academy's primary objective is to enable students to be emotionally available to learn. They provide customized educational services to individuals with neurobiological disorders, grade 3-12.

The Gersh Experience
North Tonowanda, NY 14120
Post Secondary Program
631-385-3342
www.coralrockacademy.org./index.php/schools/the-gersh-experience

The Gersh Experience provides a customized educational program that allows students with neurobiological disorders to successfully experience college life away from the home.

The LearningSpring Elementary School
247 East 20th Street
New York, NY 10003
212-239-4926
Margaret Poggi, Head of School
mpoggi@learningspring.org
www.learningspring.org

The LearningSpring elementary school uses a Cooperative Learning Paradigm, where academics is integrated with mastery of social/emotional, pragmatic language, organization and sensory-motor skills.

McCarton School
350 East 82nd Street
New York, New York 10028
212-996-9035
info@mccartonschool.org
www.mccartonschool.org

The McCarton School provides an educational program for autistic children by using an integrated one-to-one model of therapy that is grounded in Applied Behavioral Analysis (ABA) combined with speech and language therapy, motor skills training, and peer interaction.

Millwood Learning Center
12 Schumann Road
Millwood, NY 10546
914-941-1991
www.devereux.org

Located in Westchester County, the Center provides year-round, full-day, intensive educational and behavioral interventions to students with autism and other pervasive developmental disorders.

New York City Center for Autism Charter School
433 E. 100 Street
New York, NY 10029
212-860-2580

Contact: Julie Fisher, Principal
http://schools.nyc.gov/SchoolPortals/04/M337/
default.htm

This school serves grades 1 through 8 and provides special services and extra-curricular activities for children with autism.

Rebecca School
40 East 30th Street
New York, NY 10016-7374
212-810-4120
info@rebeccaschool.org
www.rebeccaschool.org

Therapeutic day school for children 4 to 18 that uses the Developmental Individual Difference Relationship-based (DIR) model in the education of children with PDD and autism.

Shema Kolainu-Hear Our Voices
4302 New Utrecht Ave.
Brooklyn, NY 11219
718-686-9600
info@skhov.org
www.shemakolainu.org

SK-HOV's mission is to hear the voices of the children and families they serve as they strive to achieve their full potential for independence, productivity and inclusion in the community. Shema Kolainu is dedicated to the education of children with autism spectrum disorders (ASD). Their vision is to provide the best opportunity offered anywhere for children with ASD to achieve recovery.

Summit Academy
150 Stahl Rd.
Getzville, NY 14068
716-629-3400
Fax: 716-629-3499
www.summited.org/early.asp

For Young Adults: 18-28
Triform Camphill Community
Hudson, New York
http://www.triform.org

Triform Camphill Community is a residential therapeutic community, founded in 1979. Triform is a growing energetic community. In the past five years, we have built a residential house and a weavery-therapy building. As a youth-guidance community, Triform endeavors to accompany young adults with special needs to adulthood, self-development, and fulfillment of their potential through education and work training. About 60 people live on 125 acres of land. The community is rich in agriculture, crafts, festivals, and arts. Triform is located in upstate New York, near the city of Hudson and the Hudson River, 2 hours from New York City, 3 hours from Boston, and 1 hour from Albany, New York State's capital as well as 10 miles from the Camphill Village in Copake, New York.

West Hills Montessori School (operated by Gersh Academy)
313 Round Swamp Road
Melville, NY 11747
631-385-3342
www.gershacademy.org

It is a private, co-educational day school that serves 100 students, ages 18 months to 12 years (Toddler through 6th grade), from both Nassau and Suffolk counties.

North Carolina:

Mariposa School for Children with Autism
The Mariposa School for Children with Autism
203 Gregson Drive
Cary, NC 27511
919-461-0600
Contact: Dr. Jacqueline Gottlieb, Head of Mariposa School
info@MariposaSchool.org
www.mariposaschool.org

The Mariposa School staff serves and teaches autistic children by reassessing their needs constantly and giving each child an individual teaching plan.

Ohio:

Autism Academy of Learning
219 Page Street
Toledo, Ohio 43620
419-865-7487
Anthony Gerke, Director of Education agerke@theautismacademy.org
www.theautismacademy.org/

The Autism Academy of Learning is structured to provide every student with Autism Spectrum Disorder an appropriate foundation in the areas of academics, behavior, daily living skills, vocational skills, and independence. Our goal is to promote a higher quality of life, and the realization of the full intellectual and social development of students with Autism Spectrum Disorder.

Haugland Learning Center
3400 Snouffer Rd.
Columbus, OH 43235
614-602-6473
hlccolumbus.com

Haugland Learning Center (HLC) serves the educational needs of over 120 children with Autism or Asperger syndrome throughout the state of Ohio, accepting students from preschool through twelfth grade (including those with behaviors) and is therefore an excellent alternative to public school. All students with an Autism or Asperger's diagnosis are eligible to receive the Autism Scholarship from the Ohio Department of Education, which can be used to pay for educational services at HLC.

Oakstone Academy
5747A Cleveland Avenue
Columbus, OH 43231
614-865-9643

The Oakstone Academy is a non-profit, fully inclusive, chartered school dedicated to serving children with autism and their families, and we are determined to use the principles of applied behavior analysis within the natural environment and implement the most effective empirically based strategies to promote language, social, behavioral, and academic competency in children with autism.

Summit Academy Schools
www.summitacademies.com

Oregon:

Building Bridges
3533 Southeast Milwaukie
Portland, OR 97202
503-235-3122
http://bridgespdx.wordpress.com
Beth Mishler, Board Certified Behavior
Analyst beth@bridgespdx.com

Building Bridges is pleased to offer three behavioral classrooms for children with language and social disorders including autism spectrum disorder: primary (ages 6-8), kindergarten (ages 5-6), and preschool (ages 3-4). The curriculum includes instruction in language arts, mathematics, science, social studies, language, social skills and graphomotor skills, and functional and play skills needed in the classroom are also taught.

The Child Development School of Oregon
12208 NW Cornell Road
Portland, OR 97229
503-646-9135
Therese Steward

Our mission is to provide state-of-the-art education for students with autism and related disabilities and to help all our students reach their full potential in school, in the community, and in life.

School of Autism
7714 N Portsmouth
Portland, OR 97203
503-283-9603
schoolofautism@yahoo.com
www.schoolofautism.com

The School of Autism is a place that families with children with autism can go to get therapy, support and education. Through play, sensory immersion and guidance by people who actually have been through the same process, families and children with autism can be treated AND educated in one place.

Pennsylvania:

Autistic Endeavors Learning Center
7340 Jackson Street
Philadelphia, PA, 19136
Barbara A. Butkiewicz Co-Founder/President
aelcinfo@yahoo.com
www.autisticendeavors.org
215-360-1569

The mission of Autistic Endeavors Learning Center is to promote independent functioning of children with Autistic Spectrum Disorders. The Center will provide an intensive instructional program using, but not limited to, methods of Applied Behavior Analysis to help children with Autism acquire effective communication and socialization skills.

For Children: Pre-K to Grade 12
Camphill Special School
Glenmoore, Pennsylvania
http://www.camphillspecialschool.org

Children, ages 5-19 years, live in an extended family with coworkers—often with their own children—and other volunteers in specially designed homes. The education program is adapted from Waldorf education focusing on experiential learning and emphasizing social, artistic and practical skills, and is supported by a variety of therapies that are available to help the child in his or her development. The community consists of approximately 90 students, 40 teachers and teacher aides, 10 therapists, 70 additional coworkers and 11 staff and is located in the same general area of southeastern Pennsylvania as Camphill Village Kimberton Hills and Camphill Soltane.

Camphill Soltane
Glenmoore, Pennsylvania
http://www.camphillsoltane.org

Camphill Soltane is a life-sharing community of 80 people, including young adults, ages 18-35, with developmental disabilities. At Soltane, we encourage self-advocacy for those with disabilities, help coworkers reach their aspirations through effective and inspiring training, and encourage teamwork in home and work areas. Soltane's mission is to build a bridge to adulthood for young people with disabilities, and our cornerstone is an attempt to actively involve every person in the process of creating community. We are located 1 hour west of Philadelphia, PA, in a semi-rural setting.

Camphill Village Kimberton Hills
Kimberton, Pennsylvania
http://www.camphillkimberton.org

Camphill Village Kimberton Hills is a 432 acre, land-based, life-sharing community located about an hour west of Philadelphia in Chester County Pennsylvania. Made up of 120 members, Kimberton Hills strives to restore vitality to our ecosystems and societal structures through Anthroposophy, the spiritual philosophy of Rudolf Steiner. Adults who have developmental disabilities live and work side by side with volunteers in family households to form a supportive community based on shared responsibilities and caring. The community features a large biodynamic CSA Garden which offers a two year apprenticeship study program, an award winning organic dairy, a café and bakery which serve the village and surrounding region, weavery and fiber arts workshops, as well as land and building maintenance programs. Kimberton Hills is known locally for its sustainable buildings and its strong cultural life of festivals, music, and art.

The Comprehensive Learning Center (CLC)
150 James Way
Southampton, PA 18966
215-322-7852

clcschool@clcschool.net
www.clcschool.net

The Comprehensive Learning Center's primary mission is to ensure that each of its students reaches their maximum potential through an intensive, comprehensive education and treatment program based on the scientifically validated procedures of applied behavior analysis.

Devereux Kanner/Kanner CARES
390 East Boot Road
West Chester, PA 19380
610-431-8100
www.devereux.org/site/
PageServer?pagename=kan_cares

Devereux Childhood Autism Research and Education Services (CARES) is a state of the science center-based, day education program for young children with autism using contemporary strategies and methodologies consistent with Applied Behavior Analysis (ABA).

The Melmark School
2600 Wayland Road
Berwyn, Pennsylvania 19312
610-325-4969
admissions@melmark.org
www.melmark.org

The Melmark School offers day and residential special education services to children and adolescents ages 5 to 21 with learning difficulties and/or challenging behaviors secondary to a diagnosis of Autism Spectrum Disorder; Acquired Brain Injury; Mental Retardation, mild to profound; Cerebral Palsy; and/or Neurological Disorders.

TALK Institute and School
(formerly Magnolia)
395 Bishop Hollow Road
Newtown Square, PA 19073
610-356-5566
www.talkinc.org/about.html
New Students
Email mikeabramson@comcast.net
Media Inquiries
Email melkot@aol.com

The Vista School
1249 Cocoa Avenue
Hershey, PA 17033
717-835-0310
Kristen Yurich, Clinical Director kyurich@
thevistaschool.org

Vista serves children with ASD ranging in age from pre-kindergarten to secondary school age from Berks, Cumberland, Dauphin, Franklin, Juniata, Lancaster, Lebanon, and Perry Counties, who are functioning on the moderate to severe end of the autism spectrum, who often display severe delays in communication skills, engage in higher rates of problematic or challenging behaviors, require assistance for activities of daily living, have little or limited ability to appropriately occupy their leisure time, and need one-on-one instruction for learning new skills.

Tennessee:

The King's Daughters' School for Autism
900 Trotwood Avenue
Columbia, Tennessee 38401
931-388-3810

The mission of The King's Daughters' School is to serve the educational and training needs of children and adults with developmental disabilities. The school strives to provide a high-quality program of personal development in a wholesome residential atmosphere aimed at allowing each person to reach his or her fullest potential as an independent and productive citizen.

Texas:

Autism Treatment Center – Dallas
10503 Metric Drive
Dallas, Texas 75243
972-644-2076
www.atcoftexas.org

The mission of the Autism Treatment Center is to assist people with autism and related disorders throughout their lives as they learn, play, work and live in the community.

Capitol School of Austin
2011 West Koenig Lane
Austin, Texas 78756
512-467-7006

The mission of Capitol School of Austin is to provide an enriched learning environment where children with speech, language, and learning differences can reach their full potential and develop skills necessary to succeed in future educational settings.

Focus On The Future Training Center
3405 Custer Rd. Suite 100
Plano, TX 75023

972-599-1400
Contact: Brenda M. Batts, Director
focussped@yahoo.com
www.focussped.com/index.html

Focus on the Future Training Center is a highly regarded Pre-K to Grade 12 private school for children with autism and other mental disabilities. They offer some of the best autism early intervention and other individualized curriculum featuring Speech Therapy, Occupational Therapy, and Music Therapy.

The Monarch School
1231 Wirt Rd.
Houston, TX 77055
713-479-0800
Contact: Sharon Duval
sduval@monarchschool.org
www.monarchschool.org
Developmental Individuarl Difference / FloorTime based program.

Newfound School
2206 Heads Lane, Suite 110
Carrollton, TX 75006
214-390-1749
www.newfoundschool.com

Newfound School is a small private school for grades PreK - 12 for children with learning and/or behavior challenges. It is designed to provide meaningful instruction and learning in a caring, nurturing atmosphere. Students are provided lifelong learning strategies for academics, behavior, and social skills.

The Westview School
1900 Kersten Drive
Houston, TX 77043
713-973-1900
Jane G. Stewart, Director
www.westviewschool.org

The Westview School is a private, non-profit school which was founded in 1981 to provide a structured, nurturing, and stimulating learning environment for children with learning differences which prevent them from being successful in regular programs.

Utah:

The Carmen B. Pingree Center for Children with Autism
780 South Guardsman

UT 84108
801-581-0194
Contact: Pete Nicholas, Director
petern@vmh.com
www.carmenbpingree.com

The Pingree Center is a preschool and kindergarten program for children with autism that uses a unique 5-step approach for a discrete trial format method of teaching.

Spectrum Academy
575 Cutler Drive
North Salt Lake, UT 84054
801-936-0318
http://spectrumcharter.org/

The Spectrum Academy is the premier charter school in Utah that tailors learning environment and curriculum to accommodate the unique needs of children with Asperger's Syndrome and other high-functioning Autism Spectrum Disorders. Our mission encompasses all children, and we are pleased to be free and offer enrollment open to the public.

Vermont:

Heartbeet
Hardwick, Vermont
http://www.heartbeet.org

Howard Center
208 Flynn Avenue Suite 3J
Burlington, Vermont 05401
802-488-6000
debs@howardcenter.org
www.howardcenter.org

The Autism Spectrum Program (ASP) at Howard Center provides intensive, specialized instructional and behavioral treatment and support services year-round to individuals with Autism Spectrum Disorders, ages 2-21 years. Services are provided in home, school, and community settings and target the teaching and shaping of essential communication, social, adaptive behavior, daily living, and functional learning skills. Multiple treatment methodologies under the principles of Applied Behavior Analysis are utilized.

INSPIRE for Autism
77 Dylan Rd.
Brattleboro, VT 05301
802-251-7301

info@inspireforautism.org
http://inspire4autism.com/

I.N.S.P.I.R.E. for Autism, Inc. will strive to maximize the potential for adolescents and young adults with Autism Spectrum Disorders to lead satisfying, self-sustaining lives in connection with their communities.

Virginia:

Alternative Paths Training School--Alexandria
5632 Mt. Vernon Memorial Highway
Alexandria, VA 22309
703-766-8708
Renee Loebs, Curriculum Specialist
rloebs@aptschool.org
www.aptschool.org

ATPS's mission is to provide students with the knowledge and practical skills essential for their successful integration into the community Locations in Alexandria and Fredericksburg.

Blue Ridge Autism Center
312 Whitwell Drive
Roanoke, VA 24019
540-366-7399
BRAC.1@juno.com
www.blueridgeautismcenter.com

BRAC is committed to providing resources and training to families and professionals throughout the Roanoke Valley and surrounding areas.

Dominion School for Autism
4205 Ravenswood Rd.
Richmond, VA 23222
804-355-1011
wendy.brown@dominionautism.org
www.dominionautism.org

The mission and educational philosophy of The Dominion School is to provide children with autism an individualized, ABA-based educational program in a loving and supportive atmosphere.

Spiritos School
400 Coalfield Road
Midlothian, Virginia 23113
804-897-7440
Janet@spiritosschool.com
www.spiritosschool.com

Our mission is to create a wealth of individualized instructional and treatment experiences that provide continual educational programming in an atmosphere of love and acceptance for children with autism and developmental delay.

The Aurora School
420 Wildman St.
Leesburg, VA 20176
540-751-1414
Courtney Deal, Program Director
cdeal@aurora-school.org

At Aurora, we believe that education works best for students and families when valid research findings from the fields of education and psychology, behavior analysis in particular, are constantly applied in the classroom, so teaching practices at the school are derived primarily from applied behavior analysis (ABA).

The Faison School
1701 Byrd Avenue
Richmond, VA 23230
804-612-1947
Dr. Kathy Mathews, Director of Education
kathy@kmaba.com
www.thefaisonschool.org

The Faison School for Autism/ACV is dedicated to giving each child the best chance he or she has to improve their life's journey by employing a three-pronged approach of empirically-driven treatment, research, and training to best serve our students. Our philosophy is a holistic one, focusing on the child, their family, and all those who touch and enrich their lives.

Virginia Institute for Autism
1414 Westwood Road
Charlottesville, VA 22901-5149
434-923-8252
information@viaschool.org
www.viaschool.org

VIA is dedicated to providing comprehensive, outcome-based education to people with autism; supporting families coping with the challenges that come with autism; and developing and supporting primary research, advocacy and training in the education of people with autism.

Washington:

DIR®/Floortime™ Summer Camp
20310 19th Ave NE
Shoreline, WA 98155
206-367-5853
Contact: Rosemary White, OTR/L, DIR® Faculty
pedptot@comcast.net

Various Locations:

Lovaas Institute
Various Locations
856-616-9442 (East Clinical Treatment Headquarters)
310-410-4450 (West Clinical Treatment Headquarters)
info@lovaas.com
www.lovaas.com

Intensive Applied Behavioral Analysis (ABA) Program that uses the Lovaas Method for autistic children ages 2 to 8 (children over the age of 5 qualify for consultative services, but not clinic-based services).

May Institute (Headquarters)
41 Pacella Park Drive
Randolph, MA 02368
781-440-0400
info@mayinstitute.org
www.mayinstitute.org

May Institute is one of the largest providers of private schools specifically serving children with autism. Our four May Centers for Child Development offer full-day, year-round educational services to children and adolescents with autism spectrum disorders (ASD) and other developmental disabilities. Schools are located in Massachusetts and California.

CANADA:

Autism Society Canada
PO Box 65
Orangeville
ON, L9W 2ZS
Canada
1-866-874-3334
info@autismsocietycanada.ca
www.autismsocietycanada.ca

Autism Society Canada's mission is to work with our many partners to address the national priorities facing the Autism community.

Camphill Communities Ontario
Angus, Ontario, Canada
http://www.camphill.on.ca

Camphill Communities Ontario, a life sharing endeavor serving people with developmental disabilities, has two locations: Camphill Nottawasaga is a rural community with adults and made up of several homes and workshops including woodwork, pottery, forestry and a vegetable garden. Our work is to care for each other, our homes, our gardens and our land. We share this work, each one according to his wishes and capabilities. The aim is to build a vital community life that offers each person the conditions for healing growth and renewal. Camphill Sophia Creek is developing residential workshop opportunities in an urban environment in the downtown core of Barrie, which is 1 hour north of Toronto.

The Cascadia Society

North Vancouver, British Columbia, Canada
http://www.cascadiasociety.org

The Cascadia Society is a life-sharing community that includes adults with special needs. Cultural, artistic and therapeutic experiences are provided through residential home care and day activities within the urban setting of Vancouver's North Shore. The Cascadia Society is dedicated to bringing healing to human beings and to the earth. Their primary task is to allow the potential in each person to unfold and to be in harmonious relationship with the environment.

The Ita Wegman Association of BC

Duncan, British Columbia, Canada
http://www.glenorafarm.com

The Ita Wegman Association of operates Glenora Farm, a rural, agriculturally based community for adults with special needs. The community operates a biodynamic farm. At Glenora Farm, those who are in need of special care, and those who provide it, relate to each other as companions, rather than as professionals and clients. In the way they live together, care for the land and in the things they make, they uphold the ideals of Camphill, in which each contributes what he or she is able to, and receives in turn what he or she needs.

St. Marcellinus School

730 Courtneypark Dr W
Mississauga, ON L5W 1L9, Canada
905-564-6614
Contact: Lynda Arsenault, Admissions
lynda.arsenault@dpcdsb.org
www.dpcdsb.org/MARCL

RECOMMENDED READING

Adams, Christina, *A Real Boy*. Berkley Books, 2005.

Bailey, Sally, *Wings to Fly: Bringing Theatre Arts to Studentswith Special Needs* (Woodbine House, 1993) and *Barrier-Free Drama*

Barbera, Mary Lynch, and Tracy Rasmussen. *The Verbal Behavior Approach: How to Teach Children with Autism and Related Disorders*. Jessica Kingsley Publishers, 2007.

Bluestone, Judith. *The Fabric of Autism: Weaving the Threads into a Cogent Theory*. The HANDLE Institute, 2004.

Bock, Kenneth, and Cameron Stauth. *Healing the New Childhood Epidemics: Autism, ADHD, Asthma, and Allergies: The Groundbreaking Program for the 4-A Disorders*. Ballantine Books, 2008.

Buckley, Julie A. *Healing Our Autistic Children: A Medical Plan*. Palgrave Macmillan 2010.

Casanova, Manuel F. Brain and *Brain, Behavior and Evolution* magazines, *Recent Developments in Autism Research* (Nova Biomedical Books, 2005), *Asperger's Disorder* (Medical Psychiatry Series) [Informa Healthcare, 2008], *Neocortical Modularity And The Cell Minicolumn* (Nova Biomedical Books, 2005)

Chauhan, Abha, Ved Chauhan, and Ted Brown, editors. *Autism: Oxidative Stress, Inflammation, and Immune Abnormalities*. CRC Press, 2009.

Chinitz, Judith Hope, *We Band of Mothers:Autism, My Son, and the Specific Carbohydrate Diet* (Autism Research Institute, 2007)

Davis, Dorinne S., *Every Day A Miracle: Success Stories through Sound Therapy*. Kalco Publishing LLC (October 6, 2004)

Davis, Dorinne. *Sound Bodies through Sound Therapy*. Kalco Publishing LLC, 2004.

Delaine, Susan K. *The Autism Cookbook: 101 Gluten-Free and Dairy-Free Recipes*. Skyhorse Publishing, 2010.

Fine, Aubrey, and Nya M. Fine, editors. *Therapeutic Recreation for Exceptional Children : Let Me In, I Want to Play*. Delta Society, 1996.

Fine and Eisen. *Afternoons with Puppy*. Purdue University Press 2008.

Fine, Aubrey. *The Handbook on Animal Assisted Therapy: Theoretical Foundations and Guidelines for Practice*. Academic Press, 1999.

Gabriels, R. "Art therapy with children who have autism and their families." *Handbook of art therapy*. Ed. C. Malchiodi. Guilford Press, 2003.

Grandin, Temple, *The Way I See It*. Future Horizons, 2011.

Goldberg, Michael J., with Elyse Goldberg. *The Myth of Autism: How a Misunderstood Epidemic Is Destroying Our Children*. Skyhorse Publishing, 2011.

Gottschall, Elaine G. *Breaking the Vicious Cycle: Intestinal Health Through Diet*. Kirkton Press, 1994.

Gillman, Priscilla, *The Anti-Romantic Child*. Harper Perennial.

Grandin, Temple and Catherine Johnson. *Animals in Translation Using the Mysteries of Autism to Decode Animal Behavior*. Houghton Mifflin Harcourt, 2005.

Greenspan, Stabley and Wieder, Serena. *Engaging Autism: Using the Floortime Approach to Help Children Relate, Communicate, and Think.* Da Capo Press, 2006.

Greenspan, Stanley, with Jacob Greenspan. *Overcoming ADHD: Helping Your Child Become Calm, Engaged, and Focused—Without a Pill.* Da Capo Lifelong Books, 2009.

Grinspoon, Lester, *Marihuana Reconsidered* (Harvard University press 1971, 1977, and American archives press classic edition, 1994) and *Marijuana, the Forbidden Medicine* (Yale University press, 1993, 1997)

Heflin, Juane, *Spectrum Disorders: Effective Instructional Practices* (Prentice Hall,2006)

Henley, D. R. *Exceptional children, exceptional art: Teaching art to special needs.* Worcester, MA: Davis Publications,1992.

Herskowitz, Valerie. *Autism & Computers: Maximizing Independence Through Technology.* AuthorHouse, 2009.

Heflin, L. Juane. *Students with Autism Spectrum Disorders: Effective Instructional Practices,* Prentice Hall, 2007.

Hogenboom, Marga. *Living with Genetic Syndromes Associated with Intellectual Disability.* Jessica Kingsley Publishers, 2001.

Jepson, Bryan Jepson. *Changing the Course of Autism: A Scientific Approach for Parents and Physicians.* Sentient Publications, 2007.

Kaufman, Barry Neil. *Son Rise: The Miracle Continues.* H J Kramer, 1994.

Kawar, Frick and Frick. *Astronaut Training: A Sound Activated Vestibular-Visual Protocol for Moving, Looking & Listening.* Vital Sounds LLC, 2006.

Kirby, David. *Evidence of Harm: Mercury in Vaccines and the Autism Epidemic: A Medical Controversy.* St. Martin's Press, 2005.

Kranowitz, Carol Stock, *The Out-of-Sync Child.* Perigee, 2005.

Lansky, Amy L. *Impossible Cure: The Promise of Homeopathy.* R.L. Ranch Press, 2003.

Lewis, Lisa. *Special Diets For Special Kids I & II.* Future Horizons, 2001.

Levinson, B. M. *Pet-oriented Child Psychotherapy.* Springfield, IL: Charles C. Thomas. 1969.

Lyons, Tony. *1,001 Tips for the Parents of Autistic Girls: Everything You Need to Know About Diagnosis, Doctors, Schools, Taxes, Vacations, Babysitters, Treatment, Food, and More.* Skyhorse Publishing, 2010.

Marohn, Stephanie. *The Natural Medicine Guide to Autism.* Hampton Roads Pub Co, 2002.

Martin, Nicole. *Art as an Early Intervention Tool for Children with Autism.* Jessica Kingsley Publishers, 2009.

Matthews, Julie. *Nourishing Hope for Autism: Nutrition Intervention for Healing Our Children, 3rd ed.* Healthful Living Media, 2008.

Maurice, Catherine. *Let Me Hear Your Voice: A Family's Triumph over Autism.* Ballantine Books, 1994.

McCandless, Jaquelyn. *Children with Starving Brains: A Medical Treatment Guide for Autism Spectrum Disorder, 4th ed.* Bramble Books, 2009.

McCarthy, Jenny and Jerry Kartzinel. *Healing and Preventing Autism: A Complete Guide.* Penguin, 2009.

McCarthy, Jenny. *Louder Than Words: A Mother's Journey in Healing Autism.* Penguin, 2007.

McCarthy, Jenny. *Mother Warriors.* Penguin, 2008.

Mehl-Madrona, Lewis, *Coyote Medicine* (Touchstone, 1998), *Coyote Healing* (Bear & Company, 2003) *Coyote Wisdom* (Bear & Company, 2005) *Narrative Medicine* (Bear & Company, 2007) and *Healing the Mind through the Power of Story: The Promise of Narrative Psychiatry* (Bear & Company (June 15, 2010)).

Noble, J. "Art as an instrument for creating social reciprocity: Social skills group for children with autism." *Group process made visible: Group art therapy.* Ed. S. Riley. Brunner-Routledge, 2001.

Pereira, Lavinia, and Solomon Michelle, *First Sound Series* by Trafford Publishing

Prizant, Barry, Amy Wetherby, Emily Rubin, Amy Laurent and P. Rydell. *The SCERTS Model: A Comprehensive Educational Approach for Children with Autism Spectrum Disorders.* Baltimore, MD: Paul H. Brookes Publishing, 2006.

Rimland, Bernard. *Infantile Autism: The Syndrome and Its Implication for a Neural Theory of Behavior.* Prentice Hall, 1964.

Rimland, Bernard, Jon Pangborn, Sidney Baker. *Autism: Effective Biomedical Treatments (Have We Done Everything We Can For This Child? Individuality In An Epidemic).* Autism Research Institute, 2005.

Rimland, Bernard, Jon Pangborn, Sidney Baker. *2007 Supplement - Autism: Effective Biomedical Treatments (Have We Done Everything We Can for This Child? Individuality In An Epidemic).* Autism Research Institute, 2007.

Robbins, Jim. *A Symphony in the Brain: The Evolution of the New Brain Wave Biofeedback.* Grove Press, 2008.

Rogers, Sally J. and Geraldine Dawson. *Early Start Denver Model For Young Children With Autism: Promoting Language, Learning, And Engagement.* Guilford Press, 2009.

Seroussi, Karyn. *Unraveling the Mystery of Autism and Pervasive Developmental Disorders.* Simon & Schuster, 2000.

Seroussi, Karyn and Lisa Lewis. *The Encyclopedia of Dietary Interventions for the Treatment of Autism and Related Disorders.* Sarpsborg Press, 2008.

Sicile-Kira, Chantal. *Autism Spectrum Disorders: The Complete Guide to Understanding Autism, Asperger's Syndrome, Pervasive Developmental Disorder, and Other ASDs.* Penguin, 2004.

Sicile-Kira, Chantal. *Adolescents on the Autism Spectrum: A Parent's Guide to the Cognitive, Social, Physical, and Transition Needs of Teenagers with Autism Spectrum Disorders.* Penguin, 2006.

Sicile-Kira, Chantal. *Autism Life Skills: From Communication and Safety to Self-Esteem and More —10 Essential Abilities Every Child Needs and Deserves to Learn.* Penguin, 2008.

Sicile-Kira, Chantal, *A Full Life with Autism.* Palgrave MacMillan, 2012.

Silva, Louisa. *Helping your Child with Autism: A Home Program from Chinese Medicine.* Guan Yin Press, 2010.

Silver, R. A. *Developing cognitive and creative skills through art: Programs for children with communication disorders or learning disabilities* (3rd ed. revised). New York: Albin Press 1989.

Siri, Kenneth, *1001 Tips for Parents of Autistic Boys.* Skyhorse Publishing, 2010.

Stagliano, Kim. *All I Can Handle: I'm No Mother Teresa: A Life Raising Three Daughters with Autism.* Skyhorse Publishing, 2010.

Theoharides, Theoharis C., *Pharmacology* (Essentials of Basic Science) (Little Brown and Company, 1992) *Essentials of Pharmacology* (Essentials of Basic Science) (Lippincott Williams & Wilkins, 1996)

Wiseman, Nancy D. *The First Year: Autism Spectrum Disorders: An Essential Guide for the Newly Diagnosed Child.* Da Capo Lifelong Books, 2009.

Wolfberg, Pamela J. *Play and Imagination in Children with Autism, 2nd ed.* Autism Asperger Publishing Company, 2009.

Woodward, Bob and Marga Hogenboom. *Autism: A Holistic Approach.* Floris Books, 2001.

Yasko, Amy. *Autism: Pathways to Recovery.* Neurological Research Institute, 2009.

Yasko, Amy. *Genetic Bypass: Using Nutrition to Bypass Genetic Mutations.* Neurological Research Institute, 2005.

REFERENCES

Chapter 1. Allergy Desensitization: An Effective Alternative Treatment for Autism, by Dr. Darin Ingels

1. Heuer L, Ashwood P, Schauer J, et al. Reduced levels of immunoglobulin in children with autism correlates with behavioral symptoms. *Autism Res.* 2008 Oct;1(5):275-83.
2. Careaga M, Van de Water J, Ashwood P. Immune dysfunction in autism: a pathway to treatment. *Neurotherapeutics.* 2010 Jul;7(3):283-92.
3. Trottier G, Srivastava L, Walker CD. Etiology of infantile autism: a review of recent advances in genetic and neurobiological research. *J Psychiatry Neurosci.* 1999;24(2):103-15.
4. Jyonouchi H. Autism spectrum disorders and allergy: observation from a pediatric allergy/immunology clinic. *Expert Rev Clin Immunol.* 2010 May;6(3):397-411.
5. Incorvaia C, Masieri S, Berto P, et al. Specific immunotherapy by the sublingual route for respiratory allergy. *Allergy Asthma Clin Immunol.* 2010 Nov 9;6(1):29.
6. Frati F, Scurati S, Puccinelli P, et al. Development of a sublingual allergy vaccine for grass pollinosis. *Drug Des Devel Ther.* 2010 Jul 21;4:99-105.
7. Scala G, Di Rienzo Businco A, Ciccarelli A, Tripodi S. An evidence based overview of sublingual immunotherapy in children. *Int J Immunopathol Pharmacol.* 2009 Oct-Dec;22(4 Suppl):23-6.
8. Pham-Thi N, de Blic J, Scheinmann P. Sublingual immunotherapy in the treatment of children. *Allergy.* 2006;61 Suppl 81:7-10.
9. Akdis CA, Barlan IB, Bahceciler N, Akdis M. Immunological mechanisms of sublingual immunotherapy. *Allergy.* 2006;61 Suppl 81:11-4.
10. O'Hehir RE, Sandrini A, Anderson GP, Rolland JM. Sublingual allergen immunotherapy: immunological mechanisms and prospects for refined vaccine preparation. *Curr Med Chem.* 2007;14(21):2235-44.

Chapter 3. Biofilm: A Cause of Chronic Gastrointestinal Issues in ASD, by Dr. John H. Hicks

1. Proal A. Understanding biofilms. *Bacteriality: Exploring Chronic Disease.* May 26, 2008. Available online at: http://bacteriality.com/2008/05/26/biofilm/
2. Parsek MR, Singh PK. Bacterial biofilms: an emerging link to disease pathogenesis. *Annu Rev Microbiol.* 2003;57:677-701.
3. Costerton JW, Stewart PS, Greenberg EP. Bacterial biofilms: a common cause of persistent infections. *Science.* 1999 May 21;284(5418):1318-22.
4. Higgins DA, Pomianek ME, Kraml CM, Taylor RK, Semmelhack MF, Bassler BL. The major Vibrio cholerae autoinducer and its role in virulence factor production. *Nature.* 2007 Dec 6;450(7171):883-6.
5. Singh PK, Schaefer AL, Parsek MR, Moninger TO, Welsh MJ, Greenberg EP. Quorum sensing signals indicate that cystic fibrosis lungs are infected with bacterial biofilms. *Nature.* 2000 Oct 12;407(6805):762-4.
6. Estrela AB, Wolf-Rainer A. Combining biofilm-controlling compounds and antibiotics as a promising new way to control biofilm infections. *Pharmaceuticals.* 2010;3(5):1374-93.
7. Cvitkovitch DG, Li YH, Ellen RP. Quorum sensing and biofilm formation in Streptococcal infections. *J Clin Invest.* 2003 Dec;112(11):1626-32.
8. Cho H, Jönsson H, Campbell K, Melke P, Williams JW, Jedynak B, et al. Self-organization in high-density bacterial colonies: efficient crowd control. *PLoS Biol.* 2007 Oct 30;5(11):e302.
9. Lewis K. Riddle of biofilm resistance. *Antimicrob Agents Chemother.* 2001 Apr;45(4):999-1007.
10. Stoodley P, Purevdorj-Gage B, Costerton JW. Clinical significance of seeding dispersal in biofilms: a response (Comment). *Microbiology.* 2005 Nov;151(11):3453.
11. Brockhurst MA, Hochberg ME, Bell T, Buckling A. Character displacement promotes cooperation in bacterial biofilms. *Curr Biol.* 2006 Oct 24;16(20):2030-4.
12. Jefferson KK. What drives bacteria to produce a biofilm? *FEMS Microbiol Letter.* 2004;236:163-73.

13. Waite RD, Struthers JK, Dowson CG. Spontaneous sequence duplication within an open reading frame of the pneumococcal type 3 capsule locus causes high-frequency variation. *Mol Microbiol.* 2001 Dec;42(5):1223-32.

14. Waterhouse JC, Perez TH, Albert PJ. Reversing bacteria-induced vitamin D receptor dysfunction is key to autoimmune disease. *Ann N Y Acad Sci.* 2009 Sep;1173:757-65.

15. Marphetia T. Chronic middle ear infections linked to resistant biofilm bacteria. Press release, Medical College of Wisconsin, July 11, 2006. Available online at: http://cmbi.bjmu.edu.cn/news/0607/41.htm.

16. Hall-Stoodley L, Costerton JW, Stoodley P. Bacterial biofilms: from the natural environment to infectious disease. *Nat Rev Microbiol.* 2004;2(2):95-108.

17. Morrison HI, Ellison LF, Taylor GW. Periodontal disease and risk of fatal coronary heart and cerebrovascular diseases. *J Cardiovasc Risk.* 1999 Feb;6(1):7-11.

18. Stewart R, Hirani V. Dental health and cognitive impairment in an English national survey population. *J Am Geriatr Soc.* 2007 Sep;55(9):1410-4.

19. Parracho HM, Bingham MO, Gibson GR, McCartney AL. Differences between the gut microflora of children with autistic spectrum disorders and that of healthy children. *J Med Microbiol.* 2005 Oct;54(10):987-91.

20. Ceri H, Olson ME, Stremick C, Read RR, Morck D, Buret A. The Calgary Biofilm Device: new technology for rapid determination of antibiotic susceptibilities of bacterial biofilms. *J Clin Microbiol.* 1999 Jun;37(6):1771 6.

21. Li YH, Lau PC, Lee JH, Ellen RP, Cvitkovitch DG. Natural genetic transformation of Streptococcus mutans growing in biofilms. *J Bacteriol.* 2001 Feb;183(3):897-908.

22. Singh PK, Parsek MR, Greenberg EP, Welsh MJ. A component of innate immunity prevents bacterial biofilm development. *Nature.* 2002 May 30;417(6888):552-5.

23. Starner TD, Shrout JD, Parsek MR, Appelbaum PC, Kim G. Subinhibitory concentrations of azithromycin decrease nontypeable Haemophilus influenzae biofilm formation and diminish established biofilms. *Antimicrob Agents Chemother.* 2008 Jan;52(1):137-45.

24. Marshall TG, Marshall FE. Sarcoidosis succumbs to antibiotics—implications for autoimmune disease. *Autoimmun Rev.* 2004 Jun;3(4):295-300.

25. Cogan NG, Cortez R, Fauci L. Modeling physiological resistance in bacterial biofilms. *Bull Math Biol.* 2005 Jul;67(4):831-53.

26. White A. *A Guide to Transfer Factors and Immune System Health*, 2nd ed. North Charleston: BookSurge Publishing, 2009.

27. Dusso AS, Brown AJ, Slatopolsky E. Vitamin D. *AJP-Renal Physiol.* 2005 Jul;289(1):F8-F28.

Chapter 4. Chelation: Removing Toxic Metals, by Dr. Michael Elice

"Treatment Options for Mercury/Metal Toxicity in Autism and Related Developmental Disabilities: Consensus Position Paper. Autism Research Institute. December 2004

Libutti, A., MD., Milivojevich, P.Eng.,M.Sc., Baker, Sidney, MD. Urinary Lead and Mercury Output with 10 versus 20mg/kg DMSA Suppositories. Unpublished Abstract

Shannon, M W, Townsend, MK. Adverse Effects of Reduced-Dose d-Penicillamine in Children With Mild-to-Moderate Lead Poisoning. Ann Pharmacotherapy. 2000;34:15-8

De Burbure, Buchet etal. Renal and Neurologic Effects of Cadmium, Lead, Mercury, and Arsenic in Children: Evidence of Early Effects of Multiple Interactions at the Environmental Exposure Levels. Environmental Health Perspectives. 5/11/2006.

Adams, J., Maral, M.,Bradstreet, J., El-Dahr, J., etal. Safety and Efficacy of Oral DMSA Therapy for Children with Autism Spectrum Disorders; Part B – Behavioral Results. BMC Clinical Pharacology 2009.9:17

Autism: A Unique Type of Mercury Poisoning. Bernard, Enayati, Roger, Binstock etal. ARC Research. 2000

Lee, BK, Schwartz, B etal. Provocative Chelation with DMSA and EDTA: Evidence for Differential Access to Lead Storage Sites. Occupational and Environmental Medicine 1995;52:1319.

Quig, DW. "Chronic Metal Toxicity: In Textbook of Natural Medicine, ed. J.E. Pizorno, 3rd edition, (2204)263-74

Gonzalez-Ramirez D, Maiorino RM, Zinga-Cahrles M. Sodium 2,3-dimercaptoptoptane-1-sulfonate challenge test for mercury in humans. J Pharmacol Exper Therapeutics. 1995;272:264-274

Markowitz ME, Rosen JF Assessment of lead stores in children: Validation of an 8-hour CANA2EDTA provocative test. J Pediatrics 1984;104: 337-341

Aposhian HV, Maiorino RM, Gonzalez-Ramirez D etal. Mobilization of heavy metals by newer, therapeutically useful chelating agents. Ann Rev Toxicol 1983;23;193-215

Grandjean P, Jacobsen IA, Jorgensen PJ. Chronic lead poisoning treated with dimercaptosuccinic acid. Pharmacol Toxicol 1991; 68:266-269

Besunder JB, Super DM, Anderson RL. Comparison of dimercaptosuccinic acid and calcium disodium ethylenediaminetetraacetic acid in children with lead poisoning. J Pediat 1997; 130: 966-971

Cory-Slecta DA, Weiss B, Cox C. Mobilization and redistribution of lead over the course of calcium disodium ehyl-enediamine tetraacetate chelation therapy. Pharmacol Exp Ther 1987;243:804-13

Cory-Slecta DA. Mobiization of lead over the course of DMSA chelation therapy and long-term efficacy. Pharmacol Exp Ther 1988; 246:84-91

Chapter 5. Enzymes for Digestive Support in Autism, by Dr. Devin Houston

1.   Ehren J, Moron B, Martin E, Bethune MT, Gray GM, Khosla C. A food-grade enzyme preparation with modest gluten detoxification properties. PLos ONE 4(7): e6313, 2009.
2.   Scalbert A, Johnson IT, Saltmarsh M. Polyphenols: antioxidants and beyond. Am. J. Clin. Nutr. 81 (S1):21, 2005.
3.   Scalbert A, Williamson G. Dietary intake and bioavailability of polyphenols. J. Nutr. 130:2073S, 2000.

Chapter 7. Flavonoid Formulation for Allergy-Like Symptoms and Brain Inflammation in Autism, by Dr. Theoharis Theoharides and Shahrzad Asadi

Akin C, Valent P, Metcalfe DD. Mast cell activation syndrome: Proposed diagnostic criteria. *J Allergy Clin Immunol.* 2010 Dec;126(6):1099-104.

Angelidou A, Alysandratos KD, Asadi S, Zhang B, Francis K, Vasiadi M, Kalogeromitros D, Theoharides TC. Brief report: "allergic symptoms" in children with Autism Spectrum Disorders. More than meets the eye? *J Autism Dev Disord.* 2011 Nov;41(11):1579-85.

Angelidou A, Asadi S, Alysandratos KD, Karagkouni A, Kourembanas S, Theoharides TC. Perinatal stress, brain inflammation and risk of autism-Review and proposal. *BMC Pediatrics.* 2012;In press.

Angelidou A, Francis K, Vasiadi M, Alysandratos KD, Zhang B, Theoharides A, Lykouras L, Sideri K, Kalogeromitros D, Theoharides TC. Neurotensin is increased in serum of young children with autistic disorder. *J Neuroinflammation.* 2010;7:48.

Asadi S, Theoharides T.C. CRH and extracellular mitochondria augment IgE-stimulated human mast cell VEGF release, which is inhibited by luteolin. *J Neuroinflammation.* 2012;In press.

Asadi S, Zhang B, Weng Z, Angelidou A, Kempuraj D, Alysandratos KD, Theoharides TC. Luteolin and thiosalicylate inhibit HgCl(2) and thimerosal-induced VEGF release from human mast cells. *Int J Immunopathol Pharmacol.* 2010;23:1015-1020.

Chen HQ, Jin ZY, Wang XJ, Xu XM, Deng L, Zhao JW. Luteolin protects dopaminergic neurons from inflammation-induced injury through inhibition of microglial activation. *Neurosci Lett.* 2008;448:175-179.

Dirscherl K, Karlstetter M, Ebert S, Kraus D, Hlawatsch J, Walczak Y, Moehle C, Fuchshofer R, Langmann T. Luteolin triggers global changes in the microglial transcriptome leading to a unique anti-inflammatory and neuroprotective phenotype. *J Neuroinflammation.* 2010;7:3.

Domitrovic R, Jakovac H, Milin C, Radosević-Stašić B. Dose- and time-dependent effects of luteolin on carbon tetra-chloride-induced hepatotoxicity in mice. *Exp Toxicol Pathol.* 2009;61:581-589.

Esposito P, Gheorghe D, Kandere K, Pang X, Connolly R, Jacobson S, Theoharides TC. Acute stress increases permeability of the blood-brain-barrier through activation of brain mast cells. *Brain Res.* 2001 Jan 5;888(1):117-127.

Formica JV, Regelson W. Review of the biology of quercetin and related bioflavonoids. *Food & Chemical Toxicology.* 1995;33:1061-1080.

Franco JL, Posser T, Missau F, Pizzolatti MG, Dos Santos AR, Souza DO, Aschner M, Rocha JB, Dafre AL, Farina M. Structure-activity relationship of flavonoids derived from medicinal plants in preventing methylmercury-induced mitochondrial dysfunction. *Environ Toxicol Pharmacol.* 2010 Nov 1;30(3):272-278.

Harwood M, Danielewska-Nikiel B, Borzelleca JF, Flamm GW, Williams GM, Lines TC. A critical review of the data related to the safety of quercetin and lack of evidence of in vivo toxicity, including lack of genotoxic/carcinogenic properties. *Food Chem Toxicol.* 2007 Nov;45(11):2179-205.

Jang S, Dilger RN, Johnson RW. Luteolin inhibits microglia and alters hippocampal-dependent spatial working memory in aged mice. *J Nutr.* 2010;140:1892-1898.

Jang SW, Liu X, Yepes M, Shepherd KR, Miller GW, Liu Y, Wilson WD, Xiao G, Blanchi B, Sun YE, Ye K. A selective TrkB agonist with potent neurotrophic activities by 7,8-dihydroxyflavone. *Proc Natl Acad Sci U S A.* 2010;107:2687-2692.

Jedrychowski W, Maugeri U, Perera F, Stigter L, Jankowski J, Butscher M, Mroz E, Flak E, Skarupa A, SowaA. Cognitive function of 6-year old children exposed to mold-contaminated homes in early postnatalperiod. Prospective birth cohort study in Poland.*Physiol Behav.* 2011 Oct 24;104(5):989-95.

Kandere-Grzybowska K, Kempuraj D, Cao J, Cetrulo CL, Theoharides TC. Regulation of IL-1-induced selective IL-6 release from human mast cells and inhibition by quercetin. *Br J Pharmacol.* 2006 May;148(2):208-15.

Kao TK, Ou YC, Lin SY, Pan HC, Song PJ, Raung SL, Lai CY, Liao SL, Lu HC, Chen CJ. Luteolin inhibits cytokine expression in endotoxin/cytokine-stimulated microglia. *J Nutr Biochem*. 2011;22:612-624.

Kawanishi S, Oikawa S, Murata M. Evaluation for safety of antioxidant chemopreventive agents. *Antioxid Redox Signal*. 2005;7:1728-1739.

Kempuraj D, Tagen M, Iliopoulou BP, Clemons A, Vasiadi M, Boucher W, House M, Wolfberg A, Theoharides TC. Luteolin inhibits myelin basic protein-induced human mast cell activation and mast cell dependent stimulation of Jurkat T cells. *Br J Pharmacol*. 2008;155:1076-1084.

Kempuraj D, Asadi S, Zhang B, Manola A, Hogan J, Peterson E, Theoharides Mercury induces inflammatory mediator release from human mast cells. *J Neuroinflamm*, in press, 2010.

Kempuraj D, Madhappan B, Christodoulou S, Boucher W, Cao J, Papadopoulou N, Cetrulo CL, Theoharides TC. Flavonols inhibit proinflammatory mediator release, intracellular calcium ion levels and protein kinase C theta phosphorylation in human mast cells. *Br J Pharmacol*. 2005 Aug;145(7):934-44.

Kempuraj D, Tagen M, Iliopoulou BP, Clemons A, Vasiadi M, Boucher W, House M, Wolfberg A, Theoharides TC. Luteolin inhibits myelin basic protein-induced human mast cell activation and mast cell-dependent stimulation of Jurkat T cells. *Br J Pharmacol*. 2008 Dec;155(7):1076-84.

Kimata M, Shichijo M, Miura T, Serizawa I, Inagaki N, Nagai H. Effects of luteolin, quercetin and baicalein on immunoglobulin E-mediated mediator release from human cultured mast cells. *Clin Exp Allergy*. 2000;30:501-508.

Li L, Gu L, Chen Z, Wang R, Ye J, Jiang H. Toxicity study of ethanolic extract of Chrysanthemum morifolium in rats. *J Food Sci*. 2010;75:T105-T109.

Middleton E Jr, Kandaswami C, Theoharides TC. The effects of plant flavonoids on mammalian cells: implications for inflammation, heart disease, and cancer. *Pharmacol Rev*. 2000 Dec;52(4):673-751.

Morgan JT, Chana G, Abramson I, Semendeferi K, Courchesne E, Everall IP. Abnormal microglial-neuronal spatial organization in the dorsolateral prefrontal cortex in autism. *Brain Res*. 2012 Mar 23.

Peters JL, Cohen S, Staudenmayer J, Hosen J, Platts-Mills TA, Wright RJ. Prenatal negative life events increases cord blood IgE: interactions with dust mite allergen andmaternal atopy. *Allergy*. 2012 Apr;67(4):545-51.

Skaper SD, Giusti P, Facci L. Microglia and mast cells: two tracks on the road to neuroinflammation. *FASEB J*. 2012 Apr 19.

Theoharides, TC. Autistic spectrum diseases and mastocytosis. *Intl J Immunopathol Pharmacol*. 2009 Oct-Dec;22(4):859-65.

Theoharides TC, Angelidou A, Alysandratos KD, Zhang B, Asadi S, Francis K, Toniato E, Kalogeromitros D. Mast cell activation and autism. *Biochim Biophys Acta*. 2012 Jan;1822(1):34-41.

Theoharides TC, Asadi S. Unwanted Interactions Among Psychotropic Drugs and Other Treatments for Autism Spectrum Disorders. *J Clinical Psychopharmacology*. In press.

Theoharides TC, Asadi S, Panagiotidou S. A case series of a luteolin formulation (Neuroprotek®) in children with autism spectrum disorders. *Int J Immunopathol Pharmacol*. In press.

Theoharides TC, Doyle R. Autism, gut-blood-brain barrier, and mast cells. *J Clin Psychopharmacol*. 2008 Oct;28(5):479-83.

Theoharides TC, Doyle R, Francis K, Conti P, Kalogeromitros D. Novel therapeutic targets for autism. *Trends Pharmacol Sci*. 2008 Aug;29(8):375-82.

Theoharides TC, Francis K, Vasiadi M, Sideri K, Chliva K, Christoni Z, Kempuraj K, Theoharides A, Kalogeromitros D. Increased serum neurotensin, IL-6 and IL-17 in young children with autism. *J Neuroimmunol*, 2010, in press.

Theoharides TC, Kalogeromitros D. The critical role of mast cells in allergy and inflammation. *Ann N Y Acad Sci*. 2006 Nov;1088:78-99.

Theoharides TC, Kempuraj D, Tagen M, Conti P, Kalogeromitros D. Differential release of mast cell mediators and the pathogenesis of inflammation. *Immunol Rev*. 2007 Jun;217:65-78.

Theoharides TC, Kempuraj D, Redwood L. Autism: an emerging 'neuroimmune disorder' in search of therapy. *Expert Opin Pharmacother*. 2009 Sep;10(13):2127-43.

Theoharides TC, Konstantinidou AD. Corticotropin-releasing hormone and the blood-brain-barrier. *Front Biosci*. 2007 Jan 1;12:1615-28.

Theoharides TC, Spanos C, Pang X, Alferes L, Ligris K, Letourneau R, Rozniecki JJ, Webster E, Chrousos GP. Stress-induced intracranial mast cell degranulation: a corticotropin-releasing hormone-mediated effect. *Endocrinology*. 1995 Dec;136(12):5745-50.

Verbeek R, Plomp AC, van Tol EA, van Noort JM. The flavones luteolin and apigenin inhibit in vitro antigen-specific proliferation and interferon-gamma production by murine and human autoimmune T cells. *Biochem Pharmacol*. 2004;68:621-629.

Zhang B, Angelidou A, Alysandratos KD, et al. Mitochondrial DNA and anti-mitochondrial antibodies in serum of autistic children. *J Neuroinflammation.* 2010;7:80.

Chapter 8. Gastrointestinal Disease: Emerging Concensus, by Dr. Arthur Krigsman

Afzal N, Murch S, Thirrupathy K, Berger L, Fagbemi A, Heuschkel R. Constipation with acquired megarectum in children with autism. Pediatrics. 2003 Oct;112(4):939–42.

Ashwood P, Wakefield AJ. Immune activation of peripheral blood and mucosal CD3+ lymphocyte cytokine profiles in children with autism and gastrointestinal symptoms. J Neuroimmunol. 2006 Apr;173(1-2):126–34.

Balzola F, Barbon V, Repici A, Rizzetto M. Panenteric IBD-like disease in a patient with regressive autism shown for the first time by the wireless capsule enteroscopy: another piece in the jigsaw of this gut-brain syndrome? Am J Gastro. 2005; 979–981.

Balzola F, Daniela C, Repici A, Barbon V, Sapino A, Barbera C, Calvo PL, Gandione M, Rigardetto R, Rizzetto M. Autistic enterocolitis: confirmation of a new inflammatory bowel disease in an Italian cohort of patients. Gastroenterology. 2005;128:Suppl.2;A–303.

Bolte ER. Autism and Clostridium tetani. Med Hypotheses. 1998 Aug;51(2):133–44.

Buie T, Campbell D, Fuchs G, Furuta G, Levy J, VandeWater J, Whitaker A, Atkins D, Bauman M, Beaudet A, Carr E, Gershon M, Hyman S, Jirapinyo P, Jyonouchi H, Kooros K, Kushak R, Levitt P, Levy S, Lewis J, Murray K, Natowicz M, Sabra A, Wershil B, Weston S, Zeltzer L, Winter H. Evaluation, Diagnosis, and Treatment of Gastrointestinal Disorders in Individuals With ASDs: A Consensus Report Pediatrics, Jan 2010; 125: S1 - S18.

Buie T, Fuchs G, Furuta G, Kooros K, Levy J, Lewis J, Wershil B, Winter H. Recommendations for Evaluation and Treatment of Common Gastrointestinal Problems in Children With ASDs Pediatrics, Jan 2010; 125: S19 - S29.

D'Eufemia P, Celli M, Finocchiaro R, Pacifico L, Viozzi L, Zaccagnini M, Cardi E, Giardini O. Abnormal intestinal permeability in children with autism. Acta Paediatr. 1996 Sep;85(9):1076–9.

Finegold SM, Molitoris D, Song Y, Liu C, Vaisanen ML, Bolte E, McTeague M, Sandler R, Wexler H, Marlowe EM, Collins MD, Lawson PA, Summanen P, Baysallar M, Tomzynski TJ, Read E, Johnson E, Rolfe R, Nasir P, Shah H, Haake DA, Manning P, Kaul A. Gastrointestinal microflora studies in late onset autism. Clin Infect Dis. 2002 Sep 1;35(Suppl 1):S6–S16.

Furlano RI, Anthony A, Day R, Brown A, McGavery L, Thomson MA, Davies SE, Berelowitz M, Forbes A, Wakefield AJ, Walker-Smith JA, Murch SH. Colonic CD8 and gamma delta T-cell infiltration with epithelial damage in children with autism. Pediatrics 2001;138:366–72.

Gonzalez L, Lopez K, Navarro D, Negron L, Flores L, Rodriguez R, Martinez M, Sabra A. Endoscopic and Histological Characteristics of the digestive mucosa in autistic children with gastrointestinal symptoms. Arch Venez Pueric Pediatr 69;1:19–25.

Horvath K, Papadimitriou JC, Rabazlan A. Gastrointestinal abnormalities in children with autistic disorder. J Pediatr 1999, 135:559–563.

Horvath K, Perman JA. Autistic disorder and gastrointestinal disease. Curr Opin Pediatr. 2002 Oct;14(5):583–7.

Jyonouchi, H, Geng, L, Ruby, A and Zimmerman-Bier, B. Dysregulated innate immune responses in young children with autism spectrum disorders: their relationship to gastrointestinal symptoms and dietary intervention. Neuropsychobiology, 2005;51(2):77-85.

Jyonouchi, H, Sun, S and Le, H. Proinflammatory and regulatory cytokine production associated with innate and adaptive immune responses in children with autism spectrum disorders and developmental regression. Journal of Neuroimmunology, 2001;120(1-2):170-179.

Knivsberg AM, Reichelt KL, Hoien T, Nodland M. A randomised, controlled study of dietary intervention in autistic syndromes. Nutr Neurosci. 2002 Sep;5(4): 251–61.

Knivsberg AM, Reichelt KL, Nodland M, Hoein T: Autistic Syndromes and Diet: a follow-up study. Scandinavian Journal of Educational Research 1995; 39: 223–236.

Knivsberg AM, Reichelt KL, Nodland M. Reports on dietary intervention in autistic disorders. Nutr Neurosci. 2001;4(1): 25–37.

Krigsman A, Boris M, Goldblatt A, Stott C. Clinical Presentation and Histologic Findings at Ileocolonoscopy in Children with Autistic Spectrum Disorder and Chronic gastrointestinal Symptoms. Autism Insights 2010:2 1–11.

Kuddo T, Nelson KB. How common are gastrointestinal disorders in children with autism. Curr Opin Pediatr 2003: 15(3); 339–343.

Kushak R, Winter H, Farber N, Buie T. Gastrointestinal symptoms and intestinal disaccharidase activities in children with autism. Abstract of presentation to the North American Society of Pediatric Gastroenterology, Hepatology, and Nutrition, Annual Meeting, October 20-22, 2005, Salt Lake City, Utah.

Melmed RD, Schneider CK, Fabes RA. Metabolic markers and gastrointestinal symptoms in children with autism and related disorders. J Pediatr Gastroenterol Nutr 2000:31(suppl 2)S31–32.

Parracho HM, Bingham MO, Gibson GR, McCartney AL. Differences between the gut microflora of children with autistic spectrum disorders and that of healthy children. J Med Microbiol. 2005 Oct;54(Pt 10):987–91.

Sandler RH, Finegold SM, Bolte ER, Buchanan CP, Maxwell AP, Vaisanen ML, Nelson MN, Wexler HM. Short-term benefit from oral vancomycin treatment of regressive-onset autism. J Child Neurol. 2000 Jul;15(7):429–35.

Song Y, Liu C, Finegold SM. Real-time PCR quantitation of clostridia in feces of autistic children. Appl Environ Microbiol. 2004 Nov;70(11):6459–65.

Torrente F, Machado N, Perez-Machado M, Furlano R, Thomson M, Davies S, Wakefield AJ, Walker-Smith JA, Murch SH. Enteropathy with T cell infiltration and epithelial IgG deposition in autism. Mol Psychiatry. 2002;7:375–382.

Torrente F, Anthony A. Heuschkel, RB, Thomson, M, Ashwood, P, Murch S. Focal-enhanced gastritis in regressive autism with features distinct from Crohn's disease and helicobacter Pylori gastritis. Am J Gastroenterol 2004 Apr;99(4):598–605.

Valicenti-McDermott M, McVicar K, Rapin I, Wershil BK, Cohen H, Shinnar S. Frequency of gastrointestinal symptoms in children with autistic spectrum disorders and association with family history of autoimmune disease. J Dev Behav Pediatr. 2006 Apr;27(2 Suppl):S128–36.

Wakefield AJ, Murch SH, Anthony A et al. Ileal-lymphoid nodular hyperplasia non-specific colitis and pervasive developmental disorder in children. Lancet. 1998;351:637–41.

Wakefield, AJ, Anthony, A, Murch, S, et al. Enterocolitis in Children with Developmental Disorders. American Journal of Gastroenterology, 2000;95(9):2285-2295.

Chapter 9. Biome Depletion, Helminths, and Autism, by Judith Chinitz

Ashwood, P., Anthony, A., Torrente, F., Wakefield, A. J. (2004). Spontaneous mucosal lymphocyte cytokine profiles in children with autism and gastrointestinal symptoms: mucosal immune activation and reduced counter regulatory interleukin-10. *Journal of Clinical Immunology, 24*(6): 664–673.

Ashwood, P., Wakefield, A. J. (2006). Immune activation of peripheral blood and mucosal CD3+ lymphocyte cytokine profiles in children with autism and gastrointestinal symptoms. *Journal of Neuroimmunology, 173*(1-2):126–134.

Bashir, M. E. H., Andersen, P., Fuss, I., Shi, H. N., Nagler-Anderson, C.

(2002). An enteric helminth infection protects against an allergic response to dietary antigen. *The Journal of Immunlogy, 169*: 3284–3292.

Becker, K. (2007). Autism, asthma, inflammation, and the hygiene hypothesis. *Medical Hypothesis,* doi:10.1016/j.mehy.2007.02.019.

Bilbo, S.D., Jones, J.P., Parker, W. (2012). Is autism a member of a family of diseases resulting from genetic/cultural mismatches? Implications for treatment and prevention. *Autism Research and Treatment*, volume 2012, article ID 910946.

Bilbo, S.D., Wray, G.A., Perkins, S.E., Parker, W. (2011). Reconstitution of the human biome as the most reasonable solution for epidemics of allergic and autoimmune diseases. *Medical Hypothesis*, 77 (2011), 494-504.

Careaga, M., Van de Water, J., Ashwood, P. (2010). Immune dysfunction in autism: a pathway to treatment. *Neurotherapeutics*, Jul;7(3):283-92.

Correale, J., Farez, M. (2007). Association between parasite infection and immune responses in multiple sclerosis. *Annals of Neurology, 61*: 97–108.

Croonenberghs, J., Bosmans, E., Deboutte, D., Kenis, G., Maes, M. (2002). Activation of the inflammatory response system in autism. *Neuropsychobiology, 45*(1):1–6.

Croese, J., O'Neil, J., Masson, J., Cooke, S., Melrose, W., Pritchard, D. Speare, R., (2006). A proof of concept study establishing Necator americanus in Crohn's patients and reservoir donors. *Gut, 55*: 136–137.

Diaz Heijtz, R., Wang, S., Anuar, F., Qian, Y., Bjork, B., Samuelsson, A., Hibberd, M.L., Forssberg, H., Pettersson, S. (2011). Normal gut microbiota modulates brain development and behavior. *Proceedings of the National Academy of Science*, [Epub ahead of print – retrieved February 12, 2011 from http://www.pnas.org/content/early/2011/01/26/1010529108.long].

Elliott, D. E., Summers, R. W., Weinstock, J. V. (2007). Helminths as governors of immune-mediated inflammation. *International Journal of Parasitology, 37*(5): 457–464.

Elliott, D. E., Summers, R. W., Weinstock, J. V. (2005). Helminths and the modulation of mucosal inflammation. *Current Opinion in Gastroenterology, 21*: 51–58.

Feillet, H., Bach, J.F. (2004). Increased incidence of inflammatory bowel disease: the price of the decline of infectious burden? Current Opinion in Gastroenterology:20(6):560–4.

Fumagalli, M., Pozzoli, U., Cagliani, R., Comi, G.P., Stefania, R., Clerici, M., Bresolin, N., Sironi, M. (2009). Parasites represent a major selective force for interleukin genes and shape the genetic predisposition to autoimmune conditions. *Journal of Experimental Medicine, 206*(6): 1395–1408.

Gupta, S., Aggarwal, S., Rashanravan, B., Lee, T. (1998). Th1- and Th2-like cytokines in CD4+ and CD8+ cells in autism. *Journal of Neuroimmunlogy, 85*(1): 106–109.

Hamilton, G. (2008). Why we need germs. The Ecologist Report. Retrieved August 4, 2008 from www.mindfullly. org/Health/We-Need-Germs.htm.

Hayes, K.S., Bancroft, A.J., Goldrick, M., Portsmouth, C., Roberts, I.S., Grencis, R.K. (2010). Explitation of the intestinal microflora by the parasitic nematode Trichuris muris. *Science,* June 11;328(5984):1391-4.

Jyonouchi, H., Sun, S., Le H. (2001). Proinflammatory and regulatory cytokine production associated with innate and adaptive immune responses in children with autism spectrum disorders and developmental regression. *Journal of Neuroimmunology: 120*(1-2):170–179.

Li, X., Chauhan, A., Sheikh, A.M., Patil, S., Chauhan, V., Li, X.M., Ji L., Brown, T., Malik, M. (2009). Elevated immune response in the brain of autistic patients. *Journal of Neuroimmunology, 207*(1-2):111–116.

Maizels, R. M., Yazdanbakhsh, M. (2003). Immune regulation by helminth parasites: cellular and molecular mechanisms. *Nature Reviews/Immunlogy,* volume 3.

Mangan, N.E., Fallon, R.E., Smith, P., van Rooijen, N., McKenzie, A.N., Fallon, P.G. (2004). Helminth infection protects mice from anaphylaxis via IL-10-producing B cells. *Journal of Immunology, 173*: 6346–6356.

Molloy, C. A., Morrow, A. L., Meinzen-Derr, J., Schleifer, K., Dienger, K., Manning-Courtney, P., Altaye, M., Wills-Karp, M. (2006). Elevated cytokine levels in children with autism spectrum disorders. *Journal of Neuroimmunlogy, 172*(1-2):198–205.

Newman, A.(1999). In pursuit of autoimmune worm cure. *The New York Times* on the Web. Retrieved March, 25, 2008 from http://query.nytimes.com/gst/fullpage.html?res=9A0DE6DB113BF932A0575BC0A96F958260&sc p=1&sq=in%20pursuit%20of%20an%20autoimmune%20cure&st=cse.

Parker, W. (2010). Reconstituting the depleted biome to prevent immune disorders. *The Evolution of Medicine Review*. Retrieved October 13, 2010 from http://evmedreview.com/?p=457 .

Parker, W. (2013). Evolutionary biology and anthropology suggest biome reconstitution as a necessary approach toward dealing with immune disorders. *Evolution, Medicine, and Public Health*, 2013, pp. 89-103.

Reddy, A., Fried, B. (2007). The use of Trichuris suis and other helminth therapies to treat Crohn's disease. *Parasitology Research, 100*: 921–927.

Rook, G. (2007). The hygiene hypothesis and the increasing prevalence of chronic inflammatory disorders. *Transactions of the Royal Society of Tropical Medicine and Hygiene, 101:* 1072–1074.

Rook, G., Lowry, C. A. (2008). The hygiene hypothesis and psychiatric disorders. *Trends in Immunology, 29*(4): 150–158.

Schnoeller, C., Rausch, S., Pillai, S., Avagyan, A., Wittig, B. M., Loddenkemper, C., Hamann, A., Hamelmann, E., Lucius, R., Hartmann, S. (2008). A helminth immunomodulator reduces allergic and inflammatory responses by induction of IL-10-producing macrophages. *The Journal of Immunology, 180*: 4265–4272.

Summers, R. W., Elliott, D. E., Qadir, K., Urban, J. F. Jr, Thompson, R., Weinstock, J. V. (2003). Trichuris suis seems to be safe and possibly effective in the treatment of inflammatory bowel disease. *American Journal of Gastroenterology Sep;*98(9):2034–2041.

Summers, R. W., Elliott, D. E., Urban, J. F. Jr, Thompson, R., Weinstock, J. V. (2005) Trichuris suis therapy in Crohn's disease. *Gut, 54*: 87–90.

Turner, J. D., Jackson, J. A., Faulkner, H., Behnke, J., Else, K. J., Kamgno, J., Boussinesq, M., Bradley, J. E. (2008). Intensity of intestinal infection with multiple worm species is related to regulatory cytokine output and immune hyporesponsiveness. *Journal of Infectious Diseases, 197*: 1204–1212.

Walk, S.T., Blum, A.M., Ewing, S.A., Weinstock, J.V., Young, V.B. Alterations of the murine gut microbiota during infection with the parasitic helminth Heligmosomoides polygyrus. *Inflammatory Bowel Disease*, Nov;16(11):1841-9.

Warren, R. P., Margaretten, N. C., Pace, N. C., Foster, A. (1986). Immune abnormalities in patients with autism. *Journal of Autism and Developmental Disorders, 16*(2):189–197.

Weinstock, J. V., Elliott, D. E. (2009). Helminths and the IBD Hygiene Hypothesis. *Inflammatory Bowel Disease, 15*(1):128–133.

Zaccone, P., Fehervari, Z., Phillips, J. M., Dunne, D. W., Cooke, A. (2006). Parasitic worms and inflammatory diseases. *Parasite Immunology, 28*: 515–523.

Zuk, Marlene. (2007). Riddled with Life: Friendly Worsm, Ladybug Sex, and the Parasites That Make Us Who We Are. Orlando: Harcourt Books.

Chapter 10. Intestine, Leaky Gut, and Autism: Is It Real and How to Fix It (Including with Probiotics), by Dr. Alessio Fasano

Fasano A. Pathological and therapeutical implications of macromolecule passage through the tight junction. *In* Tight Junctions. Boca Raton, FL: CRC Press, Inc., 2001, p. 697–722.

Fasano A. Physiological, pathological, and therapeutic implications of zonulin-mediated intestinal barrier modulation: living life on the edge of the wall. *Am J Pathol.* 173:1243–52, 2008.

White JF. Intestinal pathophysiology in Autism. *Exp Biol Med* 228:639–649, 2003.Prevalence of autism spectrum disorders - Autism and Developmental Disabilities Monitoring Network, United States, 2006. Autism and Developmental Disabilities Monitoring Network Surveillance Year 2006 Principal Investigators; Centers for Disease Control and Prevention (CDC). *MMWR Surveill Summ.* 2009; 58:1–20.

Buie T, Campbell DB, Fuchs GJ, III, et al Evaluation, Diagnosis, and Treatment of Gastrointestinal Disorders in Individuals With ASDs: A Consensus Report. *Pediatrics* 2010;125;S1–S18.

Buie T, Fuchs GJ, III, Furuta GT, Kooros K, Levy J, Lewis JD, Wershil BK, Winter H. Recommendations for Evaluation and Treatment of Common Gastrointestinal Problems in Children With ASDs. *Pediatrics* 2010;125;S19–S29

Guarner F Prebiotics, probiotics and helminths: the 'natural' solution? *Dig Dis.* 2009;27: 412–417. www.usprobiotics. org

Golnik AE, Ireland M., Complementary alternative medicine for children with autism: a physician survey. *J Autism Dev Disord.* 2009; 39: 996–1005.

Chapter 11. IVIG: Intravenous Immunoglobulin, by Dr. Michael Elice

Gupta, S, Aggarwal S., Heads, C. Dysregulated immune system in children with autism: beneficial effects of intravenous gamma globulin on autistic characteristics. J autism Dev disord 1996;26: 439–452.

Plioplys A V. Intravenous gamma globulin in children with autism. J Child Neurol 1998;13:79–82

Delgiudice-Asch G, Simon L, Schmeidler J, Cunningham-Rundles C, Hollander E. A pilot clinical triial of intravenous gamma globulin in childhood autism. *J Autism Dev Disord* 1999 199;29:157–160.

Boris M, goldblatt A, Galanko j, James J. Association of MTHFR gene variants with autism. *J Phys Surg* 2004;29:157–160.

National Institutes of Health. Intravenous immunoglobulin: prevention and treatment of disease. NIH consensus Statement 1990;8(2):1–23.

Latov N, Chaudhry V, Koski CL, Lisak RP Apatoff BR, Hahn AF, Howard AF. Use of intravenous gamma globulins in neuroimmunologic diseases. *J Allerg Clin Immunol* 2001;108:S126–132.

Comi AM, Zimmmerman AW, Frye VH, Law PA, Peeden JN. Familial Clustering of autoimmune disorders and evaluation of medical risk factors in autism. *J Child Neurol* 1999;14:388–394.

Swedo, SE. Sydenham's chorea: a model for childhood autoimmune neuropsychiatric disorders. *JAMA* 1994;272(22): 1788–1791.

Swedo SE, Rapoport JL, Cheslow DL, et al. High prevalence of obsessive-compulsive symptoms in patients with sydenham's chorea. *Am J Psychiatry.* 1989;46:335–341.

Swedo SE, Leonard HL, Garvey M, et al. Pediatric autoimmune neuropsychiatric disorders associated with streptococcal infections (PANDAS): a clinical description of the first fifty cases. Am J Psychiatry. 1998;155:264–271.

Giedd JN, Rapoport JL, Leonard HL, etal. Case study, acute basal ganglia enlargement and obsessive-compusive symptoms in an adolescent boy. J Am Acad Child Adolsc Pshychiatry. 1996;35(7):913–915

Garvey MA, Perlmutter SJ, Allen AJ, etal. A pilot study of penicillin prophylaxis for neuropsychiatric exacerbations triggered by streptococcal infections. Biol Psychiatry. 1999,45: 1564–1571

Barron KS, Sher MR, Silverman ED. Intravenous immunoglobulin therapy: magic or black magic. J Theumatol. 1992; 19:94–97

Perlmutter SJ, Leitman SF, Garvey MA etal. Therapeutic plasma exchange and intravenous immunoglobulin for obsessive-compulsive disorder and tic disorders in childhood. Lancet. 1999;50(6):429–439

Martino D, Defazio G, Giovannoni G. The PANDAS subgroup of tic disorders and childhood-onset obsessive-compulsive disorder. J Psychosom Res. 2009/Nov30;170(1):3–6

Gilbert DL, Kurlan R. PANDAS horse or zebra? Neurology. 2009 Oct 20;73(16):1252–3

Shulman ST. Pediatric autoimmune neuropsychiatric disorders associated with streptococci (PANDAS) update. Cuyrr Opin Pediatr. 2009 Feb;21(1): 127–30

Pavone P. Parano E, Rizzo R, Trifiletti RR.Autoimmune neuropsychiatric disorders associated with streptococcal infection: Sydenham chorea. PANDAS and PANDAS variants. J Child Neurol. 2006.Aug.21(8):678–689

Swedo SE, Grant PJ. Annotation: PANDAS: a model for human autoimmune disease. J child Psychol Psychiatry. 2005 Mar; 46(3): 227–34

Chapter 12. Medical Cannabis as a Treatment for Symptoms Associated with Autism Spectrum Disorders, by Nathan Coombs

The Yin and Yang of Medical Marijuana, full Text Available by: Lee, Martin A., Organica, Winter/Spring 2011, Vol. 25 Issue 71, p 9-31

The State of Clinical Cannabis Research in the United States, Full Text Available by: Stafford, Lindsay. HerbalGram, Feb-Apr 2010, Issue 85, p 64-68

A Novel Approach to the Symptomatic Treatment of Autism by: Grinspoon, Lester M.D., O'Shaughnessy's: The Journal of Cannabis in Clinical Practice, Spring 2010

Medical Marijuana 2010: It's Time To Fix the Regulatory Vacuum by: Cohen PJ, The Journal of Law, Medicine & Ethics: A Journal of Law, Medicine & Ethics: A Journal of the American Society of Law, Medicine & Ethics [J Law Med Ethics], ISSN: 1748-720X, 2010 Fall; Vol. 38 (3), pp. 654-66; PMID: 20880248

"Marijuana: An Effective Antiepileptic Treatment in Partial Epilepsy? A Case Report and Review of the Literature," by: Mortati Katherine MD., Reviews in Neurological Diseases, 2007 "Practical Strategies for Switching to Newer Atiepleptic Drugs." Reviews in Neurological Diseases, 2005

Medicalmarijuana.procon.org/view.resource.php?resourceID=000145

drugwarfacts.org/collection of categorized information on various aspects of the drug war

http://en.wikipedia.org/wiki/Controlled_Substances_Act

http://marijuana-as-medicine.org/Federal%20&%20State%20Law.html

http://autism.about.com/od/treatmentoptions/p/drugtreatments.html

http://travisithompson.net/frequentquestions/Medications%20Behavior/index.html

Chapter 13. Methyl-B$_{12}$: Myth or Masterpiece? by Dr. James Neubrander

1. Akesson B, Fehling C, Jagerstad M. Lipid composition and metabolism in liver and brain of vitamin B12-deficient rat sucklings. Br J Nutr. 1979 Mar;41(2):263-74.

2. Allen RH, Stabler SP, Lindenbaum J. Relevance of vitamins, homocysteine and other metabolites in neuropsychiatric disorders. Eur J Pediatr. 1998 Apr;157 Suppl 2:S122-6.

3. Allen RH, Seetharam B, Allen NC, Podell ER, Alpers DH. Correction of cobalamin malabsorption in pancreatic insufficiency with a cobalamin analogue that binds with high affinity to R protein but not to intrinsic factor. In vivo evidence that a failure to partially degrade R protein is responsible for cobalamin malabsorption in pancreatic insufficiency. J Clin Invest. 1978 Jun;61(6):1628-34.

4. Arnold GL, Hyman SL, Mooney RA, Kirby. RS.Plasma amino acids profiles in children with autism: potential risk of nutritional deficiencies. J Lab Clin Med. 1973 Apr;81(4):557-67.

5. Bachli E, Fehr J. [Diagnosis of vitamin B12 deficiency: only apparently child's play] Schweiz Med Wochenschr. 1999 Jun 12;129(23):861-72.

6. Banerjee R, Ragsdale SW. The many faces of vitamin B12: catalysis by cobalamin-dependent enzymes. Annu Rev Biochem. 2003;72:209-47.

7. Banerjee R. The Yin-Yang of cobalamin biochemistry. Chem Biol. 1997 Mar;4(3):175-86.

8. Berliner N, Rosenberg LE. Uptake and metabolism of free cyanocobalamin by cultured human fibroblasts from controls and a patient with transcobalamin II deficiency. Metabolism. 1981 Mar;30(3):230-6.

9. Berentsen S, Talstad I. [Homocysteine and methylmalonic acid. New tests—for what benefit?] Tidsskr Nor Laegeforen. 1996 Sep 20;116(22):2677-9.

10. Bhatt HR, Linnell JC. Vitamin B12 homoeostasis after haemorrhage in the rat: the importance of skeletal muscle. Clin Sci (Lond). 1987 Dec;73(6):581-7.

11. Bohr KC . [Effect of vitamin B12 on sleep quality and performance of shift workers] Wien Med Wochenschr. 1996;146(13-14):289-91.

12. Bolann BJ, Solli JD, Schneede J, Grottum KA, Loraas A, Stokkeland M, Stallemo A, Schjoth A, Bie RB, Refsum H, Ueland PM. Evaluation of indicators of cobalamin deficiency defined as cobalamin-induced reduction in increased serum methylmalonic acid. Clin Chem. 2000 Nov;46(11):1744-50.

13. Brandt LJ, Bernstein LH, Wagle A. Production of vitamin B 12 analogues in patients with small-bowel bacterial overgrowth. Ann Intern Med. 1977 Nov;87(5):546-51.

14. Burger RL, Schneider RJ, Mehlman CS, Allen RH. Human plasma R-type vitamin B12-binding proteins. II. The role of transcobalamin I, transcobalamin III, and the normal granulocyte vitamin B12-binding protein in the plasma transport of vitamin B12. J Biol Chem. 1975 Oct 10;250(19):7707-13.

15. Choi SW. Vitamin B12 deficiency: a new risk factor for breast cancer? Nutr Rev. 1999 Aug;57(8):250-3.

16. Csanaky I, Gregus Z. Effect of phosphate transporter and methylation inhibitor drugs on the disposition of arsenate and arsenite in rats. Toxicol Sci. 2001 Sep;63(1):29-36.

17. Culley, D.J., Raghavan, S.V., Waly, M., Baxter, M.G., Yukhananov, R., Deth, R.C. and Crosby, G. : Nitrous oxide decreases cortical methionine synthase transiently but produces lasting memory impairment in aged rats. Anesthesia and Analgesia 105: 83-88 (2007).

18. Delva MD. Vitamin B12 replacement. To B12 or not to B12? Can Fam Physician. 1997 May;43:917-22.

19. Deth, R., Muratore, C., Benzecry, J., Power-Charnitsky, V., and Waly, M. How environmental and genetic factors combine to cause autism: A Redox/Methylation Hypothesis. Neurotoxicology (Under Review).

20. Deth, R.C., Kuznetsova, A. and Waly, M.: Attention-related signaling activities of the D4 dopamine receptor in *Cognitive Neuroscience of Attention*, Michael Posner Ed., Guilford Publications Inc., New York (2004). p 269-282.

21. Deth RC., PhD, Molecular Aspects of Thimerosal-induced Autism; Congressional Testimony; October 6, 2003.

22. Deth, R.C. Molecular Origins of Attention: The Dopamine-Folate Connection Kluwer Academic Publishers (April, 2003)

23. Deth, R.C., Sharma, A. and Waly, M.: Dopamine-stimulated solid-state signaling: A novel role for single-carbon folates in human attention. In: Proc. 12th Int. Symp. Chem. Pteridines and Folates. Kluwer Academic Press (2002).

24. Donaldson, RM Jr: Intrinsic factor and the transport of cobalamin, in Johnson LR (ed): *Physiology of the Gastrointestinal Tract*, New York, Raven, 1981.

25. el Kholty S, Gueant JL, Bressler L, Djalali M, Boissel P, Gerard P, Nicolas JP. Portal and biliary phases of enterohepatic circulation of corrinoids in humans. Gastroenterology. 1991 Nov;101(5):1399-408

26. Ertel R, Brot N, Taylor R, Weissbach H. Studies on the nature of the bound cobamide in E. coli N5-methyltetrahydrofolate-homocysteine transmethylase. Arch Biochem Biophys. 1968 Jul;126(1):353-7.

27. Flippo TS, Holder WD Jr. Neurologic degeneration associated with nitrous oxide anesthesia in patients with vitamin B12 deficiency. Arch Surg. 1993 Dec;128(12):1391-5.

28. Fowler B. Genetic defects of folate and cobalamin metabolism. Eur J Pediatr. 1998 Apr;157 Suppl 2:S60-6.

29. Frenkel EP, Kitchens RL. Intracellular localization of hepatic propionyl-CoA carboxylase and methylmalonyl-CoA mutase in humans and normal and vitamin B12 deficient rats. Br J Haematol. 1975 Dec;31(4):501-13.

30. Frye R, Melnyk S, Fuchs G, Reid T, Jernigan S, Pavliv O, Hubanks A, Gaylor DW, Walters L, James SJ. Effectiveness of methylcobalamin and folinic acid treatment on adaptive behavior in children with autistic disorder is related to glutathione redox status. Hindawi Publishing Corporation, Autism Research and Treatment, Volume 2013, Article ID 609705, 9 pages; http://dx.doi.org/10.1155/2013/609705.

31. Funada U, Wada M, Kawata T, Mori K, Tamai H, Kawanishi T, Kunou A, Tanaka N, Tadokoro T, Mackawa A. Changes in CD4+CD8-/CD4-CD8+ ratio and humoral immune functions in vitamin B12-deficient rats. Int J Vitam Nutr Res. 2000 Jul;70(4):167-71.

32. Giannella RA, Broitman SA, Zamcheck N. Competition between bacteria and intrinsic factor for vitamin B 12 : implications for vitamin B 12 malabsorption in intestinal bacterial overgrowth. Gastroenterology. 1972 Feb;62(2):255-60.

33. Golenko OD, Ryzhova NI. [Transplacental effect of methylcobalamine on the growth of embryonic mouse kidney tissue in organotypic cultivation] Biull Eksp Biol Med. 1986 Apr;101(4):471-4.

34. Goto I, Nagara H, Tateishi J, Kuroiwa Y. Effects of methylcobalamin on vitamin B1- and B-deficient encephalopathy in rats. J Neurol Sci. 1987 Jan;77(1):97-102.

35. Hall CA, Begley JA, Chu RC. Methionine synthetase activity of human lymphocytes both replete in and depleted of vitamin B12. J Lab Clin Med. 1986 Oct;108(4):325-31.

36. Hall LL, George SE, Kohan MJ, Styblo M, Thomas DJ. In vitro methylation of inorganic arsenic in mouse intestinal cecum. Toxicol Appl Pharmacol. 1997 Nov;147(1):101-9.

37. Herbert V. Detection of malabsorption of vitamin B12 due to gastric or intestinal dysfunction. Semin Nucl Med. 1972 Jul;2(3):220-34.

38. Hogenkamp HP, Bratt GT, Sun SZ. Methyl transfer from methylcobalamin to thiols. A reinvestigation. Biochemistry. 1985 Nov 5;24(23):6428-32.

39. Honma K, Kohsaka M, Fukuda N, Morita N, Honma S. Effects of vitamin B12 on plasma melatonin rhythm in humans: increased light sensitivity phase-advances the circadian clock? Experientia. 1992 Aug 15;48(8):716-20.

40. Hvas AM, Ellegaard J, Nexo E. [Diagnosis of vitamin B12 deficiency—time for reflection] Ugeskr Laeger. 2003 May 5;165(19):1971-6.
41. Hvas AM, Ellegaard J, Nexo E. Vitamin B12 treatment normalizes metabolic markers but has limited clinical effect: a randomized placebo-controlled study. Clin Chem. 2001 Aug;47(8):1396-404.
42. Goto I, Nagara H, Tateishi J, Kuroiwa Y. Effects of methylcobalamin on vitamin B1- and B-deficient encephalopathy in rats. J Neurol Sci. 1987 Jan;77(1):97-102.
43. Ide H, Fujiya S, Asanuma Y, Tsuji M, Sakai H, Agishi Y. Clinical usefulness of intrathecal injection of methylcobalamin in patients with diabetic neuropathy. Clin Ther. 1987;9(2):183-92.
44. Imamura N, Dake Y, Amemiya T. Circadian rhythm in the retinal pigment epithelium related to vitamin B12. Life Sci. 1995;57(13):1317-23.
45. Isoyama R, Baba Y, Harada H, Kawai S, Shimizu Y, Fujii M, Fujisawa S, Takihara H, Koshido Y, Sakatoku J. [Clinical experience of methylcobalamin (CH3-B12)/clomiphene citrate combined treatment in male infertility] Hinyokika Kiyo. 1986 Aug;32(8):1177-83.
46. Jalaludin MA. Methylcobalamin treatment of Bell's palsy. Methods Find Exp Clin Pharmacol. 1995 Oct;17(8):539-44.
47. James SJ, Melnyk S, Jernigan S, Cleves MA, Halsted CH, Wong DH, Cutler P, Bock K, Boris M, Bradstreet JJ, Baker SM, Gaylor DW. Metabolic endophenotype and related genotypes are associated with oxidative stress in children with autism. Am J Med Genet B Neuropsychiatr Genet. 2006 Dec 5;141(8):947-56.
48. James SJ, Slikker W 3rd, Melnyk S, New E, Pogribna M, Jernigan S. Thimerosal neurotoxicity is associated with glutathione depletion: protection with glutathione precursors. Neurotoxicology. 2005 Jan;26(1):1-8.
49. James SJ, Cutler P, Melnyk S, Jernigan S, Janak L, Gaylor DW, Neubrander JA. Metabolic biomarkers of increased oxidative stress and impaired methylation capacity in children with autism. Am. J. Clinical Nutrition, Dec 2004; 80: 1611–1617.
50. Jin X, Jin X, Sheng X. Methylcobalamin as antagonist to transient ototoxic action of gentamicin. Acta Otolaryngol. 2001 Apr;121(3):351-4.
51. Kaji R, Kodama M, Imamura A, Hashida T, Kohara N, Ishizu M, Inui K, Kimura J. Effect of ultrahigh-dose methylcobalamin on compound muscle action potentials in amyotrophic lateral sclerosis: a double-blind controlled study. Muscle Nerve. 1998 Dec;21(12):1775-8.
52. Kal'nev VR, Rachkus IuA, Kanopkaite SI. [Cobalamins and tRNA methyltransferase activity in E. coli cells] Biokhimiia. 1981 Oct;46(10):1773-9.
53. Kapadia CR. Vitamin B12 in health and disease: part I—inherited disorders of function, absorption, and transport. Gastroenterologist. 1995 Dec;3(4):329-44.
54. Kasuya M. The effect of methylcobalamin on the toxicity of methylmercury and mercuric chloride on nervous tissue in culture. Toxicol Lett. 1980 Nov;7(1):87-93.
55. Kawata T, Tashiro A, Tamiki A, Suga K, Kamioka S, Yamada K, Wada M, Tadokoro T, Maekawa A. Utilization of dietary protein in the vitamin B12-deficient rats. Int J Vitam Nutr Res. 1995;65(4):248-54.
56. Kelly GS. Folates: supplemental forms and therapeutic applications. Altern Med Rev. 1998 Jun;3(3):208-20.
57. Kosonen T, Pihko H. [Development regression in a child caused by vitamin B12 deficiency] Duodecim. 1994;110(6):588-91.
58. Kiuchi T, Sei H, Seno H, Sano A, Morita Y. Effect of vitamin B12 on the sleep-wake rhythm following an 8-hour advance of the light-dark cycle in the rat. Physiol Behav. 1997 Apr;61(4):551-4.
59. Kolhouse JF, Allen RH. Recognition of two intracellular cobalamin binding proteins and their identification as methylmalonyl-CoA mutase and methionine synthetase. Proc Natl Acad Sci U S A. 1977 Mar;74(3):921-5.
60. Kubota K, Kurabayashi H, Kawada E, Okamoto K, Shirakura T. Restoration of abnormally high CD4/CD8 ratio and low natural killer cell activity by vitamin B12 therapy in a patient with post-gastrectomy megaloblastic anemia. Intern Med. 1992 Jan;31(1):125-6.
61. Kurimoto S, Iwasaki T, Nomura T, Noro K, Yamamoto S. Influence of VDT (visual display terminals) work on eye accommodation. J UOEH. 1983 Mar 1;5(1):101-10
62. Kuwabara S, Nakazawa R, Azuma N, Suzuki M, Miyajima K, Fukutake T, Hattori T. Intravenous methylcobalamin treatment for uremic and diabetic neuropathy in chronic hemodialysis patients. Intern Med. 1999 Jun;38(6):472-5.
63. Kuznetsova, A.Y., and Deth, R.C.: A model for gamma oscillations induced by D4 dopamine receptor-mediated phospholipid methylation. J. Computational Neuroscience (Under Review).
64. Lindstedt G. [Nitrous oxide can cause cobalamin deficiency. Vitamin B12 is a simple and cheap remedy] Lakartidningen. 1999 Nov 3;96(44):4801-5.
65. Linnell JC, Wilson MJ, Mikol YB, Poirier LA. Tissue distribution of methylcobalamin in rats fed amino acid-defined, methyl-deficient diets. J Nutr. 1983 Jan;113(1):124-30.

66. Linnel JC: The fate of cobalamin in vivo, in Babior BM (ed): *Cobalamin Biochemistry and Pathophysiology,* New York, Wiley, 1975, p287.

67. Maltin CA, Duncan L, Wilson AB. Mitochondrial abnormalities in muscle from vitamin B12-deficient sheep. J Comp Pathol. 1983 Jul;93(3):429-35.

68. Marsh EN. Coenzyme B12 (cobalamin)-dependent enzymes. Essays Biochem. 1999;34:139-54.

69. Masson C. [Combined sclerosis of the spinal cord «revisited»] Presse Med. 1999 Nov 27;28(37):2048-9.

70. Matthews RG. Cobalamin-dependent methyltransferases. Acc Chem Res. 2001 Aug;34(8):681-9.

71. McCaddon A, Regland B, Hudson P, Davies G. Functional vitamin B(12) deficiency and Alzheimer disease. Neurology. 2002 May 14;58(9):1395-9.

72. Mellman IS, Youngdahl-Turner P, Willard HF, Rosenberg LE. Intracellular binding of radioactive hydroxocobalamin to cobalamin-dependent apoenzymes in rat liver. Proc Natl Acad Sci U S A. 1977 Mar;74(3):916-20.

73. Metz J. Cobalamin deficiency and the pathogenesis of nervous system disease. Annu Rev Nutr. 1992;12:59-79.

74. Mikhailov VV, Rusanova AG, Chikina NA, Avakumov VM. [Effect of methylcobalamine on the processes of posttraumatic regeneration of the salivary glands] Biull Eksp Biol Med. 1984 Jul;98(7):95-7.

75. Mori K, Kaido M, Fujishiro K, Inoue N, Ide Y, Koide O. Preventive effects of methylcobalamin on the testicular damage induced by ethylene oxide. Arch Toxicol. 1991;65(5):396-401.

76. Moriyama H, Nakamura K, Sanda N, Fujiwara E, Seko S, Yamazaki A, Mizutani M, Sagami K, Kitano T. [Studies on the usefulness of a long-term, high-dose treatment of methylcobalamin in patients with oligozoospermia] Hinyokika Kiyo. 1987 Jan;33(1):151-6.

77. Nishizawa Y, Goto HG, Tanigaki Y, Fushiki S, Nishizawa Y. Induction of apoptosis in an androgen-dependent mouse mammary carcinoma cell line by methylcobalamin. Anticancer Res. 2001 Mar-Apr;21(2A):1107-10.

78. Nishizawa Y, Yamamoto T, Tanigaki Y, Kasugai T, Mano M, Ishiguro S, Fushiki S, Poirier LA, Nishizawa Y. Methylcobalamin decreases mRNA levels of androgen-induced growth factor in androgen-dependent Shionogi carcinoma 115 cells. Nutr Cancer. 1999;35(2):195-201.

79. [No authors listed] Vitamin B12, cognitive impairment, survival and HHV-6A. Posit Health News. 1998 Spring;(No 16):12-3.

80. [No authors listed] Methylcobalamin. Altern Med Rev. 1998 Dec;3(6):461 3.

81. Ohta T, Iwata T, Kayukawa Y, Okada T. Daily activity and persistent sleep-wake schedule disorders. Prog Neuropsychopharmacol Biol Psychiatry. 1992 Jul;16(4):529-37.

82. Okada K, Tanaka H, Temporin K, Okamoto M, Kuroda Y, Moritomo H, Murase T, Yoshikawa H., Methylcobalamin increases Erk1/2 and Akt activity through the methylation cycle and promotes nerve regeneration in a rat sciatic nerve injury model, Exp Neurol. 2010 Apr;222(2):191-203.

83. Okawa M, Mishima K, Nanami T, Shimizu T, Iijima S, Hishikawa Y, Takahashi K. Vitamin B12 treatment for sleep-wake rhythm disorders. Sleep. 1990 Feb;13(1):15-23.

84. Okuda K, Yashima K, Kitazaki T, Takara I. Intestinal absorption and concurrent chemical changes of methylcobalamin. J Lab Clin Med. 1973 Apr;81(4):557-67.

85. Pan-Hou HS, Imura N. Involvement of mercury methylation in microbial mercury detoxication. Arch Microbiol. 1982 Mar;131(2):176-7.

86. Pema PJ, Horak HA, Wyatt RH. Myelopathy caused by nitrous oxide toxicity. AJNR Am J Neuroradiol. 1998 May;19(5):894-6.

87. Peracchi M, Bamonti Catena F, Pomati M, De Franceschi M, Scalabrino G. Human cobalamin deficiency: alterations in serum tumour necrosis factor-alpha and epidermal growth factor. Eur J Haematol. 2001 Aug;67(2):123-7.

88. Pfohl-Leszkowicz A, Keith G, Dirheimer G. Effect of cobalamin derivatives on in vitro enzymatic DNA methylation: methylcobalamin can act as a methyl donor. Biochemistry. 1991 Aug 13;30(32):8045-51.

89. Raux E, Schubert HL, Warren MJ. Biosynthesis of cobalamin (vitamin B12): a bacterial conundrum. Cell Mol Life Sci. 2000 Dec;57(13-14):1880-93.

90. Ray JG, Cole DE, Boss SC. An Ontario-wide study of vitamin B12, serum folate, and red cell folate levels in relation to plasma homocysteine: is a preventable public health issue on the rise?. Clin Biochem. 2000 Jul;33(5):337-43.

91. Reynolds EH, Bottiglieri T, Laundy M, Stern J, Payan J, Linnell J, Faludy J. Subacute combined degeneration with high serum vitamin B12 level and abnormal vitamin B12 binding protein. New cause of an old syndrome. Arch Neurol. 1993 Jul;50(7):739-42.

92. Rosenblatt DS, Fenton WA: Inborn errors of cobalamin metabolism, in Banerjee R (ed): *Chemistry and Biology of B12*: New York, John Wiley, 1999, p. 367.

93. Scalabrino G, Buccellato FR, Veber D, Mutti E. New basis of the neurotrophic action of vitamin B12. Clin Chem Lab Med. 2003 Nov;41(11):1435-7.

94.   Scalabrino G, Tredici G, Buccellato FR, Manfridi A. Further evidence for the involvement of epidermal growth factor in the signaling pathway of vitamin B12 (cobalamin) in the rat central nervous system. J Neuropathol Exp Neurol. 2000 Sep;59(9):808-14.

95.   Scriver, Charles R., et. al, 2001. The Metabolic and Molecular Bases of Inherited Disease, 8th Edition, McGraw Hill Medical Publishing Division: New York, St. Louis, San Francisco. pp. 2164-2193; pp. 3896-3933.

96.   Seetharam B: Gastrointestinal absorption and transport of cobalamin (vitamin B12) in Johnson LR (ed): *Physiology of the Gastrointestinal Tract*, New York, Raven, 1997.

97.   Sennett C, Rosenberg LE, Mellman IS. Transmembrane transport of cobalamin in prokaryotic and eukaryotic cells. Annu Rev Biochem. 1981;50:1053-86.

98.   Sharma, A. and Deth, R.C.: Protein kinase C regulates basal and D4 dopamine receptor-mediated phospholipid methylation in neuroblastoma cells. Eur. J. Pharmacol. 427: 83-90 (2001).

99.   Sharma, A., Kramer, M., Wick, P.F., Liu, D., Chari, S., Shim, S., Tan, W.-B., Ouellette, D., Nagata, M., DuRand, C., Kotb, M. and Deth, R.C.: Dopamine D4 receptor-mediated methylation of membrane phospholipids and its implications for mental illnesses such as schizophrenia. Molecular Psychiatry 4: 235-246 (1999).

100. Shimizu N, Hamazoe R, Kanayama H, Maeta M, Koga S. Experimental study of antitumor effect of methyl-B12. Oncology. 1987;44(3):169-73

101. Small DH, Carnegie PR, Anderson RM. Cycloleucine-induced vacuolation of myelin is associated with inhibition of protein methylation. Neurosci Lett. 1981 Feb 6;21(3):287-92.

102. Sponne IE, Gaire D, Stabler SP, Droesch S, Barbe FM, Allen RH, Lambert DA, Nicolas JP. Inhibition of vitamin B12 metabolism by OH-cobalamin c-lactam in rat oligodendrocytes in culture: a model for studying neuropathy due to vitamin B12 deficiency. Neurosci Lett. 2000 Jul 21;288(3):191-4.

103. Takahashi K, Okawa M, Matsumoto M, Mishima K, Yamadera H, Sasaki M, Ishizuka Y, Yamada K, Higuchi T, Okamoto N, Furuta H, Nakagawa H, Ohta T, Kuroda K, Sugita Y, Inoue Y, Uchimura N, Nagayama H, Miike T, Kamei K. Double-blind test on the efficacy of methylcobalamin on sleep-wake rhythm disorders. Psychiatry Clin Neurosci. 1999 Apr;53(2):211-3.

104. Takase M, Taira M, Sasaki H. Sleep-wake rhythm of autistic children. Psychiatry Clin Neurosci. 1998 Apr;52(2):181-2.

105. Taniguchi H, Ejiri K, Baba S. Improvement of autonomic neuropathy after mecobalamin treatment in uremic patients on hemodialysis. Clin Ther. 1987;9(6):607-14

106. Tashiro S, Sudou K, Imoh A, Koide M, Akazawa Y. Phosphatidylethanolamine methyltransferase activity in developing, demyelinating, and diabetic mouse brain. Tohoku J Exp Med. 1983 Dec;141 Suppl:485-90.

107. Taylor RT, Weissbach H. Escherichia coli B N5-methyltetrahydrofolate-homocysteine methyltransferase: sequential formation of bound methylcobalamin with S-adenosyl-L-methionine and N5-methyltetrahydrofolate. Arch Biochem Biophys. 1969 Feb;129(2):728-44.

108. Taylor RT, Weissbach H. Escherichia coli B N5-methyltetrahydrofolate-homocysteine vitamin-B12 transmethylase: formation and photolability of a methylcobalamin enzyme. Arch Biochem Biophys. 1968 Jan;123(1):109-26.

109. Taylor RT, Weissbach H. Enzymic synthesis of methionine: formation of a radioactive cobamide enzyme with N5-methyl-14C-tetrahydrofolate. Arch Biochem Biophys. 1967 Mar;119(1):572-9.

110. Tefferi A, Pruthi RK. The biochemical basis of cobalamin deficiency. Mayo Clin Proc. 1994 Feb;69(2):181-6.

111. Tomczyk A, Helewski K, Glowacka M, Konecki J, Stepien M. [Neurological picture and selected diagnostic indices of vitamin b12 malabsorption syndrome]

112. [Neurological picture and selected diagnostic indices of vitamin b12 malabsorption syndrome] Wiad Lek. 2001;54(5-6):305-10.

113. Tomoda A, Miike T, Matsukura M. Circadian rhythm abnormalities in adrenoleukodystrophy and methyl B12 treatment. Brain Dev. 1995 Nov-Dec;17(6):428-31.

114. Toskes PP, Hansell J, Cerda J, Deren JJ. Vitamin B 12 malabsorption in chronic pancreatic insufficiency. N Engl J Med. 1971 Mar 25;284(12):627-32.

115. Tsao CS, Miyashita K, Young M. Cytotoxic activity of cobalamin in cultured malignant and nonmalignant cells. Pathobiology. 1990;58(5):292-6.

116. Tsao CS, Myashita K. Influence of cobalamin on the survival of mice bearing ascites tumor. Pathobiology. 1993;61(2):104-8

117. Turley CP, Brewster MA. Alpha-tocopherol protects against a reduction in adenosylcobalamin in oxidatively stressed human cells. J Nutr. 1993 Jul;123(7):1305-12.

118. Tsukerman ES, Korsova TL, Poznanskaia AA. [Cobalamins in normal and pathological states (review)] Vopr Med Khim. 1985 Sep-Oct;31(5):7-17.

119. Uchiyama M, Mayer G, Okawa M, Meier-Ewert K. Effects of vitamin B12 on human circadian body temperature rhythm. Neurosci Lett. 1995 Jun 2;192(1):1-4.

120. Van Hove JL, Van Damme-Lombaerts R, Grunewald S, Peters H, Van Damme B, Fryns JP, Arnout J, Wevers R, Baumgartner ER, Fowler B. Cobalamin disorder Cbl-C presenting with late-onset thrombotic microangiopathy. Am J Med Genet. 2002 Aug 1;111(2):195-201.

121. Vieira-Makings E, van der Westhuyzen J, Metz J. Both valine and isoleucine supplementation delay the development of neurological impairment in vitamin B12 deficient bats. Int J Vitam Nutr Res. 1990;60(1):41-6.

122. Vitols E, Walker GA, Huennekens FM. Enzymatic conversion of vitamin B-12s to a cobamide coenzyme, alpha-(5,6-dimethylbenzimidazolyl)deoxyadenosylcobamide (adenosyl-B-12). J Biol Chem. 1966 Apr 10;241(7):1455-61.

123. Wada M, Kawata T, Yamada K, Funada U, Kuwamori M, Endo M, Tanaka N, Tadokoro T, Maekawa A. Serum C3 content in vitamin B(12)-deficient rats. Int J Vitam Nutr Res. 1998;68(2):94-7.

124. Walker GA, Murphy S, Huennekens FM. Enzymatic conversion of vitamin B 12a to adenosyl-B 12: evidence for the existence of two separate reducing systems. Arch Biochem Biophys. 1969 Oct;134(1):95-102.

125. Waly, M, and Deth, R.C.: Glutathione and methylcobalamin-dependent methionine synthase activity in neuronal cells: Implications for neurodevelopmental and neurodegenerative disorders. (In Preparation).

126. Waly, M., Power Charnitsky, V., Deth, R.C.: Reduced activation of phospholipid methylation by the seven-repeat variant of the D4 dopamine receptor. Eur. J. Pharmacol. (Submitted).

127. Waly, M., Banerjee, R., Choi, S.W., Mason, J., Benzecry, J., Power-Charnitsky, V.A, Deth, R.C. PI3-kinase regulates methionine synthase: Activation by IGF-1 or dopamine and inhibition by heavy metals and thimerosal Molecular Psychiatry 9: 358-370 (2004).

128. Waly M, Olteanu H, Banerjee R, Choi SW, Mason JB, Parker BS, Sukumar S, Shim S, Sharma A, Benzecry JM, Power-Charnitsky VA, Deth RC. Activation of methionine synthase by insulin-like growth factor-1 and dopamine: a target for neurodevelopmental toxins and thimerosal. Mol Psychiatry. 2004 Jan 27 [Epub ahead of print]

129. Wang FK, Koch J, Stokstad EL. Folate coenzyme pattern, folate linked enzymes and methionine biosynthesis in rat liver mitochondria. Biochem J. 1967 Jan 27;346(5):458-66.

130. Watanabe F, Nakano Y. [Vitamin B12] Nippon Rinsho. 1999 Oct;57(10):2205 10.

131. Weinberg JR, Shugars DC, Sherman PA, Sauls DL, Fyfe JA. Cobalamin inhibition of HIV-1 integrase and integration of HIV-1 DNA into cellular DNA. Biochem Biophys Res Commun. 1998 May 19;246(2):393-7.

132. Weir DG, Scott JM. The biochemical basis of the neuropathy in cobalamin deficiency. Baillieres Clin Haematol. 1995 Sep;8(3):479-97.

133. Weissbach H, Taylor R. Role of vitamin B12 in methionine synthesis. Fed Proc. 1966 Nov-Dec;25(6):1649-56.

134. Yagihashi S, Tokui A, Kashiwamura H, Takagi S, Imamura K. In vivo effect of methylcobalamin on the peripheral nerve structure in streptozotocin diabetic rats. Horm Metab Res. 1982 Jan;14(1):10-3.

135. Yamadera H, Takahashi K, Okawa M. A multicenter study of sleep-wake rhythm disorders: therapeutic effects of vitamin B12, bright light therapy, chronotherapy and hypnotics. Psychiatry Clin Neurosci. 1996 Aug;50(4):203-9.

136. Yamashiki M, Nishimura A, Kosaka Y. Effects of methylcobalamin (vitamin B12) on in vitro cytokine production of peripheral blood mononuclear cells. J Clin Lab Immunol. 1992;37(4):173-82

137. Yaqub BA, Siddique A, Sulimani R. Effects of methylcobalamin on diabetic neuropathy. Clin Neurol Neurosurg. 1992;94(2):105-11.

138. Yeomans ND, St John DJ. Small intestinal malabsorption of vitamin B(12) in iron-deficient rats. Pathology. 1975 Jan;7(1):35-44.

139. Youngdahl-Turner P, Mellman IS, Allen RH, Rosenberg LE. Protein mediated vitamin uptake. Adsorptive endocytosis of the transcobalamin II-cobalamin complex by cultured human fibroblasts. Exp Cell Res. 1979 Jan;118(1):127-34.

140. Youngdahl-Turner P, Rosenberg LE, Allen RH. Binding and uptake of transcobalamin II by human fibroblasts. J Clin Invest. 1978 Jan;61(1):133-41.

141. Zakharyan RA, Aposhian HV. Arsenite methylation by methylvitamin B12 and glutathione does not require an enzyme. Toxicol Appl Pharmacol. 1999 Feb 1;154(3):287-91.

142. Zhao W, Mosley BS, Cleves MA, Melnyk S, James SJ, Hobbs CA. Neural tube defects and maternal biomarkers of folate, homocysteine, and glutathione metabolism. Birth Defects Res A Clin Mol Teratol. 2006 Apr;76(4):230-6.

143. Zhao, R., Chen, Y., Tan, W., Waly, M., Malewicz, B., Stover, P., Rosowsky, A. and Deth, R.C.: Influence of single-carbon folate and *de novo* purine synthesis pathways on D4 dopamine receptor-mediated phospholipid methylation. J. Neurochem. 78: 788-796 (2001).

Chapter 19. Transcranial Magnetic Stimulation for the Treatment of Autism, by Dr. Joshua M. Baruth, Dr. Estate Sokhadze, Dr. Ayman El-Baz, Dr. Grace Mathai, Dr. Lonnie Sears, and Dr. Manuel F. Casanova

American Psychiatric Association. (2000). Diagnostic and statistical manual of mental disorders (DSM-IV TR) (4th ed.). Washington, DC: American Psychiatric Association. (text revised).

Barker, A.T., Jalinous, R., Freeston, I.L. (1985). Non-invasive magnetic stimulation of the human motor cortex. *Lancet*, 1,1106-1107.

Baruth, J.M., Casanova, M., El-Baz, A., Horrell, T., Mathai, G., Sears, L., Sokhadze, E. (2010a). Low-frequency repetitive Transcranial Magnetic Stimulation (rTMS) modulates evoked-gamma oscillations in Autism Spectrum Disorder (ASD). *Journal of Neurotherapy*, 14, 179-194.

Baruth, J.M., Casanova, M., Sears, L., Sokhadze, E. (2010b). Early-stage visual processing abnormalities in Autism Spectrum Disorder (ASD). *Translational Neuroscience*, 1, 177-187.

Belmonte, M.K., and Yurgelun-Todd, D.A. (2003). Functional anatomy of impaired selective attention and compensatory processing in autism. *Cognitive Brain Research*, 17, 651-664.

Bloch, Y., Harel, E.V., Aviram, S., Govezensky, J., Ratzoni, G., Levkovitz, Y. (2010). Positive effects of repetitive transcranial magnetic stimulation on attention in ADHD Subjects: a randomized controlled pilot study. *World Journal of Biological Psychiatry*, 11, 755-8.

Bodfish, J.W., Symons, F.J., and Lewis, M.H. (1999). Repetitive Behavior Scale. Western Carolina Center Research Reports.

Brown, C., Gruber, T., Boucher, J., Rippon, G., Brock, J. (2005). Gamma abnormalities during perception of illusory figures in autism. *Cortex*, 41, 364-76.

Casanova, M.F., Baruth, J.M., El-Baz, A., Tasman, A., Sears, L., Sokhadze, E. (2012). Repetitive Transcranial Magnetic Stimulation (rTMS) modulates Event-Related Potential (ERP) indices of attention in autism. *Translational Neuroscience*, 3, 170-180.

Casanova, M. F., Buxhoeveden, D. P., Switala, A. E., & Roy, E. (2002a). Minicolumnar pathology in autism. *Neurology*, 58, 428–432.

Casanova, M. F., Buxhoeveden, D. P., Switala, A. E., & Roy, E. (2002b). Neuronal density and architecture (gray level index) in the brains of autistic patients. *Journal of Child Neurology*, 17, 515–521.

Casanova, M. F., van Kooten, I., Switala, A. E., van England, H., Heinsen, H., Steinbuch, H. W. M., et al. (2006a). Abnormalities of cortical minicolumnar organization in the prefrontal lobes of autistic patients. *Clinical Neuroscience Research*, 6, 127–133.

Casanova, M. F., van Kooten, I., van Engeland, H., Heinsen, H., Steinbursch, H. W. M., Hof, P. R., et al. (2006b). Minicolumnar abnormalities in autism. *Acta Neuropathologica*, 112, 287–303.

Casanova, M.F. (2007). The neuropathology of autism. *Brain Pathology*, 17, 422-33.

Charman T. (2008). Autism spectrum disorders. *Psychiatry*, 7, 331-334.

Croarkin, P.E., Wall, C.A., Lee, J. (2011). Applications of transcranial magnetic stimulation (TMS) in child and adolescent psychiatry. *International Review of Psychiatry*, 23, 445-53.

Douglas, R. J., & Martin, K. A. C. (2004). Neuronal circuits of the neocortex. *Annual Review of Neuroscience*, 27, 419–451.

Faraday M: Effects on the production of electricity from magnetism (1831), in Michael Faraday. Edited by Williams LP. New York, Basic Books, 1965, p 531.

George and Belmaker (2007) *Transcrainial Magenetic Stimulation in Clinical Psychiatry*. Arlington, VA: American Psychiatric Publishing, Inc.

George, M.S., Lisanby, S.H., Avery, D., McDonald, W.M., Durkalski, V., Pavlicova, M., Anderson, B., Nahas, Z., Bulow, P., Zarkowsk,i P., Holtzheimer, P.E. 3rd, Schwartz, T., Sackeim, H.A. (2010). Daily left prefrontal transcranial magnetic stimulation therapy for major depressive disorder: a sham-controlled randomized trial. *Archives of General Psychiatry*, 67, 507-16.

Gillberg, C., Billstedt, E. (2000). Autism and Asperger syndrome: coexistence with other clinical disorders. *Acta Psychiatrica Scandinavica*,102, 321-30.

Hoffman, R. E., & Cavus, I. (2002). Slow transcranial magnetic stimulation, long-term depotentiation, and brain hyperexcitability disorders. *American Journal of Psychiatry*, 159, 1093–1102.

Maeda, F., Keenan, J.P., Tormos, J.M., Topka, H., Pascual-Leone, A. (2000). Modulation of corticospinal excitability by repetitive transcranial magnetic stimulation. *Clinical Neurophysiolgy*, 111, 800-805.

Mountcastle, V.B. (2003). Introduction.Computation in cortical columns. *Cerebral Cortex*, 13, 2–4.

Mountcastle, V. B. (1997). The columnar organization of the neocortex. *Brain*, 120, 701–722.

Pascual-Leone, A., Valls-Sole, J., Wasserman, E.M., et al. (1994). Responses to rapid-rate transcranial magnetic stimulation of the human cortex. *Brain*, 117, 847-858.

Pascual-Leone, A., Walsh, V., Rothwell, J. (2000). Transcranial magnetic stimulation in cognitive neuroscience —virtual lesion, chronometry, and functional connectivity. *Current Opinion in Neurobiology*, 10, 232-7.

Quintana, H. (2005). Transcranial magnetic stimulation in persons younger than the age of 18. *The Journal of ECT*, 21, 88-95.

Rippon, G., Brock, J., Brown, C., & Boucher, J. (2007). Disordered connectivity in the autistic brain: Challenges for the 'new psychophysiology'. *International Journal of Psychophysiology*, 63, 164–172.

Rubenstein, J.L.R., Merzenich, M.M. (2003). Model of autism: increased ratio of excitation/inhibition in key neural systems. *Genes, Brain, and Behavior*, 2, 255–267.

Sokhadze, E., Baruth, J., Tasman, A., Sears, L., Mathai, G., El-Baz, A., Casanova, M. (2009a). Event-related potential study of novelty processing abnormalities in autism. *Applied Psychophysiology and Biofeedback*, 34, 37-51.

Sokhadze, E., El-Baz, A., Baruth, J., Mathai, G., Sears, L., Casanova, M. (2009b). Effects of low frequency repetitive transcranial magnetic stimulation (rTMS) on gamma frequency oscillations and event-related potentials during processing of illusory figures in autism. *Journal of Autism and Developmental Disorders*, 39, 619-34.

Sokhadze, E., Baruth, J., Tasman, A., Mansoor, M., Ramaswamy, R., Sears, L., Mathai, G., El-Baz, A., Casanova, M.F. (2010a). Low-frequency repetitive Transcranial Magnetic Stimulation (rTMS) affects Event-Related Potential measures of novelty processing in autism. *Applied Psychophysiology and Biofeedback*, 35, 147-61.

Sokhadze, E., Baruth, J., El-Baz, A., Horrell, T., Sokhadze, G., Carroll, T., Tasman, A., Sears, L., Casanova, M.F. (2010b). Impaired rror monitoring and correction function in autism. *Journal of Neurotherapy*, 14, 79-95.

Sokhadze, E.M., Baruth, J.M., Sears, L., Sokhadze, G.E., El-Baz, A.S., Casanova, M.F. (2012). Prefrontal neuromodulation using rTMS improves error monitoring and correction function in autism. *Applied Psychophysiology and Biofeedback*, 37, 91-102.

Sokhadze, E.M., El-Baz, A., Sears, L., Casanova, M.F. (2013). Neuromodulation based on rTMS improves electrocortical functional measures of information processing in autism. *International Society for Neurofeedback and Research Annual Conference,* Dallas Texas, September 18-22, 2013.

Wall, C.A., Croarkin, P.E., Sim, L.A., Husain, M.M., Janicak, P.G., Kozel, F.A., Emslie, G.J., Dowd, S.M., Sampson, S.M. (2011). Adjunctive use of repetitive transcranial magnetic stimulation in depressed adolescents: a prospective, open pilot study. *Journal of Clinical Psychiatry*, 72, 1263-9.

Wassermann, E.M. (1996). Risk and safety of repetitive transcranial magnetic stimulation: report and suggested guidelines from the International Workshop on the Safety of Repetitive Transcranial Magnetic Stimulation, June 5-7. *Electroencephalography and Clinical Neurophysiology*, 108, 1-16.

Whittington, M.A., Traub, R.D., Kopell, N., Ermentrout, B., Buhl, E.H. (2000). Inhibition-based rhythms: experimental and mathematical observations on network dynamics. *International Journal of Psychophysiology*, 38, 315–336.

Wu, A.D., Fregni, F., Simon, D.K., Deblieck, C., Pascual-Leone, A. (2008). Noninvasive brain stimulation for Parkinson's Disease and Dystonia. *Neurotherapeutics*, 5, 345-61.

Chapter 20. The Role of the Microbiome/Biome and Cysteine Deficiency in Autism Spectrum Disorder, by Dr. James Jeffrey Bradstreet

1. Careaga M, Van de Water J, Ashwood P. Immune dysfunction in autism: a pathway to treatment. *Neurotherapeutics.* 2010;7(3):283-92.

2. Gupta S, Samra D, Agrawal S. Adaptive and innate immune responses in autism: rationale for therapeutic use of intravenous immunoglobulin. *J Clin Immunol.* 2010;30(Suppl 1):90-6.

3. Li X, Chauhan A, Sheikh AM, Patil S, Chauhan V, Li XM, Ji L, Brown T, Malik M. Elevated immune response in the brain of autistic patients. *J Neuroimmunol.* 2009;207(1-2):111-6.

4. Weizman A, Weizman R, Szekely GA, Wijsenbeek H, Livni E. Abnormal immune response to brain tissue antigen in the syndrome of autism. *Am J Psychiatry.* 1982;139(11):1462-5.

5. Chez MG, Dowling T, Patel PB, Khanna P, Kominsky M. Elevation of tumor necrosis factor-alpha in cerebrospinal fluid of autistic children. *Pediatr Neurol.* 2007;36(6):361-5.

6. Vargas DL, Nascimbene C, Krishnan C, Zimmerman AW, Pardo CA. Neuroglial activation and neuroinflammation in the brain of patients with autism. *Ann Neurol.* 2005;57(1):67-81. Erratum in: *Ann Neurol.* 2005;57(2):304.

7. Bradstreet JJ, El Dahr J, Anthony A, Kartzinel JJ, Wakefield AJ. Detection of measles virus genomic RNA in cerebrospinal fluid of children with regressive autism: s report of three cases. *J Amer Physicians Surgeons.* 2004; 9(2):38-45.

8. Bradstreet JJ, El Dahr J, Montgomery SM, Wakefield AJ. TaqMan RT-PCR detection of measles virus genomic RNA in cerebrospinal fluid in children with regressive autism. Presented at the 2004 International Meeting for Autism Research (IMFAR), Sacramento, CA.

9. M Dubik, PA Offit. Measles virus RNA and autism revisited. *AAP Grand Rounds. 2004;*12:56-57.

10. Sandler RH, Finegold SM, Bolte ER, Buchanan CP, Maxwell AP, Väisänen ML, Nelson MN, Wexler HM. Short-term benefit from oral vancomycin treatment of regressive-onset autism. *J Child Neurol.* 2000;15(7):429-35.

11. Finegold SM, Dowd SE, Gontcharova V, Liu C, Henley KE, Wolcott RD, Youn E, Summanen PH, Granpeesheh D, Dixon D, Liu M, Molitoris DR, Green JA 3rd. Pyrosequencing study of fecal microflora of autistic and control children. *Anaerobe.* 2010;16(4):444-53.

12. James SJ, Cutler P, Melnyk S, Jernigan S, Janak L, Gaylor DW, Neubrander JA. Metabolic biomarkers of increased oxidative stress and impaired methylation capacity in children with autism. *Am J Clin Nutr.* 2004;80(6):1611-7.

13. Siesjö BK, Rehncrona S, Smith D. Neuronal cell damage in the brain: possible involvement of oxidative mechanisms. *Acta Physiol Scand Suppl.* 1980;492:121-8.

14. Jenner P. Altered mitochondrial function, iron metabolism and glutathione levels in Parkinson's disease. *Acta Neurol Scand Suppl.* 1993;146:6-13.

15. Do KQ, Trabesinger AH, Kirsten-Krüger M, Lauer CJ, Dydak U, Hell D, Holsboer F, Boesiger P, Cuénod M. Schizophrenia: glutathione deficit in cerebrospinal fluid and prefrontal cortex in vivo. *Eur J Neurosci.* 2000;12(10):3721-8.

16. Dvoráková M, Sivonová M, Trebatická J, Skodácek I, Waczulíková I, Muchová J, Duracková Z. The effect of polyphenolic extract from pine bark, Pycnogenol on the level of glutathione in children suffering from attention deficit hyperactivity disorder (ADHD). *Redox Rep.* 2006;11(4):163-72.

17. Kalebic T, Kinter A, Poli G, Anderson ME, Meister A, Fauci AS. Suppression of human immunodeficiency virus expression in chronically infected monocytic cells by glutathione, glutathione ester, and N-acetylcysteine. *Proc Natl Acad Sci U S A.* 1991;88(3):986-90.

18. Iantomasi T, Marraccini P, Favilli F, Vincenzini MT, Ferretti P, Tonelli F. Glutathione metabolism in Crohn's disease. *Biochem Med Metab Biol.* 1994;53(2):87-91.

19. Oeriu S, Tigheciu M. Oxidized glutathione as a test of senescence. *Gerontologia.* 1964;49:9-17.

20. James SJ, Melnyk S, Jernigan S, Cleves MA, Halsted CH, Wong DH, Cutler P, Bock K, Boris M, Bradstreet JJ, Baker SM, Gaylor DW. Metabolic endophenotype and related genotypes are associated with oxidative stress in children with autism. *Am J Med Genet B Neuropsychiatr Genet.* 2006;141B(8):947-56.

21. Salzman NH, Hung K, Haribhai D, Chu H, Karlsson-Sjöberg J, Amir E, Teggatz P, Barman M, Hayward M, Eastwood D, Stoel M, Zhou Y, Sodergren E, Weinstock GM, Bevins CL, Williams CB, Bos NA. Enteric defensins are essential regulators of intestinal microbial ecology. *Nat Immunol.* 2010;11(1):76-83.

22. Eisenhauer PB, Harwig SS, Szklarek D, Ganz T, Selsted ME, Lehrer RI. Purification and antimicrobial properties of three defensins from rat neutrophils. *Infect Immun.* 1989;57(7):2021-7.

23. Rowan FE, Docherty NG, Coffey JC, O'Connell PR. Sulphate-reducing bacteria and hydrogen sulphide in the aetiology of ulcerative colitis. *Br J Surg.* 2009;96(2):151-8.

24. Bäckhed F, Ley RE, Sonnenburg JL, Peterson DA, Gordon JI. Host-bacterial mutualism in the human intestine. *Science.* 2005;307(5717):1915-20.

25. Shaw SY, Blanchard JF, Bernstein CN. Association between the use of antibiotics in the first year of life and pediatric inflammatory bowel disease. *Am J Gastroenterol.* 2010;105(12):2687-92.

26. Parker W. Reconstituting the depleted biome to prevent immune disorders. *The Evolution & Medicine Review.* Web. Oct 13 2010.

27. McKay DM. The beneficial helminth parasite? *Parasitology.* 2006;132(Pt 1):1-12.

28. Elliott DE, Summers RW, Weinstock JV. Helminths as governors of immune-mediated inflammation. *Int J Parasitol.* 2007;37(5):457-64.

29. Summers RW, Elliott DE, Urban JF Jr, Thompson RA, Weinstock JV. Trichuris suis therapy for active ulcerative colitis: a randomized controlled trial. *Gastroenterology.* 2005;128(4):825-32.

30. Bager P, Arnved J, Rønborg S, Wohlfahrt J, Poulsen LK, Westergaard T, Petersen HW, Kristensen B, Thamsborg S, Roepstorff A, Kapel C, Melbye M. Trichuris suis ova therapy for allergic rhinitis: a randomized, double-blind, placebo-controlled clinical trial. *J Allergy Clin Immunol.* 2010;125(1):123-30.

31. Sewell DL, Reinke EK, Hogan LH, Sandor M, Fabry Z. Immunoregulation of CNS autoimmunity by helminth and mycobacterial infections. *Immunol Lett.* 2002;82(1-2):101-10.

32. La Flamme AC, Canagasabey K, Harvie M, Bäckström BT. Schistosomiasis protects against multiple sclerosis. *Mem Inst Oswaldo Cruz.* 2004;99(5 Suppl 1):33-6.

33. Singer HS, Morris C, Gause C, Pollard M, Zimmerman AW, Pletnikov M. Prenatal exposure to antibodies from mothers of children with autism produces neurobehavioral alterations: a pregnant dam mouse model. *J Neuroimmunol*. 2009;211(1-2):39-48.

34. Garbett K, Ebert PJ, Mitchell A, Lintas C, Manzi B, Mirnics K, Persico AM. Immune transcriptome alterations in the temporal cortex of subjects with autism. *Neurobiol Dis*. 2008;30(3):303-11.

35. Garvey J. Diet in autism and associated disorders. *J Fam Health Care*. 2002;12(2): 34-8.

36. Levy SE, Hyman SL. Novel treatments for autistic spectrum disorders. *Ment Retard Dev Disabil* Res Rev. 2005;11(2):131-42.

37. Miele E, Pascarella F, Giannetti E, Quaglietta L, Baldassano RN, Staiano A. Effect of a probiotic preparation (VSL#3) on induction and maintenance of remission in children with ulcerative colitis. *Am J Gastroenterol*. 2009;104(2):437-43.

38. Huynh HQ, deBruyn J, Guan L, Diaz H, Li M, Girgis S, Turner J, Fedorak R, Madsen K. Probiotic preparation VSL#3 induces remission in children with mild to moderate acute ulcerative colitis: a pilot study. *Inflamm Bowel Dis*. 2009;15(5):760-8.

39. Tursi A, Brandimarte G, Papa A, Giglio A, Elisei W, Giorgetti GM, Forti G, Morini S, Hassan C, Pistoia MA, Modeo ME, Rodino' S, D'Amico T, Sebkova L, Sacca' N, Di Giulio E, Luzza F, Imeneo M, Larussa T, Di Rosa S, Annese V, Danese S, Gasbarrini A. Treatment of relapsing mild-to-moderate ulcerative colitis with the probiotic VSL#3 as adjunctive to a standard pharmaceutical treatment: a double-blind, randomized, placebo-controlled study. *Am J Gastroenterol*. 2010;105(10):2218-27.

40. Guandalini S. Update on the role of probiotics in the therapy of pediatric inflammatory bowel disease. *Expert Rev Clin Immunol*. 2010;6(1):47-54.

41. Ashwood P, Anthony A, Pellicer AA, Torrente F, Walker-Smith JA, Wakefield AJ. Intestinal lymphocyte populations in children with regressive autism: evidence for extensive mucosal immunopathology. *J Clin Immunol*. 2003;23(6):504-17.

42. Bradstreet JJ, Smith S, Baral M, Rossignol DA. Biomarker-guided interventions of clinically relevant conditions associated with autism spectrum disorders and attention deficit hyperactivity disorder. *Altern Med Rev*. 2010;15(1):15-32.

43. Eggesbø M, Moen B, Peddada S, Baird D, Rugtveit J, Midtvedt T, Bushel PR, Sekelja M, Rudi K. Development of gut microbiota in infants not exposed to medical interventions. *APMIS*. 2011;119(1):17-35.

44. Adlerberth I, Wold AE. Establishment of the gut microbiota in Western infants. *Acta Paediatr*. 2009;98(2):229-38.

45. Hooper LV, Midtvedt T, Gordon JI. How host-microbial interactions shape the nutrient environment of the mammalian intestine. *Annu Rev Nutr*. 2002;22:283-307.

46. Winter HS (personal communication). MassGeneral Hospital for Children, January 2011.

47. Khoruts A, Sadowsky MJ. Therapeutic transplantation of the distal gut microbiota. *Mucosal Immunol*. 2011;4(1):4-7.

48. Russell G, Kaplan J, Ferraro M, Michelow IC. Fecal bacteriotherapy for relapsing Clostridium difficile infection in a child: a proposed treatment protocol. *Pediatrics*. 2010;126(1):e239-42.

49. Floch MH. Fecal bacteriotherapy, fecal transplant, and the microbiome. *J Clin Gastroenterol*. 2010;44(8):529-30.

50. Theoharides TC, Doyle R, Francis K, Conti P, Kalogeromitros D. Novel therapeutic targets for autism. *Trends Pharmacol Sci*. 2008;29(8):375-82.

Chapter 21. Effects of Ambient Prism Lenses and Visual-Motor Training on Heart Rate Variability and Behavioral Outcomes in Autism, by Dr. Brynn Dombroski, Dr. Melvin Kaplan, Dr. Barbara Kotsamanidis-Burg, Dr. Stephen M Edelson, Marie K Hensley, Dr. Estate M Sokhadze, and Dr. Manuel F. Casanova

American Psychiatric Association (2000). *Diagnostic and Statistical Manual of Mental Disorders,* Forth Edition, Text Revision. Washington, DC.

Aman, M. G., & Singh, N. N. (1994). *Aberrant Behavior Checklist - Community. Supplementary Manual*. East Aurora, NY: Slosson Educational Publications.

Bodfish, J. W., Symons, F. J., & Lewis, J. (1999). *Repetitive Behavior Scale*. Western Carolina Center Research Reports.

Boucsein, W. (2012). *Electrodermal activity*. New York: Springer, 2nd Edition.

Kaplan. M (2006) Seeing Through New Eyes . J.Kingley Publ., Philadelphia, PA.

Le Couteur, A., Lord, C., & Rutter, M. (2003). *The Autism Diagnostic Interview – Revised (ADI-R)*. Los Angeles, CA: Western Psychological Services.

Ming, X., Bain, J. M., Smith, D., Brimacombe, M., Gold von-Simson, G., & Axelrod, F. B. (2011). Assessing autonomic dysfunction symptoms in children: A pilot study. *J Child Neurol, 26*(4), 420-427.

Porges, S. W. (2001). The polyvagal theory: phylogenetic substrates of a social nervous system. *Int J Psychophysiol, 42,* 123-146.

Toichi, M., & Kamio, Y. (2003). Paradoxical autonomic response to mental task in autism. *J Autism Dev Disord, 33,* 417-426.

Wechsler, D. (2004). *Wechsler Intelligence Scale for Children-Fourth Edition Integrated (WISC-IV Integrated).* San Antonio, TX: Harcourt.

Chapter 22. Stem Cells and Autism, by Dr. James Jeffrey Bradstreet

1.   Bradstreet JJ. Stem cells: real possibilities in autism? *Autism Science Digest.* 2011;Issue 1:62-9.

2.   Weiner LP. Definitions and criteria for stem cells. *Methods Mol Biol.* 2008;438:3-8.

3.   Maurer MH. Proteomic definitions of mesenchymal stem cells. *Stem Cells Int.* 2011 Mar 3;2011:704256.

4.   Lampe KJ, Heilshorn SC. Building stem cell niches from the molecule up through engineered peptide materials. *Neurosci Lett.* 2012 Jan 25. [Epub ahead of print]

5.   Halme DG, Kessler DA. FDA regulation of stem-cell-based therapies. *N Engl J Med.* 2006 Oct 19;355(16):1730-5.

6.   www.emcell.com

7.   Careaga M, Van de Water J, Ashwood P. Immune dysfunction in autism: a pathway to treatment. *Neurotherapeutics.* 2010 Jul;7(3):283-92.

8.   Chez MG, Guido-Estrada N. Immune therapy in autism: historical experience and future directions with immunomodulatory therapy. *Neurotherapeutics.* 2010 Jul;7(3):293-301.

9.   Crop MJ, Baan CC, Korevaar SS, Ijzermans JN, Pescatori M, Stubbs AP, van Ijcken WF, Dahlke MH, Eggenhofer E, Weimar W, Hoogduijn MJ. Inflammatory conditions affect gene expression and function of human adipose tissue-derived mesenchymal stem cells. *Clin Exp Immunol.* 2010 Dec;162(3):474-86. Epub 2010 Sep 15.

10. Snyder EY, Macklis JD. Multipotent neural progenitor or stem-like cells may be uniquely suited for therapy for some neurodegenerative conditions. *Clin Neurosci.* 1995-1996;3(5):310-6.

11. Bradstreet JJ, Smith S, Baral M, Rossignol DA. Biomarker-guided interventions of clinically relevant conditions associated with autism spectrum disorders and attention deficit hyperactivity disorder. *Altern Med Rev.* 2010 Apr;15(1):15-32.

12. Boris M, Kaiser CC, Goldblatt A, Elice MW, Edelson SM, Adams JB, Feinstein DL. Effect of pioglitazone treatment on behavioral symptoms in autistic children. *J Neuroinflammation.* 2007 Jan 5;4:3.

13. Hayward D, Eikeseth S, Gale C, Morgan S. Assessing progress during treatment for young children with autism receiving intensive behavioural interventions. *Autism.* 2009 Nov;13(6):613-33.

14. Himmelmann K, Ahlin K, Jacobsson B, Cans C, Thorsen P. Risk factors for cerebral palsy in children born at term. *Acta Obstet Gynecol Scand.* 2011 Oct;90(10):1070-81. Epub 2011 Jul 27.

15. See http://video.today.msnbc.msn.com/today/23569985#23569985

16. Papadopoulos KI, Low SS, Aw TC, Chantarojanasiri T. Safety and feasibility of autologous umbilical cord blood transfusion in 2 toddlers with cerebral palsy and the role of low dose granulocyte-colony stimulating factor injections. *Restor Neurol Neurosci.* 2011 Jan 1;29(1):17-22.

17. Gupta S, Aggarwal S, Heads C. Dysregulated immune system in children with autism: beneficial effects of intravenous immune globulin on autistic characteristics. *J Autism Dev Disord.* 1996 Aug;26(4):439-52.

18. Chez MG, Memon S, Hung PC. Neurologic treatment strategies in autism: an overview of medical intervention strategies. *Semin Pediatr Neurol.* 2004 Sep;11(3):229-35.

19. Bradstreet JJ, Smith S, Granpeesheh D, El-Dahr JM, Rossignol D. Spironolactone might be a desirable immunologic and hormonal intervention in autism spectrum disorders. *Med Hypotheses.* 2007;68(5):979-87. Epub 2006 Dec 5.

20. Wang LW, Berry-Kravis E, Hagerman RJ. Fragile X: leading the way for targeted treatments in autism. *Neurotherapeutics.* 2010 Jul;7(3):264-74.

21. Bassi E, De Filippi C. Beneficial neurological effects observed in a patient with psoriasis treated with etanercept. *Am J Clin Dermatol.* 2010;11 Suppl 1:44-5.

22. Theoharides TC, Zhang B. Neuro-inflammation, blood-brain barrier, seizures and autism. *J Neuroinflammation.* 2011 Nov 30;8(1):168.

23. Connolly AM, Chez MG, Pestronk A, Arnold ST, Mehta S, Deuel RK. Serum autoantibodies to brain in Landau-Kleffner variant, autism, and other neurologic disorders. *J Pediatr.* 1999 May;134(5):607-13.

24. Buie T, Campbell DB, Fuchs GJ 3rd, Furuta GT, Levy J, Vandewater J, Whitaker AH, Atkins D, Bauman ML, Beaudet AL, Carr EG, Gershon MD, Hyman SL, Jırapinyo P, Jyonouchi H, Kooros K, Kushak R, Levitt P, Levy SE, Lewis JD, Murray KF, Natowicz MR, Sabra A, Wershil BK, Weston SC, Zeltzer L, Winter H.

Evaluation, diagnosis, and treatment of gastrointestinal disorders in individuals with ASDs: a consensus report. *Pediatrics*. 2010 Jan;125 Suppl 1:S1-18.

25. Panés J, García-Bosch O, Salas A, Benitez D. Cell therapies for inflammatory bowel disease. *Curr Drug Deliv*. 2011 Oct 21. [Epub ahead of print]

26. Macneil LK, Mostofsky SH. Specificity of dyspraxia in children with autism. *Neuropsychology*. 2012 Jan 30. [Epub ahead of print]

27. Tsuji O, Miura K, Fujiyoshi K, Momoshima S, Nakamura M, Okano H. Cell therapy for spinal cord injury by neural stem/progenitor cells derived from iPS/ES cells. *Neurotherapeutics*. 2011 Oct;8(4):668-76.

28. Davies SJ, Shih CH, Noble M, Mayer-Proschel M, Davies JE, Proschel C. Transplantation of specific human astrocytes promotes functional recovery after spinal cord injury. *PLoS One*. 2011 Mar 2;6(3):e17328.

29. Bernardo ME, Pagliara D, Locatelli F. Mesenchymal stromal cell therapy: a revolution in regenerative medicine? *Bone Marrow Transplant*. 2012 Feb;47(2):164-71. Epub 2011 Apr 11.

30. Ichim TE, Solano F, Glenn E, Morales F, Smith L, Zabrecky G, Riordan NH. Stem cell therapy for autism. *J Transl Med*. 2007 Jun 27;5:30.

31. Siepermann M, Gudowius S, Beltz K, Strier U, Feyen O, Troeger A, Göbel U, Laws HJ, Kögler G, Meisel R, Dilloo D, Niehues T. MHC class II deficiency cured by unrelated mismatched umbilical cord blood transplantation: case report and review of 68 cases in the literature. *Pediatr Transplant*. 2011 Jun;15(4):E80-6. Epub 2010 Mar 4.

32. Sarkar D, Spencer JA, Phillips JA, Zhao W, Schafer S, Spelke DP, Mortensen LJ, Ruiz JP, Vemula PK, Sridharan R, Kumar S, Karnik R, Lin CP, Karp JM. Engineered cell homing. *Blood*. 2011 Dec 15;118(25):e184-91. Epub 2011 Oct 27.

33. Cossetti C, Alfaro-Cervello C, Donegà M, Tyzack G, Pluchino S. New perspectives of tissue remodelling with neural stem and progenitor cell-based therapies. *Cell Tissue Res*. 2012 Feb 10. [Epub ahead of print]

34. Gallagher G, Forrest DL. Second solid cancers after allogeneic hematopoietic stem cell transplantation. *Cancer*. 2007 Jan 1;109(1):84-92.

35. Pera MF. Stem cells: the dark side of induced pluripotency. *Nature*. 2011 Mar 3;471(7336):46-7.

36. Amariglio N, Hirshberg A, Scheithauer BW, Cohen Y, Loewenthal R, Trakhtenbrot L, Paz N, Koren-Michowitz M, Waldman D, Leider-Trejo L, Toren A, Constantini S, Rechavi G. Donor-derived brain tumor following neural stem cell transplantation in an ataxia telangiectasia patient. *PLoS Med*. 2009 Feb 17;6(2):e1000029.

37. Clark P, Trickett A, Stark D, Vowels M. Factors affecting microbial contamination rate of cord blood collected for transplantation. *Transfusion*. 2011 Dec 30. [Epub ahead of print]

38. Dodd R, Kurt Roth W, Ashford P, Dax EM, Vyas G. Transfusion medicine and safety. *Biologicals*. 2009 Apr;37(2):62-70. Epub 2009 Feb 20.

39. Papadouka V, Metroka A, Zucker JR. Using an immunization information system to facilitate a vaccine recall in New York City, 2007. *J Public Health Manag Pract*. 2011 Nov-Dec;17(6):565-8.

Chapter 23. The Thyroid-Autism Connection: The Role of Endocrine Disruptors, by Dr. Raphael Kellman

1. Dayan CM, Daniels GH. Chronic autoimmune thyroiditis. *N Engl J Med*. 1996;335 (2):99-107.

2. National Institutes of Health, Autoimmune Diseases Coordinating Committee. *Progress in Autoimmune Diseases Research*. US Department of Health and Human Services, National Institutes of Health, NIH Publication No. 05-5140, March 2005.

3. Ch'ng CL, Jones MK, Kingham JGC. Celiac disease and autoimmune thyroid disease. *Clin Med Res*. 2007 October;5(3):184–92.

4. Berti I, Trevisiol C, Tommasini A, Città A, Neri E, Geatti O, Giammarini A, Ventura A, Not T. Usefulness of screening program for celiac disease in autoimmune thyroiditis. *Digest Dis Sci*. 2000 Feb;45(2):403-6.

5. Mainardi E, Montanelli A, Dotti M, Nano R, Moscato G. Thyroid-related autoantibodies and celiac disease: a role for a gluten-free diet? *J Clin Gastroenterol*. 2002 Sep;35(3): 245-8.

6. Cimino JA, Noto RA, Fusco CL, Cooperman JM. Riboflavin metabolism in the hypothyroid newborn. *Am J Clin Nutr*. 1988 Mar;47(3):481-3.

7. Giulivi C, Zhang YF, Omanska-Klusek A, Ross-Inta C, Wong S, Hertz-Picciotto I, Tassone F, Pessah IN. Mitochondrial dysfunction in autism. *JAMA*. 2010 Dec 1;304(21):2389-96.

8. Singh R Upadhyay G, Godbole MM. Hypothyroidism alters mitochondrial morphology and induces release of apoptogenic proteins during rat cerebellar development. *J Endocrinol*. 2003 Mar;176(3):321-9.

9. Wrutniak-Cabello C, Casas F, Cabello G. Thyroid hormone action in mitochondria. *J Mol Endocrinol*. 2001 Feb;26(1):67-77.

10. Porterfield SP. Vulnerability of developing brain to thyroid abnormalities: environmental insults to the thyroid systems. *Environ Health Perspect.* 1994 Jun;102(Suppl 2):125-30.

11. Porterfield SP. Thyroidal dysfunction and environmental chemicals-potential impact on brain development. *Environ Health Perspect.* 2000 Jun:108(Suppl 3):433-8.

12. Yasbak FE. Autism seems to be increasing worldwide, if not in London. *BMJ.* 2004 Jan 24;328(7433):226-7.

13. Berbel P , Mestre JL, Santamaría A, Palazón I, Franco A, Graells M, González-Torga A, de Escobar GM. Delayed neurobehavioral development in children born to pregnant women with mild hypothyroxinemia during the first month of gestation: the importance of early iodine supplementation. *Thyroid.* 2009 May;19(5):511–9.

14. Grandjean P, Landrigan PJ. Developmental neurotoxicity of industrial chemicals. *Lancet.* 2006 Dec 16; 368(9553):2167-78.

15. Zoeller RT, Rovet J. Timing of thyroid hormone function in the developing brain: clinical observations and experimental findings. *J Neuroendocrinol.* 2004 Oct;16(10):809-18.

16. Landrigan PJ. What causes autism? Exploring the environmental contribution. *Curr Opin Pediatr.* 2010 Apr;22(2):219-25.

17. Rovet JF, Ehrlich RM, Sorbara DL. Neurodevelopment in infants and preschool children with congenital hypothyroidism: etiological and treatment factors affecting outcome. *J Pediatr Psychol.* 1992 Apr;17(2):187-213.

18. Crofton KM, Craft ES, Hedge JM, Gennings C, Simmons JE, Carchman RA, Carter WH Jr, DeVito MJ. Thyroid-hormone-disrupting chemicals: evidence for dose-dependent additivity or synergism. *Environ Health Perspect.* 2005 Nov;113(11):1549-54.

19. Moriyama K, Tagami T, Akamizu T, Usui T, Saijo M, Kanamoto N, Hataya Y, Shimatsu A, Kuzuya H, Nakao K. Thyroid hormone action is disrupted by bisphenol A as an antagonist. *J Clin Endocrinol Metab.* 2002 Nov;87(11) 5185-90.

20. Viluksela M, Raasmaja A, Lebofsky M, Stahl BU, Rozman KK. Tissue-specific effects of 2,3,7,8-tetrachlorod-ibenzo-p-dioxin (TCDD) on the activity of 5'-deiodinases I and II in rats. *Toxicol Lett.* 2004 Mar;147(2):133-42.

21. Nishimura N, Yonemoto J, Miyabara Y, Sato M, Tohyama C. Rat thyroid hyperplasia induced by gestational and lactational exposure to 2,3,7,8-tetrachlorodibenzo-p-dioxin. *Endocrinology.* 2003 May;144(5):2075-83.

22. Pavuk M, Schecter AJ, Akhtar FZ, Michalek JE . Serum 2,3,7,8-tetrachlorodibenzop-dioxin (TCDD) levels and thyroid function in Air Force veterans of the Vietnam War. *Ann Epidemiol.* 2003 May;13(5):335-43.

23. Pluim J, de Vijlder JJ, Olie K, Kok JH, Vulsma T, van Tijn DA, van der Slikke JW, Koppe JG. Effects of pre- and postnatal exposure to chlorinated dioxins and furans on human neonatal thyroid hormone concentrations. *Environ Health Perspect.* 1993 Nov;101(6): 504-8.

24. Boas M, Feldt-Rasmussen U, Skakkebaek NE, Main KM. Environmental chemicals and thyroid function. *Eur J Endocrinol.* 2006 May;154(5):599-611.

25. Takser L, Mergler D, Baldwin M, de Grosbois S, Smargiassi A, Lafond J. Thyroid hormones in pregnancy in relation to environmental exposure to organochlorine compounds and mercury. *Environ Health Perspect.* 2005 Aug;113(8):1039-45.

26. Osius N, Karmaus W, Kruse H, Witten J. Exposure to polychlorinated biphenyls and levels of thyroid hor-mones in children. *Environ Health Perspect.* 1999 Oct; 107(10):843-9.

27. Khan MA, Hansen LG. Ortho-substituted polychlorinated biphenyl (PCB) congeners (95 or 101) decrease pituitary response to thyrotropin releasing hormone. *Toxicol Lett.* 2003 Sep 30;144(2):173-82.

28. Hagmar L. Polychlorine biphenyls and thyroid status in humans: a review. *Thyroid.* 2003 Nov;13(11):1021-8.

29. Koopman-Esseboom C, Morse DC, Weisglas-Kuperus N, Lutkeschipholt IJ, Van der Paauw CG, Tuinstra LG, Brouwer A, Sauer PJ. Effects of dioxins and polychlorinated biphenyls on thyroid hormone status of pregnant women and their infants. *Pediatr Res.*1994 Oct;36(4):468-73.

30. Rogan WJ, Gladen BC, Hung KL, Koong SL, Shih LY, Taylor JS, Wu YC, Yang D, Ragan NB, Hsu CC. Congenital poisoning by polychlorinated biphenyls and their contaminants in Taiwan. *Science.* 1988 Jul 15;241(4863):334-6.

31. Environmental Working Group. http://www.ewg.org/reports/thyroidthreat Last accessed June 26, 2011.

32. Miodovnik A, Engel SM, Zhu C, Ye X, Soorya LV, Silva MJ, Calafat AM, Wolff MS. Endocrine disruptors and childhood social impairment. *Neurotoxicology.* 2011 Mar;32(2):261-7.

33. Engel SM, Miodovnik A, Canfield RL, Zhu C, Silva MJ, Calafat AM, Wolff MS. Prenatal phthalate exposure is associated with childhood behavior and executive functioning. *Environ Health Perspect.* 2010 Apr;118(4):565-71.

34. Roberts EM, English PB, Grether JK, Windham GC, Somberg L, Wolff C. Maternal residence near agricul-tural pesticide applications and autism spectrum disorders among children in California of Central Valley. *Environ Health Perspect.* 2007 Oct;15(10):1482-9.

35. Jurewicz J, Hanke W. Prenatal and childhood exposure to pesticides and neurobehavioral development: review of epidemiological studies. *Int J Occup Med Environ Health.* 2008;21(2):121-32.

36. Korrick SA, Sagiv SK. Polychlorinated biphenyls, organochlorine pesticides, and neurodevelopment. *Curr Opin Pediatr*. 2008Apr;20(2):198-204.

37. Ribas-Fitó N, Torrent M, Carrizo D, Muñoz-Ortiz L, Júlvez J, Grimalt JO, Sunyer J. In utero exposure to background concentrations of DDT and cognitive functioning among preschoolers. *Am J Epidemiol*. 2006 Nov 15;164(10):955-62.

38. Román GC. Autism: transient in utero hypothyroxinemia related to maternal flavonoid ingestion during pregnancy and to other environmental anti-thyroid agents. *J Neurol Sci*. 2007 Nov 15;262(1-2):15-26.

39. Kraus RP , Phoenix E, Edmonds MW, Nicholson IR, Chandarana PC, Tokmakejian S. Exaggerated TSH response to TRH in depressed patients with "normal" baseline TSH. *J Clin Psychiatry*. 1997 Jun;58 (6):266-70.

40. Doi SA, Issac D, Abalkhail S, Al-Qudhaiby MM, Hafez MF, Al-Shoumer KA.TRH stimulation when basal TSH is within the normal range: is there "sub-biochemical" hypothyroidism? *Clin Med Res*. 2007 Oct;5(3):145–8.

41. Eldar-Geva T, Shoham M, Rösler A, Margalioth EJ, Livne K, Meirow D. Subclinical hypothyroidism in infertile women: the importance of continuous monitoring and the role of thyrotropin releasing hormone stimulation test. *Gynecol Endocrinol*. 2007 Jun;23(6):332-7.

42. Yun KH, Jeong MH, Oh SK, Lee EM, Lee J, Rhee SJ, Yoo NJ, Kim NH, Ahn YK, Jeong JW. Relationship of thyroid stimulating hormone with coronary atherosclerosis in angina patients. *Int J Cardiol*. 2007 Oct 31;122(1):56-60.

43. Larsen PR, Silva JE, Kaplan MM. Relationship between circulating and intracellular thyroid hormones: physiological and clinical implications. *Endocr Rev*. 1981 Winter;2(1):87-102.

44. Nagaya T, Fujieda M, Otsuka G, Yang JP, Okamoto T, Seo H. A potential role of NFkappa B in the pathogenesis of euthyroid sick syndrome. *J Clin Invest*. 2000 Aug;106(3): 393-402.

45. DeGroot LJ. "Nonthyroidal illness syndrome" is functional central hypothyroidism, and if severe, hormone replacement is appropriate in light of present knowledge. *J Endocrinol Invest*. 2003 Dec;26(12):1163-70.

46. Bernal J, Guadaño-Ferraz A, Morte B. Perspectives in the study of thyroid hormone action on brain development and function. *Thyroid*. 2003 Nov;13(11):1005-12.

47. Zoeller TR. Environmental chemicals targeting thyroid. *Hormones* (Athens). 2010 Jan-Mar;9(1):28-40.

Chapter 24. Hyperbaric Oxygen Therapy—Let's put the Pressure on Autism for Recovery, by Dr. James Neubrander

1. *Hyperbaric Medicine Team Training, Conducted at Nix Medical Center, San Antonio, Texas, June 4-8, 2007.*

2. *Neuro-HBOT Certification Course, IHA with ICIM, October 1-2, 2008, Pittsburg, PA.*

3. Akin, M. L., B. M. Gulluoglu, et al. (2002). «Hyperbaric oxygen improves healing in experimental rat colitis.» Undersea Hyperb Med 29(4): 279-85.

4. Alex, J., G. Laden, et al. (2005). «Pretreatment with hyperbaric oxygen and its effect on neuropsychometric dysfunction and systemic inflammatory response after cardiopulmonary bypass: a prospective randomized double-blind trial.» J Thorac Cardiovasc Surg 130(6): 1623-30.

5. Allen, K. D., J. S. Danforth, et al. (1989). "Videotaped modeling and film distraction for fear reduction in adults undergoing hyperbaric oxygen therapy." J Consult Clin Psychol 57(4): 554-8.

6. Alleva, R., E. Nasole, et al. (2005). "alpha-Lipoic acid supplementation inhibits oxidative damage, accelerating chronic wound healing in patients undergoing hyperbaric oxygen therapy." Biochem Biophys Res Commun 333(2): 404-10.

7. Al-Waili, N. S. and G. J. Butler (2006). "Effects of hyperbaric oxygen on inflammatory response to wound and trauma: possible mechanism of action." ScientificWorldJournal 6: 425-41.

8. Al-Waili, N. S., G. J. Butler, et al. (2005). «Hyperbaric oxygen in the treatment of patients with cerebral stroke, brain trauma, and neurologic disease.» Adv Ther 22(6): 659-78.

9. Al-Waili, N. S., G. J. Butler, et al. (2006). «Hyperbaric oxygen and lymphoid system function: a review supporting possible intervention in tissue transplantation.» Technol Health Care 14(6): 489-98.

10. Anderson, B., Jr. and J. C. Farmer, Jr. (1978). "Hyperoxic myopia." Trans Am Ophthalmol Soc 76: 116-24.

11. Anderson, D. C., A. G. Bottini, et al. (1991). «A pilot study of hyperbaric oxygen in the treatment of human stroke.» Stroke 22(9): 1137-42.

12. Ansari, K. A., M. Wilson, et al. (1986). «Hyperbaric oxygenation and erythrocyte antioxidant enzymes in multiple sclerosis patients.» Acta Neurol Scand 74(2): 156-60.

13. Ashamalla, H. L., S. R. Thom, et al. (1996). "Hyperbaric oxygen therapy for the treatment of radiation-induced sequelae in children. The University of Pennsylvania experience." Cancer 77(11): 2407-12.

14. Atochin, D. N., D. Fisher, et al. (2000). "Neutrophil sequestration and the effect of hyperbaric oxygen in a rat model of temporary middle cerebral artery occlusion." Undersea Hyperb Med 27(4): 185-90.

15. Atochin, D. N., D. Fisher, et al. (2001). "[Hyperbaric oxygen inhibits neutrophil infiltration and reduces post-ischemic brain injury in rats]." Ross Fiziol Zh Im I M Sechenova 87(8): 1118-25.

16. Atug, O., H. Hamzaoglu, et al. (2008). «Hyperbaric oxygen therapy is as effective as dexamethasone in the treatment of TNBS-E-induced experimental colitis.» Dig Dis Sci 53(2): 481-5.

17. Bader, N., A. Bosy-Westphal, et al. (2006). "Influence of vitamin C and E supplementation on oxidative stress induced by hyperbaric oxygen in healthy men." Ann Nutr Metab 50(3): 173-6.

18. Bader, N., A. Bosy-Westphal, et al. (2007). "Effect of hyperbaric oxygen and vitamin C and E supplementation on biomarkers of oxidative stress in healthy men." Br J Nutr 98(4): 826-33.

19. Baugh, M. A. (2000). "HIV: reactive oxygen species, enveloped viruses and hyperbaric oxygen." Med Hypotheses 55(3): 232-8.

20. Benedetti, S., A. Lamorgese, et al. (2004). «Oxidative stress and antioxidant status in patients undergoing prolonged exposure to hyperbaric oxygen.» Clin Biochem 37(4): 312-7.

21. Bennett, M. and H. Newton (2007). "Hyperbaric oxygen therapy and cerebral palsy—where to now?" Undersea Hyperb Med 34(2): 69-74.

22. Bennett, M. H., J. Wasiak, et al. (2005). «Hyperbaric oxygen therapy for acute ischaemic stroke.» Cochrane Database Syst Rev(3): CD004954.

23. Bitterman, H. (2007). "Hyperbaric oxygen for invasive fungal infections." Isr Med Assoc J 9(5): 387-8.

24. Boadi, W. Y., L. Thaire, et al. (1991). «Effects of dietary factors on antioxidant enzymes in rats exposed to hyperbaric oxygen.» Vet Hum Toxicol 33(2): 105-9.

25. Bornside, G. H., L. M. Pakman, et al. (1975). «Inhibition of pathogenic enteric bacteria by hyperbaric oxygen: enhanced antibacterial activity in the absence of carbon dioxide.» Antimicrob Agents Chemother 7(5): 682-7.

26. Bouachour, G., P. Cronier, et al. (1996). «Hyperbaric oxygen therapy in the management of crush injuries: a randomized double-blind placebo-controlled clinical trial.» J Trauma 41(2): 333-9.

27. Brady, C. E., 3rd, B. J. Cooley, et al. (1989). "Healing of severe perineal and cutaneous Crohn's disease with hyperbaric oxygen." Gastroenterology 97(3): 756-60.

28. Buchman, A. L., C. Fife, et al. (2001). «Hyperbaric oxygen therapy for severe ulcerative colitis.» J Clin Gastroenterol 33(4): 337-9.

29. Buras, J. A., D. Holt, et al. (2006). "Hyperbaric oxygen protects from sepsis mortality via an interleukin-10-dependent mechanism." Crit Care Med 34(10): 2624-9.

30. Calvert, J. W., J. Cahill, et al. (2007). «Hyperbaric oxygen and cerebral physiology.» Neurol Res 29(2): 132-41.

31. Calvert, J. W., W. Yin, et al. (2002). «Hyperbaric oxygenation prevented brain injury induced by hypoxia-ischemia in a neonatal rat model.» Brain Res 951(1): 1-8.

32. Calvert, J. W. and J. H. Zhang (2007). "Oxygen treatment restores energy status following experimental neonatal hypoxia-ischemia." Pediatr Crit Care Med 8(2): 165-73.

33. Chungpaibulpatana, J., T. Sumpatanarax, et al. (2008). "Hyperbaric oxygen therapy in Thai autistic children." J Med Assoc Thai 91(8): 1232-8.

34. Clark, J. M. and L. M. Pakman (1971). "Inhibition of Pseudomonas aeruginosa by hyperbaric oxygen. II. Ultrastructural changes." Infect Immun 4(4): 488-91.

35. Collet, J. P., M. Vanasse, et al. (2001). «Hyperbaric oxygen for children with cerebral palsy: a randomised multicentre trial. HBO-CP Research Group.» Lancet 357(9256): 582-6.

36. Colombel, J. F., D. Mathieu, et al. (1995). «Hyperbaric oxygenation in severe perineal Crohn's disease.» Dis Colon Rectum 38(6): 609-14.

37. Connor, D. J. and M. Bennett (2002). "Response to article by Buchman et al. Use of hyperbaric oxygenation in the treatment of ulcerative colitis." J Clin Gastroenterol 35(1): 98; author reply 98.

38. Daugherty, W. P., J. E. Levasseur, et al. (2004). "Effects of hyperbaric oxygen therapy on cerebral oxygenation and mitochondrial function following moderate lateral fluid-percussion injury in rats." J Neurosurg 101(3): 499-504.

39. Dave, K. R., R. Prado, et al. (2003). "Hyperbaric oxygen therapy protects against mitochondrial dysfunction and delays onset of motor neuron disease in Wobbler mice." Neuroscience 120(1): 113-20.

40. Demchenko, I. T., A. E. Boso, et al. (2000). «Hyperbaric oxygen reduces cerebral blood flow by inactivating nitric oxide.» Nitric Oxide 4(6): 597-608.

41. Demchenko, I. T., T. D. Oury, et al. (2002). "Regulation of the brain's vascular responses to oxygen." Circ Res 91(11): 1031-7.

42. Demirturk, L., M. Ozel, et al. (2002). "Therapeutic efficacy of hyperbaric oxygenation in ulcerative colitis refractory to medical treatment." J Clin Gastroenterol 35(3): 286-7; author reply 287-8.

43. Dennog, C., A. Hartmann, et al. (1996). "Detection of DNA damage after hyperbaric oxygen (HBO) therapy." Mutagenesis 11(6): 605-9.

44. Dennog, C., P. Radermacher, et al. (1999). "Antioxidant status in humans after exposure to hyperbaric oxygen." Mutat Res 428(1-2): 83-9.

45. Dole, M., F. R. Wilson, et al. (1975). «Hyperbaric hydrogen therapy: a possible treatment for cancer.» Science 190(4210): 152-4.

46. Efrati, S., J. Bergan, et al. (2007). «Hyperbaric oxygen therapy for nonhealing vasculitic ulcers.» Clin Exp Dermatol 32(1): 12-7.

47. Eftedal, O. S., S. Lydersen, et al. (2004). «A randomized, double blind study of the prophylactic effect of hyperbaric oxygen therapy on migraine.» Cephalalgia 24(8): 639-44.

48. Feldmeier, J. J., Chairman and Editor (2003). Hyperbaric oxygen 2003: indications and results: the hyperbaric oxygen therapy committee report. Kensington, MD, Undersea and Hyperbaric Medicine Society.

49. Feldmeier, J. J., N. B. Hampson, et al. (2005). «In response to the negative randomized controlled hyperbaric trial by Annane et al in the treatment of mandibular ORN.» Undersea Hyperb Med 32(3): 141-3.

50. Ferrer, M. D., A. Sureda, et al. (2007). "Scuba diving enhances endogenous antioxidant defenses in lymphocytes and neutrophils." Free Radic Res 41(3): 274-81.

51. Fry, D. E. (2005). "The story of hyperbaric oxygen continues." Am J Surg 189(4): 467-8.

52. Gill, A. L. and C. N. Bell (2004). "Hyperbaric oxygen: its uses, mechanisms of action and outcomes." QJM 97(7): 385-95.

53. Girnius, S., N. Cersonsky, et al. (2006). «Treatment of refractory radiation-induced hemorrhagic proctitis with hyperbaric oxygen therapy.» Am J Clin Oncol 29(6): 588-92.

54. Golden, Z., C. J. Golden, et al. (2006). "Improving neuropsychological function after chronic brain injury with hyperbaric oxygen." Disabil Rehabil 28(22): 1379-86.

55. Golden, Z. L., R. Neubauer, et al. (2002). «Improvement in cerebral metabolism in chronic brain injury after hyperbaric oxygen therapy.» Int J Neurosci 112(2): 119-31.

56. Gorgulu, S., G. Yagci, et al. (2006). «Hyperbaric oxygen enhances the efficiency of 5-aminosalicylic acid in acetic acid-induced colitis in rats.» Dig Dis Sci 51(3): 480-7.

57. Gosalvez, M., J. Castillo Olivares, et al. (1973). "Mitochondrial respiration and oxidative phosphorylation during hypothermic hyperbaric hepatic preservation." J Surg Res 15(5): 313-8.

58. Gottlieb, S. F. (1971). "Effect of hyperbaric oxygen on microorganisms." Annu Rev Microbiol 25: 111-52.

59. Granowitz, F. V., E. J. Skulsky, et al. (2002). «Exposure to increased pressure or hyperbaric oxygen suppresses interferon-gamma secretion in whole blood cultures of healthy humans.» Undersea Hyperb Med 29(3): 216-25.

60. Gregorevic, P., G. S. Lynch, et al. (2001). "Hyperbaric oxygen modulates antioxidant enzyme activity in rat skeletal muscles." Eur J Appl Physiol 86(1): 24-7.

61. Gulec, B., M. Yasar, et al. (2004). "Effect of hyperbaric oxygen on experimental acute distal colitis." Physiol Res 53(5): 493-9.

62. Gurbuz, A. K., E. Elbuken, et al. (2003). «A different therapeutic approach in patients with severe ulcerative colitis: hyperbaric oxygen treatment.» South Med J 96(6): 632-3.

63. Gurbuz, A. K., E. Elbuken, et al. (2003). «A different therapeutic approach in severe ulcerative hyperbaric oxygen treatment.» Rom J Gastroenterol 12(2): 170-1.

64. Gutsaeva, D. R., H. B. Suliman, et al. (2006). «Oxygen-induced mitochondrial biogenesis in the rat hippocampus.» Neuroscience 137(2): 493-504.

65. Hammarlund, C. and T. Sundberg (1994). "Hyperbaric oxygen reduced size of chronic leg ulcers: a randomized double-blind study." Plast Reconstr Surg 93(4): 829-33; discussion 834.

66. Harabin, A. L., J. C. Braisted, et al. (1990). "Response of antioxidant enzymes to intermittent and continuous hyperbaric oxygen." J Appl Physiol 69(1): 328-35.

67. Harch, P. G. (2006). "Medicine that overlooks the evidence." Arch Phys Med Rehabil 87(4): 592-3; author reply 593.

68. Harch, P. G., C. Kriedt, et al. (2007). «Hyperbaric oxygen therapy improves spatial learning and memory in a rat model of chronic traumatic brain injury.» Brain Res 1174: 120-9.

69. Hardy, P., J. P. Collet, et al. (2002). «Neuropsychological effects of hyperbaric oxygen therapy in cerebral palsy.» Dev Med Child Neurol 44(7): 436-46.

70. Hardy, P., K. M. Johnston, et al. (2007). "Pilot case study of the therapeutic potential of hyperbaric oxygen therapy on chronic brain injury." J Neurol Sci 253(1-2): 94-105.

71. Harrison, D. K., N. C. Abbot, et al. (1994). «Protective regulation of oxygen uptake as a result of reduced oxygen extraction during chronic inflammation.» Adv Exp Med Biol 345: 789-96.

72. Helms, A. K., H. T. Whelan, et al. (2007). "Hyperbaric oxygen therapy of acute ischemic stroke." Stroke 38(4): 1137; author reply 1138-9.

73. Henninger, N., L. Kuppers-Tiedt, et al. (2006). "Neuroprotective effect of hyperbaric oxygen therapy monitored by MR-imaging after embolic stroke in rats." Exp Neurol 201(2): 316-23.

74. Heuser, G., S. A. Heuser, et al. (2002). «Treatment of neurologically impaired adults and children with "mild" hyperbaric oxygenation (1.3 atm and 24% oxygen). In Hyperbaric oxygenation for cerebral palsy and the brain-injured child. Edited by Joiner JT. Flagstaff, Arizona: Best Publications.»

75. Hollis, A. L., W. I. Butcher, et al. (1992). «Structural alterations in retinal tissues from rats deficient in vitamin E and selenium and treated with hyperbaric oxygen.» Exp Eye Res 54(5): 671-84.

76. Hu, Z. Y., X. F. Shi, et al. (1991). «The protective effect of hyperbaric oxygen on hearing during chronic noise exposure.» Aviat Space Environ Med 62(5): 403-6.

77. Inamoto, Y., F. Okuno, et al. (1991). "Effect of hyperbaric oxygenation on macrophage function in mice." Biochem Biophys Res Commun 179(2): 886-91.

78. Jacobs, E. A., P. M. Winter, et al. (1969). «Hyperoxygenation effect on cognitive functioning in the aged.» N Engl J Med 281(14): 753-7.

79. Kiralp, M. Z., S. Yildiz, et al. (2004). «Effectiveness of hyperbaric oxygen therapy in the treatment of complex regional pain syndrome.» J Int Med Res 32(3): 258-62.

80. Kudchodkar, B. J., A. Pierce, et al. (2007). «Chronic hyperbaric oxygen treatment elicits an anti-oxidant response and attenuates atherosclerosis in apoE knockout mice.» Atherosclerosis 193(1): 28-35.

81. Lavy, A., G. Weisz, et al. (1994). «Hyperbaric oxygen for perianal Crohn's disease.» J Clin Gastroenterol 19(3): 202-5.

82. Leach, R. M., P. J. Rees, et al. (1998). "Hyperbaric oxygen therapy." BMJ 317(7166): 1140-3.

83. Lee, A. K., R. B. Hester, et al. (1993). «Increased oxygen tensions modulate the cellular composition of the adaptive immune system in BALB/c mice.» Cancer Biother 8(3): 241-52.

84. Lee, A. K., R. B. Hester, et al. (1994). «Increased oxygen tensions influence subset composition of the cellular immune system in aged mice.» Cancer Biother 9(1): 39-54.

85. Lou, M., Y. Chen, et al. (2006). «Involvement of the mitochondrial ATP-sensitive potassium channel in the neuroprotective effect of hyperbaric oxygenation after cerebral ischemia.» Brain Res Bull 69(2): 109-16.

86. Lou, M., J. H. Wang, et al. (2008). «[Effect of hyperbaric oxygen treatment on mitochondrial free radicals after transient focal cerebral ischemia in rats].» Zhejiang Da Xue Xue Bao Yi Xue Ban 37(5): 437-43.

87. Marois, P. and M. Vanasse (2003). "Hyperbaric oxygen therapy and cerebral palsy." Dev Med Child Neurol 45(9): 646-7; author reply 647-8.

88. Miljkovic-Lolic, M., R. Silbergleit, et al. (2003). «Neuroprotective effects of hyperbaric oxygen treatment in experimental focal cerebral ischemia are associated with reduced brain leukocyte myeloperoxidase activity.» Brain Res 971(1): 90-4.

89. Moon, R. E. and J. J. Feldmeier (2002). "Hyperbaric oxygen: an evidence based approach to its application." Undersea Hyperb Med 29(1): 1-3.

90. Neubauer, R. A. (2001). "Hyperbaric oxygenation for cerebral palsy." Lancet 357(9273): 2052; author reply 2053.

91. Neubauer, R. A. and E. End (1980). "Hyperbaric oxygenation as an adjunct therapy in strokes due to thrombosis. A review of 122 patients." Stroke 11(3): 297-300.

92. Neubauer, R. A. and S. F. Gottlieb (1993). "Hyperbaric oxygen for brain injury." J Neurosurg 78(4): 687-8.

93. Neubauer, R. A., S. F. Gottlieb, et al. (1992). «Identification of hypometabolic areas in the brain using brain imaging and hyperbaric oxygen.» Clin Nucl Med 17(6): 477-81.

94. Neubauer, R. A., S. F. Gottlieb, et al. (1994). «Hyperbaric oxygen for treatment of closed head injury.» South Med J 87(9): 933-6.

95. Neubauer, R. A. and P. James (1998). "Cerebral oxygenation and the recoverable brain." Neurol Res 20 Suppl 1: S33-6.

96. Nie, H., L. Xiong, et al. (2006). «Hyperbaric oxygen preconditioning induces tolerance against spinal cord ischemia by upregulation of antioxidant enzymes in rabbits.» J Cereb Blood Flow Metab 26(5): 666-74.

97. Pelaia, P., P. Volturo, et al. (1990). "[Mechanical ventilation in hyperbaric environment: experimental evaluation of the Drager Hyperlog]." Minerva Anestesiol 56(10): 1371.

98. Poliakova, L. V., V. L. Lukich, et al. (1991). «[Hyperbaric oxygenation and drug therapy in treatment of nonspecific ulcerative colitis and Crohn's disease].» Fiziol Zh 37(5): 120-3.

99. Qibiao, W., W. Hongjun, et al. (1995). «Treatment of children's epilepsy by hyperbaric oxygenation: analysis of 100 cases.» Proceedings of the Eleventh International Congress on Hyperbaric Medicine. Flagstaff, AZ: Best Publishing: 79–81.

100. Rachmilewitz, D., F. Karmeli, et al. (1998). «Hyperbaric oxygen: a novel modality to ameliorate experimental colitis.» Gut 43(4): 512-8.

101. Reillo, M., R. Altieri, et al. (1994). "Hyperbaric oxygen therapy to relieve chronic fatigue associated with HIV/AIDS [letter]." AIDS Patient Care 8(3): 106-7.

102. Reillo, M. R. and R. J. Altieri (1996). "HIV antiviral effects of hyperbaric oxygen therapy." J Assoc Nurses AIDS Care 7(1): 43-5.

103. Rocco, M., M. Antonelli, et al. (2001). «Lipid peroxidation, circulating cytokine and endothelin 1 levels in healthy volunteers undergoing hyperbaric oxygenation.» Minerva Anestesiol 67(5): 393-400.

104. Rockswold, G. L. and S. E. Ford (1985). "Preliminary results of a prospective randomized trial for treatment of severely brain-injured patients with hyperbaric oxygen." Minn Med 68(7): 533-5.

105. Rockswold, S. B., G. L. Rockswold, et al. (2001). "Effects of hyperbaric oxygenation therapy on cerebral metabolism and intracranial pressure in severely brain injured patients." J Neurosurg 94(3): 403-11.

106. Rossignol, D. A. (2007). "Hyperbaric oxygen therapy might improve certain pathophysiological findings in autism." Med Hypotheses 68(6): 1208-27.

107. Rossignol, D. A. (2008). The use of hyperbaric oxygen therapy in autism. Hyperbaric oxygen for neurological disorders. J. H. Zhang. Flagstaff, AZ, Best Publishing Company: 209-258.

108. Rossignol, D. A. and J. J. Bradstreet (2008). "Evidence of mitochondrial dysfunction in autism and implications for treatment." American Journal of Biochemistry and Biotechnology 4(2): 208-217.

109. Rossignol, D. A. and L. W. Rossignol (2006). "Hyperbaric oxygen therapy may improve symptoms in autistic children." Med Hypotheses 67(2): 216-28.

110. Rossignol, D. A., L. W. Rossignol, et al. (2007). «The effects of hyperbaric oxygen therapy on oxidative stress, inflammation, and symptoms in children with autism: an open-label pilot study.» BMC Pediatr 7(1): 36.

111. Rossignol DA. Hyperbaric oxygen treatment for inflammatory bowel disease: a systematic review and analysis. Med Gas Res. 2012 Mar15;2(1):6. doi: 10.1186/2045-9912-2-6.

112. Rossignol DA, Bradstreet JJ, Van Dyke K, Schneider C, Freedenfeld SH, O'Hara N, Cave S, Buckley JA, Mumper EA, Frye RE. Hyperbaric oxygen treatment in autism spectrum disorders. Med Gas Res. 2012 Jun 15;2(1):16. doi: 10.1186/2045-9912-2-16.

113. Rothfuss, A., C. Dennog, et al. (1998). «Adaptive protection against the induction of oxidative DNA damage after hyperbaric oxygen treatment.» Carcinogenesis 19(11): 1913-7.

114. Rothfuss, A., P. Radermacher, et al. (2001). "Involvement of heme oxygenase-1 (HO-1) in the adaptive protection of human lymphocytes after hyperbaric oxygen (HBO) treatment." Carcinogenesis 22(12): 1979-85.

115. Saito, K., Y. Tanaka, et al. (1991). «Suppressive effect of hyperbaric oxygenation on immune responses of normal and autoimmune mice.» Clin Exp Immunol 86(2): 322-7.

116. Sénéchal, C., S. Larivée, et al. (2007). «Hyperbaric Oxygenation Therapy in the Treatment of Cerebral Palsy: A Review and Comparison to Currently Accepted Therapies.» Journal of American Physicians and Surgeons 12(4): 109-113.

117. Sethi, A. and A. Mukherjee (2003). "To see the efficacy of hyperbaric oxygen therapy in gross motor abilities of cerebral palsy children of 2-5 years, given initially as an adjunct to occupational therapy. ." The Indian Journal of Occupational Therapy 25(1): 7-11.

118. Sheffield, P. J. and D. A. Desautels (1997). "Hyperbaric and hypobaric chamber fires: a 73-year analysis." Undersea Hyperb Med 24(3): 153-64.

119. Shi, X. Y., Z. Q. Tang, et al. (2006). «Evaluation of hyperbaric oxygen treatment of neuropsychiatric disorders following traumatic brain injury.» Chin Med J (Engl) 119(23): 1978-82.

120. Shi, X. Y., Z. Q. Tang, et al. (2003). «Cerebral perfusion SPECT imaging for assessment of the effect of hyperbaric oxygen therapy on patients with postbrain injury neural status.» Chin J Traumatol 6(6): 346-9.

121. Stoller, K. P. (2005). "Quantification of neurocognitive changes before, during, and after hyperbaric oxygen therapy in a case of fetal alcohol syndrome." Pediatrics 116(4): e586-91.

122. Sumen, G., M. Cimsit, et al. (2001). «Hyperbaric oxygen treatment reduces carrageenan-induced acute inflammation in rats.» Eur J Pharmacol 431(2): 265-8.

123. Sumen-Secgin, G., M. Cimsit, et al. (2005). "Antidepressant-like effect of hyperbaric oxygen treatment in forced-swimming test in rats." Methods Find Exp Clin Pharmacol 27(7): 471-4.

124. Takeshima, F., K. Makiyama, et al. (1999). "Hyperbaric oxygen as adjunct therapy for Crohn's intractable enteric ulcer." Am J Gastroenterol 94(11): 3374-5.

125. Thom, S. (1993). "A role for hyperbaric oxygen in clostridial myonecrosis." Clin Infect Dis 17(2): 238.

126. Thom, S. R., V. M. Bhopale, et al. (2006). «Stem cell mobilization by hyperbaric oxygen.» Am J Physiol Heart Circ Physiol 290(4): H1378-86.

127. Tomaszewski, C. A. and S. R. Thom (1994). "Use of hyperbaric oxygen in toxicology." Emerg Med Clin North Am 12(2): 437-59.

128. Vitullo, V., P. Pelaia, et al. (1990). "[The role of hyperbaric oxygenation in treatment of retinal occlusive pathology]." Minerva Anestesiol 56(10): 1379.

129. Vlodavsky, E., E. Palzur, et al. (2006). "Hyperbaric oxygen therapy reduces neuroinflammation and expression of matrix metalloproteinase-9 in the rat model of traumatic brain injury." Neuropathol Appl Neurobiol 32(1): 40-50.

130. Wada, K., T. Miyazawa, et al. (2001). "Preferential conditions for and possible mechanisms of induction of ischemic tolerance by repeated hyperbaric oxygenation in gerbil hippocampus." Neurosurgery 49(1): 160-6; discussion 166-7.

131. Wada, K., T. Miyazawa, et al. (2000). "Mn-SOD and Bcl-2 expression after repeated hyperbaric oxygenation." Acta Neurochir Suppl 76: 285-90.

132. Weber, C. A., C. A. Duncan, et al. (1990). "Depletion of tissue glutathione with diethyl maleate enhances hyperbaric oxygen toxicity." Am J Physiol 258(6 Pt 1): L308-12.

133. Weisz, G., A. Lavy, et al. (1997). «Modification of in vivo and in vitro TNF-alpha, IL-1, and IL-6 secretion by circulating monocytes during hyperbaric oxygen treatment in patients with perianal Crohn's disease.» J Clin Immunol 17(2): 154-9.

134. Wilson, H. D., J. R. Wilson, et al. (2006). "Hyperbaric oxygen treatment decreases inflammation and mechanical hypersensitivity in an animal model of inflammatory pain." Brain Res 1098(1): 126-8.

135. Xu, X., H. Yi, et al. (1997). «Differential sensitivities to hyperbaric oxygen of lymphocyte subpopulations of normal and autoimmune mice.» Immunol Lett 59(2): 79-84.

136. Yang, Z., J. Nandi, et al. (2006). «Hyperbaric oxygenation ameliorates indomethacin-induced enteropathy in rats by modulating TNF-alpha and IL-1beta production.» Dig Dis Sci 51(8): 1426-33.

137. Yang, Z. J., G. Bosco, et al. (2001). "Hyperbaric O2 reduces intestinal ischemia-reperfusion-induced TNF-alpha production and lung neutrophil sequestration." Eur J Appl Physiol 85(1-2): 96-103.

138. Yang, Z. J., C. Camporesi, et al. (2002). "Hyperbaric oxygenation mitigates focal cerebral injury and reduces striatal dopamine release in a rat model of transient middle cerebral artery occlusion." Eur J Appl Physiol 87(2): 101-7.

139. Yatsuzuka, H. (1991). "[Effects of hyperbaric oxygen therapy on ischemic brain injury in dogs]." Masui 40(2): 208-23.

140. Yildiz, S., G. Uzun, et al. (2006). «Hyperbaric oxygen therapy in chronic pain management.» Curr Pain Headache Rep 10(2): 95-100.

141. Yin, W., A. E. Badr, et al. (2002). «Down regulation of COX-2 is involved in hyperbaric oxygen treatment in a rat transient focal cerebral ischemia model.» Brain Res 926(1-2): 165-71.

Chapter 25. Cerebral Folate Deficiency in Autism Spectrum Disorders, by Dr. Richard E. Frye and Dr. Daniel A. Rossignol

1. Ramaekers VT, Husler M, Opladen T, Heimann G, Blau N. Psychomotor retardation, spastic paraplegia, cerebellar ataxia and dyskinesia associated with low 5-methyltetrahydrofolate in cerebrospinal fluid: a novel neurometabolic condition responding to folinic acid substitution. *Neuropediatrics.* 2002 Dec;33(6):301-8.

2. Ramaekers VT, Blau N. Cerebral folate deficiency. *Dev Med Child Neurol.* 2004 Dec;46(12):843-51.

3. Ramaekers VT, Rothenberg SP, Sequeira JM, Opladen T, Blau N, Quadros EV, Selhub J. Autoantibodies to folate receptors in the cerebral folate deficiency syndrome. *N Engl J Med.* 2005 May 12;352(19):1985-91.

4. Molloy AM, Quadros EV, Sequeira JM, Troendle JF, Scott JM, Kirke PN, Mills JL. Lack of association between folate-receptor autoantibodies and neural-tube defects. *N Engl J Med.* 2009 Jul 9;361(2):152-60.

5. Pineda M, Ormazabal A, Lopez-Gallardo E, Nascimento A, Solano A, Herrero MD, Vilaseca MA, Briones P, Ibanez L, Montoya J, Artuch R. Cerebral folate deficiency and leukoencephalopathy caused by a mitochondrial DNA deletion. *Ann Neurol.* 2006 Feb;59(2):394-8.

6. Ramaekers VT, Weis J, Sequeira JM, Quadros EV, Blau N. Mitochondrial complex I encephalomyopathy and cerebral 5-methyltetrahydrofolate deficiency. *Neuropediatrics.* 2007 Aug;38(4):184-7.

7. Hasselmann O, Blau N, Ramaekers VT, Quadros EV, Sequeira JM, Weissert M. Cerebral folate deficiency and CNS inflammatory markers in Alpers disease. *Mol Genet Metab.* 2010 Jan;99(1):58-61.

8. Frye RE, Naviaux RK. Autistic disorder with complex IV overactivity: A new mitochondrial syndrome. *J Ped Neurol,* 2011 9:427-434.

9. Garcia-Cazorla A, Quadros EV, Nascimento A, Garcia-Silva MT, Briones P, Montoya J, Ormazabal A, Artuch R, Sequeira JM, Blau N, Arenas J, Pineda M, Ramaekers VT. Mitochondrial diseases associated with cerebral folate deficiency. *Neurology.* 2008 Apr 15;70(16):1360-2.

10. Moretti P, Sahoo T, Hyland K, Bottiglieri T, Peters S, del Gaudio D, Roa B, Curry S, Zhu H, Finnell RH, Neul JL, Ramaekers VT, Blau N, Bacino CA, Miller G, Scaglia F. Cerebral folate deficiency with developmental delay, autism, and response to folinic acid. *Neurology.* 2005 Mar 22;64(6):1088-90.

11. Moretti P, Peters SU, Del Gaudio D, Sahoo T, Hyland K, Bottiglieri T, Hopkin RJ, Peach E, Min SH, Goldman D, Roa B, Bacino CA, Scaglia F. Autistic symptoms, developmental regression, mental retardation, epilepsy, and dyskinesias in CNS folate deficiency. *J Autism Dev Disord.* 2008 Jul;38(6):1170-7. Epub 2007 Nov 20.

12. Ramaekers VT, Blau N, Sequeira JM, Nassogne MC, Quadros EV. Folate receptor autoimmunity and cerebral folate deficiency in low-functioning autism with neurological deficits. *Neuropediatrics.* 2007 Dec;38(6):276-81.

13. Ramaekers VT, Sequeira JM, Blau N, Quadros EV. A milk-free diet downregulates folate receptor autoimmunity in cerebral folate deficiency syndrome. *Dev Med Child Neurol.* 2008 May;50(5):346-52. Epub 2008 Mar 19.

14. Ramaekers VT, Hansen SI, Holm J, Opladen T, Senderek J, Husler M, Heimann G, Fowler B, Maiwald R, Blau N. Reduced folate transport to the CNS in female Rett patients. *Neurology.* 2003 Aug 26;61(4):506-15

15. Ramaekers VT, Sequeira JM, Artuch R, Blau N, Temudo T, Ormazabal A, Pineda M, Aracil A, Roelens F, Laccone F, Quadros EV. Folate receptor autoantibodies and spinal fluid 5-methyltetrahydrofolate deficiency in Rett syndrome. *Neuropediatrics.* 2007 Aug;38(4):179-83.

16. Frye RE, Sequeira JM, Quadros EV, James SJ, Rossignol DA. Cerebral folate receptor autoantibodies in autism spectrum disorder. Mol Psychiatry. 2013 Mar;18(3):369-81. doi: 10.1038/mp.2011.175. Epub 2012 Jan 10.

17. Ramaekers VT, Quadros EV, Sequeira JM. Role of folate receptor autoantibodies in infantile autism. Mol Psychiatry. 2013 Mar;18(3):270-1. doi: 10.1038/mp.2012.22. Epub 2012 Apr 10.

18. Frye RE, Rossignol DA. Mitochondrial dysfunction can connect the diverse medical symptoms associated with autism spectrum disorders. *Pediatr Res.* 2011 May;69(5 Pt 2):41R-7R.

19. Rossignol DA, Frye RE. Mitochondrial dysfunction in autism spectrum disorders:a systematic review and meta-analysis. *Mol Psychiatry.* 2011 Jan 25. [Epub ahead of print]

20. Kriaucionis S, Paterson A, Curtis J, Guy J, Macleod N, Bird A. Gene expression analysis exposes mitochondrial abnormalities in a mouse model of Rett syndrome. *Mol Cell Biol.* 2006 Jul;26(13):5033-42.

21. Condie J, Goldstein J, Wainwright MS. Acquired microcephaly, regression of milestones, mitochondrial dysfunction, and episodic rigidity in a 46,XY male with a de novo MECP2 gene mutation. *J Child Neurol.* 2010 May;25(5):633-6. Epub 2010 Feb 8.

22. Hansen FJ, Blau N. Cerebral folate deficiency: life-changing supplementation with folinic acid. *Mol Genet Metab.* 2005 Apr;84(4):371-3. Epub 2005 Jan 22.

23. Rothenberg SP, da Costa MP, Sequeira JM, Cracco J, Roberts JL, Weedon J, Quadros EV. Autoantibodies against folate receptors in women with a pregnancy complicated by a neural-tube defect. *N Engl J Med.* 2004 Jan 8;350(2):134-42.

24. Cabrera RM, Shaw GM, Ballard JL, Carmichael SL, Yang W, Lammer FJ, Finnell RH. Autoantibodies to folate receptor during pregnancy and neural tube defect risk. *J Reprod Immunol.* 2008 Oct;79(1): 85-92. Epub 2008 Sep 18.

25. Boyles AL, Ballard JL, Gorman EB, McConnaughey DR, Cabrera RM, Wilcox AJ, Lie RT, Finnell RH. Association between inhibited binding of folic acid to folate receptor alpha in maternal serum and folate-related birth defects in Norway. *Hum Reprod.* 2011 May 15. [Epub ahead of print]

26. Molloy AM, Quadros EV, Sequeira JM, Troendle JF, Scott JM, Kirke PN, Mills JL. Lack of association between folate-receptor autoantibodies and neural-tube defects. *N Engl J Med.* 2009 Jul 9;361(2):152-60.

Chapter 26. From Preconception to Infancy: Environmental and Nutritional Strategies for Lowering the Risk of Autism, by Dr. David Berger

1. Ozonoff S, Young GS, Carter A, Messinger D, Yirmiya N, Zwaigenbaum L, et al. Recurrence risk for autism spectrum disorders: a Baby Siblings Research Consortium study. *Pediatrics.* 2011 Sep;128(3):e488-95.

2. Insel T. NIMH's response to new HRSA autism prevalence estimate. Director's blog, National Institute of Mental Health, October 15, 2009. Available online at: http://www.nimh.nih.gov/about/director/2009/nimhs-response-to-new-hrsa-autism-prevalenceestimate.shtml

3. Wang K, Zhang H, Ma D, Bucan M, Glessner JT, Abrahams BS, et al. Common genetic variants on 5p14.1 associate with autism spectrum disorders. *Nature.* 2009 May;459:528-33.

4. Bailey A, Bolton P, Butler L, Le Couteur A, Murphy M, Scott S, et al. Prevalence of the fragile X anomaly amongst autistic twins and singletons. *J Child Psychol Psychiatry.* 1993 Jul;34(5):673-88.

5. Reddy KS. Cytogenetic abnormalities and fragile-x syndrome in Autism Spectrum Disorder. *BMC Med Genet.* 2005 Jan;6:3.

6. Crawford D, Sherman SL. Fragile X syndrome: application of gene identification to clinical diagnosis and population screening. In MJ Khoury, J Little, W Burke (Eds.), *Human Genome Epidemiology: A Scientific Foundation for Using Genetic Information to Improve Health and Prevent Disease* (Chapter 23). Atlanta, GA: Centers for Disease Control and Prevention, Office of Surveillance, Epidemiology, and Laboratory Services, Public Health Genomics, revised March 2010.

7.   Li XM, Zhang YZ, Xu YX, Jiang S. [Study on the relationship of MTHFR polymorphisms with unexplained recurrent spontaneous abortion]. [Article in Chinese]. *Zhonghua Yi Xue Yi Chuan Xue Za Zhi.* 2004 Feb;21(1):39-42.

8.   Rodríguez-Guillén M del R, Torres-Sánchez L, Chen J, Galván-Portillo M, Blanco-Muñoz J, Anaya MA, et al. Maternal MTHFR polymorphisms and risk of spontaneous abortion. *Salud Publica Mex.* 2009 Jan-Feb;51(1):19-25.

9.   Klerk M, Verhoef, P, Clarke R, Blom HJ, Kok FJ, Schouten EG, et al. MTHFR 677C→T polymorphism and risk of coronary heart disease: a meta-analysis. *JAMA.* 2002 Oct;288(16):2023-31.

10.   Cortese C, Motti C. MTHFR gene polymorphism, homocysteine and cardiovascular disease. *Public Health Nutr.* 2001 Apr;4(2B):493-7.

11.   James SJ, Melnyk S, Fuchs G, Reid T, Jernigan S, Pavliv O, et al. Efficacy of methylcobalamin and folinic acid treatment on glutathione redox status in children with autism. *Am J Clin Nutr.* 2009 Jan;89(1):425-30.

12.   James SJ, Melnyk S, Jernigan S, Hubanks A, Rose S, Gaylor DW. Abnormal transmethylation/transsulfuration metabolism and DNA hypomethylation among parents of children with autism. *J Autism Dev Disord.* 2008 Nov;38(10):1966-75.

13.   Schmidt RJ, Hansen RL, Hartiala J, Allayee H, Schmidt LC, Tancredi DJ, et al. Prenatal vitamins, one-carbon metabolism gene variants, and risk for autism. *Epidemiology.* 2011 Jul;22(4):476-85.

14.   James SJ, Slikker W 3rd, Melnyk S, New E, Pogribna M, Jernigan S. Thimerosal neurotoxicity is associated with glutathione depletion: protection from glutathione precursors. *Neurotoxicology.* 2005 Jan;26(1):1-8.

15.   Martone N, Mizanur Rahman GM, Pamuku M. Determination of chromium species and mass balance in food supplements using speciated isotope dilution mass spectrometry. Pittsburgh, PA: Department of Environmental Science and Management, Duquesne University, unpublished study.

16.   Berger SL, Kouzarides T, Shiekhattar R, Shilatifard A. An operational definition of epigenetics. *Genes Dev.* 2009 Apr;23(7):781-3.

17.   Lalande M, Calciano MA. Molecular epigenetics of Angelman syndrome. *Cell Mol Life Sci.* 2007 Apr;64(7-8):947-60.

18.   Coffee B, Keith K, Albizua I, Malone T,Mowrey J, Sherman SL, et al. Incidence of fragile X syndrome by newborn screening for methylated FMR1 DNA. *Am J Hum Genet.* 2009 Oct;85(4):503-14.

19.   Nelsen DA Jr. Gluten-sensitive enteropathy (celiac disease): more common than you think. *Am Fam Physician.* 2002 Dec;66(12):2259-66.

20.   Sandhu JS, Fraser DR. Effect of dietary cereals on intestinal permeability in experimental enteropathy in rats. *Gut.* 1983 Sep;24(9):825-30.

21.   Hall EJ, Batt RM. Abnormal intestinal permeability could play a role in the development of glutensensitive enteropathy in Irish Setter dogs. *J Nutr.* 1991;121:S150-S151.

22.   Sausenthaler S, Koletzko S, Schaaf B, Lehmann I, Borte M, Herbarth O, et al. Maternal diet during pregnancy in relation to eczema and allergic sensitization in the offspring at 2 y of age. *Am J Clin Nutr.* 2007 Feb;85(2):530-7.

23.   *Physician's Desk Reference*, 65th edition. PDR Network, 2011, p. 3113.

24.   King CT, Rogers PD, Cleary JD, Chapman SW. Antifungal therapy during pregnancy. *Clin Infect Dis.* 1998 Nov; 27(5):1151-60.

25.   Shaw W. Increased urinary excretion of a 3-(3-hydroxyphenyl)-3-hydroxypropionic acid (HPHPA), an abnormal phenylalanine metabolite of Clostridia spp. in the gastrointestinal tract, in urine samples from patients with autism and schizophrenia. *Nutr Neurosci.* 2010 Jun;13(3):135-43.

26.   Braun JM, Yolton K, Dietrich KN, Hornung R, Ye X, Calafat AM, et al. Prenatal bisphenol A exposure and early childhood behavior. *Environ Health Perspect.* 2009 Dec;117(12):1945-52.

27.   Braun JM, Kalkbrenner AE, Calafat AM, Yolton K, Ye X, Dietrich KN, et al. Impact of early-life bisphenol A exposure on behavior and executive function in children. *Pediatrics.* 2011 Nov;128(5):873-82.

28.   Goldman LR, Shannon MW. Technical report: mercury in the environment: implications for pediatricians. *Pediatrics.* 2001 Jul;108(1):197-205.

29.   American Academy of Pediatrics Committee on Environmental Health. Lead exposure in children: prevention, detection, and management (AAP Policy Statement). *Pediatrics.* 2005 Oct;116(4):1036-46.

30.   US Food and Drug Administration (FDA). Mercury levels in commercial fish and shellfish (1990-2010). Available online at: http://tinyurl.com/FDA-mercury-fish

31.   Palmer RF, Blanchard S, Wood R. Proximity to point sources of environmental mercury release as a predictor of autism prevalence. *Health Place.* 2009 Mar;15(1):18-24.

32.   Palmer RF, Blanchard S, Stein Z, Mandell D, Miller C. Environmental mercury release, special education rates, and autism disorder: an ecological study of Texas. *Health Place.* 2006 Jun;12(2):203-9.

33. Sutandar M, Garcia-Bournissen F, Koren G. Hypothyroidism in pregnancy. *J Obstet Gynaecol Can.* 2007;29(4):354-6.

34. Fisher DA, Hoath S, Lakshmanan J. The thyroid hormone effects on growth and development may be mediated by growth factors. *Endocrinol Exp.* 1982 Nov;16(3-4):259-71.

35. Nambiar V, Jagtap VS, Sarathi V, Lila AR, Kamalanathan S, Bandgar TR, et al. Prevalence and impact of thyroid disorders on maternal outcome in Asian-Indian pregnant women. *J Thyroid Res.* 2011 Jul;2011:article ID 429097.

36. Brehm JM, Celedón JC, Soto-Quiros ME, Avila L, Hunninghake GM, Forno E, et al. Serum vitamin D levels and markers of severity of childhood asthma in Costa Rica. *Am J Respir Crit Care Med.* 2009 May;179(9):765-71.

37. Sorensen IM, Joner G, Jenum PA, Eskild A, Torjesen PA, Stene LC. Maternal serum levels of 25-hydroxyvitamin D during pregnancy and risk of type 1 diabetes in the offspring. *Diabetes.* 2012 Jan;61(1):175-8.

38. Vitamin D Council. Autism: introduction. Revised 2011 May 17. Available online at: http://www.vitamindcouncil.org/health-conditions/neurological-conditions/autism/introduction/

39. Vitamin D Council. Vitamin D Council statement on FNB Vitamin D Report. 2010 Nov 30. Available online at: http://www.vitamindcouncil.org/news-archive/2010/vitamin-dcouncil-statement-on-fnb-vitamin-d-report/

40. Centers for Disease Control and Prevention. Recommendations to prevent and control iron deficiency in the United States. *MMWR.* 1998 Apr;47(RR-3):1-36.

41. Latif A, Heinz P, Cook R. Iron deficiency in autism and Asperger syndrome. *Autism.* 2002 Mar;6(1):103-14.

42. Konofal E, Lecendreux M, Arnulf I, Mouren MC. Iron deficiency in children with attention-deficit/hyperactivity disorder. *Arch Pediatr Adolesc Med.* 2004 Dec;158(12):1113-5.

43. Halterma JS, Kaczorowski JM, Aligne CA, Auinger P, Szilagyi PG. Iron deficiency and cognitive achievement among school-aged children and adolescents in the United States. *Pediatrics.* 2001 Jun;107(6):1381-6.

44. Bruner AB, Joffe A, Duggan AK, Casella JF, Brandt J. Randomised study of cognitive effects of iron supplementation in non-anaemic iron-deficient adolescent girls. *Lancet.* 1996 Oct;348(9033):992-6.

45. Sever Y, Ashkenazi A, Tyano S, Weizman A. Iron treatment in children with attention deficit hyperactivity disorder. A preliminary report. *Neuropsychobiology.* 1997;35(4):178-80.

46. Milman N, Bergholt T, Eriksen L, Byg KE, Graudal N, Pedersen P, et al. Iron prophylaxis during pregnancy — how much iron is needed? A randomized dose-response study of 20-80 mg ferrous iron daily in pregnant women. *Acta Obstet Gynecol Scand.* 2005 Mar;84(3):238-47.

47. Frye RE, Rossignol DA. Cerebral folate deficiency in autism spectrum disorders. *Autism Science Digest.* 2011;Issue 2:9-15.

48. Simopoulos AP, Leaf A, Salem N. Workshop on the essentiality of and recommended dietary intakes for omega-6 and omega-3 fatty acids. *J Am Coll Nutr.* 1999 Oct;18(5):487-9.

49. Dunstan JA, Simmer K, Dixon G, Prescott SL. Cognitive assessment of children at age 2(1/2) years after maternal fish oil supplementation in pregnancy: a randomised controlled trial. *Arch Dis Child Fetal Neonatal Ed.* 2008 Jan;93(1):F45-50.

50. Helland IB, Smith L, Saarem K, Saugstad OD, Drevon CA. Maternal supplementation with very-long-chain n-3 fatty acids during pregnancy and lactation augments children's IQ at 4 years of age. *Pediatrics.* 2003 Jan;111(1):e39-e44.

51. Dunstan JA, Prescott SL. Does fish oil supplementation in pregnancy reduce the risk of allergic disease in infants? *Curr Opin Allergy Clin Immunol.* 2005 Jun;5(3):215-21.

52. Dunstan JA, Mori TA, Barden A, Beilin LJ, Taylor AL, Holt PG, et al. Fish oil supplementation in pregnancy modifies neonatal allergen-specific immune responses and clinical outcomes in infants at high risk of atopy: a randomized, controlled trial. *J Allergy Clin Immunol.* 2003 Dec;112(6):1178-84.

53. Glasson EJ, Bower C, Petterson B, de Klerk N, Chaney G, Hallmayer JF. Perinatal factors and the development of autism: a population study. *Arch Gen Psychiatry.* 2004 Jun;61(6):618-27.

54. American College of Obstetricians and Gynecologists. ACOG practice bulletin #115: vaginal birth after previous Cesarean delivery. *Obstet Gynecol.* 2010 Aug;116(2 Pt 1):450-63.

55. Kurth L, Haussmann R. Perinatal pitocin as an early ADHD biomarker: neurodevelopmental risk? *J Atten Disord.* 2011 Jul;15(5):423-31.

56. Canadian Paediatric Society. Routine administration of vitamin K to newborns. A joint position statement of the Fetus and Newborn Committee, Canadian Paediatric Society (CPS), and the Committee on Child and Adolescent Health, College of Family Physicians of Canada. *Paediatr Child Health.* 1997;2(6):429-31. Reaffirmed February 2011.

57. Fetus and Newborn Committee of the Paediatric Society of New Zealand. Vitamin K prophylaxis in the newborn. Fetus and Newborn Committee of the Paediatric Society of New Zealand, The New Zealand College of Midwives (Inc.), The New Zealand Nurses Organisation, The Royal New Zealand College of General

Practitioners, The Royal Australian and New Zealand College of Obstetricians and Gynaecologists. Prescriber Update No. 21:36-40. Available online at: http://www.medsafe.govt.nz/profs/puarticles/vitk.htm

58. National Health and Medical Research Council. Joint statement and recommendations on vitamin K administration to newborn infants to prevent vitamin K deficiency bleeding in infancy. National Health and Medical Research Council, Paediatric Division of the Royal Australasian College of Physicians, Royal Australian and New Zealand College of Obstetrics and Gynaecology, Royal Australian College of General Practitioners, Australian College of Midwives. 2010 Oct: 1. Available online at: http://www.nhmrc.gov.au/guidelines/publications/ch39

59. American Academy of Pediatrics. Breastfeeding and the use of human milk. *Pediatrics*. 2005 Feb;115(2):496-506.

60. Kramer MS, Aboud F, Mironova E, Vanilovich I, Platt RW, Matush L, et al. Breastfeeding and child cognitive development: new evidence from a large randomized trial. *Arch Gen Psychiatry*. 2008 May; 65(5):578-84.

61. Isaacs EB, Fischl BR, Quinn BT, Chong WK, Gadian DG, Lucas A. Impact of breast milk on intelligence quotient, brain size, and white matter development. *Pediatr Res*. 2010 Apr;67(4):357-62.

62. Majeed AA, Mea, Hassan K. Risk factors for type 1 diabetes mellitus among children and adolescents in Basrah. *Oman Med J*. 2011 May;26(3):189-95.

63. Gruskay FL. Comparison of breast, cow, and soy feedings in the prevention of onset of allergic disease: a 15-year prospective study. *Clin Pediatr (Phila)*. 1982 Aug;21(8):486-91.

64. Oddy WH, Holt PG, Sly PD, Read AW, Landau LI, Stanley FJ, et al. Association between breast feeding and asthma in 6 year old children: findings of a prospective birth cohort study. *BMJ*. 1999 Sep;319(7213):815-9.

65. Duncan B, Ey J, Holberg CJ, Wright AL, Martinez FD, Taussig LM. Exclusive breast-feeding for at least 4 months protects against otitis media. *Pediatrics*. 1993 May;91(5):867-72.

66. Weaver LT, Laker MF, Nelson R, Lucas A. Milk feeding and changes in intestinal permeability and morphology in the newborn. *J Pediatr Gastroenterol Nutr*. 1987 May-Jun;6(3):351-8.

67. Taylor SN, Basile LA, Ebeling M, Wagner CL. Intestinal permeability in preterm infants by feeding type: mother's milk versus formula. *Breastfeed Med*. 2009 Mar;4(1):11-5.

68. Lawrence R, Lawrence R. *Breastfeeding: A Guide for the Medical Profession*, 5th Edition. St. Louis, Missouri: Mosby Inc., 1999, pp. 117-9.

69. Fiocchi A, Assa'ad A, Bahna S. Food allergy and the introduction of solid foods to infants: a consensus document. Adverse Reactions to Foods Committee, American College of Allergy, Asthma and Immunology. *Ann Allergy Asthma Immunol*. 2006 Jul;97(1):10-20.

70. Pickering LK, Baker CJ, Kimberlin DW, Long SS (Eds.). *Red Book: 2009 Report of the Committee on Infectious Diseases*, 28th ed. Elk Grove Village, IL: American Academy of Pediatrics, 2009, p. 8.

71. Flanagan-Klygis EA, Sharp L, Frader JE. Dismissing the family who refuses vaccines: a study of pediatrician attitudes. *Arch Pediatr Adolesc Med*. 2005 Oct;159(10):929-34.

72. McDonald KL, Huq SI, Lix LM, Becker AB, Kozyrskyj AL. Delay in diphtheria, pertussis, tetanus vaccination is associated with a reduced risk of childhood asthma. *J Allergy Clin Immunol*. 2008 Mar;121(3):626-31.

73. Johnston SL, Holgate ST. *Asthma: Critical Debates*. London: Blackwell Science Ltd, 2002.

74. Marodi L. Down-regulation of Th1 responses in human neonates. *Clin Exp Immunol*. 2002 Apr;128(1):1-2.

75. Rossignol DA, Bradstreet JJ. Evidence of mitochondrial dysfunction in autism and implications for treatment. *Am J Biochem Biotechnol*. 2008;4(2):208-17.

76. Child Doe/77 v. Secretary of Health and Human Services. 2010 WL 3395654 (Fed. Cl. July 21, 2010). Available online at: http://www.uscfc.uscourts.gov/sites/default/files/CA MPBELLSMITH.%20DOE77082710.pdf

77. Rossignol DA, Frye RE. Mitochondrial dysfunction and autism spectrum disorders: a simplified approach. *Autism Science Digest*. 2011;Issue 2:20-7.

78. Cohen AD, Shoenfeld Y. Vaccine-induced autoimmunity. *J Autoimmun*. 1996 Dec;9(6):699-703.

79. Koppang EO, Bjerkås I, Haugarvoll E, Chan EK, Szabo NJ, Ono N, et al. Vaccination-induced systemic autoimmunity in farmed Atlantic salmon. *J Immunol*. 2008 Oct ; 181(7):4807-14.

80. O'Leary ST, Glanz JM, McClure DL, Akhtar A, Daley MF, Nakasata C, et al. The risk of immune thrombocytopenic purpura after vaccination in children and adolescents. *Pediatrics*. 2012 Jan 9. [Epub ahead of print]

81. Singh VK, Lin SX, Newell E, Nelson C. Abnormal measlesmumps-rubella antibodies and CNS autoimmunity in children with autism. *J Biomed Sci*. 2002 Jul-Aug;9(4):359-64.

82. Connolly AM, Chez MG, Pestronk A, Arnold ST, Mehta S, Deuel RK. Serum autoantibodies to brain in Landau-Kleffner variant, autism, and other neurologic disorders. *J Pediatr*. 1999 May;134(5):607-13.

83. Singer HS, Morris CM, Williams PN, Yoon DY, Hong JJ, Zimmerman AW. Antibrain antibodies in children with autism and their unaffected siblings. *J Neuroimmunol*. 2006 Sep;178(1-2):149-55.

84.	Gallagher C, Goodman M. Hepatitis B triple series vaccine and developmental disability in US children aged 1-9 years. *Toxicol Environ Chem.* 2008 Sep;90(5):997-1008.
85.	Gallagher CM, Goodman MS. Hepatitis B vaccination of male neonates and autism diagnosis, NHIS 1997-2002. *J Toxicol Environ Health A.* 2010;73(24):1665-77.

Chapter27. Tetrahydrobiopterin Metabolism in Autism Spectrum Disorder, by Dr. Richard E. Frye

1.	Frye RE, Huffman LC, Elliott GR. Tetrahydrobiopterin as a novel therapeutic intervention for autism. *Neurotherapeutics : the journal of the American Society for Experimental NeuroTherapeutics.* Jul 2010;7(3):241-249. PMCID: 2908599
2.	Tani Y, Fernell E, Watanabe Y, Kanai T, Langstrom B. Decrease in 6R-5,6,7,8-tetrahydrobiopterin content in cerebrospinal fluid of autistic patients. *Neuroscience letters.* Nov 7 1994;181(1-2):169-172. PMCID:
3.	Frye RE. Central tetrahydrobiopterin concentration in neurodevelopmental disorders. *Frontiers in neuroscience.* 2010;4:52. PMCID: 2906199
4.	Nakan Y, Naruse H, Hayashi T, Takesada M, Yamazaki K. Clinical effect of R-THBP on Infantile Autism. In: Naruse H, Ornitz E, eds. *Neurobiology of Infantile Autism.* New York: Elsevier Science Publishers; 1992:337-349.
5.	Naruse H, Hayashi T, Takesada M. *A preliminary study on clinical effect of tetrahydrobiopterin in infantile autism.*: Ministry of Health and Welfare;1985.
6.	Naruse H, Hayashi T, Takesada M, Nakane Y, Yamazaki K. Metabolic changes of aromatic amino acids and monoamine in infantile autism and development of new treatment related to findings. *No to Hattatu.* 1989;21:181-189. PMCID:
7.	Naruse H, Hayahi I, Takesada M, Nakane Y, Yamazaki K, Noguchi T, Watanabe Y, Hayaisho O. Therapeutic effect of tetrahydrobiopterin in infantile autism. *Proceedings of the Japan Academy.* 1987;63(231-233). PMCID:
8.	Naruse H, Takesada M, Nakane Y, Yamazaki K, Uchiyama T, Kaihara S, Ohashi T. Clinical evaluation of R-tetrahydrobiopterin (SUN 0588) on infantile autism — a double-blind comparative study using placebo as a control. *Rinsho Iyaku.* 1990;6:1343-1368. PMCID:
9.	Naruse H, Takesada M, Nagahata M, Kazamatsuri H, Nakane Y, Yamazaki K. An open clinical study of apropterin hydrochloride (R-tetrahydrobiopterin SUN 0588) in infantile autism — clinical study using a Rating Scale for Abnormal Behaviors in Children. *Rinsho Iyaku.* 1990;6:1859-1875. PMCID:
10.	Nagahata M, Kazamatsuri H, Naruse H, Yamazaki K, Takesada M, Nakane Y, Kaihara S, Ohashi T. Clinical evaluation of aproterin hydrochloride (R-THBP. SUN 0588) on infantile autism - a multicenter cooperative study. *Rinsho Iyaku.* 1990;6:1877-1899. PMCID:
11.	Nakane Y, Asuo T, Shimogawa S, Fujiwara T, Kawabata Y, Kubota J. Clinical efficacy and effects on physical development of long-term treatment of R-tetrahydrobiopterin (R-THBP, SUN 0588) for autism. . *Kiso to Rinshou.* 1990;24:4579-4598. PMCID:
12.	Takesada M, Naruse H, Nagahata M. An open clinical study of aprpterin hydrochloride (R-tetrahydrobiopterin, R-THBP) in infantile autism — clinical effects and long-term follow-up. International Symposium on Neurobiology of Infantile Autism; November 10–11, 1990; Tokyo, Japan.
13.	Danfors T, von Knorring AL, Hartvig P, Langstrom B, Moulder R, Stromberg B, Torstenson R, Wester U, Watanabe Y, Eeg-Olofsson O. Tetrahydrobiopterin in the treatment of children with autistic disorder: a double-blind placebo-controlled crossover study. *Journal of clinical psychopharmacology.* Oct 2005;25(5):485-489. PMCID:
14.	Fernell E, Watanabe Y, Adolfsson I, Tani Y, Bergstrom M, Hartvig P, Lilja A, von Knorring AL, Gillberg C, Langstrom B. Possible effects of tetrahydrobiopterin treatment in six children with autism—clinical and positron emission tomography data: a pilot study. *Developmental medicine and child neurology.* May 1997;39(5):313-318. PMCID:
15.	Frye RE, DeLatorre R, Taylor HB, Slattery J, Melnyk S, Chowdhury N, James SJ. Metabolic effects of sapropterin treatment in autism spectrum disorder: a preliminary study. *Translational psychiatry.* 2013;3:e237. PMCID: 3625913
16.	Klaiman C, Huffman L, Masaki L, Elliott GR. Tetrahydrobiopterin as a treatment for autism spectrum disorders: a double-blind, placebo-controlled trial. *Journal of child and adolescent psychopharmacology.* Jun 2013;23(5):320-328. PMCID:

Chapter 28. Observing the Autism Brain with Real-Time Imaging: the Role of Transcranial Ultrasound (TUS) in Autism, with Implications for the Brain-Immune System Link in Autism and an Exploration of Interventions, by Dr. James Jeffrey Bradstreet

Bradstreet JJ, Pacini S, Ruggiero M. A new methodology of viewing extra-axial fluid and cortical abnormalities in children with autism via transcranial ultrasonography. *Front. Hum. Neurosci.* 2014. 7:934. doi: 10.3389/fnhum.2013.00934 .

Bradstreet J, Vogelaar E, Thyer L. Initial Observations of Elevated Alpha-N-Acetylgalactosaminidase Activity Associated with Autism and Observed Reductions from GC Protein—Macrophage Activating Factor Injections. *Autism Insights.* 2012:4 31-38.

Conti P, Varvara G, Murmura G, Tete S, Sabatino G, Saggini A, Rosati M, Toniato E, Caraffa A, Antinolfi P, Pandolfi F, Potalivo G, Galzio R, Theoharides TC. Comparison of beneficial actions of non-steroidal anti-inflammatory drugs to flavonoids. *J Biol Regul Homeost Agents.* 2013 Jan-Mar;27(1):1-7.

Gesundheit B, Rosenzweig JP, Naor D, Lerer B, Zachor DA, Procházka V, Melamed M, Kristt DA, Steinberg A, Shulman C, Hwang P, Koren G, Walfisch A, Passweg JR, Snowden JA, Tamouza R, Leboyer M, Farge-Bancel D, Ashwood P. Immunological and autoimmune considerations of Autism Spectrum Disorders. J Autoimmun. 2013 Aug;44:1-7. doi: 10.1016/j.jaut.2013.05.005. Epub 2013 Jul 15.

Ruggiero M, Magherini S, Fiore M, Chiarelli B, Morucci G, Branca J, Gulisano M, Pacini S. Transcranial sonography: a technique for the study of the temporal lobes of the human and non-human primate brain. *Italian Journal of Anatomy and Embryology,* [S.l.], v. 118, n. 3, p. 241-255, Dec. 2013. ISSN 2038-5129.

Shen MD, Nordahl CW, Young GS, Wootton-Gorges SL, Lee A, Liston SE, Harrington KR, Ozonoff S, Amaral DG. Early brain enlargement and elevated extra-axial fluid in infants who develop autism spectrum disorder. *Brain.* 2013 Sep;136(Pt 9):2825-35. doi: 10.1093/brain/awt166. Epub 2013 Jul 9.

Siniscalco D, Bradstreet JJ, Sych N, Antonucci N. Perspectives on the Use of Stem Cells for Autism Treatment. *Stem Cells Int.* 2013;2013:262438. Epub 2013 Oct 10.

Siniscalco D, Cirillo A, Bradstreet JJ, Antonucci N. Epigenetic findings in autism: new perspectives for therapy. *Int J Environ Res Public Health.* 2013 Sep 11;10(9):4261-73. doi: 10.3390/ijerph10094261.

Theoharides TC, Asadi S, Panagiotidou S. A case series of a luteolin formulation (NeuroProtek®) in children with autism spectrum disorders. *Int J Immunopathol Pharmacol.* 2012 Apr-Jun;25(2):317-23.

Theoharides TC, Kempuraj D, Iliopoulou BP. Mast cells, T cells, and inhibition by luteolin: implications for the pathogenesis and treatment of multiple sclerosis. *Adv Exp Med Biol.* 2007;601:423-30. Review.

Chapter 29. Chlorine Dioxide's Role in Healing Autism, by Kerri Rivera

1.   Gupta S, Kumar S, Satapathy A, Ray U, Chatterjee S, Choudhury TK. Ascaris lumbricoides: an unusual aetiology of gastric perforation. 2012. *J of Surgical Case Reports.* doi:10.1093/jscr/rjs008.

2.   Chawala A, Patwardhan V, Maheshwari M, Wasnik A. 2003. Primary ascaridial perforation of the small intestine: Sonographic diagnosis. *Clinical Ultrasound.* 31(4): 211-213.

3.   Rivera, Kerri and Kimberly McDaniel. *Healing the Symptoms Known as Autism.* Chicago: AutismO2, 2012.

4.   United States. Department of Health and Human Services, Food and Drug Administration, Code of Federal Regulations. 2012 ed. Title 21, Pt. 173, Volume 3. Web. 20 Nov 2013.

5.   Ekiel A, Aptekorz M, Kazek B, Wiechuła B, Wilk I, Martirosian G. 2010. Intestinal microflora of autistic children. *Med Dosw Mikrobiol.* 62:237-243.

6.   Kałużna-Czaplińska J, Błaszczyk S. 2012. The level of arabinitol in autistic children after probiotic therapy. *Nutrition.* 28:124-126.

7.   Bradstreet J, Vogelaar E, Thyer L. 2012. Initial observations of elevated alpha-N-acetylgalactosaminidase activity associated with autism, and observed reductions from Gc protein – macrophage activating factor injections. *Autism Insights.* 4:31–38.

8.   Mohamad SB, Nagasawa H, Uto Y, Hori H. 2002. Tumor cell alpha-N-acetylgalactosaminidase activity and its involvement in GcMAF-related macrophage activation. *Comp Biochem Phys Part A.* 132:1-8.

9.   Bransfield RC. 2009. Preventable cases of autism: relationship between chronic infectious diseases and neurological outcome. *Pediatric Health.* 3(2):125-140.

10.   Ion Exchange: Water Tech. 2012. Chlorine Dioxide – The Disinfectant of Choice No. 12. http://www.ionindia.com/pdf/water_tech/WATERTECH%20January%202011%20-%20Final.pdf.

11. Noszticzius Z, Wittman M, Kály-Kullai, Beregvári Z, Kiss I, Rosivall L Szegedi J. Demonstrating that cholorine dioxide is a size-selective antimicrobial agent and high purity ClO2 antiseptic. Submitted to *Quantitative Biology* Apr 2013.
12. Volinsky AA, Gubarev NV, Orlovskyaya GM, Marchenko EV. Human anaerobic intestinal "rope" parasites. Submitted to *Quantitative Biology* Jan 2013.

Chapter 30. Repetitive Transcranial Magnetic Stimulation and Magnetic Resonant Therapy™ for Autism, by Dr. James Jeffrey Bradstreet

Enticott PG, Rinehart NJ, Tonge BJ, Bradshaw JL, Fitzgerald PB. A preliminary transcranial magnetic stimulation study of cortical inhibition and excitability in high-functioning autism and Asperger disorder. *Dev Med Child Neurol.* 2010 Aug;52(8):e179-83. doi: 10.1111/j.1469-8749.2010.03665.x. Epub 2010 Mar 29.

Geller V, Grisaru N, Abarbanel JM, Lemberg T, Belmaker RH. Slow magnetic stimulation of prefrontal cortex in depression and schizophrenia. *Prog Neuropsychopharmacol Biol Psychiatry.* 1997 Jan;21(1):105-10.

Hughes JR, Daaboul Y, Fino JJ, Shaw GL. The "Mozart effect" on epileptiform activity. *Clin Electroencephalogr.* 1998 Jul;29(3):109-19.

Lubar JF, Swartwood MO, Swartwood JN, O'Donnell PH. Evaluation of the effectiveness of EEG neurofeedback training for ADHD in a clinical setting as measured by changes in T.O.V.A. scores, behavioral ratings, and WISC-R performance. *Biofeedback Self Regul.* 1995 Mar;20(1):83-99.

Puzzo I, Cooper NR, Cantarella S, Fitzgerald PB, Russo R. The effect of rTMS over the inferior parietal lobule on EEG sensorimotor reactivity differs according to self-reported traits of autism in typically developing individuals. *Brain Res.* 2013 Dec 6;1541:33-41. doi: 10.1016/j.brainres.2013.10.016. Epub 2013 Oct 22.

Sokhadze EM, El-Baz A, Baruth J, Mathai G, Sears L, Casanova MF. Effects of low frequency repetitive transcranial magnetic stimulation (rTMS) on gamma frequency oscillations and event-related potentials during processing of illusory figures in autism. *J Autism Dev Disord.* 2009 Apr;39(4):619-34. doi: 10.1007/s10803-008-0662-7. Epub 2008 Nov 22.

Thompson L, Thompson M. Neurofeedback combined with training in metacognitive strategies: effectiveness in students with ADD. *Appl Psychophysiol Biofeedback.* 1998 Dec;23(4):243-63.

Chapter 33. Augmentative and Alternative Communication, by Patti Murphy

"Study of nonverbal autism must go beyond words, experts say." Retrieved November 9, 2013 from http://sfari.org/news-and-opinion/news/2013/study-of-nonverbal-autism-must-go-beyond-words-experts-say.

Millar, D.C. (2009). Effects of AAC on the natural speech development of individuals with autism spectrum disorders. In Mirenda, P. & Iacono, T. (Eds.) Autism Spectrum Disorders and AAC (pp. 171-192). Paul H. Brookes Publishing Co.

Light, J., Roberts, B., DiMarco, R., & Greiner, N. (1998). Augmentative and alternative communication to support receptive and expressive communication for people with autism. Journal of Communication Disorders, 31, 153-180.

Peeters, C. & Gillberg, C. (1999). Autism: Medical and educational aspects. London: Whurr

Silverman, F.H. (1980). Communication for the Speechless (3rd ed.). Needham Heights, MA: Allyn & Bacon.

Berry, J.O. (1987). Strategies for involving parents in programs for young children using augmentative and alternative communication. Augmentative and Alternative Communication, 3: 90-93.

Daniels, M. (1994). The effect of sign on hearing children's language. Communication Education, 43: 291-98.

Mesibov, G. B., Adams, L. W., & Klinger, L. G. (1997). Autism: Understanding the disorder. New York: Plenum Press.

Cafiero, J. (2004). AAC supports for engaging students with autism spectrum disorders (ASD) in group instruction, Closing the Gap, 23(4),

Partner Augmented Input, Instructional Video, Retrieved October 30, 2013 from http://www.dynavoxtech.com/training/toolkit/details.aspx?id=261,

Chain of Cues, Instructional Video, Retrieved October 30, 2013 from http://www.dynavoxtech.com/training/toolkit/details.aspx?id=280,

Positive Communication Environment, Instructional Video, Retrieved October 30, 2013 http://www.dynavoxtech.com/training/toolkit/details.aspx?id=254,

The National Professional Development Center on Autism Spectrum Disorders – Evidence-Based Practice: Social Narratives, Retrieved November 30, 2010 from http://autismpdc.fpg.unc.edu/content/social-narratives

Gray, C.A. (1995). Teaching child with autism to read social situations. In K.A. Quill (Ed.), Teaching children with autism: Strategies to enhance communication and socialization (pp. 219-242). New York: Delmar.

Bellini, S. (2008). *Building social relationships: A systematic approach to teaching social interactions skill to children and adolscents with autism spectrum disorders and other social difficulties.* Kansas: AAPC Textbooks.

Murdock, L. C., & Hobbs, J. Q. (2011). Tell me what you did today: A visual cueing strategy for children with ASD. *Focus on Autism and Other Developmental Disabilities, 26*(3), 162-172.

About Positive Behavioral Supports, Instructional Video, Retrieved December 1, 2013 from http://youtu.be/PKyTc-qaq27w

Hatch, P., Erickson, K., Dennis, A., & Cummings, M. (2012). A core issue: A core vocabulary for the Common Core. Retrieved December 3, 2013from http://www.med.unc.edu/ahs/clds/files/conference-hand-outs/ASHA2012CoreVocabularyPost.pdf

Chapter 38. Specific Carbohydrate Diet (SCD), by Judith Chinitz

1. Buie, T, Fuchs, GJ 3rd, Furuta, GT, Kooros, K, Levey, J, Lewis, JD, Wershil, BK, Winter, H. Recommendations for evaluation and treatment of common gastrointestinal problems in children with ASDs. Pediatrics 2010 Jan:125 Supple 1:S19-29.

2. Walker, SJ, Fortunato, J, Gonzalex, LG, Krigsman, A. Identification of unique gene expression profile in children with regressive autism spectrum disorder (ASD) and ileocolitis. PLoS ONE 2013;8(3): e58058.

3. Williams, BL, Hornig, M, Buie, T., Bauman, M, Cho Paik, M, Wick, I, Bennett, A, Jabado, O, Hirschberg, DL, Lipkin, WI. Impaired Carbohydrate digestion and transport and mucosal dysbiosis in the intestines of children with autism and gastrointestinal disturbances. PLoS ONE 6(9): e24585.

4. Gottschall, E. Breaking the Vicious Cycle. Kirkton Press: Baltimore Ontario. 1994.

5. Yap, I.K.S, Angley, M., Veselkov, K.A., Holmes, E., Lindon, J.C., Nicholson, J.K. (2010). Urinary metabolic phenotyping differentiates children with autism, from their unaffected siblings and age-matched controls. *Journal of Proteome Research.*

6. Gomez-Llorente, C., Munoz, S., Gil, A. (2010). Role of Toll-like receptors in the development of the immunotolerance mediated by probiotics. Proceedings of the Nutrition Society, 69(3): 381-9.

7. Heijtz, R.D., Wang, S., Anuar, F., Qian, Y., Bjorkholm, B., Samuelsson, A., Hibberd, M.L., Forssberg, H., Pettersson, S. (2011). Normal gut microbiota modulates brain development and behavior. *Proceedings of the National Academy of Science,* as yet unpublished.

8. Riazi, K., Galic, M.A., Kuzmiski, J.B., Ho, W., Sharkey, K.A., Pittman, Q.J. (2008). Microglial activation and TNFalpha production mediate alterned CNS excitability following perifpheral inflammation. Proceedings of the National Academy of Science, 105(44): 17151-6.

9. Vargas, D.L., Nascimbene, C., Krishnan, C., Zimmerman, A.W., Pardo, C.A. (2005). Neuroglial activation and neuroinflammation in the brain of patients with autism. *Annals of Neurology, 57*(1):67-81.

10. Parracho, H.M.R.T., Bingham, M.O., Gibson, G.R., McCartney, A.L. (2005). Differences between the gut microflora of children with autistic spectrum disorders and that of healthy children. *Journal of Medical Microbiology,* 54, 987-991.

11. Finegold, S.M., Dowd, S.E., Gontcharova, V., Liu, C., Henley, K.E., Wolcott, R.D., Youn, E., Summanen, P.H., Granpeesheh, D., Dixon, D., Liu, M., Militoris, D.R., Green, J.A 3rd. (2010). Pyrosequencing study of fecal microflora of autistic and control children, Anaerobe Aug:16(4):444-53.

12. Goldstein, R., Braverman, D., Stankiewicz, H. (2000). Carbohydrate malabsorption and the effect of dietary restriction on irritable bowel syndrome and functional bowel complaints. *Israeli Medical Association Journal,* Aug,2(8):683-7.

13. Reif, S., Klein, I., Lubin, F., Farbstein, M., Hallak, A., Gilat, T. (1997). Pre-illness dietary factors in inflammatory bowel disease. *Gut,* June;40(6):754-60.

14. Gibson, P.R., Barrett, J.S. (2010). The concept of small intestine bacterial overgrowth in relation to functional gastrointestinal disorders. *Nutrition* 11-12: 1-38-43.

15. Quiros, J.A, Sankaran, S., Pan, J., Rolston, M., Li, J., Bauman, S., Andersen, G.L., DeSantis, T.Z., Prindiville, T., Dandekar, S. (2011). Impact of Diet in Fecal Microbial Diversity in Patients with Crohn's Disease. Presented at The 15th International Congress of Mucosal Immunology (ICMI 2011), Paris, France.

16. Chinitz, J. (2007). *We Band of Mothers: Autism, My Son and The Specific Carbohydrate Diet.* San Diego: Autism Research Institute.

Chapter 40. The Healing Power of Fermented Foods, by Dr. John H. Hicks and Betsy Hicks

1. Adams C. *Probiotics—Protection Against Infection: Using Nature's Tiny Warriors to Stem Infection and Fight Disease*. Wilmington, DE: Sacred Earth Publishing, 2009.
2. Lammers KM, Helwig U, Sweenen E, Rizzello F, Venturi A, Caramelli E, Kamm MA, Brigidi P, Gionchetti P, Campieri M. Effect of probiotic strains on interleukin 8 production by HT29/19A cells. *Am J Gastroenterol*. 2002 May;97(5):1182-6.
3. Isolauri E, Salminen S. Probiotics, gut inflammation and barrier function. *Gastroenterol Clin North Am*. 2005 Sep;34(3):437-50,viii.
4. Madsen K, Cornish A, Soper P, McKaigney C, Jijon H, Yachimec C, Doyle J, Jewell L, De Simone C. Probiotic bacteria enhance murine and human intestinal epithelial barrier function. *Gastroenterology*. 2001 Sep;121(3):580-91.
5. Adams C. *Oral Probiotics: The Newest Way to Prevent Infection, Boost the Immune System and Fight Disease*. Wilmington, DE: Sacred Earth Publishing, 2010.
6. Huffnagle GB, Wernick S. *The Probiotics Revolution: The Definitive Guide to Safe, Natural Health Solutions Using Probiotic and Prebiotic Foods and Supplements*. New York: Bantam Books, 2007.

Chapter 43. CARD eLearning™ and Skills®: Web-based Training, Assessment, Curriculum, and Progress Tracking for Children with Autism, by Dr. Doreen Granpeesheh and Dr. Adel C. Najdowski

Dixon, D.R., Tarbox, J., Najdowski, A.C., Wilke, A.E. & Granpeesheh, D. (2011). A comprehensive evaluation of language for early behavioral intervention programs: the reliability of the SKILLS™ language index. *Journal of Research in Autism Spectrum Disorders, 5,* 506-511.

Jang, J., Dixon, D.R., Tarbox, J., Granpeesheh, D., Kornack, J., & de Nocker, Y. (2012). Randomized trial of an elearning program for training family members of children with autism in the principles and procedures of applied behavior analysis, *Journal of Research in Autism Spectrum Disorders, 6,* 852-856.

Granpeesheh, D. (2008). Recovery from autism: learning why and how to make it happen more. *Autism Advocate, 50,* 54-58.

Granpeesheh, D., Tarbox, J., Dixon, D.R., Carr, E., & Herbert, M. (2009). Retrospective analysis of clinical records in 38 cases of recovery from autism. *Annals of Clinical Pyschiatry, 21(4),* 195-204.

Granpeesheh, D., Tarbox, J., Dixon, D.R., Peters, C.A., Thompson, K., & Kenzer, A. (2010). Evaluation of a learning tool for training behavioral therapists in academic knowledge of applied behavior analysis. *Journal of Research in Autism Spectrum Disorders, 4,* 11-17.

Chapter 44. Drama Therapy, by Sally Bailey

Attwood, T. (1998). *Asperger's syndrome: A guide for parents and professionals*. London: Jessica Kingsley Publishers.

Bailey, S. (2009a). Performance in drama therapy. In D.R. Johnson & R. Emunah (Eds.), *Current approaches in drama therapy, 2nd. ed.* (pp. 374-392) Springfield, IL: Charles C. Thomas Publisher.

Bailey, S. (2009b). Theoretical reasons and practical applications of drama therapy with clients on the autism spectrum. In S.L. Brooke (Ed.), *The use of the creative therapies with autism spectrum disorders* (pp. 303-318). Springfield, IL: Charles C. Thomas Publisher.

Bailey, S. (2006). Ancient and modern roots of drama therapy. In S.L. Brooke (Ed.), *Creative Arts Therapies Manual: A Guide to the History, Theoretical Approaches, Assessment, and Work with Special Populations of Art, Play, Dance, Music, Drama, and Poetry Therapy* (pp. 214-222). Springfield, IL: Charles C. Thomas Publisher.

Bolding, G. (2007, November 9) Student overcomes autism with acting. *The Kansas State Collegian*, p. 3.

Blair, R. (2008). *The actor, image, and action: Acting and cognitive neuroscience*. London: Routledge.

Chasen, L.R. (2011). *Social skills, emotional growth and drama therapy: Inspiring connection on the autism spectrum*. London: Jessica Kingsley Publishers.

Grandin, T. (2002). Teaching tips for children and adults with autism. [Electronic Version]. *Center for the Study of Autism*. Retrieved on August 2, 2005 from http://www.autism.org/temple/tips.html.

Iacoboni, M. & Dapretto, M. (2006, December 7). The mirror neuron system and the consequences of its dysfunction. *Nature Reviews: Neuroscience, 942-951,* Retrieved on July 27, 2008 from www.csulb.edu/~cwallis/cscenter/mnc/abstracts/nn2024.pdf.

Iacoboni, M., Molnar-Szacks, I., Gallese, V., Buccino, G., Mazziotta, J.C., & Rizzolatti, G. (2005). Grasping the intentions of others with one's own mirror neuron system. *PLoS Biology*, 3(3) 79e. Retrieved January 23, 2006 from www.plosbiology.org.

Jensen, E. with Dabney, M. (2000). *Learning smarter: The new science of teaching.* San Diego, CA: The Brain Store.

Martinovich, J. (2005). *Creative Expressive Activities and Asperger's Syndrome: Social and Emotional Skills and Positive Life Goals for Adolescents and Young Adults.* London: Jessica Kingsley Publishers.

McConachie, B. (2008). *Engaging audiences: A cognitive approach to spectating in the theatre,* NY: Palgrave Macmillan.

Posner, M., Rothbart, M.K., Sheese, B. E., & Kieras, J. (2008). How arts training influences cognition. In C. Ashbury & B. Rich (Eds.), *Learning, Arts, and the Brain* (pp. 1-10). New York: Dana Press.

Oberman, L.M. & Ramachandran, V.S. (2007). The simulating social mind: The role of the mirror neuron system and simulation in the social and communicative deficits of autism spectrum disorders. *Psychological Bulletin,* 133(2), 310-327.

Ramachandran, V.S. & Oberman, L.M. (2006, November) Broken mirrors: A theory of autism. *Scientific American,* 63-69.

Regan, T. (Director). (2007). *Autism: The musical.* [Motion picture]. United States: Bunim-Murray Productions.

Chapter 46. Integrated Play Groups® (IPG) Model, by Dr. Pamela Wolfberg

American Speech-Language-Hearing Association. 2006. "Guidelines for Speech-Language Pathologists in Diagnosis, Assessment, and Treatment of Autism Spectrum Disorders Across the Life Span." http://www.asha.org/policy/GL2006-00049.htm.

Bottema-Beutel, K. (2010). The negotiation of footing and participation structure in a social group of teens with and without autism spectrum disorder. *Journal of interactional research in communication disorders,* 2(1), 61-83.

Bottema-Beutel, K. (in review). A mixed methods analysis of a social group intervention for adolescents with social disabilities and their typically developing peers. *American journal on intellectual and developmental disabilities.*

Bottema-Beutel, K. & Smith, N. (in review). The interactional construction of identity: An adolescent with autism in interaction with peers. *Linguistics and education.*

DiSalvo, C., & Donald O. (2002) "Peer-Mediated Interventions to Increase the Social Interaction of Children with Autism: Consideration of Peer Expectancies." Focus on Autism and Other Developmental Disabilities 17:198–207.

Fuge, G & Berry, R. (2004) *Pathways to Play! Combining Sensory Integration and Integrated Play Groups. Theme-based activities for children with Autism Spectrum and Other Sensory Processing Disorders.* Shawnee Mission, KS: Autism Asperger Publishing Company

Gonsier-Gerdin, J. (1992). *Elementary school children's perspectives on peers with disabilities in the context of Integrated Play Groups: "They're not really disabled, they're like plain kids."* (unpublished study) UC Berkeley-San Francisco State University-CA.

Iovannone, R. Dunlop, G, Huber, H. & Kincaid, D. (2003). Effective educational practices for students with ASD. *Focus on Autism and Other Developmental Disabilities,* 18 (3), 150-165

Julius, H., Wolfberg, P. Jahnke, I., & Neufeld, D., (2012) *Integrated Play and Drama Groups for Children and Adolescents on the Autism Spectrum. Alexander von Humboldt Foundation TransCoop Program: Transatlantic Cooperation in the Humanities, Social Sciences, Law, and Economics. (2009-2012).*

Lantz, J.F., Nelson, J.M. & Loftin, R.L. (2004) Guiding Children with Autism in Play: Applying the Integrated Play Group Model in School Settings. *Exceptional Children,* 37 (2), 8-14.

Mikaelan, B. (2003) *Increasing language through sibling and peer support play.* Unpublished Master Thesis, San Francisco State University, CA.

National Research Council (2001) *Educating Children with Autism.* Committee on Educational Interventions for Children with Autism: Division of Behavioral and Social Sciences and Education, National Academy Press: Washington, D.C.

National Autism Center (2009) *National standards project report- findings and conclusions: Addressing the need for evidence-based practice guidelines for Autism Spectrum Disorder.* Integrated Play Groups™ (IPG) model identified as "Established" practice within category of "Peer Intervention Package" based on studies reviewed; cited on p. 14, 30, & 50.

O'Connor, T. (1999). *Teacher perspectives of facilitated play in Integrated Play Groups.* Unpublished Master Thesis, San Francisco State University, CA.

Richard, V, & Goupil, G. (2005). Application des groupes de jeux integres aupres d'eleves ayant un trouble envahissant du development (Implementation of Integrated Play Groups with PDD Students). *Revue quebecoise de psychologie, 26(3),* 79-103

Vygotsky, L. (1966). Play and its role in the mental development of the child. Soviet Psychology, 12, 6-18 (Original work published in 1933).

Vygotsky, L. S. (1978). *Mind in society: The development of higher psychological processes.* Cambridge, MA: Harvard University Press.

Wolfberg, P. J. (1988). *Integrated play groups for children with autism and related disorders.* Unpublished master's field study, San Francisco State University.

Wolfberg, P.J. (1994). *Case illustrations of emerging social relations and symbolic activity in children with autism through supported peer play* (Doctoral dissertation, University of California at Berkeley with San Francisco State University). *Dissertation Abstracts International,* #9505068.

Wolfberg, P.J., & Schuler, A.L. (1992). *Integrated play groups project: Final evaluation report* (Contract # HO86D90016). Washington, DC: Department of Education, OSERS.

Wolfberg, P.J. (2009). *Play and imagination in children with autism.* (second edition) New York: Teachers College Press, Columbia University.

Wolfberg, P. J. (1988). *Integrated play groups for children with autism and related disorders.* Unpublished master's field study, San Francisco State University.

Wolfberg, P.J. (2003) *Peer play and the autism spectrum: The art of guiding children'socialization and imagination.* Shawnee, KS: Autism Asperger Publishing Company.

Wolfberg, P., Bottema-Beutel, K. & DeWitt, M. (2012) Including children with autism in social and imaginary play with typical peers: Integrated Play Groups model, *American Journal of Play. 5, 1,* 55-80.

Wolfberg, P., Turiel, E., DeWitt, M., Bottema-Beutel, K., Young, G., & Nguyen, T. (2012). *Integrated Play Groups: Promoting symbolic play, social engagement and communication with peers across settings in children with autism.* Autism Speaks Treatment Grant (2008-2011).

Wolfberg, P.J., & Schuler, A.L. (1992). *Integrated play groups project: Final evaluation report* (Contract # HO86D90016). Washington, DC: U.S.Department of Education, OSERS.

Wolfberg, P.J., & Schuler, A.L. (1993). Integrated Play Groups: A model for promoting the social and cognitive dimensions of play in children with autism. *Journal of Autism and Developmental Disorders, 23*(3), 467-489.

Yang, T., Wolfberg, P.J., Wu, S, Hwu, P. (2003) Supporting children on the autism spectrum in peer play at home and school: Piloting the Integrated Play Groups model in Taiwan. *Autism: The International Journal of Research and Practice.* 7(4) 437–453.

Zercher, C., Hunt, P., Schuler, A.L., & Webster, J. (2001). Increasing joint attention, play and language through peer supported play. *Autism: The International Journal of Research and Practice, 5,* 374-398.

Chapter 47. Integrative Educational Care, by Dr. Mary Joann Lang

1. Humphreys A, Post T, Ellis A. (1981). *Interdisciplinary methods: A thematic approach.* Santa Monica, CA: Goodyear Publishing Company.
2. Palmer J. (1991). Planning wheels turn curriculum around. *Educational Leadership.* 49(2);57-60.

Chapter 49. Relationship Development Intervention, by Laura Hynes

Gutstein, S., Burgess, A. & Montfort, A. (2007). Evaluation of the Relationship Development Intervention Program. *Autism,* 11, 397.

Hobson, J.A. (2011, October). *Engaging with a child with autism: A research perspective.* Presentation to Annual Conference on Relationship Development Intervention, Houston TX.

Hobson, J. A., & Hobson, R. P. (2011, May). *Emotional regulation in autism: A relational, therapeutic perspective.* Poster presented at the International Meeting for Autism Research, San Diego.

Chapter 50. Asynchronous Telehealth Technology for Autism Spectrum Disorder, by Dr. Mary Joann Lang and Ronald Oberleitner

1. *What is Telemedicine.* (n.d.). Retrieved from http://www.americantelemed.org/learn/what-is-telemedicine
2. *Bill Text - AB-809 Healing arts: telehealth.* (n.d.). Retrieved from http://leginfo.legislature.ca.gov/faces/billNavClient.xhtml?bill_id=201320140AB809
3. Retrieved from http://www.apapracticecentral.org/ce/guidelines/telepsychology-guidelines.pdf
4. Reischl U, Oberleitner R. Development of a Telemedicine Platform for the Management of Children with Autism. *German Journal for Young Researchers* 2009/1(1)
5. Ibid.
6. Oberleitner R. NIMH 9R44MH099035-05 Progress Report, On file with National Insttitute of Mental Health July, 2013
7. Reischl U, Oberleitner R, Colby C, Hamilton A. (2009) Association for Behavior Analysis International, Annual Conference, Phoenix, AZ. 2009
8. Oberleitner R. Reischl U. Lacy T. Goodwin M. Spitalnick JS. Commun Med Care,*Compunetics* (2011) 1: 93-104. doi: 10.1007/8754_2010_5

Chapter 53. Houston Homeopathy Method for Autism and ASDs: Sequential Homeopathy and Beyond, by Julianne Adams, Lynn Rose Demartini, Cindy L. Griffin, and Lindyl Lanham

Cole, Jean; Dyson, Roger; Classical Homoeopathy Revisited; West Wickham, Kent; 1997, Reprinted 2000
Elmiger, Jean; Rediscovering Real Medicine, Shaftesbury, Dorset; 1998
Hahnemann, Samuel; Ed. O'Reilly Organon of the Medical Art, Palo Alto, 1996

Chapter 55. Living Energy: Using Therapeutic Grade Essential Oils in the Treatment of Autism, by Dr. Shawn K. Centers

Badia P, Wesensten N, Lammers W, Culpepper J, Harsh J. Responsiveness to olfactory stimuli presented in sleep. *Physiol Behav*. 1990 Jul;48(1):87-90.
Bremner JD, Randall P, Vermetten E, Staib L, Bronen RA, Mzure C, et al. MRI-based measurement of hippocampal volume in posttraumatic stress disorder related to childhood physical and sexual abuse: a preliminary report. *Biol Psychiatry*. 1997;41(1):23-32.
Buchbauer G, Jirovetz L, Jäger W, Dietrich H, Plank C. Aromatherapy: evidence for sedative effects of the essential oil of lavender after inhalation. *Z Naturforsch C*. 1991 Nov- Dec;46(11-12):1067-72.
Buchbauer G, Jirovetz L, Jäger W, Plank C, Dietrich H. Fragrance compounds and essential oils with sedative effects upon inhalation. *J Pharm Sci*. 1993 Jun;82(6):660-4.
Chevrier MR, Ryan AE, Lee DYW, Zhongze M, Wu-Yan Z, Via CS. Boswellia carterii extract inhibits TH1 cytokines and promotes TH2 cytokines in vitro. *Clin Diagn Lab Immunol*. 2005 May;12(5):575-80.
Hardy M, Kirk-Smith MD, Stretch DD. Replacement of drug treatment for insomnia by ambient odour. *Lancet*. 1995 Sep;346(8976):701.
LeDoux JE. Emotion circuits in the brain. *Annu Rev Neurosci*. 2000;23:155-84.
LeDoux JE. Emotional colouration of consciousness: how feelings come about. In L Weiskrantz & M Davies (Eds.), *Frontiers of Consciousness: The Chichele Lectures*. Oxford: Oxford University Press, 2008.
Lis-Balchin M, Hart S. Studies on the mode of action of the essential oil of lavender (Lavandula angustifolia P. Miller). *Phytother Res*. 1999 Sep;13(6):540-2.
Maddocks-Jennings W. Critical incident: idiosyncratic allergic reactions to essential oils. *Complement Ther Nurs Midwifery*. 2004 Feb;10(1):58-60.
Masago R, Matsuda T, Kikuchi Y, Miyazaki Y, Iwanaga K, Harada H, et al. Effects of inhalation of essential oils on EEG activity and sensory evaluation. *J Physiol Anthropol Appl Human Sci*. 2000 Jan;19(1):35-42.
Moussaieff A, Rimmerman N, Bregman T, Straiker A, Felder CC, Shoham S, et al. Incensole acetate, an incense component, elicits psychoactivity by activating TRPV3 channels in the brain. *FASEB J*. 2008 Aug;22(8):3024–34.
Price S, Price L. *Aromatherapy for Health Professionals*, 4th edition. New York, NY: Churchill Livingstone, 2011.
Schultz V, Hubner WD, Ploch M. Clinical trials with phyto-psychopharmacological agents. *Phytomedicine*. 1997;4:379-87.
Schnaubelt K. *Advanced Aromatherapy: The Science of Essential Oil Therapy*, US edition. Rochester, VT: Healing Arts Press, 1998. Translation of *Neue Aromatherapie*, Cologne, 1995, vgs verlagsgesellschaft.
Sigurdsson T, Doyère V, Cain CK, LeDoux JE. Long-term potentiation in the amygdala: a cellular mechanism of fear learning and memory. *Neuropharmacology*. 2007 Jan;52(1):215-27.
Tramer MR. Treatment of postoperative nausea and vomiting. *BMJ*. 2003 Oct;327(7418):762-3.
Young DG, Lawrence RM. *Essential Oils Integrative Medical Guide: Building Immunity, Increasing Longevity, and Enhancing Mental Performance with Therapeutic-Grade Essential Oils*. Orem, UT: Life Science Publishing, 2003.

Chapter 57. Osteopathy: A Philosophy and Methodology for the Effective Treatment of Children with Autism, by Dr. Shawn K. Centers

Balan P, Kushnerenko E, Sahlin P, Huotilainen M, Näätänen R, Hukki J. Auditory ERPs reveal brain dysfunction in infants with plagiocephaly. *J Craniofac Surg*. 2002;13(4):520-5.
Ballaban-Gil K, Tuchman R. Epilepsy and epileptiform EEG: association with autism and language disorders. *Ment Retard Dev Disabil Res Rev*. 2000;6:300–8.
Breggin P. *Brain-disabling Treatments in Psychiatry: Drugs, Electroshock, and the Psychopharmaceutical Complex*. New York: Springer Publishing Co., 2007.
Breggin P, Stern E (Eds.). Spearheading a transformation. Co-published simultaneously in *The Psychotherapy Patient*, 1996;9(3/4): 1-7; and *Psychosocial Approaches to Deeply Disturbed Persons*, Binghamton, NY: The Haworth Press, Inc., 1996:1-7.

Cohen JA. Association of American Medical Colleges. A Word from the President: "Filling the Workforce Gap." *AAMC Reporter*. April 2005.

Culbert KM, Breedlove SM, Burt SA, Klump KL. Prenatal hormone exposure and risk for eating disorders: a comparison of opposite-sex and same-sex twins. *Arch Gen Psychiatry*. 2008;65(3):329-36.

Fernández-Guardiola A, Martínez A, Valdés-Cruz A, Magdaleno-Madrigal VM, Martínez D, Fernández-Mas R. Vagus nerve prolonged stimulation in cats: effects on epileptogenesis (amygdala electrical kindling): behavioral and electrographic changes. *Epilepsia*. 1999;40(7):822-9.

Frymann VM. Learning difficulties of children viewed in the light of the osteopathic concept. *J Am Osteopath Assoc*. 1976;76(1):46-61.

Frymann VM, Carney RE, Springall P. Effect of osteopathic medical management on neurologic development in children. *J Am Osteopath Assoc*. 1992;92(6):729-44.

Gevitz N. *The DOs: Osteopathic Medicine in America*. Baltimore, MD: John's Hopkins University Press, 1982.

Glasson EJ, Bower C, Petterson B, de Klerk N, Chaney G, Hallmayer JF. Perinatal factors and the development of autism: A population study. *Arch Gen Psychiatry*. 2004;61(6): 618-27.

Hadjivassiliou M, Gibson A, Davies-Jones GA, Lobo AJ, Stephenson TJ, Milford-Ward A. Does cryptic gluten sensitivity play a part in neurological illness? *Lancet*. 1996 Feb 10;347(8998):369-71.

Kaplan M, Rimland B, Edelson SM. Strabismus in autism spectrum disorder. *Focus Autism Other Dev Disabl*. 1999;14(2):101-5.

McNeil TF, Cantor-Graae E, Weinberger DR. Relationship of obstetric complications and differences in size of brain structures in monozygotic twin pairs discordant for schizophrenia. *Am J Psychiatry*. 2000;157(2):203-12.

Miller RI, Clarren SK. Long-term developmental outcomes in patients with deformational plagiocephaly. *Pediatrics*. 2000;105(2):E26.

Moskalenko YE, Kravchenko TI, Gaidar BV, Vainshtein GB, Semernya VN, Maiorova NF, et al. Periodic mobility of cranial bones in humans. *Human Physiol*. 1999;25(1):51-8.

Moskalenko YE, Frymann V, Weinstein GB, Semernya VN, Kravchenko TI, Markovets SP, Panov AA, Maiorova NF. Slow rhythmic oscillations within the human cranium: phenomenology, origin, and informational significance. *Human Physiol*. 2001;27(2):171-8.

Moskalenko YE, Frymann VM, Kravchenko T. A modern conceptualization of the functioning of the primary respiratory mechanism. In King HH (Ed.), Proceedings of international research conference: Osteopathy in Pediatrics at the Osteopathic Center for Children in San Diego, CA, 2002. Indianapolis, IN: American Academy of Osteopathy, 2005, pp. 12-31.

Murch SH, Thomson MA, Walker-Smith JA. Author's reply. *Lancet*. 1998;351(9106),908.

Nichols DS, Thorn BE, Berntson GG. Opiate and serotonergic mechanisms of stimulation-produced analgesia within the periaqueductal gray. *Brain Res Bull*. 1989;22(4):717-24.

Rossiter TR, La Vaque TJ. A comparison of EEG biofeedback and psychostimulants in treating attention deficit/hyperactivity disorders. *J Neurotherapy*. 1995;1(1):48-59.

Reichelt KL, Knivsberg A-M, Lind G, Nødland M. Probable etiology and possible treatment of childhood autism. *Brain Dysfunct*. 1991; 4:308-19.

Rutgers University, New Jersey Agricultural Station. Variation in mineral composition of vegetables. Reprinted from *Soil Science Society of America Proceedings* 1948, Volume 13, pp. 380-4. Madison, Wisconsin: The Soil Science Society of America, 1949. Available at http://njaes.rutgers.edu/pubs/bearreport/.

Sims JM. *The Story of My Life*. New York: Appleton, 1889.

Stein D, Weizman A, Ring A, Barak Y. Obstetric complications in individuals diagnosed with autism and in healthy controls. *Compr Psychiatry*. 2006;47(1):69-75.

Still AT. *Philosophy and Mechanical Principles of Osteopathy*. Hudson-Kimberly Pub. Co., 1902.

Still AT. *Osteopathy, Research and Practice*. Kirksville, MO: American School of Osteopathy, 1910.

Whiteley P, Rodgers J, Savery D, Shattock P. Research: a gluten-free diet as an intervention for autism and associated spectrum disorders: preliminary findings. *Autism*. 1999;3(1):45-65.

Chapter 58. NAET Explained, by Geri Brewster

1. Merriam-Webster [Internet]. Meridian. Merriam-Webster, Inc., 2011 [cited 2011 June 22]. Available at: http://www.merriam-webster.com/dictionary/meridians.

2. Nambudripad DS. *Say Good-bye to Illness*, 3rd ed. Buena Park, CA: Delta Publishing, 2002.

3. Schmitt WH Jr, Leisman G. Correlation of applied kinesiology muscle testing findings with serum immunoglobulin levels for food allergies. *Int J Neurosci*. 1998 Dec;96(3-4):237-44.

4. Ericsson AD, Pittaway K, Lai R [Internet]. ElectroDermal analysis. Biomeridian Innovations in Health, 2011 [cited 2011 June 23]. Available at: http://www.biomeridian.com/electrodermal-analysis.htm.

5. Nambudripad's Allergy Research Foundation. NAET screening for food allergy, sensitivity and intolerances using IgE-specific antigen test and NST- NAET®. In: ClinicalTrials.gov [Internet]. Bethesda, MD: National Library of Medicine, National Institutes of Health [cited 2011 June 22]. Available at: http://www.clinicaltrials. gov/ct2/results?term=NCT00275795

6. Masuda H, Saito Y, Moosad M, Nambudripad RA. The importance of avoidance of the desensitized allergen for the following 25 hours of the initial NAET® to derive satisfactory results after each NAET® TX. *JNECM*. 2010;6(2):1439-52.

7. Nambudripad DS. NAET protocols and modalities. Part 1: basics. *JNECM*. 2005;1(1):19-28.

8. Shelton BH. Introducing the NAET®/DesBio homeopathic protocol. Deseret Biologicals, Inc., 2006 – 2009 [cited 2011 June 22]. Available online from: http://www.desbio.com/NAET.html

9. Nambudripad's Allergy Research Foundation. Treatment of autistic children using NAET procedures. In: ClinicalTrials.gov [Internet]. Bethesda, MD: National Library of Medicine, National Institutes of Health [cited 2011 June 22]. Available at: http://www.clinicaltrials.gov/ct2/results?term=NCT00277407

10. Nambudripad's Allergy Research Foundation. An autism study using Nambudripad's food allergy elimination treatments. In: ClinicalTrials.gov [Internet]. Bethesda, MD: National Library of Medicine, National Institutes of Health [cited 2011 June 22]. Available at: http://www.clinicaltrials.gov/ct2/results?term=NCT00247156

11. Nambudripad DS. *Say Good-bye to Allergy Related Autism*. Buena Park, CA: Delta Publishing, 1999.

12. Nambudripad's Allergy Research Foundation. Milk allergy elimination through NAET® (Nambudripad's Allergy Elimination Techniques). In: ClinicalTrials.gov [Internet]. Bethesda, MD: National Library of Medicine, National Institutes of Health [cited 2011 June 22]. Available at: http://www.clinicaltrials.gov/ct2/results?term=NCT00328731

Chapter 59. CranioSacral Therapy and Autism, by Tami A. Goldstein

[1]John E Upledger, D.O., F.A.A.O and Jon D. Vredevoogd, M.F.A, *Craniosacral Therapy* (Seattle Washington, East-Land Press, 2004) p.5.

[2]Dr. Upledger testified on the topic of autism before the Government Reform Committee of the US House of Representatives, 106th Congress (1999-2000). The daylong session features testimonies from leaders in autism research and treatment as well as from parents of autistic children. Transcript of Dr. Upledger's presentation, April 6, 2000.

[3,4]Amen Clinic, "Functional Neuroanatomy," accessed December 22, 2013. http://www.amenclinics.com/about-us-23/the-science-2/spect-gallery/item/functional-neuroanatomy, For additional reading:

The Inner Physician and You by Dr. John Upledger

The Autistic Brain by Temple Grandin

Chapter 60. Dance/Movement Therapy, by Mariah Meyer LeFeber

Adler, J. (2003). From autism to the discipline of authentic movement. *American Journal of Dance Therapy, 25*(1), 5–16.

American Dance Therapy Association. (2008). Retrieved October 28, 2008 from www.adta.org/about/factsheet.cfm.

Berrol, C. (2006). Neuroscience meets dance/movement therapy: Mirror neurons, the therapeutic process and empathy. *The Arts in Psychotherapy, 33*, 302–315.

Canner, N. (1968). *And a Time to Dance*. Boston: Beacon Press.

Erfer, T. (1995). Treating children with autism in a public school system. In F. J. Levy, J. P. Fried, & F. Leventhal (Eds.), *Dance and Other Expressive Arts therapies* (pp. 191–211). New York: Routledge.

Hartshorn, K., Olds, L., Field, T., Delage, J., Cullen, C., & Escalona, A. (2001). Creative movement therapy benefits children with autism. *Early Child Development & Care, 166*, 1–5.

Kestenberg, J. A., Loman, S., Lewis, P., & Sossin, K. M. (1999). *The meaning of movement: Developmental and clinical perspectives of the Kestenberg Movement Profile*. New York: Brunner-Routledge.

Levy, F. (2005). *Dance Movement Therapy: A Healing Art*. Reston, VA: National Dance Association.

Loman, S. (1995). The case of Warren: A KMP approach to autism. In F. J. Levy, J. P. Fried, & F. Leventhal (Eds.), *Dance and Other Expressive Arts Therapies: When Words Are Not Enough* (pp. 213–224). New York: Routledge.

Meekums, B. (2002). *Dance Movement Therapy: A Creative Psychotherapeutic Approach*. London: Sage Publications.

Wolf-Schein, E., Fisch, G., & Cohen, I. (1985). A study of the use of nonverbal systems in the differential diagnosis of autistic, mentally retarded and fragile x individuals. *American Journal of Dance Therapy, 8*(1985), 67–80.

Chapter 64. The Listening Program®: An Effective Treatment for Autism, by Alex Doman

1. John Esteves, Sheri Stein-Blum, Jonathan Cohen, Allison Tischler, "Indentifying the effectiveness of a music-based auditory stimulation method on children with sensory integration and auditory processing concerns: A pilot study" *Music that works: Contributions of biology, neurophysiology, psychology, sociology, medicine and musicology.* Haas, Roland; Brandes, Vera (eds.) (Springer 2009).

2. Alex Doman, "Which brain areas are most involved in music listening" http://alexdoman.com/2013/06/06/which-brain-areas-are-involved-in-music-listening/ (last accessed 23, November, 2013).

3. Lillian Stiegler, Rebecca Davis, "Understanding sound sensitivity in individuals with autism spectrum disorders". *Focus on Autism and Other Developmental Disabilities,* June 2010, vol. 25 no. 2 67-75

4. Jay Lucker, Alex Doman, "Auditory hypersensitivity and autism spectrum disorders: An emotional response" *Autism Science Digest,* vol.4, 2012.

5. Jay Lucker, Alex Doman, *Autism Science Digest,* issue 4, 2012.

6. Learn more about Waves™, the multi-sensory audio system optimized for The Listening Program at http://advancedbrain.com/waves (last accessed 23, November, 2013).

7. Jay Lucker, Alex Doman, *Autism Science Digest,* vol.4, 2012.

8. Learn more about TLP SPECTRUM and how to get your child started at http://advancedbrain.com/spectrum (last accessed 23, November, 2013).

9. TLP Online is a subscription based service and is not available in all areas. Learn more at http://tlp.advancedbrain.com (last accessed 23, November, 2013).

10. "A Parent's Guide to Toileting for Children with Autism" *Autism Speaks, Autism Treatment Network, Autism Intervention Research Network on Physical Health,* http://www.autismspeaks.org/docs/sciencedocs/atn/atn_air-p_toilet_training.pdf (last accessed 24, November, 2013).

11. K.A. Kroeger, Rena Sorensen- Burnworth, "Toilet training individuals with autism and other developmental disabilities: A critical review" *Research in Autism Spectrum Disorders,* 3 (2009) 607-618.

12. Gwenyth Jeyes, "A study to establish whether the use of The Listening Program® is effective in improving auditory skills for children with autism" http://www.advancedbrain.com/pdf/research/jeyes_study_autism.pdf (last accessed 24, November, 2013).

13. June Rogers, "A pilot investigation into the effects of listening to modified classical music, including bone conduction, in improving toilet training outcomes for children with learning difficulties" http://www.advancedbrain.com/pdf/research/tlp_research10_10_rogers.pdf, (last accessed 24, November, 2013).

14. "Insufficient sleep is a public health epidemic". *Centers for Disease Control and Prevention,* http://www.cdc.gov/features/dssleep/ (last accessed 24, November, 2013).

15. "Kids with autism may have poorer sleep" http://www.huffingtonpost.com/2013/10/01/autism-sleep_n_4018215.html (last accessed 25, November, 2013).

16. Joanna S Humphreys et al "Sleep patterns in children with autistic spectrum disorders: A prospective cohort study" *Archives of Disease in Childhood,* September 2013, doi:10.1136/archdischild-2013-304083.

17. For more information on TLP SLEEP including white papers, interviews, and audio samples visit http://advancedbrain.com/sleep (last accessed 24, November, 2013).

18. To review completed research, case studies, and studies in progress visit The Listening Program Science. http://advancedbrain.com/science (last accessed 23, November, 2013).

Chapter 65. NACD's Targeted Neurodevelopmental Intervention: Perspectives and Interventions for Those on the Autism Spectrum, by Bob Doman

"The Autism Spectrum," *NACD Journal,* Vol. 17 No. 1, 2004 (www.nacd.org/journal/autismspectrum.php).

"The Autistic Child," *NACD Journal,* Vol. 6 No. 11, 1986 (www.nacd.org/journal/article3.php).

"Neurodevelopmental Perspectives on Autism and Asperger's Syndrome," *NACD Journal,* Vol. 22 No. 10, 2008 (www.nacd.org/journal/0909_autism_spectrum.php).

"Philosophy and Rationale," *NACD Journal,* Vol. 10 No. 5, 1996 (www.nacd.org/journal/article20.php).

Testimonial—"Gregge," www.nacd.org/testimonials/autism_gregge.php

Testimonial—"Celeste's Story," www.nacd.org/testimonials/autism_celeste.php

Testimonial—"Marcus," www.nacd.org/testimonials/autism_marcus.php

NACD Autism Spectrum Workshop on YouTube: http://www.youtube.com/watch?v=mQKx1uovIPQ&list=PLFC29382970708250

Chapter 66. Animals in the Lives of Persons with Autistic Spectrum Disorder (ASD): Companions to Co-Therapists, by Dr. Aubrey H. Fine

American Pet Products Association (2012). Industry statistics & trends. from: http://www.americanpetproducts.org/press_industrytrends.asp.

American Pet Products Association. (2009). *Industry statistics & trends.* Retrieved August 16, 2009 from: http://www.americanpetproducts.org/press_industrytrends.asp

Barol, J. (2006) *The Effects of AAT on a child.* Unpublished Thesis. New Mexico Highland University.

Dayton, L. (2010, January 23). Pets are a natural remedy for owners' health. *The Australian (Sydney, Australia).*

Delta Society. (1996). *Standards of practice in animal-assisted activities and therapy.* Bellevue, WA: Delta Society

Fine, A. H. (2014) Our Faithful Companions: Revealing the Essence of Our Kinship with Animals. Crawford, CO. Alpine Publications

Fine, A.H (2010) (Ed.), *Handbook on animal-assisted therapy: Theoretical foundations and guidelines for practice.* USA: Academic Press.

Fine, A. H., & Eisen, C. (2008). *Afternoons with Puppy: Inspirations from a therapist and his therapy animals.* West Lafayette, Indiana: Purdue University Press.

Foxall, E. L. (2002). The use of horses as a means of improving communication abilities of those with autism spectrum disorders: An investigation into the use and effectiveness of the horse as a therapy tool for improving communication in those with autism. Unpublished manuscript, Coventry, UK: Conventry University.

Friedmann, E., Locker, B. Z., & Lockwood, R. (1990). Perception of animals and cardiovascular responses during verbalization with an animal present. *Anthrozoos, 6*(2), 115-134.

Frewin, K. & Gardiner, B. (2005). New age or old sage? A review of equine assisted psychotherapy. In *The Australian Journal of Counseling Psychology,* 6, pp. 13-17.

Gabriels, R, Agnew, J., Holt. K., Shoffner, A., Zhaoxing, P., Ruzzano, S., Clayton, G., and Mesbiov, G. (2012) Pilot study measuring the effects of therapeutic horseback riding on school-age children and adolescents with autism spectrum disorder. *Research in Autism Spectrum Disorders* 6 (2012) 578–588.

Grandin, T. (2011). The roles that animals can play with individuals with autism. In P McCardle, S McCune, J. Griffin, L Esposito, & L Freund, *Human–Animal Interaction in Family, Community, and Therapeutic Settings.* Baltimore, MD: Brookes Publishing, 183-195.

Grandin, T., Fine, A., & Bowers, C. (2010). The use of therapy animals with individuals with autism. In A. Fine (Ed.) *The Handbook on Animal-Assisted Therapy: Theoretical Foundations and Guidelines for Practice (3rd Edition).* New York: Elsevier Science Press.

Grandin, T., & Johnson, C. (2005). *Animals in translation.* New York, NY: Scribner.

Journal of the American Veterinary Medical Association. (1998). Statement from the committee on the human-animal bond. *Journal of the American veterinary medical association, 212*(11), 1675.

Levinson, B. (1969). *Pet oriented child psychotherapy.* Springfield, IL: Charles C. Thomas Publisher.

Martin, F. & Farnum, J. (2002). Animal assisted therapy for children with pervasive developmental disorders. *Western Journal of Nursing Research, 24,* 657-670.

Mason, M. A. (2004). Effects of therapeutic riding in children with autism. Unpublished dissertation. Minneapolis, MN: Capella University.

O'Haire, M.E. (2013). Animal-assisted intervention for autism spectrum disorder: A systematic literature review. *Journal of Autism and Developmental Disorders, 43*(7), 1606-1622.

The North American Riding for the Handicapped Association (NARHA) (2010).

Equine-facilitated psychotherapy and equine-facilitated learning FAQ. [Online]. Available: http://www.narha.org/faq#efp.

McNicholas, J. & Collis, G. M. (2000). Dogs as catalysts for social interactions: robustness of the effect. *British Journal of Psychology,* 91, 61-70.

McNicholas, J., & Collis, G. (2006). Animals as supports. Insights for understanding animal assisted therapy. In A. Fine (Ed.) *Handbook on animal assisted therapy (2nd Edition,* pp. 49-71). San Diego, CA: Academic Press.

Ming Lee Yeh, A. (2008). Canine AAT model for autistic children. At Tawian International Association of Human-Animal Interaction International Conference, Tokyo Japan, 10/5-8/2008.

Odenthal, J., & Meintjes, R. (2003). Neurophysiological correlates of affiliative behavior between humans and dogs. *Veterinary Journal,165,* 296-301.

Olmert, M. D. (2009). *Made for each other.* Philadelphia: De Capo Press.

Silva, K., Correia, R., Lima, M., Magalhães, A., & de Sousa, L. (2011). Can dogs prime autistic children for therapy? Evidence from a single case study. *Journal of Alternative and Complementary Medicine, 17*(7), 1-5.

Viau, R., Arsenault-Lapierre, G., Fecteau, S., Champagne, N., Walker, C., & Lupien, S. (2010). Effect of service dogs on salivary cortisol secretion in autistic children. *Psychoneuroendocrinology, 35*(8), 1187-1193.

Wells, D. L. (2009). The effects of animals on human health and well-being. *Journal of social issues, 65*(3), 523-543.

Chapter 67. Architecture and Autism: Creating a Toxic-Reduced Environment for Your Autistic Child, by Catherine Purple Cherry

1. California's Proposition 65, State of California, Environmental Protection Agency, Office of Environmental Health Hazard Assessment, September 2, 2011.
    http://www.oehha.ca.gov/prop65/prop65_list/Newlist.html.
    Substances are placed on the Proposition 65 list of chemicals "known to the state of California to cause reproductive toxicity" if an independent science advisory board has concluded they possess sufficient evidence of such toxicity in animals or humans, or if an authoritative organization such as the National Toxicology Program have reached a similar conclusion, or if a federal regulatory agency requires a reproductive toxicity warning label. Also, the Proposition 65 list identifies whether a chemical is a developmental toxicant.
2. *Health Effects, Scorecard: The Pollution Information Site, 2005.* http://scorecard.goodguide.com/health-effects/references.tcl?short_hazard_name=cancer
3. US Environmental Protection Agency, Indoor Air Division, 2011.
    http://www.epa.gov/radon/healthrisks.html
4. ToxTown, National Library of Medicine, NIH, 2011.
    http://toxtown.nlm.nih.gov/text_version/chemicals.php?id=31
5. Mold, Centers for Disease Control and Prevention, 2011.
    http://www.cdc.gov/mold/faqs.htm
6. PFOAs, US Environmental Protection Agency, Office of Pollutant Protection and Toxics, 2011.
    http://www.epa.gov/oppt/pfoa/index.html
7. New Study: Autism Linked to Environment, Scientific American, January 9, 2009
    http://www.scientificamerican.com/article.cfm?id=autism-rise-driven-by-environment&page=2
8. *Mind, Disrupted: How Toxic Chemicals May Change How We Think and Who We Are, A Biomonitoring Project with Leaders of the Learning and Developmental Disabilities Community*, Stephenie Hendricks February 4, 2010.
    http://www.minddisrupted.org/media.php
9. *Toxic Effects, Everyday Exposures*, Metametrix Inc., 2011.
    http://www.everydayexposures.com
10. Pollution in People Report, May 2006
    http://pollutioninpeople.org/results/download
11. Home Safe Fact Sheets, Washington Toxics Coalition,
    http://watoxics.org/publications

Chapter 68. Art Therapy Approaches to Treating Autism, by Nicole Martin and Dr. Donna Betts

American Art Therapy Association (2009a). *About art therapy.* Retrieved January 6, 2010 from www.arttherapy.org/aboutart.htm.
American Art Therapy Association (2009b). *How did art therapy begin?* Retrieved January 6, 2010 from www.arttherapy.org/faq.htm#howbegin.
Betts, D. J. (2003). Developing a projective drawing test: Experiences with the Face Stimulus Assessment (FSA). *Art Therapy: Journal of the American Art Therapy Association*, 20(2), 77–82.
Betts, D. J. (2009). Introduction to the Face Stimulus Assessment (FSA). In E. Horovitz & S.
Eksten (Eds.), *Art Therapy Handbook: Assessment, Diagnosis, and Counseling.* Springfield, IL: Charles C. Thomas.
Evans, K., Dubowski, J. (2001). *Art Therapy with Children on the Autistic Spectrum: Beyond Words.* London: Jessica Kingsley.
Gilroy, A. (2006). *Art therapy: Research and Evidence-Based Practice.* London, UK: Sage Publications. (Reviews research on ASD from pages 144–146.)
Kramer, E. (1979). *Childhood and Art Therapy: Notes on Theory and Application.* New York: Schocken Books.
Martin, N. (2008). Assessing portrait drawings created by children and adolescents with autism spectrum disorder. *Art Therapy: Journal of the American Art Therapy Association*, 25(1), 15–23.
Martin, N. (2009a). *Art as an Early Intervention Tool for Children with Autism.* London: Jessica Kingsley.
Martin, N. (2009b). Art therapy and autism: Overview and recommendations. *Art Therapy: Journal of the American Art Therapy Association*, 26(4), 187–190.
Stack, M. (1998). Humpty Dumpty's shell: Working with autistic defense mechanisms in art Therapy. In M. Rees (Ed.), (1998), *Drawing on Difference: Art Therapy with People Who Have Learning Difficulties.* London: Routledge.

Chapter 72. Vision Therapy, by Dr. Jeffrey Becker

Becker, J. (2009). Vision Therapy Can Help Spectrum Children With Visual Dysfunctions. *The Autism File USA* 33, 76–81

Cohen, A. H., Lowe, S.E., Steele, G.T., Suchoff, I.B., Gottlieb, D.D., & Trevorrow, T.L. (1988). The efficacy of optometric vision therapy, *Journal Of The American Optometric Association, 59*(2), 95–105.

Holmes, J., Rice, M., Karlsson, V., Nielsen, B., Sease, J., & Shevlin, T. (2008). The best treatment determined for childhood eye problem. *Archives of Ophthalmology, 126*(10) 1336–1349. HTS Inc. (2009). 6788 S. Kings Ranch Rd., Gold Canyon, AZ 85118. NeuroSensory Centers of America. (2009). 300 Beardsley Road, Austin, TX 78746

Kawar, M.J., Frick, S.M., & Frick, R. (2005). *Astronaut training: A sound activated vestibular-visual protocol.* Vital Links: Madison, WI.

Taub, M.B., & Russell, R. (2007). Autism spectrum disorders: A primer for the optometrist. *Review of Optometry. 144*(5). 82–91

Trachtman, J.N. (2008). Background and history of autism in relation to vision care, *Optometry, 79*(7), 391–396.

INDEX

Adaptive Behavior, 149, 318, 336, 353, 354, 355, 358, 366, 385, 386, 461, 469, 470, 477, 478, 518, 544, 546, 547, 604, 619

Adams, Julianne, 400

Aggression, 32, 47, 48, 49, 69, 201, 213, 225, 242, 246, 329, 337, 405, 446, 461, 557

Allergic,
  diseases, 54, 451, 615, 639, 640
  disorders, 36, 62, 134
  non-allergic triggers, 35, 37
  reaction(s), 3, 4, 7, 11, 13, 37, 39, 415, 449, 451, 454, 529, 530
  response, 37, 407, 454, 615, 616
  rhinitis, 37, 626
  sensitivity, 53, 451
  sensitization, 638
  substance, 3, 4, 38, 450–52, 454–55
  symptomatology, 36, 37,
  symptoms, 3, 4, 37, 451, 612
  triggers, 3, 4, 37, 39, 200
  -type reactions, 34, 108, 110

Allergies, 195, 196, 203, 205, 206, 312, 358, 407, 454, 534
  cause of, 36, 37, 38, 101, 200, 206, 207
  environmental, 37, 313, 450
  food, 4, 29, 37, 111, 207, 209, 223, 298, 313, 450. See also Food Intolerance
  history of, 7, 36, 37, 196, 209, 300
  inhalant, 4, 530
  respiratory, 134
  symptoms of, 2, 3, 37, 499
  treatment of, 3, 5, 224, 309, 313, 406, 450, 454–55, 530

Allergy,
  -associated symptoms, 51

desensitization, 2, 3, 450–52, 454
elimination, 449, 450, 451, 454, 650
elimination programs, 449, 450
elimination techniques, 449, 450
extracts, 3
food, 3, 37, 101, 640. See also Food Intolerance
injections, 3, 4, 5
-like symptoms, 35, 36, 37
milk, 454, 650
reactions, 3, 451
-related, 454
risk of, 3, 39, 40, 200, 534, 639
shots, 3
symptoms (of), 2, 3, 4, 134, 452
test(s)(ing), 3, 4, 5, 34, 37, 454
treatment, 2, 3, 4, 34, 54, 55, 402, 449, 450, 452, 454
vaccine, 207

Ambient Prism Lenses, 139–50

American Academy of Allergy, Asthma, and Immunology(AAAI), 36, 37

American College of Allergy, Asthma, and Immunology, 207

Animal-Assisted,
  activities (AAA), 515
  interventions (AAI), 513, 515–22
  therapy (AAT), 513, 652

Antibiotics
  effects of, xviii, 21, 136, 196, 307, 440, 441
  exposed(ure) to, 133, 196, 207
  prophylactic, 66, 68, 633
  resistant(ce) to, 16, 19, 20, 21, 24
  responses to, 133, 406
  use of, ix, xvi, xviii, 21, 52, 66, 68, 105, 108, 136, 196, 227, 294, 441

Antiepileptic,
  drugs, 7–12, 76
  medication(s), 7, 9–13 76
  treatments, 6–13, 76

Antifungal Medication,

use of, 52, 58, 200, 223, 307
prescription, 52, 105
resistant to, 16, 23, 24
Antihistamines, 40
prescription oral, 3
Anthroposophy, 602
Antiviral Therapy, 223, 227, 312
Applied Behavior Analysis (ABA),
xxi, xxii, 118, 157, 160–61, 230,
316–23, 334, 335, 338, 342, 358,
361, 377–83, 413, 480, 532, 578,
580, 589–605
Applied Verbal Behavior (AVB), 321 ,
Arranga, Teri, xi, xvi, 573, 576,
Art Therapist, 532, 533, 534, 535
Art Therapy, 532–36, 607, 609
Asadi, Shahrzad, 35, 612
Asynchronous Telehealth Technology,
377–83
Augmentative and Alternative
Communication (AAC), 236–37,
245–55, 275–77, 279
AutisMate, 236–39

Bailey, Sally, 339, 607, 645
Baruth, Joshua M., 120, 624
Beacon Day School, 353–54, 359, 377,
382, 590
Becker, Jeffrey, 565, 654
Berkley, Alison, 324
Berard Auditory Integration Training,
537–42, 557
Berger, David, 195, 637
Betts, Donna, 532, 653
Biofilm, 14–24, 224, 309, 611
Biome Depletion Theory, 50–56,
133–37, 292
Bleecker, Tim, 343
Bradstreet, James Jeffrey, xii, xiv, xvi,
131, 151, 214, 228, 573, 611, 620,
625, 628, 642, 643
Brain Inflammation, 35–41, 51, 58,
133, 134, 137, 157, 192, 230,
292–93, 296, 409
Brewster, Geri, 449, 649
Brockett, Sally, 537
Buri da Cunha, Jennifer, 384

Camp Ramapo, 384–90
Camphill Communities, The, 590, 596,
599, 600, 601, 602, 605, 606
Cannabis, 71–77, 574
Casanova, Manuel F., 121, 139, 230,
234, 573, 608, 627
Center for Autism and Related
Disorders (CARD), 317, 322,
333–34, 578
eLearning, 333–38, 645
Centers, Shawn K., 414, 435, 648
Chelation, 25–27, 58, 114, 201–2, 422,
611
agents, 26–27
Cherry, Cathy Purple, 523, 653, 608,
644
Chinitz, Judith, 50
Chiropractic Therapy, 395, 450, 459,
588
Chlorine Dioxide, 223–27, 642
Clark, Jenifer, 361
Coombs, Nathan, 72, 618
Community-Based Speech Language
Pathology, 272–77
Core Muscle Weakness, 355–56, 482
Coyle, Mary, 409
Craniosacral Therapy, 458–62, 650
Crohn's Disease, 19, 44, 47, 48, 134,
135, 156, 296, 615, 616, 626, 632,
634, 635, 636, 644
Cuevas, Allan, 480

Dairy, 29, 59, 60, 61, 80, 106, 204, 207,
224, 296, 305, 312
allergies. 224, *See also* Allergies
-free diet, 106, *See also* Diet

intolerance, 29
products, 29, 80, 207, 296
Dance/Movement Therapy (DMT),
    463–67
Davis, Dorinne, 554, 607
Davis Model of Sound Intervention,
    554–64
Dawson, Geraldine, 609
Demartini, Lynn Rose, 400, 648
Denver Model, 609
Detoxification, 17, 26–27, 78, 111–14,
    180, 195, 412, 421
    detoxifiers, 114
    detoxify, 19, 24, 111, 114, 313, 421
    detoxing, 413, 563
Development(al), 85, 141–42, 144–46,
    148, 150, 300, 343, 344, 348, 363,
    365, 370, 466
    ladder, 343–44, 348
    milestones, 85, 300, 344, 370
    models, 361, 363, 365
    perceptual motor, 465
    sensorimotor, 466
    visuo-motor, 141–42, 144–46, 148,
        150
Diet(s), 9–10, 13, 29, 32–33, 86, 105,
    113, 451, 507, 608, 620
    dairy-free., 106 *See also* Dairy
    elimination(s), 10, 451
    gluten-free, 105, 422
    ketogenic, 9, 13, 86, 88
    low carbohydrate, 9, 13, 86, 200, 298
    restricted(ive),
    restrictions, 534
    sensory, 356, 545, 552,
    Specific Carbohydrate Diet, 50, 105,
        137, 200, 290–97
    yeast-free, 23, 30, 105
Dietary, 9–10, 30, 31, 58, 59, 63, 105–7,
    109, 294, 298, 644
    changes, 137
    modulation, 294
    options, 58

restriction, 294, 298, 644
supplement(s), 30, 31, 59, 63, 105–7,
    109
treatment, 9–10
Digestive, 23–34, 28–29, 31, 32, 33, 34,
    51, 55, 80, 87, 104, 105, 107–9,
    112, 201, 292, 295, 305–6, 394,
    431, 433
    discomforts, 109
    disorders, 394, 431, 433
    disturbances, 104
    enzyme(s). *See also* Enzyme 28–34,
        80, 105, 107–109, 112, 201, 305–6
    functioning, 55
    issues, 292
    problems, 31, 87, 394
    process(es), 29, 107, 394
    sensitivities, 32, 34
    support, 28–29, 31
    system(s), 34, 51, 104, 292, 295
    tract, 29, 33, 51, 104, 107, 305
Discrete Trial Training (DTT), 318
Dogris, Nicholas, 115
Doman, Alex 498
Doman, Bob 505
Dombroski, Brynn, 138
Drama Therapy, 339–42
Drugs,
    antiepileptic. *See also* Antiepileptic,
        6–13, 76
    antifungal, 16, 23–24, 52, 58, 105,
        200, 223, 307
    antipsychotic, 76, 85
    risperidone (Risperdal), xxi, 48
    hypnotic, 623
    long-term effects of, 11, 66, 83
    pharmaceutical, 16, 18, 56, 71,
        75–76, 105, 409, 415
    psychotropic, 48, 76, 536
    steroid, 3, 9–10, 12, 85, 132, 157

Early Intervention Program, 92, 255,
    265, 303, 378, 480–90, 546, 588,

591, 603

Edelson, Stephen, 138, 538, 627

El-Baz, Ayman, 121, 624

Elice, Michael, 25, 64, 611, 617

Emerge & See, 324, 327–28

Emotional Vocal Exploration (EVE), 324–32

EnListen, 559–60

Enzymes, 22–24, 26, 79, 86, 172, 175–76, 197, 211, 421, 451

digestive, 29–31, 32–34, 58, 105, 107, 109, 112, 290, 295, 305–6, 309, 313, 394, 410. (*see also* Digestive)

Enzymatic System, 410

Equine Assisted Therapy, 513, 516–17, 520–21, 582, 589 ,

Fasano, Alessio, 57, 617

Fast ForWord, 561,

Feeding Therapy, 256–63, 299–303

Fermented Foods, 59–63, 296, 304–13

Fernandez, Isauro, 491

Fine, Aubrey H., 512, 608, 652

Flavonoid, 35–41

Floortime, 342, 327–28, 343–48, 603, 605

Folate, 96, 167, 198, 204, 209, 211–12

cerebral folate deficiency, 8, 9, 86, 186–94, 204

cycle, 80–81

Food Intolerance, 29, 34, 309

feeding disorders, 259

food allergy, 29, 209. *See also* Allergy

food selectivity, 39

Freilich, Mark, xxvi

Friedman, Amanda, 324

Frye, Richard E., 6, 84, 186, 210, 636, 641

Functional Communication Training (FCT), 319

Gastrointestinal, (GI), 184, 306

abnormalities, 85, 86

ailments, 44

cause, 529–30,

complaint(s), 43

disease, 42–49

disorders, 12

disturbances, 105

dysfunction, 442, 527

evaluation, 105, 109

function, 74, 178

inflammation, 132

issues, xiv, xv, xvi, 14–34, 109, 110, 118, 459

pain, 109

pathology, 44–45

problem(s), xx, 3, 9, 29, 43, 108, 119, 290, 529–30

side-effects, 11

stress, 309

symptoms, 11, 42–43, 47, 58, 140, 290

system, 19, 34, 85, 87

tract, 17, 51, 104, 108, 193, 208, 305–6, 446

treatments, 9, 12, 21–24, 48–49, 58, 104–14, 119, 178, 291, 305–13, 443–44

ulceration, 12, 109

Gemmotherapy, 405

Geslak, David, 468

Gluten, 29, 101, 166–67, 199, 308, 394.

-free diet, 9, 29, 58, 105, 137, 167, 207, 224, 305, 422, 534, 608, *See also* Diet

Goldberg, Michael, 608

Goldberg, Jessica, 278

Goldstein, Tami, 458, 650

Gonzalez, Kristin Selby, 33

Goss Goldstein, Erica, 300

Granpeesheh, Doreen, 316, 333, 645

Greenspan, Jake, 344

Griffin, Cindy, 400, 648
Grinspoon, Lester, 608
Gut-Brain Connection, xvi, 104, 133
Gut Inflammation, 29, 135, 162, 292,
    294

Heflin, L. Juane, 608
Helminthic Therapy, 53, 55, 56, 134
    helminths, 50–56, 137, 225, 290
Hensley, Marie, 138, 627
Herskowitz, Valerie, 608
Hicks, Betsy, 305, 645
Hicks, John H., 15, 305, 610, 645
Hippotherapy, 516
Hogenboom, Marga, 608, 609
Holistic Approach to
    Neurodevelopment and
    Learning Efficiency, The
    (HANDLE), 393–99, 608
Homeopathy, 408, 412, 417, 452, 608
    homeopathic remedies, 23, 411–12,
    452
    Houston Homeopathy Method,
    400–7, 574
    sequential, 400–5
Homeostasis, 170, 172, 292, 401, 403,
    440–41
Homotoxicology, 404, 408–13
Horse(s), 516, 520–22. *See also*
    Equine-Assisted Therapy and
    Therapeutic Horseback Riding,
Houston, Devin, 28, 612
Human BioAcoustics, 563
Hygiene Hypothesis, 52–53
Hynes, Laura, 370, 647
Hyperbaric Oxygen Therapy, xiii,
    180–85, 226

Immune, 16–18
    aberrations, 131
    abnormalities, 50–56, 65, 607, 616
    activation, 132, 193, 213
    activity, 134

allergic response, 37
balance, 22–23, 137
barrier function, 108
benefit, 34, 135–36
biasing, 134
boosting nutrients, 23, 111
    cells, 36, 38, 50, 54, 98, 219, 293
cytokines, 18, 50–55
defenses, 16, 17, 21
deficiencies, 110
disorder(s), 20, 26, 36, 75, 176–77
dysfunction, 2–3, 18–19, 85, 106,
    409, 499, 524, 527
dysregulation, 67, 131, 135–36, 156,
    195, 219, 221
function(ing), 2–3, 21, 26, 51, 87, 97,
    110, 133, 203, 291, 411, 429
inflammatory cells, 58
inflammatory condition, 196
issues, 108–9
mechanisms, 3
pathways, 54
problems, xvii, 111
process, 191, 221
programming, 135
reactions, 5, 162, 207, 224
regulation, 215, 220–21
related, 54, 110
response(s), 37, 107, 111, 114, 132,
    137, 157, 208, 212, 291, 293, 308,
    312–13
signaling, 51, 101, 326
stimulation, 24, 51, 53
Immunotherapy, 3–5
    subcutaneous, 3–5
    sublingual, 3–5
Individualized Education Program
    (IEP), 253, 354, 377, 469, 510, 535
Ingels, Darin, 2, 610
Integrated Play Groups, 349–52
Integrative(Integrated) Educational,
    353–60
    care, 353–60

model, 353–60
Interactive Metronome, 50, 290, 562
Intravenous Immunoglobulin (IVIG),
    3, 9, 12, 64–70, 132, 157, 206
iPrompts, 277
Izak, Jonathan, 236

Jarrow, Markus, 543
Joint Action Routines (JARs), 278–87

Kamara, Lerone, 278
Kaplan, Melvin, 138, 142, 627, 631, 649
Kellman, Raphael, 165, 629
Krigsman, Arthur, 42, 614, 644
Kunin, Mike, 384, 385

Lang, Mary Joann, 353, 376, 647
Lanham, Lindyl, 400, 574, 648
Leaky Gut, xxi, 21, 57–63, 108, 112,
    109, 206, 311, 313
Listening Program The, 498–504, 509,
    537, 538, 560
Lovaas Therapy, 139, 316, 320, 321, 333
Low Dose Naltrexone (LDN), 227
Low Muscle Tone, 115, 394

Magnetic Resonant Therapy, 228–29,
    231, 233, 573
Martial art therapy, 491–95
Martin, Nicole, 532, 608
Mast Cell Activation, 36–39
    idiopathic mast cell activation
        disorder, 37
Mastocytosis, 36
Medication(s), 7–12, 71, 74, 200, 307
    antiepileptic. *See also* Antiepileptic,
        7–12
    antifungal. *See also* Antifungal
        Medication , 200, 307
    medicinal marijuana, 71, 74
Mehl-Madrona, Lewis, 608
Melatonin, 109, 420, 503

Mentalization Enhanced Remediation
    Integrated Treatment (MERIT),
    361–65, 367–68
Methyl-B12, 78–83, 184
Meyer LeFeber, Mariah, 463
Microbiome, 58–59, 131–37, 219, 296
Mitochondrial Dysfunction, 6, 84–88,
    166, 168, 186, 189–91, 204, 208,
    210
Mukhopadhyay, Soma, 240
Murphy, Patti, 245
Music Therapy, 499, 555,

Najdowski, Adel C., 333, 645
Nambudripad Allergy Elimination
    Technique (NAET), 449–55
Natural Environment Training
    (NET), 15, 277, 302, 318, 379,
    386, 534
Neubrander, James, 78, 180, 618, 620,
    626, 631
Neurofeedback, 89–95, 115–19, 136,
    229, 499
NeuroField, 115–20
Neuroimmune Dysfunction, 36, 156
Newman, Larry, 103, 592, 616
Nourizadeh, Karen, 429
Nutrigenomics, 95–102
Nuyens, Carolyn, 392

Oberleitner, Ronald, 376, 647
Occupational Therapy, 273, 275, 303,
    337, 340, 354, 363, 395, 460, 469,
    479, 499, 501, 543–53, 566
Oligotherapy, 405
Oral-Motor Therapy, 394
Osteopathy, 435–48, 459
Othmer, Siegfried, 89
Othmer, Susan F., 89

pEMF, 115–19
Parasite Therapy, 58

Pereira, Lavinia, 609

Pet Therapy. *See also* Animal-Assisted Therapy, Animal-Assisted Intervention, Equine-Assisted Intervention, Therapeutic Horseback Riding

Physical Therapy, 273, 275, 356, 363, 469, 479–90, 557, 565

Picture Exchange Communication System (PECS), 276–79, 231

Pivotal Response Training (PRT), 318, 321

Probiotics, xvi, 24, 57, 59, 60, 62, 63, 76, 105, 108, 109, 135, 137, 200, 294, 295, 305–13, 447

Proloquo2Go, 276

Psychotropic Medications, 48, 76, 536

PROMPT (Prompts for Restructuring Oral Muscular Phonetic Targets) Treatment, 240–55, 299, 307, 318, 428

Rapid Prompting Method (RPM), 240–44, 327

Relationship Development Intervention, 369–75

Rezvani, Alpin, 256, 272, 278, 279

Rivera, Kerri, 222, 573, 642

Rogers, Sally J., 609

Rossignol, Daniel A., 182, 183, 186, 627, 628, 635–40

Samonas Method, The, 560, 561

Sapropterin, 213, 641

Schneider, Harry, 264, 615, 619, 635

Sears, Lonnie, 120, 624, 625

Sensory, xix, 32, 65, 92, 98, 115, 118, 123, 129, 139, 140, 142, 195, 228, 231, 242, 257–59, 278, 299–303, 325, 327, 344–49, 355, 356, 363, 392–98, 442, 447, 458, 461, 465, 469, 474, 497–522, 534, 539–63, 570

gym 544–46

integration therapy, 32, 115, 118, 140, 142, 195, 228

Sensory-Based Antecedent Interventions, 137, 380, 382

Sensory Learning Program, 335

Sequential Therapy, 250, 253, 400, 408, 506, 509, 561, 565

Shiwbalak, Debbie 256

Siri, Ken iv, vii, xix, xxiv, 574

Sleep, 7, 8, 13, 27, 32, 55, 67–69, 83, 85, 109, 213, 396, 398, 405–7, 412, 420, 427, 432, 454, 461, 470, 498, 502–4, 515, 557, 562

disturbances, 13, 32, 55, 83, 85, 213, 420, 432

regulation, 27, 109

Sokhadze, Estate, 120, 138, 624, 625, 627, 643

Solomon, Michelle, 609

Sound-Based Therapies, 272–77

Speech-Language, 245, 248, 255, 256, 264, 272–79, 299, 351, 501

therapy,

pathologist, 248, 255, 256, 264, 272–79, 299, 501

Stem Cells, 131, 151–64, 214, 220, 221, 228

Sulfation, 107, 111, 112, 201

Suliteanu, Marlene, 392

Tarbox, Jonathon, 316, 645

Tazartes, Lisa, 384

Technological-Based Interventions, 247, 264, 323

Tetrahydrobiopterin Treatment, 74, 86, 167, 187, 188, 191, 192, 198, 210–13

Theoharides, Theoharis, 35, 220, 221, 609, 612, 613, 642

Therapeutic Grade Essential Oils, 414–28

Therapeutic (Horseback) Riding. *See*

also Animal-Assisted Intervention, Animal-Assisted Therapy, Equine-Assisted Therapy, Pet Therapy

Thyroid, 87, 97, 165–79, 191, 202, 203, 209, 309, 455, 460
    hypothyroidism, 87, 165–79, 202, 203, 209
Tomatis Method, The, 447, 554–64
Transcranial Direct-Current Stimulation (tDCS), 265, 266
Transcranial Magnetic Stimulation, 116, 120–30, 228–34, 264
Transcranial Ultrasound, xiv, 214–27, 537
TSO, 55, 56, 134, 137

Verbal Behavior Analysis (VBA), 321
Vision Therapy, 149, 150, 565–71

Wolfberg, Pamela, 349, 609, 613, 646, 647

Yasko, Amy, 95, 100
Yoga Nidra, 429–34
Yoga therapy, 491–95